The Physiological and Technical Basis of Electromyography

William F. Brown, M.D., F.R.C.P.(C)

Associate Professor of Neurology,
University of Western Ontario Faculty of Medicine
Director, EMG Laboratory, and
Consultant Neurologist, University Hospital, London, Ontario

With a Foreword by Roger W. Gilliatt, D.M., F.R.C.P.

Professor of Clinical Neurology and Chairman,
Department of Clinical Neurology,
Institute of Neurology,
The National Hospital, London, U.K.

BUTTERWORTH PUBLISHERS
Boston • London
Sydney • Wellington • Durban • Toronto

Every effort has been made to ensure that the drug dosage schedules within this text are accurate and conform to standards accepted at time of publication. However, as treatment recommendations vary in light of continuing research and clinical experience, the reader is advised to verify drug dosage schedules herein with information found on product information sheets. This is especially true in cases of new or infrequently used drugs.

Library of Congress Cataloging in Publication Data

Brown, William F. (William Frederick), 1939–
   The physiological and technical basis of electromyography.

   Includes index.
   1. Electromyography. I. Title.
RC77.5.B76   1984   616.7′407547   84–7752
ISBN 0–409–95042–4

Butterworth Publishers
80 Montvale Avenue
Stoneham, MA 02180

10 9 8 7 6 5 4 3 2 1

Printed in the United States of America.

CONTENTS

FOREWORD

In his Oliver Sharpey lectures of 1925 on the "Interpretation of the Electromyogram," Dr. E.D. Adrian wrote: 'The subject of these lectures is not one in which striking advances have been made in the last few years. It is one which raises many more questions than it solves, and it may turn out in the end to have little or no importance in practical medicine.'

At that time recordings from muscle were made through surface electrodes and gave little information about the behavior of individual muscle fibers or groups of fibers. Nothing was known about the discharge frequency of either nerve or muscle fibers during voluntary effort or whether one followed the other. This was also before the concept of the motor unit had been developed by Sherrington, who later defined it as "an individual motor nerve fibre with the bunch of muscle fibres it activates" (Sherrington, 1929).

By 1929 Adrian and Bronk had developed the concentric needle electrode with its restricted pickup range; by recording from the human triceps they were able to show that during voluntary contraction the gradation in force was brought about by changes in the discharge frequency of individual motor units and also by changes in the number of units in action. Papers by Smith (1934) and by Lindsley (1935a, b) on the electrical activity of human motor units followed, including the ob-

servation by Lindsley that in severe neurogenic atrophy the discharge frequency of surviving motor units was not reduced. In 1938 Denny-Brown and Pennybacker published their classic study of fasciculation, followed by a study of myotonia (Denny-Brown and Nevin, 1941). Also in 1941 Buchthal and Clemmesen published their pioneer studies of "single oscillations" in neurogenic muscular atrophy, and Harvey and Masland combined nerve stimulation with muscle recording to study myasthenia gravis. Human nerve action potentials had been recorded by Eichler as early as 1937, but his work did not become generally known until Jung drew attention to it many years later (Dawson, 1950).

Important as these papers were for the future of the subject, at first they made little impact on the practice of clinical neurology since the necessary apparatus was only available in a few centers and technical difficulties tended to limit the examination of patients. The wider application of electromyography to clinical problems had to wait for the technical advances in electronics which followed the Second World War.

After the passage of many years we tend to forget the myths and uncertainties surrounding clinical practice in the 1930s. Since he did not have the aid of myelography or nerve conduction studies, a clinician of that period can be forgiven for believing that cervical and lumbar disc syndromes were due to intrinsic inflammation of peripheral nerves or that the carpal tunnel syndrome was due to irritation of the brachial plexus. Although muscle responses to faradism and galvanism were known to change after denervation, the clinical distinction between disuse atrophy and denervation, or between neuropathy and myopathy, was difficult even for the expert.

To illustrate, one may cite the Barnes family, published in *Brain* in 1932, as an example of dominantly inherited distal myopathy. Forty years later, EMG studies of survivors and descendants showed them to be suffering from neurogenic atrophy and not from myopathy (Riddoch, 1974). For other examples one need only turn to textbooks in use at the time; in the 1933 edition of Russell Brain's *Diseases of the Nervous System* the list of infective conditions causing polyneuritis included septicemia; puerperal, typhoid, paratyphoid, and scarlet fevers; influenza; tuberculosis; syphilis; gonorrhea; mumps; typhus; and malaria. This illustrates the difficulty that must have existed in distinguishing neurogenic muscle weakness from the generalized weakness and cachexia associated with severe infections.

We can be justly proud of the way in which neurophysiological studies have contributed to the certainty of diagnosis at the present time, and there is no sign that the tempo of advance is slowing down. Newer techniques such as single-fiber electromyography and the use of somatosensory evoked potentials are already proving to be important additions to our diagnostic repertoire. As a practicing neurologist I have always taken the view that electrodiagnostic studies are best done by clinicians, but the range and variety of available techniques are now such that one must ask whether a clinician can be expected to have a sufficient background in physiology to make him a good "do-it-yourself" electromyographer. It is for this reason that I particularly value the book that Dr. William Brown has written. Here is the physiological and technical background of electromyography, summarized and interpreted with admirable clarity and simplicity by someone who is himself an acknowledged master of the subject. To each and every reader let me emphasize that it is only through an understanding of this basic physiological detail that the clinical EMG examination will come alive and lead to the discoveries of the future.

Roger W. Gilliatt

References

Adrian ED. Interpretation of the electromyogram. Lancet 1925;1:1229.

Adrian ED, Bronk DW. The discharge of impulses in motor nerve fibres. Part II. The frequency of discharge in reflex and voluntary contractions. J Physiol 1929;67:119–51.

Barnes S. A myopathic family: with hypertrophic, pseudo-hypertrophic, atrophic and terminal (distal in upper extremities) stages. Brain 1932;55:1–46.

Brain WR. Diseases of the nervous system. London: Oxford University Press, 1933.

Buchthal F, Clemmesen S. On the differentiation of muscle atrophy by electromyography. Acta Psychiatr Neurol 1941;16:143–81.

Dawson GD. Cerebral responses to nerve stimulation in man. Br Med Bull 1950;6:326–29.

Denny-Brown D, Nevin S. The phenomenon of myotonia. Brain 1941;64:1–16.

Denny-Brown D, Pennybacker JB. Fibrillation and fasciculation in voluntary muscle. Brain 1938; 61:311–32.

Eichler W. Über die Ableitung der Aktionspotentiale vom menschlichen Nerven in situ. Z Biol 1937;98:182–214.

Harvey AM, Masland RL. Method for study of neuromuscular transmission in human subjects. Bull Johns Hopkins Hosp 1941;68:81–93.

Lindsley DB. Electrical activity of human motor units during voluntary contraction. Am J Physiol 1935a;114:90–99.

Lindsley DB. Myographic and Electromyographic studies of myasthenia gravis. Brain 1935b;58: 470–82.

Riddoch D. Barnes' myopathy: a reappraisal. Paper read to the Association of British Neurologists, November 1974.

Sherrington CS. Some functional problems attaching to convergence. Proc Roy Soc B 1929;105: 332–62.

Smith Olive C. Action potentials from single motor units in voluntary contraction. Am J Physiol 1934;108:629–38.

PREFACE

This book was written to help the clinician involved in the study of diseases of the peripheral nervous system and muscle to better understand the pathophysiological basis for many of the observations derived from electromyography and nerve conduction studies. The book is intended not only for practicing electromyographers but also for those neurologists and physiatrists who, although they may not practice electromyography, have an interest in neuromuscular diseases and the place of electromyography in the analysis of these disorders.

Neuromuscular diseases are common. Kurtzke (Neurology 1982; 32:1207–1214) has recently shown statistically what many neurologists already know from their practice: that the prevalence of all neuromuscular disorders, taken together, clearly exceeds even the most common of other neurological disorders such as cerebrovascular disease in the general population. Some neuromuscular disorders— for example, the root entrapment syndromes and mononeuropathies—are particularly widespread, while others, such as the polyneuropathies, primary disorders of neuromuscular transmission, and polymyositis, are much less common.

The last two decades have seen important advances in our understanding of the basic pathophysiological mechanisms of several of these diseases, including myasthenia gravis, the Eaton-Lambert syndrome, and the primary demyelinating and compressive neuropathies. These advances have, in some cases, led to promising new treatment options and made it all the more important for the physician to establish the correct diagnosis. In this book I have attempted to aid the clinician in this endeavor. At the same time, I have sought to engender a healthy sense of caution in the interpretation of electrophysiological studies in health and disease through an appreciation of the pitfalls of these techniques.

The experience of writing this book has made me only too painfully aware of my own deficiencies in experience and knowledge. My hope is that what is gained in continuity of approach throughout the text will offset what may have been lost through less expert treatment of some subjects than would be found in a multiauthored book. It was not my intention to provide a hands-on guide for carrying out the various electromyographic tests. For this, several excellent sources are now available, including the recent books by Ludin (*Electromyography in Practice,* Thieme-Stratton, New York, 1980), Ludin and Tackmann (*Sensory Neurography,* Thieme-Stratton, New York, 1981), Swash and Schwartz (*Neuromuscular Diseases,* Springer-Verlag, New York, 1981), and Kimura (*Electrodiagnosis in*

Diseases of Nerve and Muscle, F.A. Davis, Philadelphia, 1983) and the instructional programs put out by the American Association of Electromyography and Electrodiagnosis. Rather, the emphasis here is on the underlying pathophysiological changes in peripheral nerves and muscles as well as the principles on which the various currently available electrophysiological techniques for studying neuromuscular disorders in man are based.

Throughout the preparation of this book, I was continually reminded of the enormous debt all electromyographers owe to figures such as Professors F. Buchthal, E.H. Lambert, R.W. Gilliatt and E. Stålberg, who have helped to shape the field of electrophysiology as applied to nerve and muscle disease. My own maturation as an electromyographer owes much to what I learned from Geoffrey Rushworth, in whose Oxford laboratory I spent a year as a McLaughlin fellow in 1970, as well as from my associations with other electromyographers and neurophysiologists whom it has been my pleasure to know and to learn from over the years. My clinical colleagues in London have helped me to keep electromyography in its proper perspective as a diagnostic tool while at the same time they have challenged me to exploit the techniques to improve our understanding of the pathophysiology of some of the neuromuscular disorders we see every day. In my home base, Drs. Charles Bolton, Thomas Feasby, Angelika Hahn, Joseph Gilbert, and Arthur Hudson have greatly enriched the neuromuscular environment in which I work, both by their own endeavors and through the accompanying free exchange of experience and ideas which has characterized this group. I also gratefully acknowledge and especially thank Stephen Yates, who has contributed so much to the clinical investigative studies of this EMG laboratory, and Mark Davis, whose technical expertise has had much to do with the success of our laboratory.

A strong effort has been made in this book to provide first-rate illustrations, and whatever success we have had in meeting this objective can be credited to the fine artwork of George Moogk and the photographic reproductions of Stephen Mesjaric.

Mrs. Kathy Stead has provided very able secretarial help and has been a source of patient good humor throughout the many corrections and modifications to the text.

Finally, I wish to thank my wife Janet and children Tim and Martha for their endurance and support throughout the seemingly endless hours when I was immersed in the preparation of this book.

W.F.B.

INTRODUCTION: THE LIMITATIONS OF ELECTROPHYSIOLOGICAL TESTING

The considerable progress of recent years in understanding and treating many of the neuromuscular diseases has broadened the range of clinical possibilities for the physician. With the increased capacity for managing patients afflicted with these disorders has come stronger emphasis on rapid and accurate diagnosis. Present electrophysiological methods have established an important place in the diagnostic workup for diseases of muscle and nerve. If these tests are to be used to best advantage, however, their role and their limitations must be understood.

Despite the many conceptual and methodological advances of recent years, the clinical examination remains the best single tool for analysis of neuromuscular diseases. In the case of peripheral neuropathies, for example, it should be possible to establish whether the basic pattern of the peripheral neuropathy is primarily distal or proximal, is symmetrical or asymmetrical, or is best explained by multiple local lesions affecting peripheral nerve. The examination should also predict the likely types of nerve fibers involved (motor, sensory, autonomic) and even give some indication of whether demyelination, axonal degeneration, or both are prominent characteristics of the neuropathy. Moreover, only the history can tell us about the presence or absence of abnormal spontaneous activity in sensory nerve fibers. The presence of such activity, reported as paresthesias, dysesthesias, or pain, often provides the earliest clue to the nature and localization of a lesion in the peripheral or root compression syndromes.

The place of electrophysiological testing in the assessment of neuromuscular diseases is to act as an extension of the neurological examination. Specifically, the pattern of the pathophysiological changes seen in the electromyogram (EMG) and on nerve conduction studies (NCS) can shed light on the location of the lesion and on the nature of the underlying processes in the nerve or muscle (or both). These electrophysiological techniques provide evidence as to whether neuronal (or axonal) degeneration has taken place, whether any substantial degree of demyelination is present, and whether there is a disorder affecting neuromuscular transmission or one primarily affecting the muscle fibers. Additionally, the tests can provide important clues to the localization of lesions affecting the peripheral nerves and an indication of the severity of the lesions. Electrophysiological tests thus provide a sort of physiological biopsy of the peripheral nervous system and muscle. For example, degeneration of neurones or axons may be indicated by a number of alterations in the NCS and EMG, as outlined in Table 1 and discussed in detail in Chapters 2, 3, 6, 8 and 10. Table 2 lists the alterations to be expected in an established primary demyelinating neuropathy and Table 3, the indications of a focal nerve lesion.

As any neurological clinician or experienced electromyographer knows, all abnormalities observed in NCS and the EMG must be interpreted in the light of the history and findings on examination. For example, increases in fiber density, the appearance of fibrillation potentials, and abnormalities in neuromuscular transmission may all be seen in primary muscle diseases. In these disorders, portions of muscle fibers may become denervated and collateral reinnervation may later take place, with concomitant alteration in the innervation patterns of muscle fibers and formation of new neuromuscular junctions. Likewise, characteristic features such as conduction slowing and desynchronization of nerve and muscle potentials, ordinarily seen in demyelinating neuropathies, may be absent, for example, early in the course of Guillain-Barré polyneuropathy. At the same time, conduction block may not be apparent unless the very proximal portions of the peripheral nervous system are included in the study.

Even in diseases in which axons undergo degeneration, fibrillation may be difficult to detect or even absent if the degeneration has been very recent or the disease is progressing

TABLE 1.   Indicators of Neuronal-Axonal Degeneration*

Loss of nerve fibers
  Motor
    ↓ Maximum M-potential amplitude (area)
    ↓ Recruitment
    ↓ Motor unit estimates
  Sensory
    ↓ Amplitude of nerve action potential
Denervation of muscle (no equivalent for sensory fibers)
  Fibrillation potentials
  Positive sharp waves
Reinnervation (no equivalent for sensory fibers)
    ↑ M-potential amplitude
    ↑ Fiber density
    ↑ Amplitude and duration of motor unit potentials
  ± ↑ Territory of motor unit (potential)
    ↑ Incidence of linked potentials
  Neuromuscular ↑ jitter ± blocking
  Axonal blocking
Conduction velocities
  Normal or only minimally reduced

*See Chapters 2, 3, 6, 8, and 10.

TABLE 2.   Indicators of Demyelination*

Substantial reduction in conduction velocities of motor/sensory nerve fibers
Desynchronization of compound nerve and muscle action potentials
Conduction block

*See Chapters 2 and 3.

TABLE 3.   Indication of a Focal Nerve Lesion*

At the site of the lesion
  Slowing of conduction in excess of that proximal or distal to the lesion
  Desynchronization of impulses transmitted through the lesion
  ± Conduction block
Proximal to the lesion
  ± Reduction of conduction velocity (real or apparent)
Distal to the lesion
  ± Evidence of degeneration of motor or sensory fibers beyond the site of the lesion
  ± Slowing of conduction

*See Chapter 2.

slowly. Furthermore, in some severe late-stage neuronopathies such as the neuronal type of Charcot-Marie-Tooth disease (HMSN type II), so few motor axons may remain that a motor conduction velocity determination is based on less than 5 percent of the normal number of motor axons. In the extreme, it could represent only the last surviving motor axon and could fall well below the 2 standard deviation lower limit for healthy maximum motor conduction velocities. Such a result could indicate abnormally slow conduction in a normally faster conducting nerve fiber because of associated demyelination, axonal shrinkage, or both; or, theoretically at least, it could represent normal conduction in a motor axon that ordinarily conducts more slowly. In such a case, the conduction velocity may be so low as to mistakenly suggest a primary demyelinating neuropathy. More normal conduction velocities in less affected motor nerves, as well as electromyographic signs of denervation and reinnervation, help to establish the predominant pathological alteration in the nerve fibers to give a more accurate picture of the clinical situation.

Critical to a proper appreciation of the role of EMG and NCS is a clear understanding of what these studies do *not* tell us and the biases inherent in many of the techniques. For example, conduction velocities as conventionally measured assess conduction in the fastest-conducting motor axons, while there is known to be a 30 to 50 percent range in the conduction velocities of alpha motor axons in man. Inherent in studies of sensory conduction is a similar bias toward the faster-conducting nerve fibers. In these studies, the compound nerve action potential is generated primarily by fibers with conduction velocities between 30 and 65 meters per second, more slowly conducting and numerous smaller-diameter fibers making relatively little contribution except to the later components of the compound nerve action potential.

On the other hand, needle electromyographic studies, whether utilizing conventional concentric needle electrodes or the more recently introduced macro or single-fiber needle electrodes (see Chapter 7) are biased as well. In these studies, the bias is toward the lowest-threshold motor units recruited in muscle contractions. From earlier investigations in normal human subjects, it is known that such lower-threshold motor units generate the least tensions and that the conduction velocities of their axons are slower compared with higher-tension, higher-recruitment-threshold motor units having faster-conducting motor axons and larger-amplitude motor unit potentials as recorded with surface electrodes (Chapter 5). Thus, while maximum motor conduction velocity determinations probably reflect primarily the contributions of the higher-tension, larger-amplitude motor units, studies of motor unit potentials based on the first few potentials recruited at each recording site in the course of a voluntary contraction are probably weighted toward the smaller motor units with slower-conducting motor axons (Fig. 1). It seems likely too, based on the range of motor unit tensions and amplitudes in normal subjects, that the maximum M-potential primarily reflects the contributions of the larger-amplitude motor unit potentials. The fastest-conducting motor axons, however, probably constitute a minority of the whole population of motor unit potentials.

Needle electromyographic studies share yet another bias: they reflect the activities of only those muscle fibers in motor units lying within the pickup territory of the recording electrode. While the size of this pickup zone varies appreciably with the surface area and shape of the recording electrode, all conventional concentric needle electrodes see but a part of the whole motor unit at least in respect to the spike components of the motor unit potential. The amplitude of the potentials recorded is

FIGURE 1.   Relationship between the size of a motor unit as measured by the tension or voltage it generates and the threshold at which motor units are recruited (see Chapter 5). In all studies carried out to date in humans, the lowest-threshold motor units are those generating the least tension. These same motor units have slower conduction velocities compared to the larger-tension, larger-voltage motor units recruited only in stronger contractions. The latter are precisely those motor units which, because of their faster conduction velocities, are responsible for the maximum motor conduction velocities (MCV) measured throughout the various somatic motor nerves in the body; they are probably not the same motor units whose potentials (MUPs) are recruited in weak voluntary contractions and studied by electromyography.

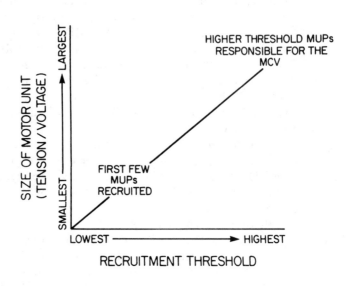

determined predominantly by the number of muscle fibers sharing the same innervation within the spike detection zone of the electrode. Such studies, while reflecting the innervation patterns of motor units, provide no indication of the overall anatomical or physiological size of the motor unit (innervation ratio and tension).

Another blind spot in conventional NCS is the proximal portion of the peripheral nervous system. This area is much more difficult to assess electrophysiologically than are the intermediate or distal portions of peripheral nerves. Lesions affecting the lumbosacral or brachial plexuses or nerve roots are probably best localized by looking for denervation in muscles supplied by the affected root(s) or component(s) of the plexus. Wallerian degeneration must, a priori, have taken place in sufficient numbers of motor axons for fibrillation to develop and be detected in these muscles. The assessment of conduction across the root or plexus, however, is much more difficult. Indirect methods exist, such as the use of F-response applicable to motor fibers (Chapter 3) and evoked potential techniques for assessing proximal conduction in sensory fibers (Chapters 3 and 4). Still, it is not possible except with direct stimulation of the roots or plexus to directly assess conduction across the affected regions. In more peripheral nerve entrapments, in contrast, the abnormal region can be bridged by recording and stimulation sites on both sides of the lesion.

The preceding examples should make it apparent that all these electrophysiological techniques have certain inherent limitations in the kinds of information they can provide. Errors in application of the techniques may further degrade the value of the assessments. Despite these difficulties, electrophysiological testing in peripheral nerve and muscle diseases, when thoroughly understood and correctly utilized, is unquestionably a valuable diagnostic tool. The purpose of this book is to aid the clinician in proper understanding and application of electromyographic methods in disorders of muscle and nerve.

The Physiological and Technical Basis of Electromyography

1 THE NORMAL TRANSMEMBRANE POTENTIAL AND IMPULSE CONDUCTION

Peripheral nerves are the communication links between the periphery and the central nervous system (CNS). In this role, nerves transmit to the CNS knowledge of the present state of the internal and external environments and the instructions of the CNS to muscles, other tissues, and organs. These transmissions are carried by transient electrical impulses that begin in various receptor end organs or in the neurons themselves and propagate toward their target cells at velocities between 0.3 and 100 m/s. Passage of these impulses is accompanied by brief reversals of the transmembrane potential by as much as 120 to 130 mV.

The principal role of the peripheral nervous system (PNS) as a communication link can be disturbed by diseases that:

1. Destroy motoneurons, dorsal root ganglion cells, or their respective peripheral processes and terminals
2. Block transmission of impulses in their axons, even though the axons themselves are intact
3. Upset the normal temporal coding of impulses necessary to mediate a particular response (Figure 1.1)
4. Block transmission at central or peripheral (neuromuscular) synapses
5. Lead to ectopic impulse generation or ephaptic transmission
6. Produce abnormal regeneration patterns

Electrophysiological tests can reveal many of these abnormalities in peripheral nerves. The proper use and interpretation of these tests depends on a working knowledge of the properties of excitable membranes, impulse generation, and conduction, the subjects of this chapter. Expert and clear treatment of these subjects is available in a number of standard texts, monographs, and reviews (Woodbury, 1965; Hodgkin, 1967; Hille, 1977; Kuffler and Nicholls, 1976; Woodbury, 1976; Costantin, 1977; Barchi, 1980; Mountcastle, 1980; Armstrong, 1981). This chapter is intended to provide enough basic background knowledge to enable the reader to understand the pathophysiological mechanisms covered in subsequent chapters.

FIGURE 1.1. (A) Vibratory stimulus to pacinian corpuscles and the resultant more or less synchronous volleys of action potentials at 7- to 8-ms intervals passing along the peripheral and central afferent pathways.

(B) Tendon tap-evoked afferent volleys in primary spindle afferents, which in turn evoke monosynaptic excitatory postsynaptic potentials in motoneurons innervating the muscle(s) in which the receptors reside. Discharge of the motoneurons leads to contraction of the peripherally related complements of muscle fibers supplied by each of the discharged motoneurons and the visible contraction and shortening of the muscle. The afferent volley may be somewhat asynchronous in this case because of differences in the distances between the spinal cord and the receptor end-organs, especially in long muscles.

(C) Hypothetical reconstruction of what could be the impact of greater degrees of temporal dispersion among the arrival times of impulses in Ia afferents on whether or not the motoneurons discharge. In cat lumbosacral motoneurons, impulses in as many as 100 or more Ia afferents must sum to generate a compound excitatory postsynaptic potential large enough to discharge the motoneuron (Mendell and Henneman, 1971). In this simple model, however, the unitary excitatory postsynaptic potentials of only five Ia afferents are shown, and on the left in the normal case, despite minor degrees of desynchronization between their arrival times at the motoneuron, the compound postsynaptic potential is still large enough to discharge the motoneuron. When, however, as on the right, the arrival times of the impulses in the five Ia

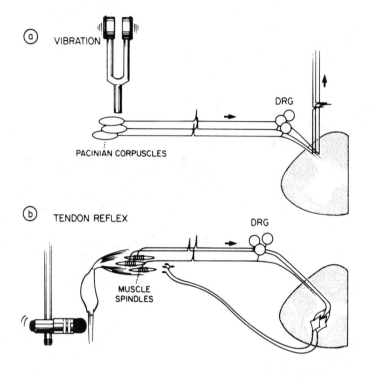

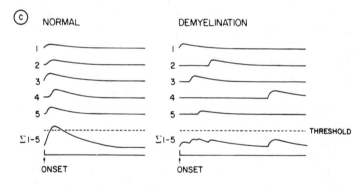

afferents are too dispersed with respect to one another to depolarize the motoneuron beyond threshold, the motoneuron will fail to fire. Such excessive degrees of temporal dispersion could be expected in demyelinating neuropathies and may be one reason for the loss of tendon or H reflexes in these diseases.

TRANSMEMBRANE POTENTIAL

The interior of excitable cells is electronegative (-70 to -90 mV) with respect to the extracellular compartment. This transmembrane potential (TMP) is a product of the selective permeability properties of the cell membrane and the relative concentrations of the various charged particles, in this instance ions, in the intracellular and extracellular compartments. The membrane is therefore a logical place to begin.

The Membrane

Biological membranes are complex (see reviews by Singer and Nicholson, 1972; Singer, 1974; Armstrong, 1975; Pfenninger, 1978; Waxman and Foster, 1980). They are 50 to 100 Å thick and consist of a bilayer of phos-

pholipid molecules and protein. The lipid molecules are polar, containing at one end a *hydrophilic* or water-soluble glycerol phosphate grouping and at the other end a *hydrophobic* or nonwater-soluble hydrocarbon acyl chain. Artificial membranes can be constructed by mixing such phospholipid molecules in water, the molecules spontaneously linking together into a bilayer. The water-soluble polar groups are oriented to the outside of the membrane and the hydrocarbon chains toward the interior of the membrane (Figure 1.2). There is a remarkable degree of spontaneous movement of individual phospholipid molecules both side to side and about their long axis, although there is little movement between the layers.

The phospholipid membrane is impermeable to ions because the charged ion must pass through the hydrophobic interior of the membrane. Inserted into the lipid matrix of the

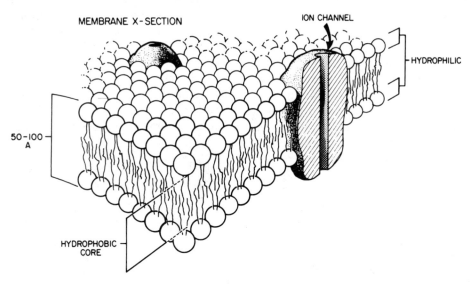

FIGURE 1.2.   Illustration of a cell membrane shows the bilayer of phospholipid molecules. The outer (extracellular) and inner (intracellular) surfaces are hydrophobic and the inner core region of the sandwich is hydrophilic. Inserted in the membrane at intervals much more widely spaced than shown are macromolecular proteins, some of which serve as channels for the passage of ions through the membrane. Some are voltage gated and others act as more passive ion channels.

membrane, however, are protein macromolecules that act as channels to the passage of ions when the channels are in the so-called open state. Some channels are open all the time irrespective of the TMP, while others open or close depending on the magnitude and polarity of the TMP. The ion-permeant properties of the latter channels are hence spoken of as voltage dependent or *voltage gated*. These proteinaceous ion channels in the membrane are also selective for the type of ion that can be passed through even in the open state, some channels being selective for sodium, others for potassium ions, and still others for calcium ions. Some are linked to receptors that combine with specific neurotransmitter substances such as acetylcholine, to be discussed later.

In the mammalian unmyelinated axolemmal membrane and the membranes of muscle fibers, there are both sodium and potassium channels. These are by and large uniformly distributed throughout the membrane. The same is true in the membrane of the squid axon. Hodgkin (1975) has suggested that there is an optimal density of sodium channels at which conduction velocity is maximal in the squid axon. In myelinated mammalian nerve fibers, however, there is a very high concentration of sodium channels but no potassium channels in the nodal axolemmal membrane. This contrasts with the internodal membrane, including the paranodal region, where there are potassium channels but only a small number of sodium channels (Table 1.1).

There have been enormous strides in the last decade in localization and quantification of the various ion channels as well as in biophysical and pharmacological investigation of the properties of these channels (see Waxman and Ritchie, 1981; Armstrong, 1981; Ulbricht, 1981; Culp and Ochoa, 1982). There have been recent attempts to isolate and purify channels. The introduction of the so-called patch clamp technique has also made possible the measurement of membrane currents in

TABLE 1.1. Concentrations of Sodium Channels in Muscle and Nerve Fibers

Fibers	Channels per Micrometer
Muscle	
Frog	200–400
Rat	200
Nerve	
Unmyelinated	
Squid	500
Rabbit	100
Myelinated	
Rabbit	
Nodal membrane	10,000
Internodal membrane	25

From Ritchie (1979).

single channels and the investigation, in detail, of the kinetics of these channels (Hamil, Marty, Neher, Sakmann, and Sigworth, 1981).

The concentrations of the various ions in muscle and nerve cells are dissimilar in the intracellular and extracellular compartments (Table 1.2). In the mammalian muscle cell, the concentration of K^+ in the intracellular compartment is approximately 30 times that in the extracellular compartment; conversely, sodium concentration in the extracellular compartment is 12 times higher. It is the rel-

TABLE 1.2. Ion Concentration (μmoles/cm^3) in Mammalian Skeletal Muscle and in the Extracellular Space

	Intracellular	Extracellular
Cations		
Na^+	12	145
K^+	155	4
H^+	13×10^{-5}	3.8×10^{-5}
Anions		
Cl^-	4	120
HCO_3^-	8	27
Other	155	7

From Woodbury (1965).

ative intracellular and extracellular concentrations of these two ions and their respective membrane permeabilities that primarily control the active and passive properties of the membrane. The membrane is not permeable to organic anions, however. In general, the chloride and bicarbonate permeabilities do not contribute to the transmembrane potential. The membrane, because of the protein macromolecules within its lipid matrix, is very permeable to water, and the numbers of moles of dissolved particles per unit volume (osmolarity) are therefore equal in the intracellular and extracellular compartments.

In solution, all molecules are in random motion. The intensity of this activity depends on temperature. The rate of *diffusion* is much lower through a membrane compared to an equal thickness of water, even when the membrane is partially permeable to the molecules. When a permeable membrane separates two solutions that have equal concentrations of a particular molecule, the rates of outward *(efflux)* and inward *(influx)* flux through the membrane are equal and the net movement or *flux* is zero. When the concentrations of the molecule are not equal, the flux will be proportional to the magnitude of the difference between the concentrations of the ion on the two sides of the membrane. The ease with which a molecule can traverse the membrane is called its *permeability.*

Flux = permeability
   × (concentration inside
   − concentration outside)
or
$$p \times ([x]_i - [x]_o),$$

where p = permeability,
   x = molecular species,
   i = inside, and
   o = outside.

This is the chemical equivalent of Ohm's law in electricity, namely:

$$Current = voltage \times \frac{1}{resistance} \quad or$$
$$Current = voltage \times conductance.$$

Conductance is the reciprocal of resistance.

If the molecules do not carry a charge, their net movement across a membrane is solely dependent on the relative concentrations of the molecular species on the two sides of the membrane, net movement being toward the solution with the lowest concentration. In solution, ionic molecules have a charge. Their movement is therefore controlled not just by whatever concentration gradient there may be across the membrane, but by the polarity and magnitude of any electrical potential acting across the membrane. Depending on the polarities of the TMP and the ionic species involved, the TMP can act to oppose or move in the same direction as the concentration gradient.

The TMP comes about because of separation of charge, which in turn is a product of the selective permeability properties of the membrane. For example, when a membrane permeable only to potassium (K^+) separates two neutral but unequal concentrations of K^+ in solution, a TMP will develop. This happens because there is a net movement of potassium ions to the solution with the lowest K^+ concentration. This makes the solution with the highest K^+ concentration electronegative with respect to the solution with the lower concentration of K^+ ion. In mammalian cells, the interior K^+ ion concentration is much higher than the corresponding concentration of K^+ in the extracellular space. This inequality leads to a net movement of K^+ outward across the membrane. Because the membrane is impermeable to the negative (anion) charge in the interior, the net movement of positive charge to the exterior is not balanced by an equivalent outward movement of negative charge. This leads to the interior of the cell becoming electronegative with respect to the exterior. The resultant charge separation and imbalance are responsible for the TMP. This net leakage of K+ cannot continue to the point at which the potassium concentrations are equal in the solutions because the developing TMP, in turn, more and more resists the leakage of K+ to the exterior. This resistance is the result of the increasing accumulation of positively charged ions on the exterior of the membrane, attracted and held there by the equivalent accumulation of negatively charged ions on the interior membrane.

The more electronegative charges that accumulate near the interior surface, the larger the number of positive ions per unit area of membrane that can be attracted and held on the outside. It is this increase in concentration of positive charges on the outside that resists the further net movement of the positive K+ ions through the membrane despite the steep concentration gradient of this ion acting to drive K+ ions out through the membrane. The work required to move positive charges through the membrane is directly related to the concentration of charge on the membrane, and this in turn is a function of the ability or capacity of the membrane to hold charge on its surface.

The capacity to store charge is a product of the thickness of the membrane. The thinner the membrane, the less distance that separates the charges on its two sides and the greater the force the extra negative charge on the interior surface can bring to bear on the opposite positive charges on the outside surface. The consequence is that larger numbers of like charges can be held close together on the surface of the membrane despite the forces of repulsion between these like charges. Positively charged ions can therefore move onto the intracellular surface and other positive ions can be displaced away from the outside or extracellular surface of the membrane. Negative charges move in the opposite direction. Hence even though no charge moves directly through

the membrane, current can flow between the intracellular and extracellular spaces. In this manner the membrane functions like a capacitor, acting as the insulator between the intracellular and extracellular conductors.

When there is no charge on the membrane, resistance to the movement of ions across the membrane is determined solely by its permeability to various ions. With increasing charge separation and the progressive accumulation of charge, however, there is increasing resistance to movement of more positive charge through the membrane. The electrical potential across the membrane is proportional to the work necessary to move positive charges through the membrane and, as pointed out before, this is related to the capacity of the membrane to store charge. The magnitude of the transmembrane voltage (E_m) is therefore directly related to the quantity of positive charge on and capacitance (C) of the membrane; that is:

$$E_m = Q \times \frac{1}{C},$$

where E_m = transmembrane voltage,
   Q = total membrane charge, and
   C = capacitance.

Eventually, a balance is struck in the cell when the outward transmembrane movement of potassium propelled by inequalities in potassium concentration is checked by the equal and opposite-acting TMP. The TMP at which this electrochemical equilibrium is reached is the *equilibrium potential*. The net movement of an ion across the membrane is zero at its equilibrium potential.

For any species of ion, it is expressed by the *Nernst equation*. The equilibrium potential is simply the transmembrane potential at which the net outward and inward movement of a particular species of ion is zero. The work (W_E) required to move a mole of ion (X) against the transmembrane potential (electrical work) must equal the work (W_C) exerted by the concentration gradient (chemical work or concentration potential energy difference) acting in the opposite direction from the equilibrium potential for the ion under consideration. It turns out that the work (W_E) to move one mole of ion (X) across a membrane at any particular value of the transmembrane potential (E_m) is:

$$W_C = Z_X \times F \times E_m,$$

where Z = valence of the ion,
X = the ion species,
F = number of coulombs per mole of charge,
E_m = transmembrane potential (joules per coulomb), and
W_C = work.

Similarly, the work (W_C) exerted on an ion (X) to move it through the membrane is proportional to the difference between the logarithm of the intracellular (i) and extracellular (o) concentrations of the ion, or:

$$W_C = RT \times (log_e\ [X^Z]_i - log_e\ [X^Z]_o) \quad \text{or}$$
$$W_C = RT\ log_e \frac{[X^Z]_i}{[X^Z]_o}$$

where R = universal gas constant,
T = absolute temperature, and
e = base of the natural logarithm = 2.718.

Now to return to the Nernst equation: at the equilibrium potential, the chemical and electrical works acting on the ion must be equal, and therefore $Z_X \times F \times E_m$ must equal $RT\ log_e\ [X^Z]_i/[X^Z]_o$. At the equilibrium potential for ion Y, $W_E + W_C$ must equal zero, or:

$$Z_X \times F \times E_m + RT\ log_e \frac{[X^Z]_i}{[X^Z]_o} = 0$$

Solving for E_m:

$$E_m = \frac{RT}{Z_XF} \times log_e \frac{[X^Z]_o}{[X^Z]_i}.$$

If the ion is K, then E_m is E_K, and solving for E_K:

$$E_K = 61\ log_{10} \frac{[K^+]_o}{[K^+]_i}.$$

By using the K^+ ion intracellular and extracellular concentrations listed in Table 1.2, $E_K = -97$ mV for a mammalian muscle cell.

The E_K is close to but exceeds by about 20 or more mV the resting TMP (-60 to -80 mV) of the TMP in mammalian muscle cells.

The difference between the two values is explained by the fact that the membrane is permeable not just to potassium but to sodium ions as well. The sodium equilibrium potential, calculated by the Nernst equation and based on the intracellular and extracellular concentrations of this ion (see Table 1.2) is between $+30$ and $+50$ mV. Sodium ions are therefore a long way from their equilibrium potential at the resting TMP of -60 to -80 mV.

The resting membrane is somewhat permeable to sodium ions, although the ratio of potassium to sodium permeabilities is between about $50:1$ and $100:1$. Because sodium flux is opposite in direction to potassium, the net charge separation is a little less than would be the case if potassium were the only migrant ion. Calculation of the TMP must therefore take account not just of the concentration of potassium but of the concentrations of sodium ions and the relative permeabilities of the two ions. These relationships are expressed by the *Goldman-Hodgkin-Katz* voltage equation (Hille, 1977), namely:

$$E_m = RT\ log_e \frac{pK\ [K^+]_o}{pK\ [K^+]_i} + \frac{pNa\ [Na^+]_o}{pNa\ [Na^+]_i}$$
$$+ \frac{pCl\ (Cl^-)_o}{pCl\ (Cl^-)_i} + \frac{pX\ [X^Z]_o}{pX\ [X^Z]_i},$$

where p = the permeability coefficient of the various ions and
X = other permeant ions.

Since in mammalian nerve and skeletal muscle fibers the only important permeant ions are sodium and potassium, the above can be rewritten and simplified as:

$$E_m = 60 \times \log_e \frac{(K^+)_o}{(K^+)_i} + 0.01 \times \frac{(Na^+)_o}{(Na^+)_i}.$$

For a muscle cell $\dfrac{pNa}{pK} = \dfrac{1}{100}$ and
$$E_m = -90 \text{ mV}.$$

For a nerve cell $\dfrac{pNa}{pK} = \dfrac{1}{50}$ and
$$E_m = -70 \text{ mV}.$$

If the above processes continued unchecked, eventually, over hours the difference in concentration in sodium and potassium across the membrane would disappear. Even so, isolated nerve can continue to initiate and propagate thousands of action potentials before the TMP deteriorates in an anoxic environment. Indeed, in squid axons, the axoplasm can be replaced by artificial solutions, and provided the membrane permeability characteristics are intact and the relative concentrations of sodium and potassium are maintained, action potentials can be generated in the isolated nerve in the absence of an energy source.

To maintain the ionic concentrations constant requires work because of the continual inward movement of potassium and outward movement of sodium across the membrane. These constant passive losses are balanced by an energy-dependent pumping mechanism that pumps potassium inward and sodium outward. This *sodium-potassium pump* is slightly electrogenic in that it pumps out more sodium than potassium passes inward. Metabolic poisons can block the pump and cause gradual uncompensated leakage of sodium into the interior of the cell, making the interior less electronegative relative to the exterior and in this way reducing the TMP. When the TMP reaches about -30 mV, action potentials can no longer be generated.

The equivalent sodium-potassium pumping mechanism at the nodal region of myelinated fibers could be dependent on the Schwann cells, the cytoplasm of which contains many more mitochondria than the nearby nodal axoplasm (Ritchie, 1982). Even more speculative is the suggestion that some of the sodium channels themselves may be located in the Schwann cell membrane.

ELECTRICAL PROPERTIES OF EXCITABLE MEMBRANES

Before discussing the electrochemical events that operate in the action potential, it is necessary to review the passive electrical properties of excitable cell membranes. The membrane has both a capacitive element, because of its insulating and charge-separation properties imposed by the ion-impermeable regions of the membrane, and a parallel resistive element corresponding to those membrane regions where even at rest the membrane is partially permeable to ions (channel and other glycoprotein insertion sites in the membrane).

Figure 1.3 illustrates the equivalent circuit for a membrane. If there were no capacitive element in the membrane, the TMP would be directly and instantaneously proportional to the resistive element if the transmembrane current were constant. If, however, there is a capacitor included in parallel with the resistance element in the membrane, the TMP will not be directly proportional to the current at least initially, but will change in an exponential manner (Figure 1.3). Inclusion of the capacitive element increases the time required for E_m to reach a constant level in response to the constant transmembrane current because it requires time for the charge on the capacitor to discharge. The magnitude of E_m

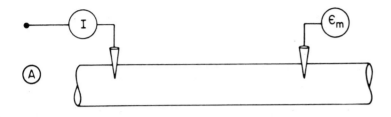

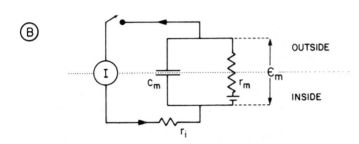

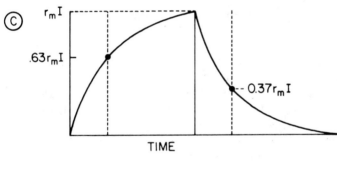

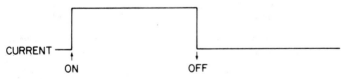

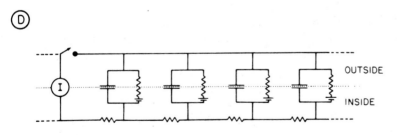

FIGURE 1.3. Electrical properties of the cell membrane and its response to an imposed transmembrane current.

(A) Current is injected into the fiber membrane (left) and the resultant change in the transmembrane potential is recorded by an intracellular electrode (outside reference) (right).

(B) The electrical circuit equivalent of the above is to consider the membrane as having, in parallel, the properties of a resistor and a capacitor (an RC circuit). Also, because of the finite diameter of the cell, there may be appreciable resistance to the passage of current through the interior (r_i), the resistance outside the fiber being considered negligible by comparison.

(C) The resultant time course of the change in transmembrane potential (E_M) resulting from the square current pulse is determined by the values of the resistance and capacitive elements in the RC circuit. The higher the capacitance, the longer the current must flow for the transmembrane potential to reach a steady-state value. The *time constant* is the time taken for the E_M to reach 0.63 of its steady-state value when the current pulse is turned on or off.

(D) The equivalent circuit of the membrane may be modeled by distributed parallel resistive and capacitive elements in the membrane linked in series with one another through the internal longitudinal resistive element of the axoplasmic core of the muscle fiber. The membrane in the figure is indicated by the interrupted line.

at any instant is proportional to the concentration of charge per unit area of membrane at that time, but not directly to the magnitude of the current. Even though there are no actual ionic currents passing through the membrane capacitive element alone, charge accumulates or is lost on the surfaces of the capacitor, and as a consequence, current flows up to and away from the surfaces of the membrane.

Axons and muscle cells are long and their diameters small by comparison. Conduction therefore takes place along the length of what amounts to a cable. The equivalent circuit for this type of cable is illustrated in Figure 1.3. When as in Figure 1.3 an inward transmembrane current is passed by way of an intracellular electrode across the membrane at one end, the inward current passes longitudinally down the interior of the axoplasm (the *internal longitudinal current,* ILC) and outward through the membrane (the *transverse membrane current,* TMC) to return by way of the extracellular space to the stimulus cathode (the *external longitudinal current,* ELC).

The resultant TMPs at various distances and times following onset of the transmembrane stimulus current are illustrated in Figure 1.4. The two most important observations are:

1. The TMP (E_m) at any time is proportional to the distance between the site of origin of the transmembrane stimulus current and the site at which E_m is measured and to the internal longitudinal resistance (ILR). The ILR in turn is inversely proportional to the cross-sectional area of the cylinder (r^2) and the specific resistance of the axoplasm. Ignoring the specific resistance of the axoplasm, the magnitude of TMP at a point distant from the site of the stimulus is proportional to $d \times r^2$, where d = distance between the current source and the recording electrode. The transverse resistance per unit area of membrane remains constant (except in myelinated nerve) along the length of the membrane. Except when the nerve or muscle fiber is immersed in a high-resistance medium such as air or oil, the external longitudinal resistance is negligible with respect to the internal longitudinal resistance.

2. The magnitude of the TMP at any particular distance is related to the interval between onset of the stimulus current and the time when E_m is measured. This time lag in turn reflects the distributed membrane capacitance and resistance between the stimulus and the point where the TMP is measured, and increases as the longitudinal distance increases away from the stimulus source. The magnitude of this time lag is expressed by the *time constant.* By definition, the time constant of the membrane is the time taken for the TMP to decay to 1/C or 0.37 of the initial TMP when the source current stops. The time constant is proportional to $R_m \times C_m$ (see Figure 1.3).

Note that increasing the distance between the origin of the stimulus and the point at which the TMP is measured causes the total distributed capacitance between them to increase (Figure 1.3). Hence the time necessary for the TMP at any point to reach its constant and maximum value increases as the distance is increased between the site of stimulation and the recording site. The reason for this is that when current passes through the membrane, it initially attempts to return to the source by passing outward through the adjacent membrane where the ILR is least (shortest current path).

The initial transmembrane current through successive newly depolarized regions of the membrane is capacitive. The resultant progressive accumulation of positive charge on the inner side of the membrane, however, progressively impedes further outward capacitive current flow to the point where the limit on outward current flow in this region of membrane is set solely by the relatively high

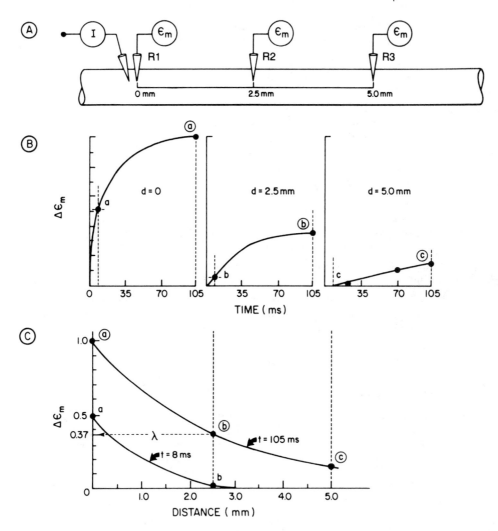

FIGURE 1.4.   Longitudinal extension of transmembrane potential changes (ΔE_m) in response to a steadily applied inward current beginning at time zero in a single skeletal muscle fiber.

(A) Experimental arrangement: intracellular recording electrodes R1-3 record the E_m at 0, 2.5, and 5.0 mm away from the current injection site.

(B) The time courses of the ΔE_m at the three recording sites. Note the rate of rise of the ΔE_m slows and the final steady-state E_m is lower the more longitudinally distant from the current injection site is the recording site.

(C) Replot of data in B to show the magnitudes of the E_m at the three recording sites at 8 and 105 ms following onset of the stimulus current. Beyond 105 ms there was no further significant change in E_m at any of the recording sites. At this time the *length constant* (λ) may be calculated and is equal to the longitudinal distance along the fiber at which the steady-state E_m is 0.37 of its initial value at R1.

Note also that at shorter times, here, for example, 8 ms, there is less spatial extension of the ΔE_m than later.

Redrawn and adapted from Ruch, Patton, Woodbury, Towe (1965).

resistive elements of the membrane. The latter forces more and more of ILC to seek a lower resistance path to the outside by passing further down the core of the cylindrical cell outward transversely through the next most distalward region of the membrane. At successively more distal levels the magnitude of ILC falls off because of the transverse leakage currents through the intervening membrane. In the above manner the return current distributes itself in time and space down the length of the muscle or nerve fiber membranes.

Obviously, the larger the diameter of the cylinder or nerve fiber, the less the ILR and the further down the axoplasmic core the ILC will spread. The relationship between the ILR and the transverse (or radial) membrane resistance is expressed by the *length constant* (also called space constant), which is the length of a fiber for which the ILR equals the total transverse resistance of the membrane at that length.

The length constant is equal to

$$\left(\frac{R_m \times r}{2R_c} \right) \text{½},$$

where R_m = specific membrane resistance in ohms per cm^2,
R_c = cytoplasmic resistivity in ohms per cm, and
r = radius of the fiber in cm.

The magnitude of the change in TMP at any point imposed by the passage of a constant transmembrane current is thus a function of the total distributed capacitance and resistance of the membrane between the recording electrode and the site of stimulation, as well as the interval between onset of stimulus and the time when the recording is made.

The preceding concepts are important because the action potential is initiated by just such a local outward capacitive current that depolarizes the inactive membrane. There-

fore the lower the capacitance of the membrane and the lower the ILR, the shorter the time needed to depolarize the membrane to the required critical level necessary to trigger the action potential and the shorter the conduction time per unit length of nerve or muscle.

Behavior of Ion Channels

It was pointed out earlier that membrane channels provide a much lower resistance pathway for the passage of certain ions through the membrane than does the surrounding lipid matrix. Sodium and some potassium channels also exhibit voltage-dependent changes in their permeability properties. For example, at the resting transmembrane potential of -70 mV in the squid axon, only about 1 percent of the sodium channels are open. A step depolarization of the membrane to -50 mV, however, leads to a sharp increase in the proportion of sodium channels that are open (activation of the sodium channels), a corresponding sharp increase in sodium membrane conductance (leakiness to sodium ions), and to an inward sodium current driven by the electrochemical gradient of sodium toward the sodium equilibrium potential. This sequence is terminated in the squid axon by the slower processes of inactivation of the sodium channels and activation of the potassium channels. The latter leads to an increase in potassium conductance and, because at this point the transmembrane potential is far from the potassium equilibrium potential, to an outward potassium ion current.

Models of the behavior of the sodium and potassium channels were proposed by Hodgkin and Huxley (see review by Hodgkin, 1967). These have served to predict the proportions and rates at which these channels open and close in response to changes in the TMP. Hodgkin and Huxley postulated that for the sodium channel there were four independent gating mechanisms. Three, called m gates, were closed at the resting transmembrane potential but opened in response to depolarization of the membrane, each opening in about one-tenth of the time necessary for the fourth gate (h) to close. The later h gate was postulated to be open at the resting TMP but to close slowly in a voltage-dependent manner as depolarization of the membrane progressed. In this model m represents the probability that a single gate is in the open position and all three m gates must be open at once.

The magnitude of the resultant sodium channel current is equal to (Hille, 1977):

$$m^3 \times h \times \overline{G}_{Na} (E_m - E_{Na}),$$

where $\overline{G}_{Na}$ = sodium conductance,
$\quad E_m$ = transmembrane potential, and
$\quad E_{Na}$ = equilibrium potential for
$\qquad$ sodium.

It has been suggested that these m gates are negatively charged particles whose negative poles are oriented toward the outside when the channel is closed. To open the channel would then require that all three negatively charged particles alter their orientation toward the inner surface of the channel for the channel to conduct and be open (Armstrong, 1981). This type of change in the spatial orientation of molecules is spoken of as a change in conformation. Hodgkin and Huxley proposed that the inactivation process was not dependent on m events. Recent evidence, however, suggests that the two processes are dependently linked or coupled, that is, that inactivation can only continue when preceded by activation of the channel (Armstrong, 1981).

Whether or not the proportion of sodium channels open changes in response to depolarization depends on how slowly depolarization develops. If depolarization is too slow, the normally slower inactivation process can better keep pace with activation, and the

membrane can then accommodate to the slow depolarization without developing enough open channels to trigger and sustain an action potential. The kinetics of sodium and potassium channels in response to step depolarizations are illustrated by Figure 1.5.

For the potassium channel, Hodgkin and Huxley postulated the presence of four independent but similar gates (n), all of which had to be open at once to open the channel. The potassium channels open more slowly than sodium channels, the proportion of open potassium channels increasing in an S-shaped manner. Depolarization is accompanied by an exponential decline in the number of open potassium channels, although there is no "active" inactivation process as in the sodium channel.

The magnitude of the resultant potassium current would be equal to (Hille, 1977):

$$n^4 \times \overline{G}_K (E_m - E_K),$$

where $\overline{G}_K$ = potassium conductance,
$\quad E_m$ = transmembrane potential, and
$\quad E_k$ = equilibrium potential
$\qquad$ for potassium.

Agents that Block Channels

Large numbers of chemical substances exist in nature, some of which are naturally occurring toxins, which can block various types of ion channels. These agents have provided important tools for the study of the numbers, locations, and properties of ion channels (Ritchie and Chiu, 1981; Ulbricht, 1981). Often these substances act in more than one manner (Strichartz, 1981; Strichartz, Hahin, and Cahalan, 1982). Nonetheless, it is possible to divide them into various groups depending on their primary actions (Table 1.3).

Channel occluders are agents that reduce the permeability of the membrane to sodium irrespective of transmembrane voltage. The effect is to reduce the number of available channels and the conductance per channel as

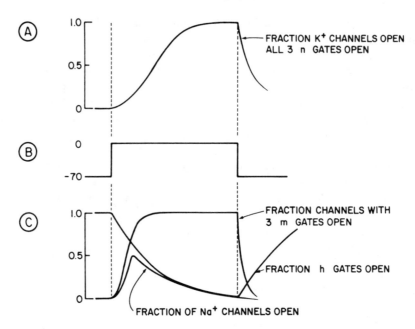

FIGURE 1.5. Kinetics of the potassium (K+) and, in the membrane in sodium (Na+) channels, response to an imposed step depolarization of the membrane from −70 to 0 mv (B).
(A) The fraction (0 to 1) of the K+ channels at which all three n gates are open, the necessary precondition for opening of the potassium channels.
(C) The fractions of Na+ channels at which all three m gates and at which the h gates are open, and the resultant fraction of Na+ channels at which both conditions are met, namely, all three m gates and h gates together are open; the necessary precondition for opening of the sodium channel itself. Note that as more and more h channels close, the fraction of open Na+ channels falls.

if the channels were partially or completely plugged. The binding sites of tetrodotoxin (TTX) and saxitoxin (STX) are on the outside of the channel. These binding sites are not present in sodium channels of denervated muscle membrane. Activators act to increase the proportion of sodium channels open at any particular transmembrane potential. The three naturally occurring alkaloids veratroidine, aconitine, and batrachotoxin are soluble in the membrane. The latter two agents also change the ion-permeability properties of the mem-brane, making the sodium channels more leaky to other, generally larger, monovalent cat-ions.

The scorpion toxins are low-molecular-weight polypeptides and fall into two groups. The north African and Middle Eastern vari-eties have been shown to slow and inhibit the inactivation process and hence substantially prolong the duration of the action potential. The toxin of the sea anemone acts in a similar nonvoltage-dependent manner to block the inactivation process. The American genus

TABLE 1.3.   Agents that Alter Channel Function

Sodium Channel Blockers
  Channel occluders
    Tetrodotoxin (TTX)
    Saxitoxin (STX)
  Channel activators
    Veratroidine
    Aconitine
    Batrachotoxin
    Centruroides (American scorpion)
    Sea anemone
  Blockers of inactivation (stabilizers)
    Androctonus ⎤
    Buthus | (North African and Middle
    Leiurus   ⎦ East scorpions)
    Marine mollusk (genus *Conus*)
  Local anesthetics
  Nonspecific channel modulators
Potassium Channel Blockers
  Tetraethylammonium (TEA)
  4-Aminopyridine (4-AP)

Based on Strichartz, Hahin, and Cahalan (1982).

Centruroides, by contrast, acts as a voltage-dependent channel activator, depolarization increasing the proportion of open channels.

Local anesthetics act to occlude channels and alter the voltage-dependent properties of the sodium channels. These agents are lipid soluble and act from the axoplasmic side of the membrane. Some, such as lidocaine and procainamide, produce a *frequency-dependent block* because of their ability to block trains of impulses, the first few getting through but subsequent impulses in the train blocking because access of the agents to the channels depends on prior activity in the channels.

Still other agents act on sodium channels in a nonspecific manner by altering the charge on the membrane. Normally, cell membranes carry a net negative charge on both the outer and inner surfaces as a result of negatively charged groups in the membrane phospholipids. The positive cations, especially multi-

valent ones, are attracted to these negative charges on the membrane and alter the membrane properties. Lowering concentrations of extracellular calcium ions can cause spontaneous impulse generation, which can be reversed by the addition of calcium ions or other bivalent ions, probably because of the stabilizing effects of these cations on the channel. Increasing tissue pH has an effect similar to that of low calcium levels, possibly by neutralizing negatively charged acidic groups on the membrane.

Potassium channels are blocked by both tetraethylamonium (TEA) and 4-aminopyridine (4-AP), which produce voltage-dependent block; indeed, 4-AP has been used to prove the presence of a late outward potassium current in demyelinated nerve fibers. Both TEA and 4-AP have been shown to prolong the durations of action potentials in unmyelinated nerve fibers, proving the presence of potassium currents in these fibers (see review by Bostock, 1982).

ACTION POTENTIAL

The direction and time courses of the transmembrane ionic currents at the time of the action potential have been analyzed by the voltage clamp technique and selective pharmacological blockade of ion channels by various toxins (Hodgkin, 1967; Hille, 1977). Figure 1.6 illustrates the relative time courses and directions of the TMP, membrane ionic currents, and the changes in membrane conductances in the course of the squid axon action potential. In *phase 1,* there develops depolarization of the membrane by an outward transmembrane capacitive current generated by an adjacent inward ionic current. The transmembrane ionic current through the inactive membrane is low at this point. In *phase 2,* however, the threshold value of the TMP is

FIGURE 1.6. Summary of membrane events in the course of the squid axon impulse. The time courses of the ionic Na+ and K+ currents (B), conductance changes in the membrane to these ion species (C), capacitative membrane currents (D), and the fraction of m, n, and h values open at various times in the course of the action potential cycle (A) of the squid axon. Adapted from Hille (1977).

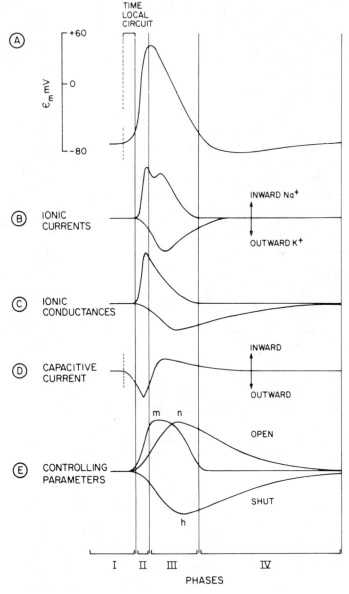

exceeded, and in the Hodgkin and Huxley models there is an abrupt increase in the proportion of m gates open and therefore sodium channels open. The respective potassium n gates and sodium h gates are slower to open and close respectively. The large proportion of open sodium channels substantially increases the sodium permeability of the membrane, and because sodium is far from its equilibrium potential, a large rapid inward sodium current develops accompanied by a subsequent reversal of the TMP toward the sodium equilibrium potential (E_{Na}). At this point the inward ionic current begins to depolarize the adjacent membrane by an outward capacitive current (the local circuit).

Reversal of the TMP is terminated by inactivation or closure of the sodium channels because of the increasing proportion of h gates shut by the depolarization *(phase 3)*. This lowers the sodium conductance and transmembrane current. The increase in potassium conductance is slower to develop because of the slower kinetics of n gate openings. The increase in the proportion of potassium channels open increases the membrane conductance to potassium. There is a consequent large increase in the outward potassium ionic current because the TMP at this point is much nearer to the sodium than the potassium equilibrium potential (E_K).

Finally, in *phase 4* the membrane becomes hyperpolarized because, even though the increase in sodium conductance has come to an end, the increase in membrane conductance to potassium has not. The TMP is therefore driven toward the potassium equilibrium potential only to return to the resting level when the increase in the potassium conductance terminates.

The action potential is thus the result of:

1. Inequalities in concentrations of sodium and potassium between the interior and exterior of the cell
2. Voltage-dependent gating properties of the sodium and potassium channels
3. Relative kinetics of sodium and potassium channel gates
4. The regenerative nature of the sodium conductance (Figure 1.7)

The membrane does not return to normal immediately following the passage of the spike (Figure 1.8). There is an initial period, lasting about 1 to 2 ms, in which no stimulus, however intense, can initiate a second impulse. This period is called the *absolute refractory period* and lasts until the process of sodium channel inactivation terminates and, in the Hodgkin and Huxley models, the h gates begin to reopen. Between the beginning of the latter period and the time when all h gates return to the open position, the membrane remains relatively refractory (the *relative refractory period*). To initiate a second impulse in this period the stimulus must be more intense to overcome the remaining outward potassium current and sodium inactivation process and retrigger the cycle once more. In the relative refractory period the velocity of a second impulse is lower than normal.

Following the relative refractory period there is a *supranormal period* that lasts 100 to

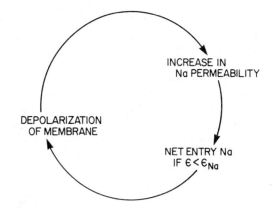

FIGURE 1.7. The regenerative nature of the increase in sodium permeability in the course of the action potential. Depolarization of the membrane increases the proportion of sodium channels open and thence the membrane permeability to sodium ions; this in turn further depolarizes the membrane. This resultant cascade is brought in check by the progressive closure of the h components of the sodium channels and the lessened electrical gradient for sodium as the membrane potential approaches the sodium equilibrium potential.
Redrawn from Hodgkin (1967).

INCREASE IN Na PERMEABILITY

DEPOLARIZATION OF MEMBRANE

NET ENTRY Na IF $\epsilon < \epsilon_{Na}$

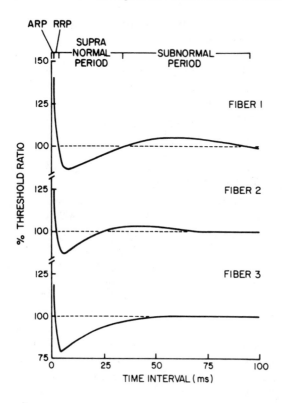

FIGURE 1.8. Excitability changes in single human motor axons (median or ulnar) following a single conditioning percutaneous stimulus. Threshold was defined as the least intensity of stimulus that would evoke five consecutive responses of the motor axon as indicated by the "all" response of the corresponding motor unit potential recorded with surface electrodes over the respective intrinsic hand muscles.

Changes in excitability are expressed as the ratio of the threshold current of the test pulse when conditioned by a preceding pulse to the threshold value of test pulse delivered alone.

The recovery period after a single conditioning pulse is characterized by the *absolute refractory period* (ARP), the *relative refractory period* (RRP), a *supranormal period*, and a late phase of subnormality ending by about 100 ms and absent here in fiber 3. Trains of conditioning stimuli tend to abolish the supranormal period and enhance the period of subnormality.

Redrawn from Bergmans (1970, figure 4A–C).

300 ms. In this period the threshold is lower than normal and the propagation velocity is increased. This period has been observed in human motor axons (Bergmans, 1970). The mechanism is unknown, but may involve an increase in the extracellular potassium concentration.

The supranormal period is followed by a *subnormal period* in which excitability and propagation velocity are lower. This is especially evident in unmyelinated nerve fibers following repetitive stimulation. The mechanism is not understood but may result from the slight electrogenic nature of the sodium-potassium pump, in which the outward flux of sodium slightly exceeds the inward flux of potassium and causes a slight hyperpolarization of the membrane.

Despite the large displacement in TMP in the course of the action potential and the accompanying transmembrane ionic movements, there is usually no substantial change in concentrations of intracellular ions because the actual number of ions that must cross the membrane is very small with respect to their intracellular concentrations. Therefore the concentration gradients for sodium and potassium remain unchanged. This is true even when there have been hundreds of action potentials and the sodium-potassium pump has been blocked.

In electrochemical terms, *threshold* is that level of TMP at which a little depolarization in TMP will trigger an irreversible escalation in the proportion of open sodium channels (the sodium regenerative cycle) (Figure 1.9). Threshold is normally between -55 and -60 mV in mammalian muscle. This level is related to the rate at which the membrane is depolarized, the necessary membrane displacement being a little less when the rate of depolarization is more rapid. This last phenomenon is termed *accommodation*. If the inward transmembrane current produced by the

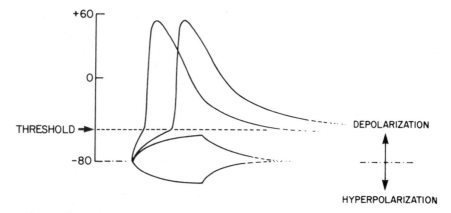

FIGURE 1.9. Intracellularly recorded action potential. Threshold (*interrupted horizontal line*) is the level of depolarization, which if exceeded, triggers the regenerative sodium cycle and produces the action potential.

stimulus lasts too long and is too weak, the sodium channels are shut or inactivated rather than opened, and in excitable membranes where there are potassium channels there is an increase in potassium permeability. This suggests that higher proportions of h gates are closed than m gates are opened in the sodium channels.

Propagation of the Action Potential

The action potential is preceded by a local and outward capacitive transmembrane current that depolarizes the adjacent inactive membrane to threshold and propagates without decrement in a continuous manner along the membrane away from the site of its origin. Such continuous conduction is characteristic of muscle and unmyelinated nerve fibers. The velocity with which the action potential propagates can be calculated simply by dividing the distance between two successive recording sites by the time difference for the impulse to pass between the sites.

Important factors that determine conduction velocity include:

1. Internal longitudinal resistance (ILR); this is related to the diameter of the cylinder and resistance of the core plasm
2. Membrane capacitance

In the case where the membrane capacitance is increased, the local outward transmembrane current must flow longer to discharge the greater charge on the membrane. This prolongs the time required for depolarization to reach threshold and so slows the conduction of the action potential. Conversely, decreasing the membrane capacitance will tend to increase the speed of conduction of the action potential. The capacitance of the membrane is effectively reduced, in the case of myelinated nerve, by the multilaminated myelin sheath.

In muscle fibers, the transverse tubular system has the effect of increasing the overall membrane capacitance. This tends further to slow the overall conduction velocity of the action potential along the outside of the muscle fiber despite the relatively low ILR, because of larger diameter muscle fibers relative to nerve fibers. In theory, changes in resistance of the core plasm of excitable cells could be an important determinant of ILR, but there is no direct evidence to date that conduction is slower in any disease because of an increase in the resistance of the core plasm per se.

The diameter of the excitable cell (see earlier discussion of the electrical properties of the membrane) is a vital factor determining the speed of conduction of action potentials. In unmyelinated nerve fibers the conduction velocity can only be increased by an increase in the diameter of the fiber. There is, however, a practical limit to this solution. For example, the squid unmyelinated axon, which has a conduction velocity of about 25 m/s, has a diameter of about 500 µ. Such an increase in diameter is thus one evolutionary solution to the need to increase conduction velocity and meets the needs of lower animals with less complex nervous systems. This solution is not a very satisfactory one in more complex nervous systems where space is at a premium. To achieve conduction velocities in unmyelinated nerve fibers equivalent to those in the more rapidly conducting myelinated nerve fibers, the diameters of the unmyelinated nerve fibers would have to be so large as to impose an enormous and unacceptable increase in the bulk of the peripheral nerves in order to transmit the equivalent volume of impulse traffic. For this reason alone, increasing the diameter of unmyelinated nerve fibers is a poor means of increasing conduction velocities in peripheral nerves and central tracts. Moreover, because conduction is continuous and the entire membrane is open to extracellular space in unmyelinated nerve fibers, the total active and passive ionic movements through the membrane are larger in comparison to myelinated nerve fibers. This imposes substantially higher metabolic loads on the sodium-potassium

pump mechanism. Therefore the biological limitations imposed on unmyelinated nerve fibers in the mammalian nervous system relative to myelinated nerve fibers are their higher metabolic demands and slower conduction velocities.

Action Potential Generation and Conduction in Myelinated Nerve

The action potential of the squid axon is a reasonable model of action potential conduction for mammalian unmyelinated nerve fibers in that in both, the early inward sodium current is followed by the slower development of an outward potassium current. In mammalian myelinated nerve fibers, however, the nodal membranes contain few if any potassium channels. Indeed, the outward potassium current is probably less necessary in myelinated nerve fibers because of the higher speed of inactivation of sodium channels in the nodal region and the larger leakage currents in these fibers compared to the squid axon. Late outward potassium currents in mammalian myelinated nerve fibers have been shown where the paranodal membrane has been bared by treatments designed to loosen the attachment of the paranodal myelin, the axolemma, or break down the myelin sheath in this region (Chiu and Ritchie, 1980, 1981; Sherratt, Bostock, and Sears, 1980; Bostock, Sears, and Sherratt, 1981; Bostock, 1982; Waxman, 1983).

The evidence is excellent that in normal myelinated nerve, conduction of the action potential is discontinuous or saltatory (Figure 1.10). Active membrane ionic currents are limited to the nodal membrane (Figure 1.10), the internode membrane behaving like a short cable segment with a distributed capacitance through which the transmembrane currents are only outward and passive. Demonstration of the above current pattern in myelinated nerve

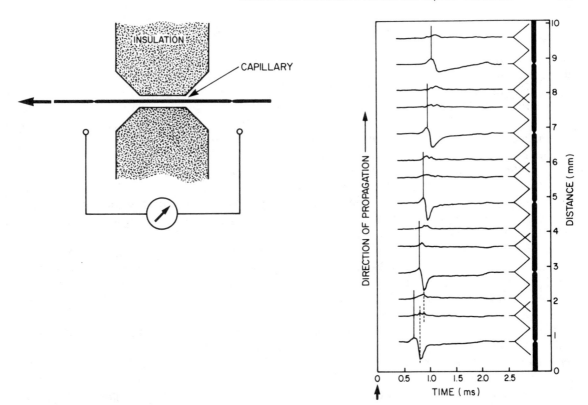

FIGURE 1.10. (Left) Single myelinated nerve fiber being drawn through a fine capillary whose width is somewhat less than the internode length of the fiber. The external longitudinal currents across the short segment of the nerve fiber enclosed by the capillary will be proportional to the difference in potential across the capillary segment. The external longitudinal currents across successive segments of the nerve fiber may be examined by drawing the fiber through the capillary.

(Right) Saltatory conduction in a frog myelinated nerve fiber. Shown are the membrane currents (currents outward through the membrane are shown as up) derived by subtraction of successive adjacent external longitudinal currents. Note that the largest currents are inward and occur opposite the nodal regions. Between adjacent nodal regions, the direction of the transmembrane currents is outward. Note also the stepwise increase in latency of the membrane currents at each successive node and next adjacent internodal segment. Onsets of the inward currents are indicated by solid vertical bars. The two interrupted vertical lines indicate the outward membrane currents through one internode segment produced by the inward nodal currents at the nodes immediately proximal and distal to this internodal segment.

Redrawn from Huxley and Stämpfli (1949a, figures 3 and 12).

fibers was established by Tasaki and Takeuchi (1942), Tasaki (1953), and later Huxley and Stämpfli (1949a, 1949b), and has been reviewed by Rogart and Stämpfli (1982). Because the modified method of Huxley and Stämpfli has been employed in examinations

of conduction in demyelinated nerve fibers, the original method is reviewed here.

In this method, in order to limit the extension of the external longitudinal current pathway to the immediate extracellular space, single myelinated nerve fibers were drawn through a short (less than one internode length) glass capillary tube (Figure 1.10 left). Measurement of the potential across the capillary segment provides a measure of the external longitudinal current and changes in the latter with time and passage of the nerve impulse. It was pointed out earlier that beyond a stimulus current source, the internal longitudinal current diminishes with distance because of the series internal longitudinal resistance and the outward (or transverse) current leakages through the intervening membrane. For like reasons, the magnitude of the external longitudinal current progressively falls off as the longitudinal distance increases between the site of origin of the current and the site where the current is measured.

If the external longitudinal currents are measured over adjacent segments, that part of the internal longitudinal current that has leaked transversely through the membrane can be calculated by subtraction of the external longitudinal currents measured over successive short segments of nerve fiber. The resultant serial transmembrane currents are outward along the internode segment but diminish with increasing distance from the proximal node. At the nodal region, however, the initial outward and capacitive current is terminated by a larger inward current, evidenced by a reversal in the direction of the current trace (Figure 1.10). The TMP can be obtained by integration of the current with distance. Because the internode segment behaves like a passive cable with a high transverse resistance and low capacitance, the transmembrane potential at the mid-internode level approximates the mean of the equivalent levels at the two adjacent nodal regions.

Special note should be made of the abrupt increase in latency of the external longitudinal current at the beginning of successive internode segments. This time delay is present because:

1. There is a slight time delay in progression of the transmembrane current down the internode segment; this in turn is the product of distributed internode membrane capacitance.
2. The time is required for the outward transmembrane current at the nodal region to reach threshold for generation of the inward sodium regenerative current. Potassium channels, as mentioned earlier, are absent in the nodal membrane, although present in the internodal membrane in myelinated nerve fibers.

The number of internode segments per action potential and the internode conduction time are more or less constant irrespective of the diameters of the nerve fibers in any particular species. Among species, however, the internode conduction time varies between 70 μsec in the cat to 25 μsec in the rat.

The original method pioneered by Huxley and Stämpfli was subsequently modified by Rasminsky and Sears (1972) and later Bostock and Sears (1978) to investigate conduction in single myelinated nerve fibers in an intact multifiber spinal root preparation in the rat (Figure 1.11). In this preparation the unbranched root was presumed to be a uniform linear conductor. Single nerve fibers were excited by microstimulation at a more distal level, and the voltage differences between a closely spaced pair of electrodes (interelectrode distances were less than the internode length) were measured at intervals along the length of the root. The potential difference was assumed to be proportional to the external longitudinal current generated by the underlying nerve impulse. For example, $V = I$ (external longitudinal current) times R, where R equals the resistance between the recording electrodes and is assumed to be relatively constant.

Unlike the original Huxley-Stämpfli

methood, the whole-root preparation precludes measurement of the absolute values of the external longitudinal current because the actual interelectrode resistances along the root are not constant. The distinction is minor, however, because the method still makes it possible to establish the general pattern and direction of the membrane currents by subtraction of adjacent external longitudinal currents and measurement of the latencies of the respective external longitudinal and transmembrane currents.

The external longitudinal current measured over the internode has two peaks corresponding to their origins from their respective proximal and distal nodal regions. The above method has the outstanding advantage of being able to record the membrane currents in undissected and therefore minimally disturbed fibers in various experimental peripheral nerve lesions. Although propagation of the inward membrane current is saltatory and jumps from node to node, propagation of the action potential is continuous. Depolarization and repolarization progress down the internode segment at an even rate, the value of the TMP at the mid-internode being the mean of the potentials at the proximal and distal nodal regions. This even progression of TMP down the length of the internode is purely a reflec-

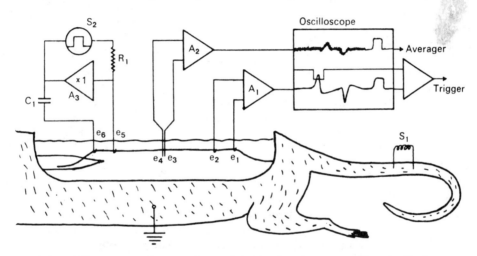

FIGURE 1.11. (Above) Experimental arrangement for recording the external longitudinal currents accompanying conduction of impulses in single myelinated nerve fibers of a multifiber root. In this modification of the original method reported by Rasminsky and Sears (1972), single motor axons in the rat's tail are excited by a fine pair of stimulating electrodes inserted into the tail. Antidromic potentials in the corresponding ventral root fibers were recorded by electrode pair e_1-e_2 and the intensity of the stimulus was adjusted to be just above threshold for evoking a single all-or-nothing biphasic spike at e_{1-2}. The later spike served to trigger an electronic averager, which in turn served to average the potential difference recorded by a second pair of electrodes e_3-e_4 on which the ventral root was mounted. The electrodes in this pair were close to one another (120 to 140 μ apart). The later potential drop across the gap between the e_3 and e_4 electrodes is proportional to the external longitudinal current, the resistance between e_3 and e_4 being considered constant for practical purposes. By subtraction of such successively recorded external longitudinal currents, the transmembrane currents and their direction may be derived. Electronic averaging of these recordings is necessary because of the high impedance presented by such fine recording electrodes.

(continued)

FIGURE 1.11. *(continued)*

The second stimulator circuit (S_2), also receiving its trigger pulse from the spike recorded at e_1-e_2, puts out a known current pulse for calibrating the potentials recorded at e_3-e_4. This allows the experimenter to take account of variations in interelectrode e_3-e_4 resistance and so rescale the derived membrane currents as the electrode pair is moved along the ventral root. In this way the membrane currents over successive short segments of the myelinated nerve fibers may be measured. A time-calibrated pulse (x) is also put out by amplifier A_3 when the impulse reaches e_5. A constant conduction time between e_1 and e_5 helps to ensure that the experimental conditions have not changed in the course of the procedure. This calibration pulse, like the calibrated current pulse, extends along the root to be picked up at e_4-e_3 and e_2-e_1.

(Right) Illustrative recordings of the averaged external longitudinal currents (A) as measured over successive short intervals of a single myelinated nerve fiber in a healthy rat plotted against time (ms) and position along the fiber (mm). (B) The corresponding derived transmembrane currents obtained through subtracting successive adjacent external longitudinal membrane currents are shown. Inward currents are shown as down; the impulse propagates from below upward. Note the current calibration pulse on the right of the external longitudinal current recordings.

From Bostock and Sears (1978, figures 1 and 3).

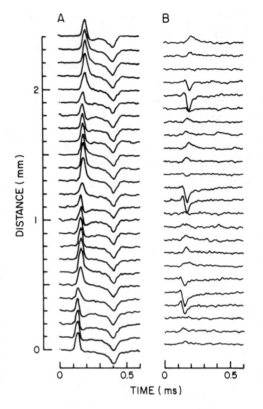

tion of the passive cable properties of the internode. There is, however, a progressive increase in the rise time of the potential as it progresses down the internode toward the next node. This is because of the distributed capacitance of the internode segment, with refreshment of the potential near the terminal end of the internode due to renewal of the inward transmembrane current at the next node.

Many nodal regions are active at once, the nerve impulse extending over as many as 10 to 30 internodes (Figure 1.12). The length of the nerve fiber over which the impulse extends is a product of the duration and conduction velocity of the impulse. Thus the wavelength of the impulse (in millimeters) equals spike duration (in milliseconds) times conduction velocity (in millimeters per millisecond). For example, the length occupied by an impulse in a myelinated nerve fiber that has a conduction velocity of 60 m/s is about 20 mm or more. In this example, over 20 internodes are active at one instant. The length of nerve fiber occupied by the impulse in a smaller nerve fiber that has a lower conduction velocity is correspondingly less (Table 1.4).

The conduction velocity of myelinated nerve fibers, like unmyelinated nerve fibers, is directly related to the ILR, especially that part related to axon diameter, the cable properties of the membrane (both capacitance and resistance), internode length, and temperature.

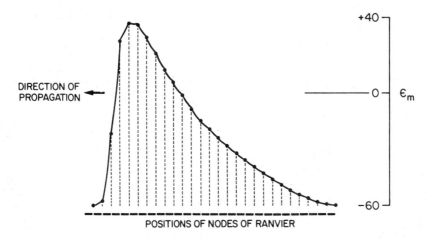

FIGURE 1.12.   Longitudinal distribution of the action potential in a single myelinated nerve fiber whose successive internode segments are indicated by successive dashes in the horizontal line at the base. Note that in this hypothetical nerve fiber the action potential actually extends over 27 successive internodes and the active inward sodium currents over three to four successive nodes.
Adapted from Rogart and Ritchie (1977, figure 13).

The importance of these factors in the conduction of the nerve impulse in abnormal nerve is stressed in later chapters.

In normal myelinated fibers, optimal relationships exist among myelin thickness, axon diameter, and internode length to achieve the maximum impulse velocity. For example, leakages of transmembrane current across the internodal myelin and axonal membrane can be reduced by increasing the thickness of the myelin sheath by increasing the number of myelin lamellae. For a given outside diameter

TABLE 1.4.   Physiological Characteristics of Action Potentials in Myelinated and Unmyelinated Nerve Fibers

Type of Nerve Fiber	Duration of Spike (ms)	CV (m/s)	Length Occupied by the Spike (mm)	ARP	RRP	Blocking Frequency (Hz)
Large myelinated to Small myelinated	0.2–0.5	30–120	30	0.7–1.0	2–3	100
Unmyelinated	About 1.0	<1.0	1	10–20		10

Adapted from Paintal (1966).
ARP = absolute refractory period.
RRP = relative refractory period.

TABLE 1.5.   Scaling Factors in Relation to the Diameters of Nerve Fibers in Various Species

Species	Investigators	Nerve Fiber Diameter (μ)	Scaling Factor
Cat	Boyd and Kalu (1979)	10–20	5.7
		3–10	4.6
Primate	McLeod and Wray (1967)	17–18	5.2
Human	Buchthal and Rosenfalck (1966)	7–12	5.7

of a nerve fiber, however, the effect is to reduce the axonal diameter and thus increase the ILR, thereby limiting the longitudinal spread of the ILC. The optimal ratio of axonal diameter to overall nerve fiber diameter is approximately 0.6 (Rushton, 1951).

In mammalian myelinated nerve, the magnitude of the conduction velocity is related to the diameter and internode length of the nerve fiber. The precise relationships between the outside diameters of nerve fibers and their conduction velocities are not constant but vary somewhat with species and fiber size. The relationship between fiber diameter and conduction velocity is expressed by the scaling factor:

Scaling factor

$$= \frac{\text{conduction velocity of the nerve fiber   (in m/s)}}{\text{outside diameter of the nerve fiber (in μ)}}.$$

The scaling factor values for various species and diameters of nerve fibers are illustrated in Table 1.5.

Conduction velocities in myelinated nerve are also related to the internode length (IL), the optimal ratio of IL to outside diameter varying with the species (Table 1.6). In human sural nerve the range of internode lengths is between 0.2 mm in the smallest- to 2.0 mm in the largest-diameter myelinated fibers.

One of the most important determinants of conduction velocity is environmental temperature. In cat nerve, the velocity falls by about 2 m/s per degree centigrade as the temperature is lowered (Paintal, 1965a, 1965b, 1973) (Figure 1.13). Equivalent values have been observed in man (DeJong, Hershey, and Wagman, 1966; Buchthal and Rosenfalck, 1966; Denys, 1980). The slower velocities are probably the result of slower opening times for sodium channels at lower temperatures. It therefore takes longer for the outward current at the next nodal region to depolarize the nodal membrane to threshold and begin the sodium regenerative cycle.

There may also be a slower rate of sodium inactivation. These changes in sodium channel kinetics would be expected to prolong the duration and slow the rise time of the action potential as well as possibly increase its am-

TABLE 1.6.   Ratio of Internode Length to Outside Diameter in Various Species

Species	Ratio IL:OD
Cat	90
Rabbit	59–72
Rat	175
Human	100

IL = internodal length.
OD = outside diameter.

FIGURE 1.13. Changes in conduction velocity of two myelinated nerve fibers in the same filament of the cat saphenous nerve. Changes are expressed as a percentage of their maximum velocity at 36°C, over the temperature range between 4 and 36°C (left). Note similar relative changes in conduction in both fibers whose normal conduction velocities were widely dissimilar. The absolute declines in conduction velocity are of course much greater in the larger, faster-conducting nerve fibers (right). Adapted from Paintal (1965b, figure 2).

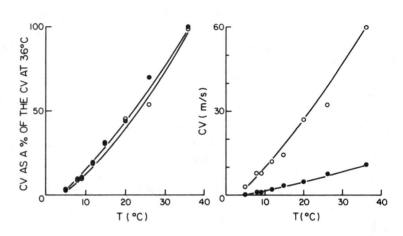

plitude (Hodgkin and Katz, 1949) (Figure 1.14). Also, the slower sodium channel inactivation times could explain the progressive lengthening of the absolute refractory period observed at lower environmental temperatures (Paintal, 1965a, 1965b). The absolute refractory period is notably longer in slower-conducting than in faster-conducting nerve fibers (Paintal, 1973).

The longer transmembrane currents at lower temperatures no doubt explain the restoration of saltatory conduction in some de-

myelinated nerve fibers where these impulses have been blocked at higher temperatures (Rasminsky, 1973). In healthy myelinated nerve, the impulses block at temperatures of over 44°C and below 5 to 10°C (Paintal, 1973; Schauf and Davis, 1974). Unmyelinated nerve fibers are said to block at even lower temperatures.

Conduction blocks in amphibian myelinated nerve fibers at about 30°C, whereas in some mammalian nerve fibers it may continue up to 48°C, at which point the block becomes

FIGURE 1.14. Changes in the shape of the action potential in the squid axon at temperatures between 32.5°C action potential on the left and 3.6°C action potential on the right. Note the higher amplitude and much longer duration of the action potential at the lower temperatures. The two action potentials in between were recorded at 20.2° and 9.8°C respectively. Redrawn from Hodgkin and Katz (1949, figure 4).

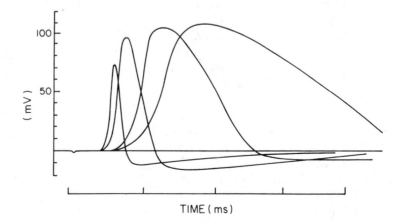

irreversible. Conduction block at higher temperatures probably develops because as the temperature increases, the rate of sodium channel inactivation increases to a level at which inactivation so reduces the inward current that the latter is no longer adequate to depolarize the membrane (Rogart and Stämpfli, 1982).

The relationship of the time course and amplitudes of impulses to their conduction velocities is important. The larger the diameter of a nerve fiber and the faster its conduction velocity, the longer the peak-to-peak (p-p) duration and the higher the p-p amplitude of its action potential recorded by extracellular techniques, the amplitude of the extracellularly recorded nerve fiber action potential being proportional to the square of its conduction velocity.

ELECTRICAL EVENTS IN MUSCLE FIBERS

The preceding reviews of the TMP and generation of the action potential were based primarily on observations in nerve fibers. Muscle fibers as excitable cells have some important and unique characteristics (Costantin, 1977). For example, they have an extensive transverse tubular system (TTS), which consists of tubules open to the extracellular space.

This tubular network is flanked on both sides by vesicles that belong to the sarcoplasmic reticulum. The myofibrils are surrounded by both tubular and sarcoplasmic reticulum elements, the latter extending from Z line to Z line and taking the shape of the cisternae in the region of the I band. The number of contacts between the sarcoplasmic reticulum and transverse tubular junctions is higher in faster-contracting muscles.

The total membrane area in contact with the extracellular space is enormously increased by the tubular network, this more than doubling the membrane capacitance of the

outside membrane alone with which it is in series. One consequence of the high capacitance in muscle fibers is slowing of conduction to a velocity well below that which would be observed in a squid axon, even if allowances are made for differences between their diameters and internal conductivities.

The action potential in a muscle membrane originates at the postsynaptic region, from which region it propagates, without decrement, in opposite directions toward the ends of the muscle fiber. The potential spreads inward at intervals along the transverse tubular network toward the interior of the muscle fiber. Inward conduction has been demonstrated to be active and not electrotonic (or passive). By unknown mechanisms the depolarization in the transverse tubular membrane leads to release of calcium ions from the cisternae of the sarcoplasmic reticulum into the myoplasm. This triggers the repetitive cycle of attachment and reattachment of cross-bridge linkages between the actin and myosin myofilaments, and progressive movement of actin filaments inward on the myosin filaments to shorten the muscle fiber. The sequence is terminated by reuptake of the calcium ions by adenosinetriphosphate-dependent mechanisms in the cisternae. Although the velocity of muscle shortening is independent of the degree of overlap in the myofilaments, the force generated is proportional to the number of cross bridges between the myofilaments.

The impulse in muscle fibers is similar in its voltage-time characteristics to the impulse in the squid axon. The negative afterpotential lasts much longer in muscle, however. The reasons are not clear at this time, but possibilities include:

1. Potassium accumulation in the transverse tubular system (there is no direct evidence for this)
2. Earlier inactivation of potassium conductance when the transmembrane po-

tential is within 20 mV of resting TMP, the subsequent repolarization being slowed to the time course of the time constant of the muscle fiber (about 20 ms)

The chloride conductance of the transverse tubular system is limited, a point that will be returned to in a later chapter when the myotonic phenomenon is reviewed. Furthermore, the permeability of muscle fiber membrane to potassium has the rectifying property of passing potassium ions much better in one direction than the other, the magnitude of the potassium current depending on the direction of the current.

ELECTRICAL STIMULATION OF NERVE AND MUSCLE

Stimulation of muscle and nerve has been reviewed by Ranck (1981), Swett and Bourassa (1981), and Mortimer (1981). Direct passage of current through the membrane can be achieved by introduction of one electrode of a pair into the interior of the cell. Provided there is no appreciable leakage of current

about the puncture site, the nearby membrane can be depolarized by making the intracellular electrode positive with respect to an extracellular electrode, the return current passing outward through the membrane. Biologically, current is carried by ions and is conventionally in the direction of the positive ions. Such direct transmembrane stimulation is only possible by means of microelectrodes.

In all human situations where it is necessary to stimulate nerve or muscle, both stimulating electrodes must be extracellular. The electrode arrangement may be monopolar, in which case a small cathode is placed near the desired site of stimulation. A larger remote electrode, often in the longitudinal axis of the nerve trunk or muscle, serves as the anode. More often the arrangement is bipolar (or bifocal) and one in which both electrodes, cathode and anode, are positioned near one another with the cathode nearest the recording electrode. This method has less associated stimulus artifact than does the monopolar technique, but it does have disadvantages (discussed in Chapter 3).

Figure 1.15 illustrates direction and path of current in the course of extracellular stimu-

FIGURE 1.15. Percutaneous stimulation of an underlying nerve fiber. (A) At the outset the current path shown by the lines passing through the underlying tissues between the anode (+) and cathode (−) pass mostly outside the nerve fiber, very little current going through the underlying membranes.

(B) As the stimulus intensity is increased, more and more of the current passes into the fiber beneath the anode, hyperpolarizing its membrane, then continues longitudinally down the core of the fiber to exit through the membrane underlying the anode. The membrane beneath the cathode is depolarized, and should this exceed threshold, an action potential will be generated at this site.

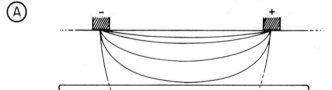

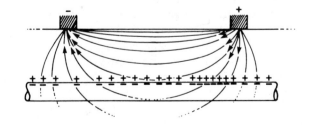

lation of an unmyelinated nerve fiber. When the stimulus pulse is turned on, the current distributes itself throughout the extracellular space and seeks the path of least resistance between the anode and cathode. At low stimulus intensities all the current will be extracellular. If the current intensity is increased, however, part of the current will pass through the membrane beneath the anode, and traverse the interior of the fiber to exit beneath the cathode. Beneath the cathode there is movement of positive ions toward and onto the interior surface of the membrane. This releases positive charges on the external surface previously held there by the net negative charge on the interior. These positive charges on the external surface are now free to move toward the cathode. The initial transmembrane current is therefore capacitive.

The TMP at rest is directly proportional to the charge concentration on the membrane surface. The initial transmembrane outward capacitive current beneath the cathode is not paralleled by a proportional change in the transmembrane voltage because relatively little work is required to discharge the charge on the membrane. Shortly, however, there is a progressive increase in the work required to bring more positive charge onto the interior membrane surface because of a progressive increase in the concentration of positive charge on the inner membrane surface. At some point the membrane begins to depolarize, and as the current continues, the level of this depolarization approximates more and more the applied current as the work required to bring more positive charge onto the membrane approaches the work required to move ions directly through the membrane (resistive current). The level of depolarization eventually reaches the critical level at which there is an abrupt change in the permeability of the membrane to sodium, and generation of the all-or-nothing impulse follows.

In a similar manner, the outward capacitive transmembrane current that precedes the all-or-nothing impulse depolarizes the membrane just ahead of the impulse. This outward current is termed the *local circuit*. The longitudinal extent of this local circuit depolarization is limited primarily by the ILR.

In myelinated nerves the current most easily enters the nerve fiber at the nodal regions. It is the relative magnitudes of ILRs that primarily govern the excitabilities or *thresholds* of nerve fibers of various diameters. The larger the diameter of the nerve fiber, the smaller the axoplasmic core resistance to the passage of the ILC (ILR is proportional to the square of the diameter). Larger-diameter nerve fibers also have longer length constants (the length of the fiber at which the transverse membrane resistance equals the internal longitudinal resistance, or ILR) and shorter time constants. The last property is primarily a product of the lower membrane capacitance of the internode segments in the more thickly myelinated larger nerve fibers. In healthy myelinated nerve fibers the length constant is approximately equal to two internode lengths.

Differences in the relative excitabilities of nerve fibers of differing diameters are well illustrated by a comparison of their strength/duration curves. The strength/duration curve is a plot of the least stimulus intensities at various stimulus durations that are capable of exciting a nerve. The curve expresses the relationship between threshold current and stimulus pulse duration for a given single fiber or group of fibers. Figure 1.16 illustrates the curves for nerve fibers of differing diameters (outside). In this type of plot, *rheobase* is theoretically the least current required to stimulate a fiber with a stimulus pulse of infinitely long duration. Very long stimulus pulses, however, cause accommodation and loss of excitability. For this reason, the longest stimulus pulses employed are somewhat shorter (1 to 2 ms) and another measurement, the chronaxie, is used to describe the relative excita-

FIGURE 1.16.   Relationships between stimulus intensity in milliamperes (ma) and pulse duration for excitation of myelinated nerve fibers of different diameters based on calculations using Frankenhaeuser-Huxley equations for myelinated axons. Note the higher relative thresholds for smaller-diameter fibers.
Courtesy of Mortimer (1981, figure 18).

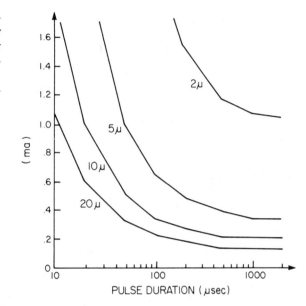

PULSE DURATION (μsec)

bilities of nerve or muscle fibers. *Chronaxie* is the duration of a stimulus whose current is double rheobase and which just stimulates the nerve fiber or muscle fiber. Table 1.7 illustrates the differences in chronaxie between myelinated and unmyelinated nerve fibers.

The larger the nerve fiber, the shorter the chronaxie. The best separation between thresholds of nerve fibers is achieved by stimulus pulses about 100 μsec in duration. Because of their large capacitance and despite their large diameters, muscle fibers have much higher chronaxie values than do nerve fibers.

TABLE 1.7.   Chronaxie Values of Nerve Fibers in Peripheral and Central Nervous Systems

	Chronaxie (ms)
Peripheral nervous system	
A alpha fibers	0.020
C fibers	1.500
Central nervous system	
Myelinated fibers	0.050–0.100
Unmyelinated fibers	0.156–0.380

From Ranck (1981).

In human investigations it is also important to employ as brief a stimulus as possible, because the longer the stimulus duration the more uncertainty as to the exact time the impulse was initiated beneath the cathode. There is a minimum period, shorter than the stimulus duration, in which the local current must flow before the impulse is initiated. Therefore the time between onset of stimulus and when the impulse reaches a position beneath the recording electrode is equal to the time required for the local current to depolarize the membrane to threshold plus the actual conduction time between where the impulse was initiated and its arrival beneath the recording electrode.

If the time the local current must flow is too long in relation to conduction time, a substantial error may be introduced in measurement of conduction velocity (Figure 1.17). Two ways to avoid this error include:

1.   Use of the briefest stimulus possible, with an intensity 10 to 20 percent supramaximal to initiate the impulse

FIGURE 1.17. (A) Model of a single nerve fiber (or muscle fiber) into which two recording electrodes $(E_m)_1$ and $(E_m)_2$ are inserted a distance d_2 apart for the purpose of recording the transmembrane potential (E_m). If a current (1) is injected into the fiber, the membrane in the region of E_{m_1} becomes depolarized. The more intense the current pulse, the brisker the depolarization and the sooner threshold is exceeded and the action potential generated at E_{m_1} (B). The arrival times (t 1-3) of the action potential at $(E_m)_2$ depend not only on the conduction distance (d) and the conduction velocity between the two recording electrodes, but on the time interval between onset of the stimulus pulse and subsequent generation of the action potential. For maximum accuracy in the measurement of conduction times (and velocities) it is important therefore to use brief suprathreshold stimulus pulses. Moreover, the conduction velocity over d is best calculated by measuring the interval between onset or arrival of the spike at E_{m_1} and E_{m_2}, and not the interval between onset of the stimulus and the arrival of the action potential, because the later time includes an obligatory activation time.

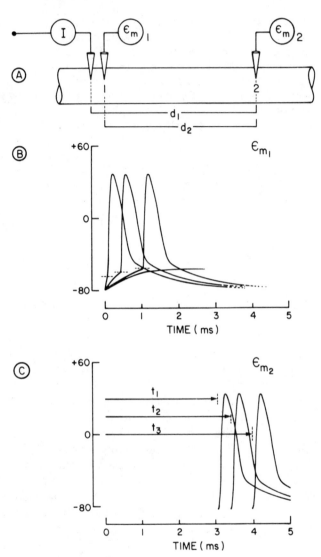

2. Measurement of the conduction velocity between two recording points along the length of the nerve beyond the stimulating electrode

When the stimulus is too high, *anodal block* may develop in the vicinity of the anode because of hyperpolarization of the membrane at this site. *Break excitation* in the same region may occur at the termination of the stimulus pulse. Both problems may produce errors and artifacts in human electrophysiological investigations of peripheral nerve, especially in situations in which thresholds of peripheral nerve fibers are very high and bipolar stimulating electrodes are employed.

References

Armstrong CM. Ionic pores, gates and gating current. Q Rev Biophys 1975;7:179–210.

Armstrong CM. Sodium channels and gating currents. Physiol Rev 1981;61:644–83.

Barchi RL. Excitation and conduction in nerve. In: Sumner, AJ, ed. The physiology of peripheral nerve disease. Philadelphia: WB Saunders, 1980.

Bergmans J. The physiology of single human nerve fibers. Louvain, Belgium: Vander, 1970.

Bostock H. Conduction changes in mammalian axons following experimental demyelination. In: Culp WJ, Ochoa J, eds. Abnormal nerve and muscles as impulse generators. Oxford: Oxford University Press, 1982:236–52.

Bostock H, Sears TA, Sherratt RM. The effects of 4-amionopyridine and tetraethylammonium ions on normal and demyelinated mammalian nerve fibers. J Physiol 1981;313:301–15.

Bostock H, Sears TA. The internodal axon membrane: electrical excitability and continuous conduction in segmental demyelination. J Physiol 1978;280:273–301.

Boyd IA, Kalu KU. Scaling factor relating conduction velocity and diameter for myelinating afferent nerve fibers in the cat hind limb. J Physiol 1979;289:277–97.

Buchthal F, Rosenfalck A. Evoked action potentials and conduction velocity in human sensory nerves. Brain Res 1966;3:1–122.

Chiu SY, Ritchie JM. Evidence for the presence of potassium channels in the internodal region of acutely demyelinated mammalian nerve fibers. J Physiol 1981;313:415–37.

Chiu SY, Ritchie JM. Potassium channels in nodal and internodal axonal membrane of myelinated fibers. Nature 1980;284:170–71.

Costantin LL. Activation in striated muscle. In: Handbook of physiology. Section I: The nervous system. Vol. 1. Cellular biology of neurons. Bethesda, Md.: American Physiological Society, 1977:215–59.

Culp WJ, Ochoa J, eds. Abnormal nerves and muscles as impulse generators. Oxford: Oxford University Press, 1982.

DeJong RH, Hershey WN, Wagman IH. Nerve conduction during hypothermia in man. Anaesthesiology 1966;27:805–10.

Denys EH. The role of temperature in electromyography. Minimonograph 14. Rochester, Minn.: American Association of Electromyography and Electrodiagnosis, 1980.

Hamil OP, Marty A, Neher E, Sakmann B, Sigworth FJ. Improved patch-clamp techniques for high-resolution current recording from cells and cell-free membrane patches. Pflügers Arch 1981;391:85–100.

Hille B. Ionic basis of resting and action potentials. In: Kandel ER, ed. Handbook of physiology. The nervous system. Vol. 1. Cellular biology of neurons. Bethesda, Md.: American Physiological Society, 1977:99–136.

Hodgkin AL. The conduction of the nervous impulse. Liverpool: Liverpool University Press, 1967.

Hodgkin AL. The optimal density of sodium channels in an unmyelinated nerve. Philos Trans R Soc Lond [Biol] 1975;270:297–300.

Hodgkin AL, Katz B. The effect of temperature on the electrical activity of the giant axon of the squid. J Physiol 1949;109:240–49.

Huxley AF, Stämpfli R. Evidence for saltatory conduction in peripheral myelinated nerve fibers. J Physiol 1949a;108:315–39.

Huxley AF, Stämpfli R. Saltatory transmission of the nervous impulse. Arch Sci Physiol 1949b;3:435–48.

Kuffler SW, Nicholls JG. From neuron to brain. Sunderland, Mass.: Sinauer Associates, 1976:1–486.

McLeod JG, Wray SH. Conduction velocity and fiber diameter of the median and ulnar nerves of the baboon. J Neurol Neurosurg Psychiatry 1967;30:240–47.

Mendell LM, Henneman E. Terminals of single Ia fibers: locations, density and distribution within a pool of 300 homonymous motoneurons. J Neurophysiol 1971;34:171–87.

Mortimer JT. Motor prostheses. In: Brooks VB, ed. Handbook of physiology. The nervous system. Vol 2. Motor control. Bethesda, Md.: American Physiological Society, 1981.

Mountcastle VB. Medical physiology. Baltimore: CV Mosby, 1980.

Paintal AS. Block of conduction in mammalian myelinated nerve fibers by low temperatures. J Physiol 1965a;180:1–19.

Paintal AS. Effects of temperature on conduction in single vagal and saphenous myelinated nerve fibers of the cat. J Physiol 1965b;180:20–49.

Paintal AS. The influence of diameter of medullated nerve fibers of cats on the rising and falling phases of the spike and its recovery. J Physiol 1966;184:791–811.

Paintal AS. Conduction in mammalian nerve fibers. In: Desmedt JE, ed. New developments of electromyography and clinical neurophysiology. Basel: Karger 1973:19–41.

Pfenninger KH. Organization of neuronal membranes. Ann Rev Neurosci 1978;1:445–71.

Ranck JB. Extracellular stimulation. In: Patterson M, Kesner RP, eds. Electrical stimulation research techniques. New York: Academic Press, 1981:2–36.

Rasminsky M. The effects of temperature on conduction in demyelinated single nerve fibers. Arch Neurol 1973;28:287–92.

Rasminsky M, Sears TA. Internodal conduction in undissected demyelinated nerve fibers. J Physiol 1972;227:323–50.

Ritchie JM. Sodium channels in muscle and nerve. In: Aguayo AJ, Karpati G, eds. Current topics in nerve and muscle research. Amsterdam, Oxford: Excerpta Medica, 1979:210–19.

Ritchie JM, Chiu SY. Distribution of sodium and potassium channels in mammalian myelinated nerve. In: Waxman SG, Ritchie JM, eds. Demyelinating disease: basic and clinical electrophysiology. New York: Raven Press, 1981:329–42.

Ritchie JM. On the relation between fiber diameter and conduction velocity in myelinated nerve fibers. Proc R Soc Lond 1982;217:29–35.

Rogart RB, Ritchie JM. Physiological basis of conduction in myelinated nerve fibers. In: Morell P, ed. Myelin. New York, London: Plenum Press, 1977:117–159.

Rogart RB, Stämpfli R. Voltage-clamp studies of mammalian myelinated nerve. In: Culp WJ, Ochoa H, eds. Abnormal nerves and muscles as impulse generators. Oxford: Oxford University Press, 1982:193–210.

Ruch TC, Patton HD, Woodbury JW, Towe AL. Neurophysiology. Philadelphia: WB Saunders, 1965.

Rushton WAH. A theory of the effects of fiber size in medullated nerve. J Physiol 1951;115:101–22.

Schauf CL, Davis FA. Impulse conduction in multiple sclerosis: a theoretical basis for modification by temperature and pharmacological agents. J Neurol Neurosurg Psychiatry 1974;37:152–61.

Sherratt RM, Bostock H, Sears TA. Effects of 4-aminopyridine on normal and demyelinated mammalian nerve fibers. Nature 1980;283:570–72.

Singer SJ. The molecular organization of membranes. Ann Rev Biochem 1974;43:805–33.

Singer SJ, Nicholson GL. The fluid mosaic model of the structure of cell membranes. Science 1972;175:720–31.

Strichartz G. Pharmacological properties of sodium channels in nerve membranes. In: Waxman SG, Ritchie JM, eds. Demyelinating disease: basis and clinical electrophysiology. New York: Raven Press, 1981:343–56.

Strichartz G, Hahin R, Cahalan M. Pharmacological models for sodium channels producing abnormal impulse activity. In: Culp WJ, Ochoa J, eds. Abnormal nerves and muscles as impulse generators. Oxford: Oxford University Press, 1982:98–127.

Swett JE, Bourassa CM. Electrical stimulation of peripheral nerve. In: Patterson MM, Kesner RP, eds. Electrical stimulation research techniques. New York: Academic Press, 1981:244–98.

Tasaki I. Nervous transmission. Springfield, Ill.: Charles C Thomas, 1953.

Tasaki I, Takeuchi, T. Weitere Studien über den Aktionsstrom der markhaltigen Nervenfaser und über die elektrosaltatorische Übertragung des Nervenimpulses. Pfluegers Arch Ges Physiol 1942;245:764–82.

Ulbricht W. Kinetics of drug action and equilibrium results at the node of Ranvier. Physiol Rev 1981;61:785–828.

Waxman S. Action potential propagation and conduction velocity—new perspectives and questions. Trends in neurosciences. Vol. 6. New York: Elsevier North-Holland, 1983:157–61.

Waxman SG, Foster RE. Ionic channel distribution and heterogeneity of the axon membrane in myelinated fibers. Brain Res Rev 1980;2:205–34.

Waxman SG, Ritchie JM. Demyelinating disease:

basic and clinical electrophysiology. New York: Raven Press, 1981.

Woodbury JW. Action potential: properties of excitable membranes. In: Ruch TC, Patton HD, eds. Neurophysiology. Philadelphia: WB Saunders, 1965:26–72.

Woodbury JW. Recent advances in membrane physiology. Rochester, Minn.: American Association of Electromyography and Electrodiagnosis, 1976.

2 CONDUCTION IN ABNORMAL NERVE

This chapter examines the basic and clinical physiological consequences of the main patterns of injury and repair affecting the peripheral nervous system. In such studies it is often impossible to establish precise correlations between the observed conduction abnormalities and the corresponding structural alterations in the nerve fibers. This is particularly so where there is much variability in the structural changes seen among the various nerve fibers or even within the same nerve fiber throughout its course between the spinal cord and its peripheral site of termination. The problem of correlating physiological and morphological studies is compounded further by the impossibility of establishing the functional identity of the nerve fibers from the appearance or size of the fibers alone. Moreover, nerve biopsies, of necessity, examine but a short segment of the nerve, and this at a relatively distal site.

Except where clinical studies of conduction examine the region of the nerve biopsied or direct in vitro electrophysiological studies are carried out on the same or an equivalent fascicle of the biopsied nerve, precise correlations between conduction studies and morphological alterations in the nerve are difficult to establish.

The problems of correlating disordered morphology and physiology are to some extent overcome in experimental studies where the lesions are relatively uniform in appearance (Ochoa, Fowler, and Gilliatt, 1972; Smith and Hall, 1980). Even so, means do not yet exist for directly visualizing the same nerve fibers subjected to the physiological studies, and uncertainties must therefore remain about the precise relationship of structure to function in abnormal nerve fibers. Indeed, alterations in conduction are not always accompanied by obvious changes in the appearance of the nerve fibers (Sharma and Thomas, 1974) and perhaps reflect changes in the kinetics of the sodium channels in the nodal membrane, although of course this is pure speculation.

To the clinical electrophysiologist, the basic pathological changes in peripheral nerves that are most amenable to testing and measurement are those that alter conduction velocities and reduce the numbers of axons. These changes can be the result of either block in the transmission of their impulses or degeneration and actual loss of the axons.

To emphasize these basic priorities, the patterns of injury and repair in the peripheral nervous system have been divided as shown in Table 2.1. There are available several ex-

TABLE 2.1.   Basic Patterns of Injury and Repair in the Peripheral Nervous System

---

Demyelination and remyelination
Wallerian degeneration
Neuronopathies
Axonopathies
Physical injuries
Ischemia
Cold

---

cellent, authoritative guides to the pathology of peripheral neuropathies (Dyck, Thomas, and Lambert, 1975; Dyck, Thomas, Lambert, and Bunge, 1984; Urich, 1976; Allt, 1976; Weller and Cervos-Navarro, 1977; Asbury and Johnson, 1978).

DEMYELINATION AND REMYELINATION

Demyelination may be primary or secondary to neuronal or axonal degeneration. In *primary demyelination* the main injury is to the Schwann cell or myelin. Examples of human primary demyelinating neuropathies include diphtheritic polyneuropathy (Fisher and Adams, 1956); Guillain-Barré polyneuropathy (Asbury, Arnason, and Adams, 1969) and metachromatic leukodystrophy (Dayan, 1967). Degenerative changes in axons may be present in these neuropathies, but they are in general much less prominent.

Secondary demyelination is common in degenerative neuronal and axonal disease. It is a common accompaniment of axons undergoing degeneration and is most complete and extensive toward the extremities of the degenerating axons. In both the primary and secondary varieties, myelin retraction and breakdown occur near the nodal regions, producing paranodal demyelination. Later the demyelination becomes more extensive and may come to occupy the whole internode segment to produce so-called segmental demyelination (Figure 2.1).

In response to the breakdown of myelin and

FIGURE 2.1.   Single myelinated nerve fibers teased in epon from (A) normal subject. Successive portions of the same fiber are shown, there being a little overlap in adjacent photomicrographs. Shown are normal nodes of Ranvier and the Schmidt-Lanterman's clefts (asterisk).
(B) Demyelination extending over the whole length of one internode segment (bar). There is no indication of remyelination.
(C) Demyelinated internode segment (bar). Portions of this internode appear to have been thinly remyelinated.
(D) Example of demyelination confined to the paranodal region (bar).
(E) Successive segments of one fiber undergoing wallerian degeneration. Shown are the linear rows of ovoids.
   All these fibers were taken from the superficial peroneal nerve, except that in E, which was from the deep peroneal nerve.
Courtesy of Dr. A. Hahn.

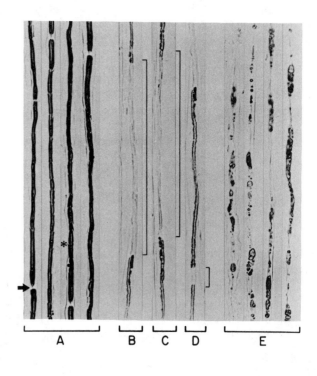

in some cases destruction of the Schwann cells themselves, the remaining Schwann cells proliferate, each one coming to remyelinate the region of the axon in its immediate vicinity. In primary demyelination, such remyelinated segments are often shorter than the adjacent, more normal internode segments, producing a pattern of widely varying internode segments and new nodal regions. This contrasts with the situation in regenerating axons where the new internodes are much more uniform in length, although shorter than normal.

Demyelination is a common and important morphological characteristic of many peripheral neuropathies, and indeed, of central demyelinating diseases. Its physiological cost depends on its extent and severity and the types of nerve fibers involved. The physiological consequences of demyelination are listed in Table 2.2.

Demyelination impairs the transmission of impulses primarily by changing the properties of the paranodal and internodal membranes. The loss of myelin increases capacitance and diminishes transverse resistance in the paranodal and internodal regions. In so doing, it increases the outward leakage currents through these regions (Koles and Rasminsky, 1972; Rasminsky and Sears, 1972; Bostock and Sears, 1978; 1981; Lafontaine, Rasminsky, Saida, and Sumner, 1982; Sumner, Saida, Saida, Silberberg, and Asbury, 1982) (Figures 2.2 and 2.3). The larger leakage currents increase the time the internal longitudinal current (ILC) must flow in order to depolarize

the next nodal membrane to threshold. This increases the internodal conduction time and slows transmission of the impulse. If the transverse current leakages are excessive, not enough current may be available to depolarize the nodal membrane to threshold (safety factor <1.0) and the impulse blocks. The safety factor for transmission of the impulse is the ratio of the current available to the current required to depolarize the next nodal mem-

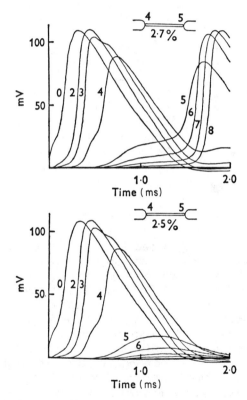

FIGURE 2.2.   Computer simulation of a conducted action potential in a myelinated nerve fiber in conditions in which (Top) the myelin thickness of the internode segment between nodes 4 and 5 was reduced to 2.7 percent of the normal thickness. Note the long delay before onset of the action potential again at node 5. (Bottom) Here the internodal myelin thickness was further reduced to 2.5 percent of normal thickness. As a consequence, the impulse blocks at node 5.
From Koles and Rasminsky (1972, figuré 3).

TABLE 2.2.   Physiological Consequences of Peripheral Demyelination

---

Increases in internodal conduction times
Impulse block
Reduced ability to transmit a second impulse after
    a short interval or a train of impulses
Continuous conduction
± Spontaneous impulse generation
± Ephaptic transmission

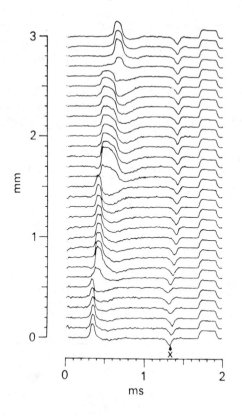

FIGURE 2.3. Averaged external longitudinal currents at 0.1-mm intervals along the length of a diphtheria toxin-demyelinated rat ventral root fiber. The downward pulse (X) and the square pulse following X provide the respective time and current calibration pulses (see Figure 1.11). The ordinate indicates the distance along the nerve fiber where these currents were obtained. Zero distance and time are arbitrary. Successive traces beginning at the bottom show progression of the impulse along the fiber.

Note, in comparison to Figure 1.11 (bottom), substantial time delays between regeneration of the impulse at successive nodal regions. These delays were in some cases as much as ten times longer than normal intervals between the regeneration of the impulse at successive nodes of Ranvier.

Note in particular the prolonged external longitudinal current in the second internode segment from the top necessary prior to regeneration of the action potential at the next (top) internode.

From Bostock and Sears (1978, figure 8A).

brane to just beyond threshold for generation of the impulse.

Demyelination in the paranodal region is thought to be particularly critical because retraction of the myelin sheath and Schwann cell processes here would increase the available nodal membrane and dilute the available outward current over a large membrane surface (Koles and Rasminsky, 1972; Rasminsky and Sears, 1972; Bostock and Sears, 1978) (Figures 2.2 and 2.3). Moreover, although potassium channels do not exist in the normal nodal region, they are present in the nearby paranodal axolemmal membrane, and these could be exposed by paranodal demyelination (Bostock, Sears, and Sherratt, 1981; Chiu and Ritchie, 1981). The resultant slow but outward potassium current could diminish and shorten the inward current and in the process reduce the safety factor for transmission even more.

The magnitude of the internal longitudinal current available to depolarize the next node(s) may also be reduced by increasing the temperature (Figure 2.4). Such increases in temperature are thought to shorten the period of increased sodium conductance (Hodgkin and Katz, 1949; Paintal, 1965; Rasminsky, 1973; Schauf and Davis, 1974; Davis, Schauf, Reed, and Kesler, 1975; Bostock, Sherratt, and Sears, 1978). The resultant shorter-lasting ILC may no longer be sufficient to overcome the excessive transverse leakage currents through critically demyelinated regions, so that the current available to depolarize the next node(s) may fall below that necessary to trigger an impulse and further progression of the impulse is arrested or blocked at this point.

Demyelinated nerve fibers are less tolerant of higher temperatures than normal fibers are, their impulses blocking at progressively lower temperatures, the more severe the degree of demyelination (Schauf and Davis, 1974). In multiple sclerosis, our best model of a human central demyelinating disorder, increases in the body temperature by as little as 0.5°C can

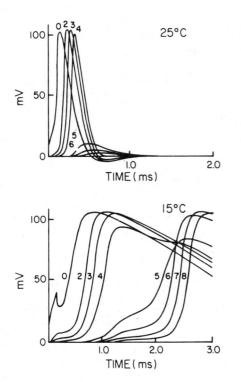

FIGURE 2.4.   Computer simulations of conduction of action potentials in a myelinated nerve fiber at successive nodes. In this fiber, paranodal demyelination is present proximal to node 5. In the top the potentials were computed for 25°C. Note the failure of the impulse to be regenerated at node 5. Conduction was restored, however, by lowering the temperature (here 15°C). Note the more prolonged nature of the action potentials at 15°C, reflecting greatly prolonged, underlying transmembrane ionic currents. Sometimes reductions of as little as 0.5°C are sufficient to restore conduction to a critically demyelinated fiber.

From Koles and Rasminsky (1972, figures 5e and f).

worsen visual field defects and produce or aggravate other neurological signs (McDonald, 1974), probably through increasing the degree of conduction block present in the related portions of the optic nerves and central tracts. Conversely, cooling the body or affected limb may improve clinical signs in multiple sclerosis and partially reverse a conduction block in some peripheral demyelinating disorders.

Conduction block in human hereditary demyelinating neuropathies is much less common than in the acute demyelinating neuropathies, despite the sometimes very slow conduction in the former, possibly because of the insertion of new sodium channels in the paranodal and internodal axolemmal membranes. Such remodeling of the axolemmal membrane would tend to increase the available sodium current and possibly provide refreshment for the impulse in its passage between successive nodal regions. Otherwise the impulse would be forced to conduct passively through the bared paranodal or internodal membrane regions. The resultant larger leakage currents could, in critically demyelinated regions, block the impulse. Such a formation of new sodium channels has not yet been directly shown experimentally.

Basic mechanisms by which transmission of impulses can be blocked in the absence of axonal degeneration are shown in Table 2.3.

Other mechanisms (Table 2.3) could contribute to the development of conduction block. For example, when the load on the available ILC is increased by increasing the area of the membrane through which the ILC is able to pass, the result may be to dilute the available current in the manner similar to that mentioned earlier with respect to paranodal demyelination. Examples of such *impedance mismatches* (Waxman, 1977, 1978, 1980; Swadlow, Kocsis, and Waxman, 1980) in normal nerve include the large amyelinated initial segments of motoneurons, branch points in myelinated nerve fibers where the branches impose extra loads on the available ILC originating at or proximal to the branch points, and sites of transition between the proximal myelinated and the terminal amyelinated segments of nerve fibers. The normally lower safety factor for transmission of impulses at the above makes transmission at these sites

TABLE 2.3.   Mechanisms by which Conduction Can Be Blocked

Increases in the load on the available internal longitudinal current
    Paranodal and internodal demyelination operate to
        Increase nodal membrane area and dilute the available current over a wider area
        Increase the transverse leakage currents through the internodal region by increasing
        capacitance and reducing resistance of the membrane(s)
    Increases in the internal longitudinal resistance (ILR)
        Increase in specific resistivity of the axoplasm
        Reduction in axon diameter
    Axon branching
Reductions in the current available to depolarize the next nodal region(s)
    Blocking of available sodium channels
        ?Blocking agents (e.g., tetrodotoxin[1])
        Hypercalcemia
        Lower pH
    Shortening activation time of sodium channels by increases in environmental
        temperature
    Shortening of inward current time by imposition of an outward potassium current, in
        turn the result of exposure of potassium channels in the paranodal region

---

[1]See Lafontaine, Rasminsky, Saida, and Sumner (1982).

even more susceptible to conduction block than adjoining regions in the presence of demyelination.

Theoretically, sodium channels could be blocked or even destroyed by humerol agents or toxins in various diseases, and this could contribute to or produce conduction block in these diseases. There is no evidence to support this hypothesis in human demyelinating neuropathies. Temporary worsening of the safety factor for transmission could also be produced by altering the concentrations of certain ions, such as calcium, potassium, and sodium, or the pH in the region of the sodium channels, because these are all known to alter membrane conductances and currents.

The longitudinal extension of the ILC depends on the resistivity of the axoplasm, the magnitude of the ILC, the transverse leakage currents, and the diameter of the axon. Factors altering the available ILC transverse leakage currents have been discussed. There is no evidence that the resistivity values of the axoplasm are changed in demyelinating neu-

ropathies. There is evidence, however, that the diameters of axons in a demyelinated zone may shrink somewhat (Denny-Brown and Brenner, 1944; McDonald, 1963). Such a change would increase the internal longitudinal resistance (ILR) but at the same time reduce transverse leakage currents because of the smaller membrane area available through which these currents must pass (Figure 2.5).

One other important physiological consequence of demyelination is the reduced ability to transmit impulses at short intervals (Rasminsky and Sears, 1972; Smith and Hall, 1980; McDonald, 1982). The least interval at which two impulses can be transmitted is the *refractory period of transmission* (RPT). Linked to the increase in RPT is the reduced inability to transmit trains of impulses. The least intervals between impulses in a train at which impulses block is somewhat longer than the RPT. The reason for the increase in the RPT is not clear, although the impaired inability to transmit trains of impulses is possibly explicable by the accumulation of sodium ions beneath the nod-

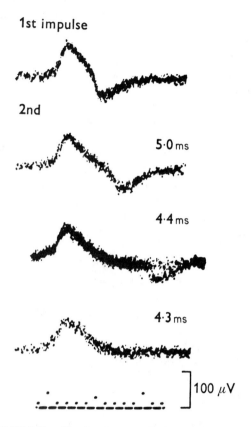

1st impulse

2nd

5·0 ms

4·4 ms

4·3 ms

]100 μV

FIGURE 2.5.   Demonstration of the refractory period of transmission (RPT) in a rat single ventral root fiber demyelinated by diphtheria toxin. The records consist of about 20 superimposed tracings of the external longitudinal currents as recorded at one site. In the top trace, successive phases of the current recording signal the change in direction of the external longitudinal current as it traverses two successive internodes. In the next and subsequently lower traces are shown the current traces which correspond to a second impulse following the first (top) at progressively shorter time intervals. Note that at 4.4 ms, not only is the current trace corresponding to the external longitudinal current in the next internode strikingly delayed, but sometimes it is absent, indicating that the impulse has intermittently blocked between the two internodes. When the interval was shortened still further, the second impulse failed to cross to the second internode completely. Records time scale pips are at 0.1 ms intervals. The study was done at 30°C. From Rasminsky and Sears (1972, figure 9).

al membrane. The latter, by reducing the inward sodium current could reduce the available ILC below that necessary to generate an impulse at the next node.

The preceding discussions have outlined the major costs of demyelination, namely, slowing of conduction, conduction block, and a reduced capacity to transmit pairs and trains of impulses. Now we turn our attention to mechanisms that can restore conduction (Table 2.4). Some of these, such as the effects of changes in temperature and reduced the extracellular concentration of calcium in the vicinity of the nerve, have been attended to in preceding sections.

Conduction may be restored to nerve fibers whose impulses were previously blocked by demyelination by several mechanisms. Theoretically, some of the original conduction block may have been caused by a direct action of circulating toxins or antibodies on the sodium channels themselves, although this has never been shown to be the case in the human or experimental demyelinating neuropathies. In such cases, however, recovery of previously blocked sodium channels or the insertion of new channels could help to restore conduction.

TABLE 2.4.   Mechanisms by which Conduction may be Restored in Demyelination

Increasing the current available to depolarize the next nodal region(s)
Blocking the outward potassium current
Reducing environmental temperature
Reducing extracellular calcium ion concentration
Increasing local pH
Increasing number of available sodium channels
Reducing load on available current
Remyelination
Shortening internode length
Continuous conduction, including possible insertion of new sodium channels into the bared paranodal or internodal membrane

Much more important, however, as a means of restoring conduction is remyelination of the bared regions of the nerve fibers. Koles and Rasminsky (1972) have pointed out previously, based on their computer simulation studies, that conduction may block beyond a single demyelinated internode where the myelin thickness in the affected internode is reduced to less than 2.7% of normal. Conversely, remyelination need not proceed far to restore conduction (Koles and Rasminsky, 1972; Saida, Sumner, Saida, Brown, and Silberberg, 1979).

Remyelination, by increasing the transverse resistance and reducing the capacitance, reduces the transverse current leakages through the affected internodal and especially paranodal regions. The result is that more of the internal longitudinal current originating in nodal membranes proximal to the critically demyelinated regions is made available to depolarize the nodal region distal to the region of the block, and this may be sufficient to restore conduction. Remyelination in the paranodal region is probably additionally important because the outward potassium currents that accompany the impulse when the potassium channels in the paranodal region are exposed through retraction or breakdown of the myelin sheath shorten and reduce the internal longitudinal current available for depolarizing succeeding nodal regions. Indeed, Bostock, Sears, and Sherratt (1978) have shown that blocking such outward potassium currents in experimentally demyelinated nerve fibers by applying 4-aminopyridine or tetraethylammonium to the affected fibers is able to restore conduction to previously blocked fibers.

Repair of demyelinated regions of nerve fibers is accompanied by proliferation of Schwann cells and the formation of new shorter internodes, each internode corresponding to the territory of a single Schwann cell. In the process, new nodes of Ranvier are established, and at these sites, new sodium channels must have been inserted in the membrane.

Whether the densities of such sodium channels in the newly formed nodal region correspond to those at the older established nodes is unknown. By decreasing the distance between adjacent nodes, the shorter internodes possibly increase the overall safety factor for transmission along such fibers, although they may act in the mature and recovered fiber to slow conduction somewhat because of increased transverse current leakages through the greater number of nodes.

Koles and Rasminsky (1972) and Waxman (1977, 1978) stress the importance of the condition of the internode segments that immediately precede the demyelinated segments in possibly restoring conduction. For example, the interposition of a short internode(s) just proximal to the demyelinated segment can restore conduction through the later segment by increasing the current available to the nodal membrane(s) beyond the demyelinated segment.

In regions where demyelination is incomplete, restoration of conduction can occur by the development of *continuous conduction* across the bare segment (Bostock and Sears, 1978) (Figure 2.6). This phenomenon has been observed in experimental diphtheritic neuritis (Bostock and Sears, 1978); regenerating myelinated nerve fibers prior to their remyelination (Feasby, Pullen, and Sears, 1981; Feasby, Bostock, and Sears, 1981); and in roots of dystrophic mice, many of which have no myelin at all (Rasminsky and Kearney, 1976; Rasminsky, Kearney, and Aguayo, 1978; Bostock and Rasminsky, 1983). Such continuous conduction represents an important way of restoring conduction in regions where the myelin sheath has been partially or completely absent.

The precise mechanisms by which such continuous conduction develops are unknown, but in all likelihood these involve the

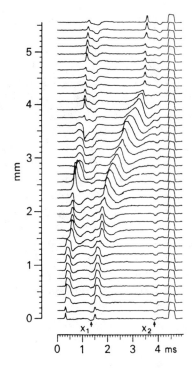

FIGURE 2.6.   The external longitudinal currents are recorded at successive 0.1-mm intervals from a demyelinated rat ventral root fiber 14 days after injection of diphtheria toxin. Here it was possible to record impulses in two independent nerve fibers: x_1 and x_2 represent the times when the impulses successively reached the e_5 electrode (see Figure 1.11).

Note that for the more rapidly conducting of the two impulses (left), conduction remained saltatory despite abnormal increases in the time intervals between regeneration of the impulse at successive nodal regions. In the second fiber, conduction became continuous over a distance of about 2 mm (2.2- to 4.2-mm mark). Over this last segment (within the resolution of this technique), the inward transverse membrane current appeared to move continuously along the fiber without interruption or apparent saltation. Recording at 30°C.

From Bostock and Sears (1978, figure 12A).

creation of new sodium channels in the bared axolemmal membrane. It is not clear whether, in some cases, what looks to be continuous conduction may not be saltatory conduction between patches of excitable membrane at very short intervals. The last cannot be excluded as a theoretical possibility by present electrophysiological techniques, but it is well to point out that patches of high concentrations of sodium channels have not been demonstrated either.

Consequences of Demyelination in Human Peripheral Neuropathies

The most common of the primary demyelinating peripheral neuropathies in man is Guillain-Barré polyneuropathy. This disease serves as a good model for illustrating the correlations among the clinical disturbances, clinical electrophysiological observations, what is known about structural changes in peripheral nerves in this disorder, and what has been reviewed about basic pathophysiological mechanisms in demyelination in the preceding section. The characteristic clinical physiological disorders in Guillain-Barré polyneuropathy include paralysis, loss of tendon reflexes, paresthesia, and often some loss of somatic sensation, as well as, in some patients, various autonomic disorders. The most plausible explanation for the negative symptoms and signs, namely, the paralysis and to some degree the losses of sensation, include:

1.   Conduction block
2.   Inability to transmit trains of impulses
3.   Axonal degeneration

The force of a voluntary muscle contraction depends primarily on the numbers of motor units (MUs) recruited, their rates of discharge, and muscle length. The precise timing of the discharges of the active MUs with respect to one another is probably not an important factor governing the force generated by the contraction. Hence, although slowing the conduction velocities of some motor axons relative to others might well be expected to upset the timing of the discharges of their MUs relative to one another, it is unlikely that any appreciable degree of weakness would result on this basis alone. Indeed, in the early phase of Guillain-Barré polyneuropathy when the paralysis is greatest, the maximum motor conduction velocities are often normal and temporal dispersion in excess of normal may not be apparent (Brown and Feasby, 1984).

The more likely causes of the weakness are conduction block, commonly demonstrable in one or more motor nerves beginning with the onset of paralysis (Figures 2.7 and 2.8), and axonal degeneration. The morphological correlates of early conduction block have not been so easy to establish. Obviously, paranodal and internodal demyelination is reason enough and is well documented, at least in later stages of the disease (Asbury, Arnason, and Adams, 1969; Asbury and Johnson, 1978). Whether a direct blocking of nodal sodium channels by circulating agents in this disease also occurs is unknown. Nor has this concept been dealt with by recent experiments in which demyelination in rat nerve has been produced by the intraneural injection of serum from patients with Guillain-Barré polyneuropathy (Feasby, Hahn, and Gilbert, 1980). Sometimes it is possible to demonstrate a temperature-reversible component to the conduction block in Guillain-Barré neuropathy.

Inability to transmit trains of impulses, especially when the intervals between successive impulses are short, could theoretically contribute to the weakness (McDonald, 1982), but only where the firing rates of the MUs approach rates equivalent to those where impulse blocking could occur. This seems unlikely because the firing rates of MUs are, in most instances, too low (up to 50 Hz) for such frequency-dependent blocking to occur. The safety factor for impulse transmission and

ability to transmit trains of impulses may be somewhat lower distally in the terminal and preterminal motor axon branches where frequency-dependent conduction block could possibly occur at lower firing frequencies. The higher RPT characteristic of demyelinated nerves could also prevent the catchlike increments in force produced by double discharges of MUs at very short intervals (Burke, 1980).

Degeneration and loss of motoneurons or their axons could also contribute to the weakness. Reactive changes and sometimes degeneration of motoneurons and wallerian degeneration in peripheral nerve fibers have all been observed in Guillain-Barré polyneuropathy (Haymaker and Kernohan, 1949; Asbury, Arnason, and Adams, 1969; Asbury and Johnson, 1978). In keeping with this, denervation has been recorded in some patients with this disease (Eisen and Humphreys, 1974; McLeod, Walsh, Prineas, and Pollard, 1976; Brown and Feasby, 1984) and in diphtheritic polyneuropathy, another primary demyelinating neuropathy (Kurdi and Abdul-Kader, 1979). Axonal lesions have also been shown in experimental antiserum-mediated demyelination (Saida, Saida, Saida, and Asbury, 1981). Such axonal degeneration is probably the major source of persistent weakness and wasting in this disease. In the early paralytic stage prior to the appearance of denervation, it may be impossible to distinguish between the conduction block of motor axons undergoing degeneration but in which conduction has not ceased completely (Erlanger and Schoepfle, 1946) and the demyelinative type of block in which the axons are intact (Figures 2.9 and 2.10).

Because the degree of slowing is not the same in all nerve fibers, slowing of conduction and the resultant temporal dispersion could contribute to reductions or losses of tendon reflexes and vibration sense. Both of these no doubt depend on a high degree of temporal

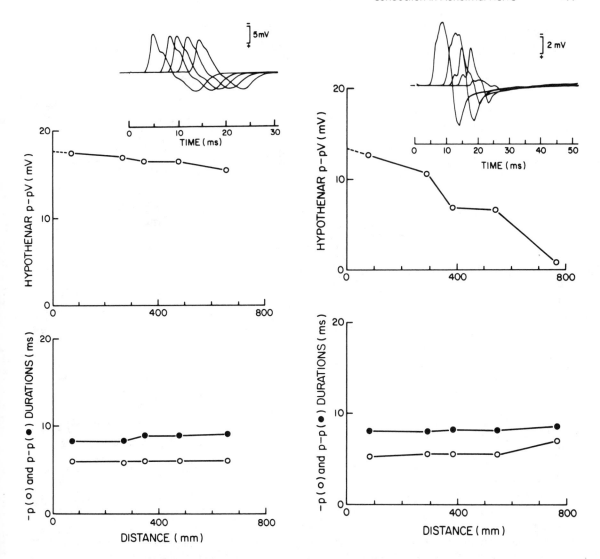

FIGURE 2.7.   (Left) Successive surface-recorded hypothenar maximum M-potentials elicited by just supra-maximal stimuli at Erb's point, the proximal upper arm, just proximal and distal to the elbow (embracing the retroepicondylar and transcubital tunnel segments), and the wrist. There was no more than 15 percent increase in the peak-to-peak (p-p) and negative peak (−p) durations, and less than 20 percent decline in p-p amplitude between Erb's point and the wrist (see accompanying plots).

(Right) Patient with Guillain-Barré polyneuropathy examined 14 days following onset of paralysis. Methods were the same as at the left, but note the decline (approximately 90 percent) in the p-p amplitude of the hypothenar maximum M-potential, which was accompanied by no more than 15 percent (upper limit of controls) increase in −p or p-p duration between Erb's point and the wrist. This strongly suggests the presence of conduction block in many of the hypothenar motor axons. Major declines in the size of the M-potential were seen across the elbow and transaxillary segments.

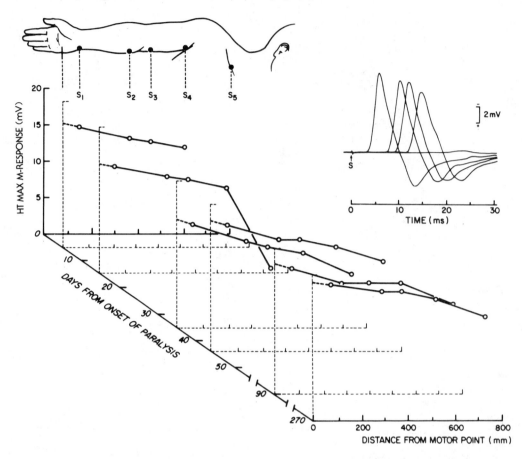

FIGURE 2.8.   Proximal conduction block in a patient with Guillain-Barré polyneuropathy 14 days following onset of paralysis.

(Inset) Shown are the maximum hypothenar M-potentials successively elicited at Erb's point (S5), the proximal arm (S4), just proximal (S3), and distal (S2) to the elbow and wrist (S1) levels by percutaneous supramaximal stimuli delivered to the ulnar nerve. Note that in comparison to the maximum M-potential evoked by stimulation at the proximal arm, the potential elicited by stimulation, about 200 mm more proximally at Erb's point, was much smaller. That this indicated conduction block in a high proportion of the hypothenar nerve fibers was supported by the lack of any accompanying increase in the M-potential duration (p-p, −p, or total) to suggest an increase in the degree of temporal dispersion among the motor axon impulses.

Also shown are serial plots of these changes in M-potential (amplitude) at various times following onset of paralysis. Note recovery from the proximal block by the time of the next study at 35 days.

coincidence in the arrival times of their respective afferent volleys at the central nervous system and could be impaired by temporal dispersion alone, although conduction block

probably contributes to the impairments at least in the early paralytic stage.

Ectopic discharges similar to those observed in demyelinated peripheral nerves

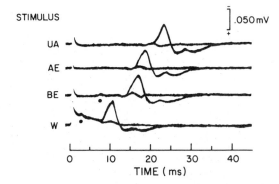

STIMULUS

].050 mV

UA

AE

BE

W

| | | | | |
0   10   20   30   40
TIME (ms)

FIGURE 2.9.   A 60-year-old patient with Guillain-Barré polyneuropathy examined four days following onset of paralysis. Shown are the only two remaining excitable and detectable all-or-nothing hypothenar MUPs (recorded here with surface electrodes) that could be elicited by incremental stimulation at the wrist (W) below the elbow (BE), above the elbow (AE), and at the proximal upper arm. The motor terminal latency was more than twice normal, but the proximal conductions were within the 2-SD lower limit of controls, indicating that these surviving motor units were among the fastest of the ulnar motor axons of this muscle group.

This patient went on to develop fibrillation potentials in these and other muscles. Even at six months following onset of paralysis, the M-potentials in the most distal muscles remained very small.

The solid dot indicates the sensory prepotential which precedes the M-potentials in the bottom two traces.

(Burchiel, 1980) and dystrophic roots devoid of myelin (Rasminsky, 1978, 1982, 1983) could clearly explain the paresthesia observed in the primary demyelinating peripheral neuropathies in man (see Chapter 9 and review by Culp and Ochoa, 1982). This type of abnormal spontaneous activity could, perhaps through collisions between naturally and ectopically originating impulses in the same nerve fibers, block the transmission of some of the impulses. Such ectopic impulses could also alter the excitabilities and thresholds of the nerve fibers in which they originate, and so possibly further reduce the safety factor for

transmission of naturally occurring impulses in the same fibers, possibly blocking or slowing conduction of their impulses.

The main clinical electrophysiological abnormalities in Guillain-Barré polyneuropathy are listed in Table 2.5 and illustrated by Figures 2.7 through 2.9.

In the chronic acquired and sometimes relapsing type of inflammatory polyneuropathy, demyelination and remyelination and various degrees of onion bulb formation are found (see reviews by Asbury and Johnson, 1978; Schaumburg, Spencer, and Thomas, 1983). In the relapsing variety, conduction block is characteristically most prominent during the relapse and improves as the degree of weakness apparent on clinical examination improves. Even between relapses, the maximum conduction velocities are often very reduced (<20 m/s) (Figure 2.11) and abnormal temporal dispersion may be very striking despite, in some cases, apparently normal strength. The last observation gives weight to the contention that even very slow conduction velocities in motor axons are quite compatible with normal strength. Tremor, the amplitude of which is sometimes very large, may reappear or be exacerbated in periods of relapse, only to disappear or substantially improve as the patient's strength improves.

Demyelination is often a prominent feature of entrapment neuropathies (see later section), and acute and chronic conduction block may be observed in these disorders as well.

TABLE 2.5.   Clinical Electrophysiological Abnormalities in Guillain-Barré Polyneuropathy

Conduction block (Figures 2.7 and 2.8)
Reductions in conduction velocities
  Reductions in the maximum motor and sensory
      conduction velocities
  Increased temporal dispersion
  Prolonged F-response latencies
Denervation

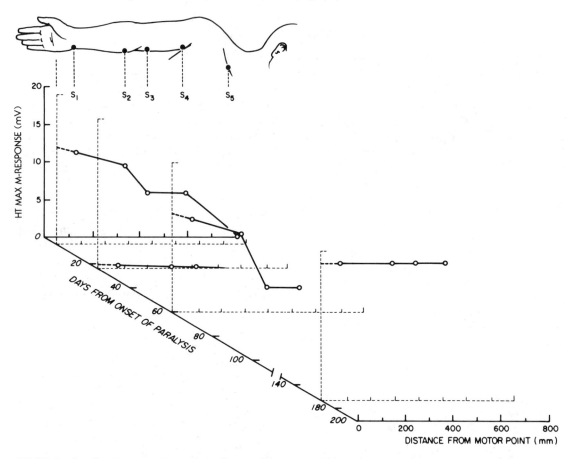

FIGURE 2.10.   Study in a patient with Guillain-Barré polyneuropathy illustrates changes in amplitude of the maximum M-potential at various times following onset of paralysis.

Serial plots of the changes in the maximum hypothenar M-potential were elicited by stimulation as in Figure 2.8. Note the severe reduction in the maximum M-potential to stimulation as distally as the wrist at 18 days following onset of paralysis. Usually, when elicited by distal stimulation, such low-amplitude M-potentials indicate a poor prognosis and probable subsequent development of substantial spontaneous denervation activity in the muscle because of degeneration of many of the axons or their terminals. Here, however, denervation activity did not appear, and at 60 days the M-potential elicited distally had returned to within the 2-SD control lower limit. This suggests that the low, distally elicited M-potentials in this case were due to a primary demyelinative type of block rather than to prior degeneration of the motor axons or conduction block in axons undergoing degeneration (Erlanger and Schoepfle, 1946).

There was a disproportionate reduction in the amplitude of the M-potential and reduction in the conduction velocity across the elbow compared to the segment proximal and distal to the elbow. This suggested the presence of a compression injury to the nerve at this common entrapment site in addition to the more general peripheral neuropathy. Such local changes at the common entrapment site occur frequently in acute generalized peripheral neuropathies such as Guillain-Barré polyneuropathy.

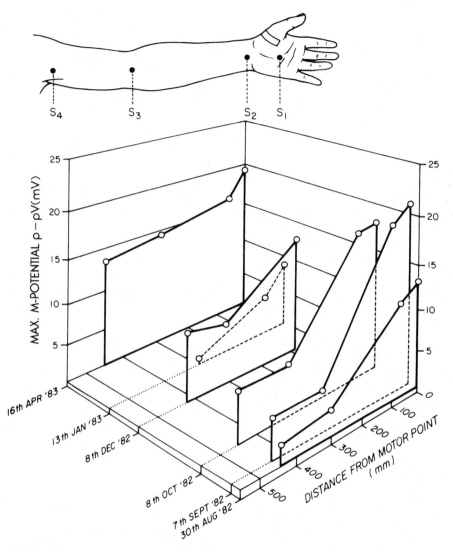

FIGURE 2.11.   Patient with chronic, relapsing, biopsy-proved inflammatory and de-myelinating polyneuropathy. Shown are successive plots of the peak-to-peak am-plitude of the maximum thenar compound action potentials as recorded with surface electrodes and elicited by supramaximal stimuli delivered to the median nerve at the proximal upper arm (S4), elbow (S3) just proximal to the wrist (S2), and in all but one instance, just distal to the flexor retinaculum. The studies were carried out at irregular intervals but clearly illustrate not only the steep decline in amplitude (paralleled by changes in the area of the respective M-potential) as the distance increased between the site of stimulation and the motor point, indicating conduction block; examples being 30 Aug. 1982, 7 Sept. 1982, 8 Oct. 1982, and 13 Jan. 1983, but the changes in the degree of block apparent at successive studies. The study on 16 April 1983 was recorded when the patient was at his best and on 13 January when he was the most weak in the period of study embraced by the above recordings.

WALLERIAN DEGENERATION

Wallerian degeneration is a term used to cover structural alterations in normal nerves distal to a crush injury or transection of the nerve. These structural changes and the subsequent repair processes have been the subjects of a number of recent reviews (Lieberman, 1971, 1974; Joseph, 1973; Thomas, 1974; Dyck, 1975; Urich, 1976; Allt, 1976; Sunderland, 1978, 1979, 1980; Asbury and Johnson, 1978; Selzer, 1980). In this chapter, emphasis is on the physiological abnormalities that accompany the early degenerative and subsequent regenerative processes both proximal and distal to the level of the injury.

Physiological alterations distal to the injury site are identical in crush and transection injuries. There are, however, important distinctions between the injuries in the course of the subsequent repair and regenerative processes. Table 2.6 lists the earliest abnormalities that develop subsequent to a crush injury severe enough to interrupt axonal continuity or to transection of the nerve.

Proximal to the Transection

Even in clean transections, retrograde degeneration in the axon can extend backward several millimeters and even further in more extensive injuries. So-called reactive changes such as central chromatolysis develop in the parent motoneurons or dorsal root ganglion cells, the intensities of these reactions being related to how near the transection is to the neuron and to the age of the subject (Sunderland, 1978). These reactive changes in the neuron cell bodies are paralleled by physiological changes.

In motoneurons, these include resting membrane depolarizations, partial all-or-nothing potentials, lower thresholds (Eccles, Libet, and Young, 1958), reduced responsiveness of the motoneurons to Ia inputs, and lower amplitudes and shorter rise times of excitatory postsynaptic potentials (EPSPs) of the same origin (Eccles, Libet, and Young, 1958; McIntyre, Bradley, and Brock, 1959; Kuno and Linás, 1970; Mendell, Munson, and Scott, 1976). These last phenomena are pos-

TABLE 2.6.   Early Abnormalities Following Crush Injury with Interruption of Axonal Continuity or Nerve Transection

Proximal to Injury	Distal to Injury
Axon	Neuromuscular junction
Degeneration	Block in neuromuscular transmission
Reduction in axon diameter	Axon
Reduction in conduction velocities	Impulse block
Neuron	Degeneration and breakdown in axon and
Reactive changes (nucleus, cytoplasm)	myelin
Partial neuronal depolarization	Later, Schwann cell proliferation
Dendritic all-or-nothing potentials	Muscle
Retraction of input to the neuron	Depolarization
	Tetrodotoxin-resistant action potentials
	Increased contraction time
	Fibrillation
	Extension of ACh receptors to extrajunctional
	sites

sibly explicable by retraction of the input terminals away from the motoneuron membranes (Sumner, 1975, 1976).

Proximal (up to 70 mm) to experimental transection or crush injuries, conduction velocities may slow (Cragg and Thomas, 1961; Kuno, Miyata, and Muñoz-Martinez, 1974a, 1974b; Mendell, Munson, and Scott, 1976), perhaps because of the shrinkages in axonal diameters noted proximal to these injuries (Cragg and Thomas, 1961; Aitkin and Thomas, 1962) and perhaps the nodal lengthening and internodal demyelination seen in association with the axonal atrophy proximal to the site of a transection (Dyck, Lais, Karnes, Sparks, Hunder, Low, and Windeback, 1981). Similar reductions in conduction velocities proximal to compressive or transection injuries have been reported in man (Gilliatt, 1973; Stöhr, Schumm, and Reill, 1977; McComas, Sica, and Banerjee, 1978). Slower maximum conduction velocities proximal to a compression may be more apparent than real where measurement of the proximal conduction velocities depends on transmission through the site of compression and transmission in the more rapid fibers has been blocked by the compression.

Distal to the Transection

In the rat hemidiaphragm preparation, the earliest degenerative changes distal to transection of the parent phrenic nerve develop in the motor axon terminals and the end-plate (Miledi and Slater, 1970). About the same time, neuromuscular transmission blocks at the end-plates and end-plate potentials (EPPs) and miniature end-plate potentials (MEPPs) stop. The latent period of these developments is proportional to the length of the distal stump (Miledi and Slater, 1970). The progressive block of neuromuscular transmission precedes the subsequent development of a progressive

block in impulse transmission in the nerve distal to the transection site (Miledi and Slater, 1970; Gilliatt and Hjorth, 1972; Wilbourn, 1977). For the most part, conduction velocities of impulses in the degenerating axons remain normal up to the point when transmission blocks, although some have claimed that conduction velocities may be somewhat slower just prior to complete loss of excitability (Gilliatt and Hjorth, 1972; Wilbourn, 1977). In degenerating axons transmission of impulses may block at multiple points distal to the site of injury (Erlanger and Schoepfle, 1946). In the human, the nerve distal to a transection becomes inexcitable within three to seven days (Gilliatt, 1973; Wilbourn, 1977).

The earliest degenerative changes include breakdowns in the structures of the neurofilaments, microtubules, and endoplasmic reticulum, and swelling of the mitochondria. Later the degenerating axons develop a beaded appearance. The breakdown products of the axons and myelin subsequently become digested by the Schwann cells and macrophages. The Schwann cells divide and become collected into longitudinal columns, the bands of Bunger, within their original endoneural tubes to await invasion of the regenerating axons.

In the early postdenervation period, partial depolarization of the muscle membrane develops accompanied by the appearance of tetrodotoxin-resistant action potentials and probable changes in the kinetics of the sodium channels (Thesleff, 1974; also see Chapter 1). Shortly thereafter, the extrajunctional regions of the membrane become much more sensitive to acetylcholine (ACh), indicating the development of much larger numbers of ACh receptors in the extrajunctional membrane.

Denervated muscle membranes are more irritable. This is evident in the increased and prolonged insertional activity, evoked by insertion, and movement of an intramuscular needle electrode. *Fibrillation,* spontaneous action potentials in single muscle fibers, soon develops. The latent period between the injury and the appearance of fibrillation is proportional to the length of the motor axons distal to their sites of interruption. For example, in C8–T1 root or lower brachial plexus injuries in man, three to four weeks may pass before abnormal spontaneous activity develops in the hand muscles, whereas only one to two weeks may pass between interruptions of the C5–6 roots or upper brachial plexus and the appearance of fibrillation potentials in the rhomboid, spinatus, or deltoid muscles. Similarly, seven to ten days following acute lumbar or sacral root compressions in which wallerian degeneration develops distal to the compression, fibrillation develops earliest, preceded by increased insertional activity in the paraspinal muscles (seven to ten days) and only much later (two to four weeks) in more distal muscles in the territory of the affected roots. These abnormal insertional and spontaneous activities in denervated muscle develop much later than do failures of neuromuscular transmission and impulse transmission and loss of excitability in the nerve distal to the trauma.

Provided some part of the motor innervation is spared, within a short time, the remaining intact motor axons begin to sprout terminal and preterminal collateral branches. These proceed to reinnervate those muscle fibers that have lost their innervation. This process changes the innervation patterns in the muscle (see Chapter 8).

Changes in distribution patterns of MUs and probably innervation ratios as well account for changes in motor unit potentials (MUPs) seen in the course of reinnervation in man (Kugelberg, Edström, and Abbruzzese, 1970; Kugelberg, 1973; Stålberg and Ekstedt, 1973; Stålberg and Trontelj, 1979; also see Chapter 8). The characteristic electromyographic (EMG) abnormalities help to identify denervation and reinnervation, although similar changes can sometimes be seen in some muscle diseases (see Chapters 7 and 8).

Following acute interruption of the axonal continuity by crush or transection injuries, axonal regeneration in the proximal stump begins within the initial 24 hours. The major events that characterize nerve regeneration are shown in Table 2.7. Figure 2.12 illustrates the temporospatial progression of regeneration in a previously severed cat nerve.

Sprouts and *growth cones* develop at the proximal cut ends of axons, sometimes within 24 hours. Some sprouts appear to spring from nodal regions proximal to the injury site.

One important distinction between crush and transection injuries is the interruption of the Schwann cell basement membranes (part of the neurilemmal sheath) (see Asbury and Johnson, 1978) in the latter, and its preservation in all but the most severe crush injuries. These basement membrane tubes are continuous between the roots and the distal terminal axonal branches, and serve as guides to the regenerating axon. Where these tubes are intact, axon sprouts stand the best chance of crossing the injury site in the least time and reaching their intended targets (muscle or sense organs) by growing down their own tubes with their contained proliferated Schwann cell columns.

Destruction of basement membrane tubes creates severe problems because many sprouts are unable to cross the injury site, and many of those that succeed do not reach the basement membrane tubes in the distal stump that match their assigned target tissues. The resulting faulty regeneration patterns can result in permanent weakness, sensory impairment, and bizarre innervation patterns (see Chapter 11). Injuries that extend over any appreciable length of a nerve and those in which there is excessive connective response also add to the time necessary for axons to cross the injury site and reduce the quantitative success of such regeneration (Sunderland, 1978).

Characteristically, axon sprouts are multiple, and sometimes two or more are able to regenerate toward the periphery contained

TABLE 2.7.   Physiological and Structural Changes in Regenerating Nerve Fibers

Structural	Physiological
Early sprout and growth cone formation	Electrophysiological characteristics of the axons include Low conduction velocities (<1–2 m/s at distal end) (Figure 2.14) Very high thresholds to electrical stimulation (Figure 2.13) Continuous conduction
Subsequent regeneration across the injury zone. The latent periods in experimental lesions to cross are: Nerve crush 1–3 days Nerve transection 5+ days and progressive increase in number of axons that cross site of injury (Figure 2.12)	Subsequent progressive maturation Establishment of saltatory conduction Progressive reduction in thresholds (Figure 2.13) Progressive increases in conduction velocities Progressive reduction in degree of temporal dispersion in the compound nerve potential (Figure 2.12)
Progressive (proximal to distal) increases in axonal diameter and degree of myelination	Characteristics of early MUPs Low amplitude, long durations, and hypercomplex (Figure 2.16) Abnormal neuromuscular transmission Very prolonged latencies Axonal block
In motor axons, reinnervation is accompanied by progressive Extension of innervation to more and more of the denervated muscles End-plate maturation Increases in diameters and myelination of axon terminal and preterminal branches	Subsequent progressive maturation of MUPs Increases in numbers of MUPs that can be detected Increases in amplitudes and shorter durations of MUPs More normal neuromuscular transmission

within a single basement membane tube. Provided both branches mature and are able to regenerate, such multiple axon sprouts are possible sources of abnormal axon reflexes (see Chapter 8).

Early regenerating axons are very thin and possess no myelin sheaths. Their stimulus thresholds are high (Figures 2.13 and 2.14) and the velocities of their impulses very low (<1 to 2 m/s) (Berry, Grundfest, and Hinsey, 1944; Devor and Govrin-Lippmann, 1979) (Figure 2.14). The impulses in these very immature axons have sometimes been shown to propagate in a continuous manner, although discontinuous conduction between high concen-trations of sodium channels spaced very close to one another could not be excluded (Feasby, Bostock and Sears, 1981). Some of these loci could become nodal regions. Once myelination becomes established, inward currents are limited to the nodal regions as in normal nerve (Feasby, Pullen, and Sears, 1981; Feasby, Bostock, and Sears, 1981). Progressive distal regeneration is accompanied by progressive increases in the diameters of the axons and in the thickness of their myelin sheaths. These two processes proceed in a proximal to distal manner. Lower stimulus thresholds (Figure 2.13) and progressive increases in impulse velocities parallel the structural maturations.

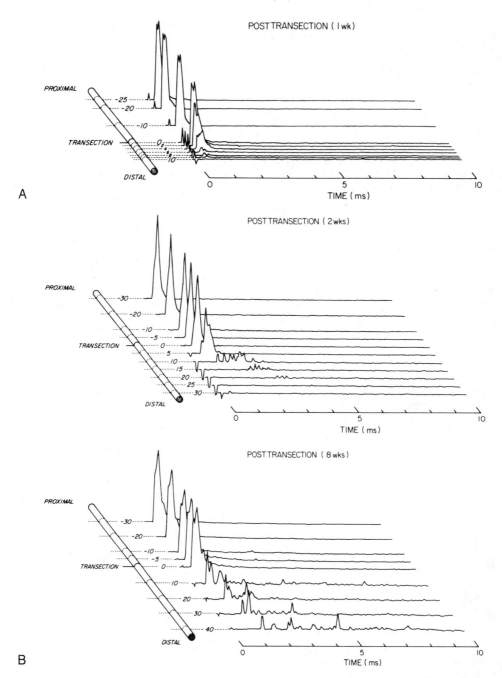

FIGURE 2.12.   Experimental transection and immediate suture of the lateral (peroneal) division of the sciatic nerve in the cat. Shown are the monophasic dorsal root potentials (DRPs) recorded in oil in response to stimulation of the nerve proximal and distal to the transection site. The nerve was mounted on a tripolar stimulating electrode (cathode central) and attached to a horizontal calibrated drive, which made it possible to stimulate the nerve at intervals as short as one mm. The exposed nerve in the thigh was kept in warm (37°C) mineral oil.

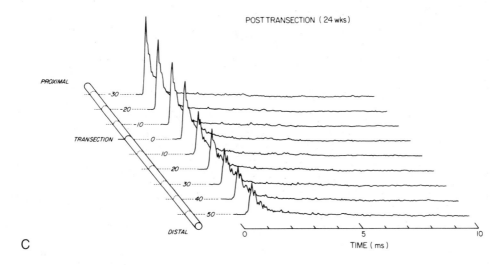

POST TRANSECTION (24 wks)

PROXIMAL

-30
-20
-10

TRANSECTION   0

10
20
30
40
50

DISTAL

0   5   10

TIME (ms)

C

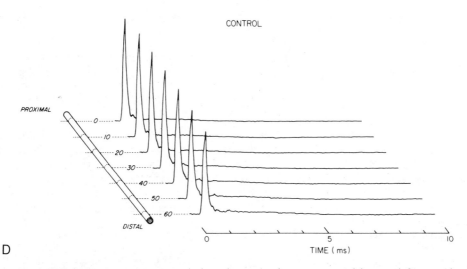

CONTROL

PROXIMAL

0
10
20
30
40
50
60

DISTAL

0   5   10

TIME (ms)

D

(A) At one week following transection, note the absence of any potential beyond 8 mm distal to the transection site. The large potentials at two and four minutes are probably partly the result of stimulus spread up the core of the nerve trunk to the much lower-threshold regions just proximal to the transection.

(B) The DRPs at two and eight weeks respectively. Note that while a few nerve fibers have reached as far as 25 mm beyond the site of transection, the main body has not progressed nearly so far. At eight weeks many more fibers have progressed much further peripherally; indeed, at this time reinnervation of the peroneal innervated muscles just below the knee is beginning, preceded by a substantial reduction in fibrillation activity in these muscles.

(C) At 24 weeks many more fibers have reached the periphery and the size of the DRP is much larger, approaching values elicited proximal to the transection. Note also the lesser degree of temporal dispersion apparent in the DRP at 24 weeks reflecting increasing axonal diameter and myelination of the regenerating nerve fibers at this stage.

(D) Comparable serial DRP in a control nerve.

(From Brown, Hurst, and Routhier, 1982).

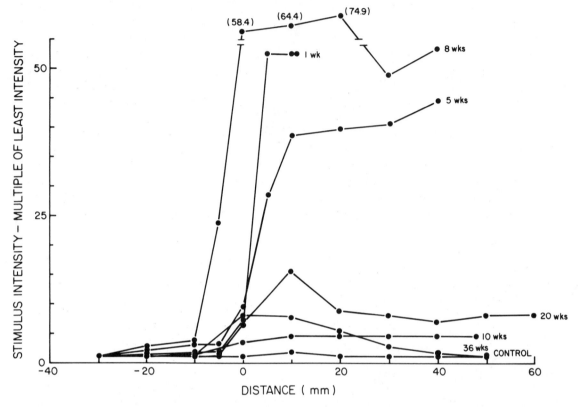

FIGURE 2.13.   Plot of the changes in stimulus intensity required to evoke a maximum DRP at various distances proximal and distal to the site of transection and reunion at 1 to 36 weeks following transection (same study as described in figure 2.12). Intensities are plotted as multiples of the least current required to elicit a maximum DRP between 0 and 30 mm proximal (−) to the transection site.

Note that in the early period (one to eight weeks posttransection) stimulus intensities were sometimes 10 × 100 those required to excite the nerve proximal to the transection. By ten or more weeks, the intensities necessary were much closer to normal.

(From Brown, Hurst, and Routhier, 1982).

At maturity, conduction velocities approach and sometimes reach normal value (Berry, Grundfest, and Hinsey, 1944; Sanders and Whitteridge, 1946; Berry and Hinsey, 1947; Cragg and Thomas, 1964; Devor and Govrin-Lippmann, 1979). Failure to reach normal values may be explained by the earlier multiplication of Schwann cells and subsequently shorter internode lengths and the often smaller diameters of the axons, and proportionately thinner myelin sheaths in the regen-

erated nerve fibers. In the human, maximum conduction velocities can reach values within 80 or even 100 percent of the normal mean (Hodes, Larrabee, and German, 1948; Struppler and Huckauf, 1962; Ballantyne and Campbell, 1973; Donoso, Ballantyne, and Hansen, 1979; Buchthal and Kühl, 1979).

In man, the latent period to the earliest detectable reinnervation is close to the expected, based on regeneration at a rate of 1 to 3 mm per day (Jasper and Penfield, 1946;

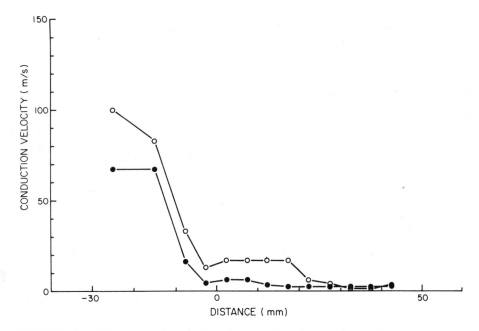

FIGURE 2.14.   Changes in the conduction velocities of two afferents in the cat, one a group I afferent *(open circles)* and the other a group II afferent; both had been sectioned three weeks previously (same study as Figure 2.12). Note the reduction in their conduction velocities just proximal to the transection (10 to 20 mm) and the very low conduction velocities at their distal extremities beyond the transection where the velocities were on the order of 1 to 2 m/s. The latter indicates that the fibers at this point must have been unmyelinated or at the most, very poorly myelinated. Their axons were probably very thin as well at this level. The actual axon tips probably extend a short distance beyond the distal limits shown here, because to demonstrate the distal extremity of axons by these techniques requires that not only the impulse be generated by the electrical stimulus delivered to the nerve, but that the impulse, once initiated, must be able to conduct without interruption all the way to the dorsal root recording site. Continuous conduction in the most distal extremities of such axons seems likely and has been demonstrated experimentally (Feasby, Bostock, and Sears, 1981). (From Brown, Hurst, and Routhier, 1982).

see review by Sunderland, 1978). For example, when the median nerve is transected at the level of the wrist, the earliest detectable motor responses in the thenar muscles to electrical stimulation proximal to the transection are seen at 120 days or more (Figure 2.15). When allowances are made for the times necessary to cross the transection site and establish enough working end-plates to produce a detectable M-potential, and when account is taken of the distance between the muscle and the transection site, the estimated maximum rate of regeneration is about 1 to 2 mm per day. Not all axons reach the target tissues at the same time; indeed, there can be very appreciable lags between the arrivals of the first few axons and the bulk of the remainder. It is not known whether this range reflects vari-

FIGURE 2.15. Previous transection of the human median nerve by a glass cut at the wrist. The nerve was resutured within 24 hours. The records taken five (bottom) and six (top) months following surgical repair illustrate the first three detectable MUPs evoked by electrical stimulation of the median nerve a few centimeters proximal to the transection.

Note the very long latencies (three to four times normal) and very high thresholds. Stimulus currents required to activate each of the MUPs in turn are listed on the right, and are at least 10 to 20 times normal. The latencies were shorter and the required stimulus intensities somewhat less one month later.

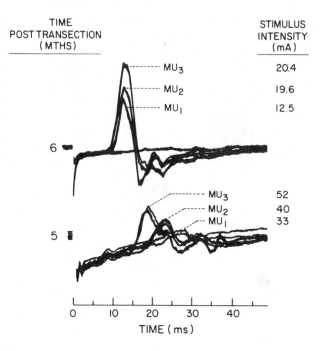

TIME POST TRANSECTION (MTHS)		STIMULUS INTENSITY (mA)
	MU$_3$	20.4
	MU$_2$	19.6
	MU$_1$	12.5
6		
	MU$_3$	52
	MU$_2$	40
5	MU$_1$	33

TIME (ms)

ations in the rate of regeneration among individual axons or a wide range in times necesary to cross the injury site.

Bare axons can be seen by silver impregnation techniques, sometimes well ahead of the distal levels at which their presence can be detected by present electrophysiological techniques (Jacobson and Guth, 1965). Even though continuous conduction in myelin-bare regenerating axons has been shown (Feasby, Bostock, and Sears, 1981), it is not known how close to the tip of the axon such a capacity to generate and propagate an impulse begins. Moreover, the smaller the diameter of the axon, the "smaller" the amplitude of its extracellularly recorded action potential. This, and the small numbers of regenerating axons at the leading edge of the regeneration, their very slow conduction velocities, and the resultant temporal dispersion of their potentials makes the recording of the compound nerve action potential proximal to the site of an in-

jury (crush or transection), in response to stimulation at various sites distal to the injury, wholly unsatisfactory. The same is also true in the case of attempts to record the nerve action potential at progressively more distal sites beyond the injury, the site of stimulation being proximal to the injury, as a means of attempting to determine the distal extent of regeneration in nerve fibers. Direct stimulation of the nerve distal to the site of transection and recording the cortical evoked potential response to such stimulation is a sensitive way of determining the distal extent of regeneration in the cat, but has not proved worthwhile in man (Brown, Hurst, and Routhier, 1982). In addition, the very high thresholds to electrical stimulation characteristic of immature regenerating nerve fibers makes any electrophysiological technique that depends on such stimulation unsatisfactory because such stimuli are commonly very uncomfortable, associated with excessive stimulus artifact. In addition, sometimes there is unwanted extension of the stimulus current to excite nearby nerves and muscles that have normal and relatively much lower thresholds than the affected nerve.

The rate of axonal regeneration is not constant, but decreases with distal progression of the regeneration. It is possibly less in nerve transections than in crush injuries (Sunderland, 1978).

Neuromuscular transmission at new and immature neuromuscular junctions often fails because the end-plate potentials are subthreshold. Moreover, in the immature axon terminals and preterminal branches, which characteristically have low conduction velocities, impulses may intermittently block, particularly at branch points. With time and progressive maturation, presynaptic conduction and neuromuscular transmission become more secure.

The earliest MUPs are frequently very short in duration, but soon their durations become characteristically much longer than normal and the potentials themselves are often hypercomplex because of the wide temporal dispersion in the timing of the discharges of their component muscle fibers (Figure 2.16). Such temporal dispersion could contribute to the prolonged contraction times of MUs when these have been elicited by indirect stimulation. Later, increases in the diameters and degree of myelination of the presynaptic nerve fibers lead to better synchronization between the activities of the component muscle fiber potentials contributing to the MUPs. As a consequence, the durations of the latter become shorter and their amplitudes increase as do the maximum M-potentials elicited by supramaximal motor nerve stimulation progressively (Figure 2.17).

Equivalent maturation in sensory axons is much harder to detect. For example, it is possible to detect the presence of even one motor axon once innervation of a number of muscle fibers has taken place. There is, however, no equivalent possible in regenerating sensory fibers whose potentials are much too small and temporally dispersed to detect even with near-nerve needle electrode recording techniques (Donoso, Ballantyne, and Hansen, 1979; Buchthal and Kuhl, 1979).

The increasing numbers of regenerating motor axons that reach the muscle progressively innervate more and more of the denervated muscle fibers. One of the earliest signs of this is a progressive reduction in the number of fibrillation potentials seen. The overall effect is to increase the size of the compound M-potential as well as the force generated by the muscle in response to a supramaximal stimulus delivered to the presynaptic nerve (Figure 2.18). There follows a progressive increase in the number of MUs that can be recruited by voluntary contraction, even though the order of recruitment may be somewhat upset following a previous transection of a nerve (Milner-Brown, Stein, and Lee, 1974).

The tips of growing axons are abnormally sensitive to mechanical deformation, and respond by repetitive discharges. This is probably the basis for the clinically well-described Tinel's sign in which the peripheral extent of a regenerating nerve may be estimated by tapping the skin along the course of the peripheral nerve. The approximate location of the leading edge of the regenerating nerve is signaled by finding the site along the nerve at which tapping provokes paresthesias referred to the peripheral cutaneous territory of the regenerating nerve (see Sunderland, 1978 for a review of Tinel's sign).

In circumstances in which nerve fibers are frustrated in their attempts to reach their peripheral target tissues, sectioned nerves may end in a tangled ball or neuroma. Spontaneous discharges have been clearly shown in such experimental neuromas (Wall and Gut-

FIGURE 2.16. Recordings of the maximum M-potential as recorded with subcutaneous electrodes positioned over the anterolateral compartment muscles, and the corresponding intramuscularly recorded (concentric needle electrode) potentials as elicited by supramaximal stimulation of the common peroneal nerve. The studies were carried out in the cat following prior transection and resuture of the lateral division of the sciatic nerve.

(Top) Early stage. Within four weeks following the expected arrival of the earliest motor axons in the muscle. At this stage the maximum M-potential is still very small and the intramuscular record shows frequent triphasic fibrillation potentials occurring randomly in respect to the stimulus. Both surface and intramuscularly recorded potentials are briefer than normal.

(Bottom) Later stage. About six weeks following the expected arrival of the motor axons in the muscle. Here the amplitude of the surface recorded maximum M-potential is still less than 10 percent of normal, but its duration is prolonged (about 50 ms) corresponding to the temporally dispersed polyspike potential recorded intramuscularly at the same time. The prolonged duration of the MUPs at this stage of reinnervation in humans or in these experiments in cats probably reflects the immature nature of the collateral axon sprouts and, to a lesser extent perhaps, a wider range among the conduction velocities of the component muscle fibers and the increased spatial scatter of the newly established end-plates in the reconstituted motor units at this stage. Note also the fluctuation in the size and shape of the surface-recorded M-potential reflecting abnormal jitter and impulse block in some of the linked potentials (not shown here). (From Brown, Hurst, and Routhier, 1982).

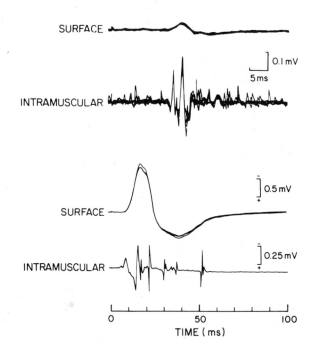

nick, 1974a, 1974b; Devor and Bernstein, 1982). Such spontaneous afferent barrages in human neuromas may, in part at least, explain the pains, paresthesias, and phantom limb sensations experienced by these patients.

NEURONOPATHIES AND AXONOPATHIES

The wallerian degeneration that follows transection or crush injuries of a nerve is not representative of the types of degeneration seen

FIGURE 2.17.   Previous division and suture of the lateral division (peroneal) of the sciatic nerve 8, 12, and 36 weeks prior to these recordings of the maximum tibialis anterior M-potentials (surface-recorded) evoked by just supramaximal stimulation of the nerve at intervals beginning proximal to and moving distally beyond the previous (bottom to top) transection.

Note the very prolonged duration and the complexity of the falling-off phase of the M-potential at eight weeks following the transection. Progressive maturation of the reinnervation process was accompanied by an increasing degree of synchronization and shorter overall duration of the M-potential, although even at 36 weeks the peak-to-peak duration of the M-potential still exceeded that of any control cat muscle. The peak-to-peak amplitudes of the M-potentials recorded at 8, 12, and 36 weeks and in the control muscle were 0.063, 5.4, 37.0, and 37.0 mV respectively (the latter two being in the normal range).

(From Brown, Hurst, and Routhier, 1982).

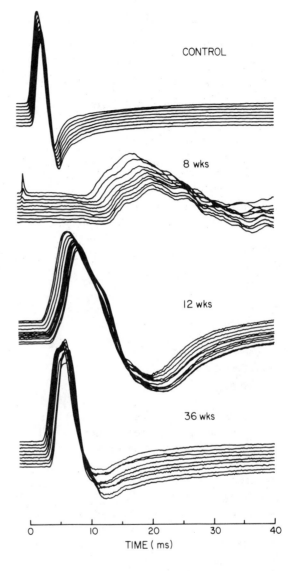

in more slowly progressive primary axonal peripheral neuropathies. Traumatic interruption of the axon leads to a shutdown in all those metabolic and structural processes in the distal stump that depend on the parent cell body and axoplasmic transport to the periphery of substances originating in the cell body. This contrasts with the situations in degenerative neuronal and axonal neuropathies where abnormalities could reside in only a part of the metabolic or transport processes. Moreover, in traumatic injuries the cell bodies and proximal axons are not directly injured and, except in very proximal axonal lesions, are able to sustain repair and regeneration of the axon. By comparison, in degenerative neuronal and

FIGURE 2.18. Comparison of the surface-recorded maximum M-potentials and maximum twitch contractions of the tibialis anterior muscle of the cat following transection of the lateral division of its sciatic nerve eight weeks previously (left) and the corresponding potential and twitch on the normal side (right). Note that at eight weeks the maximum M-potential on the transected side was not only much more reduced in amplitude, but more dispersed and its duration much more prolonged with respect to the normal M-potential. The longer duration of the surface-recorded potential was matched by an equally dispersed intramuscularly recorded potential (left middle trace). The twitch contraction time was very prolonged and was much smaller in size compared to the normal twitch at this stage. The prolongation of the twitch is partly explained on the basis of the greatly desynchronized actions of the muscle fibers contributing to the twitch.

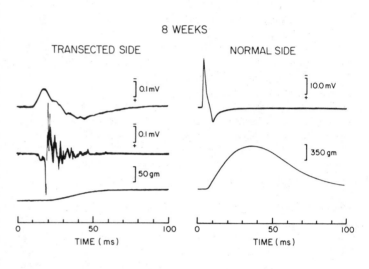

axonal neuropathies, the cell bodies or axons may well be less able to regenerate and sustain their end organs, peripheral synaptic connections, or postsynaptic cells. There is as yet no direct evidence for this last hypothesis. Repair processes such as collateral sprouting and reinnervation and hypertrophy of muscle fibers are able also to mask the severity of axon loss in the axonopathies or neuronopathies because of the comparatively much slower pace of these disorders in contrast to that of traumatic lesions.

The distinctions between the *neuronopathies,* where the primary injury is thought to be in the cell body, and *axonopathies,* where the injury site is thought to be to the peripheral axonal process, is at best arbitrary. Too little is known about the basic mechanisms involved to make this clear distinction more than speculative in any disease. The term *"dying-*

back" neuropathy was introduced by Greenfield (1954) and Cavanagh (1964) to describe those diseases in which the primary abnormalities were thought to reside in the cell bodies. In response to dysfunctional changes in the cell bodies, the earliest degenerative changes begin at the distal extremities of the axonal processes (both central and peripheral) and progress toward the parent cell bodies, leading as the terminal event to degeneration and loss of the neuron.

This hypothesis receives support in the apparent characteristic centripetal progression of the degeneration in peripheral nerves and central tracts seen in several diseases. These include the spinocerebellar degenerations and human triorthocresyl phosphate poisoning, and similar patterns can develop in the wake of exposure to various intoxicants such as acrylamide, isoniazid, and certain hexacarbons, for example, *n*-hexane and methyl *n*-butyl-ketone.

Detailed examination of experimental and human toxic neuropathies has led, however, to questions about the dying-back hypothesis (see review by Spencer and Schaumburg, 1976). These authors claimed the patterns of axonal degeneration seen in these intoxications are not what would be expected in a dying-back neuropathy. For example, were the neuron the primary site of the attack, the earliest and most severe degeneration should begin at the distal extremities of those neurons that have the largest peripheral volume to maintain (and perhaps the largest metabolic load). Degeneration should begin earliest at the distal extremities of those neurons that have the longest and largest-diameter peripheral axons. This simple view has not turned out to be true, at least in some toxic neuropathies in which degeneration begins not at the axon terminals, but at multiple preterminal sites. Spencer and Schaumburg (1976) also pointed out that although the degeneration does primarily involve the longest and thickest myelinated axons, exceptions were revealed in experimental models.

For example, in experimental acrylamide neuropathy, pacinian corpuscles begin to degenerate prior to primary endings of muscle spindles (Schaumburg, Wisniewski, and Spencer, 1974). Moreover, in experimental *n*-hexane neuropathy, nerve fibers that innervate the calf muscles degenerate before nerve fibers of equivalent diameter but longer length, such as those that innervate the feet (Spencer and Schaumburg, 1976, 1980).

Whatever their precise mechanism(s), whether neuronal or axonal in origin, the general pattern of these degenerations is common to a wide variety of peripheral neuropathies (Spencer and Schaumburg, 1980; Spencer, Sabri, Schaumburg, and Moore, 1978). The accompanying electrophysiological abnormalities have been documented in the various experimental models and human examples of some of these. They include:

1. Early receptor failures. For example, abnormal responses in muscle stretch receptors have been observed prior to conduction abnormalities in the more proximal axons (Sumner and Asbury, 1975; Lowndes, Baker, Cho, and Jortner, 1978; Lowndes, Baker, Michelson, and Vincent-Ablazey, 1978).

2. Selective losses of the largest-diameter myelinated axons. These losses explain reductions in maximum conduction velocities in acrylamide neuropathy (Hopkins and Gilliatt, 1971).

3. Progressive terminal disconnection. As the degeneration progresses toward the neuron, the most distal levels at which impulses can be generated and able to conduct proximally, propagate shrink back toward the cell body (Figure 2.19). The thresholds to electrical stimulation are highest at the extremities of the degenerating fibers.

4. Preferential involvement of certain physiological types of axons and relative sparing of other axons of equivalent diameter. For example, in acrylamide neuropathy, sensory nerve fibers having equivalent diameter and length to motor nerve fibers are more involved than the motor axons (Sumner, 1980).

Although human peripheral nerves cannot be examined with the same precision as is possible in experimental models, equivalent electrophysiological abnormalities have been observed in the human neuronopathies and axonopathies. These include:

1. Maximum conduction velocities that are in the normal range or just below the normal lower limit of controls. In those cases where maximum conduction velocities are below the

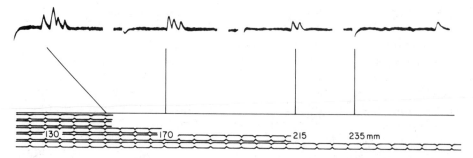

FIGURE 2.19.   Experimental acrylamide neuropathy in the cat.
    Dorsal root potentials recorded from S1 filaments in response to supramaximal stim-
ulation of the sural nerve 130, 170, 215, and 235 mm distant from the recording
electrode site. Note that as the site of stimulation was moved proximally, additional
MUPs appeared in the dorsal root record as their excitable tips were each in turn reached.
In each instance, the next fiber to be excited conducted at a faster velocity than those
excited at more distal sites along the nerve. This provides electrophysiological evidence
for the presence of axons undergoing progressive centripetal degeneration (see Sumner, 1980, figure 11.5).

normal range, several explanations are possible. For example, there may have been selective degeneration and loss of the fastest-
conducting nerve fibers or high enough losses
of nerve fibers in general, that even on a random basis the fastest-conducting nerve fibers
were lost. In these two cases the slower conduction velocities may simply reflect the velocities of the remaining, normally slower-
conducting nerve fibers. In this regard it is
well to remember that there is about a 50 percent range in the conduction velocities of motor axons in normal human motor nerves. Alternatively, the slower velocities may indicate
slowing of conduction in normally more rapid-
conducting nerve fibers. Slowing of conduction in such primary axonal or neuronal diseases could develop because of progressive reductions in axonal diameters (Baba, Fowler,
Jacobs, and Gilliatt, 1982) and secondary demyelination. For these reasons, one must be
cautious in interpreting maximum impulse velocities because even maximum conduction
velocities as low as 20 to 30 m/s could be seen

at the late stages of primary axonal or neuronal diseases in the absence of primary demyelination.
    2. Disproportionate increases in terminal
conduction times. In these disorders, the earliest structural abnormalities begin at or near
the terminal extremities of the central and peripheral processes of the sensory and motoneurons (Spencer and Schaumburg, 1976).
These degenerative changes lead to paranodal
and segmental demyelination and later, shorter
internodes. Such structural changes would slow
the conduction velocities and would explain
the disproportionate prolongations in distal
latencies observed in some human metabolic
and toxic neuropathies, although in some diseases such as alcoholic neuropathy this has
not been observed (Behse and Buchthal,
1977). Progressive centripetal degeneration
described by Sumner (1980) in acrylamide
neuropathy would be a better explanation for
the centripetal progressive loss of excitability
in sensory nerve fibers reported by Casey and
LeQuesne (1972) in alcoholic neuropathy.

3. Denervation and reinnervation. These phenomena are simply a direct consequence of the axonal degeneration and, in general, are more severe in distal than in proximal muscles.

Other neurological disorders characterized by primary involvement of the neuron are the motoneuron diseases of which amyotrophic lateral sclerosis (ALS) is the most common example. The etiology of these disorders is not known. The electrophysiological abnormalities in ALS are similar to those in the primary axonopathies, except in ALS the "upper" motoneurons as well as the bulbar and spinal motoneurons are among the primary targets (Hudson, 1981).

Physiological abnormalities in diseases of the motoneuron include:

1. Denervation and reinnervation of muscle
2. Normal or nearly normal maximum motor conduction velocities (the previous comments on conduction velocities in axonopathies are relevant here)
3. Preservation of sensory fibers and presumably their neurons until, in some cases, later stages in the diseases
4. Evidence of spontaneous impulse generation in motor axons or possibly the motoneurons themselves (see Chapter 9)

As a consequence of all the above, weakness, wasting, fasciculation, and denervation are prominent in ALS because in most patients the clinical course is relatively short.

COMPRESSION INJURIES OF PERIPHERAL NERVE

Compression is the most common cause of injury to human peripheral nerves (see reviews by Gilliatt, 1975, 1980a, 1980b). The effects, namely, paresthesias, numbness, and some-

times weakness, are temporary and reverse completely when the compression is brief, as when the legs are crossed or the subject is seated on a hard seat. In these instances, once the legs are uncrossed or the subject shifts his weight or stands, the tingling, numbness, and loss of strength in the peripheral territory of the compressed nerve disappear within a few moments. Some consider these transient disorders as primarily ischemic (Gilliatt, 1975). Sometimes, however, if the compression and possibly angulation last too long, the deficits may last much longer. Indeed, some persons may be especially susceptible to such injuries because they have a hereditary predisposition to such so-called pressure palsies (Madrid and Bradley, 1975; Urich, 1976), although such a predisposition is also seen in other hereditary and metabolic peripheral neuropathies. Often compressive injuries of peripheral nerves occur at particular sites where the nerves are especially vulnerable to direct compression or angulation because they are closer to the surface at that point, or must pass through a tight canal or over a sharp edge. The sites of these types of neuropathies, often called *entrapment neuropathies,* may be peripheral in location. Examples are the median nerve in the carpal tunnel, the ulnar nerve at the cubital tunnel or retroepicondylar space, or a more central area such as the intervertebral foramina where the nerve roots themselves may be compressed. The lesions in the entrapment neuropathies are most often recurrent and chronic. Sometimes, however, the injuries can be acute as in the median neuropathies that may develop in people who, in a short space of time, do some task that requires very forceful gripping, especially when this is combined with some wrist flexion.

Compression injuries can be divided into three main categories: (1) brief compression or percussion injuries, (2) short- to intermediate-term compression, and (3) chronic with or without repetitive compression injuries.

Brief Percussion Injuries

Transient sensations resembling electric shock and paresthesia are common when a nerve is struck by a blunt instrument. The shocklike sensation and paresthesia are expressed in the distribution of the nerve beyond the site of percussion. When the percussive blow is not very strong, the disturbance is transient. Too heavy a blow, however, can crush the nerve and lead to the train of events outlined in the section on nerve transection and crush (Richardson and Thomas, 1979) (Figure 2.20). The injury is equivalent to a crush lesion in which the basement membrane tubes remain intact (Sanders and Whitteridge, 1946; Collins, O'Leary, Hunt, and Schwartz, 1955; Cragg and Thomas, 1964; Devor and Govrin-Lippmann, 1979). It is not known whether or not transient and reversible structural abnormalities accompany the transient paresthesia and impulse block experienced in the mildest percussion injuries.

Short- to Intermediate-term Compression Injuries

Here the nerves are compressed for longer periods, sometimes as long as several hours (Figure 2.21). Characteristic human examples include the peroneal and radial neuropathies that result when these nerves are pressed for example against hard surfaces in sleep or coma. Here the resulting conduction block may sometimes last up to several months. Some evidence of wallerian degeneration almost invariably develops distal to the site of the compression (Trojaborg, 1970; Harrison, 1976; Gilliatt, 1980a, 1980b).

In experimental investigations of such short-term compressive injuries it can sometimes be very hard to distinguish between the effects of ischemia and those of direct compression at the level of the compression. This happens because pressures that exceed systolic pressure occlude the blood supply to the nerve. Even in experiments where the nerve is directly compressed in a chamber, the distributions of pressure and ischemia may be very uneven. For example, the territory of the ischemia could be restricted somewhat by diffusion of oxygen into the compressed zone from nearby uncompressed and normally oxygenated regions of the nerve or nearby tissues (Bentley and Schlapp, 1943). Moreover, in experiments where the nerves are compressed by tourniquets placed about the limb, not only are the nerves and other tissues rendered ischemic distal to the tourniquet, but the pressures registered immediately adjacent to the nerve may be well below that registered by the tourniquet, at least in some instances (Denny-Brown and Brenner, 1944; Lundborg, 1970; Rudge, 1974).

Despite misgivings about the tourniquet as a good model of short-term compression of peripheral nerve, there is considerable value in examining the physiological effects of such tourniquet use. This model can tell us much about direct compressive injuries to the nerve and the pathophysiology of peripheral nerve ischemia. It can also help to explain the occasional peripheral nerve lesions that attend use of the pneumatic tourniquet in man.

When the pneumatic pressure is below systolic pressure, no neurological impairment develops. Once above systolic pressure, however, weakness and sensory loss develop in a centripetal direction beginning at the distal extremity and progressing toward the tourniquet.

Even though the acute effects on nerve conduction are dominated by ischemia, disproportionate conduction abnormalities do develop at the proximal and distal tourniquet border zones, and may persist when the tourniquet is released (Yates, Hurst, and Brown,

FIGURE 2.20.   A 20-year-old male fell on his elbow while playing hockey. Shown are the maximum hypothenar (HT) M-potentials recorded with surface electrodes and elicited by just supramaximal stimulation of the ulnar nerve at the levels of the wrist, just distal to the cubital tunnel, proximal to the medial epicondyle, and in the proximal upper arm. The number of days following the injury are noted on the left. The sizes of the various maximum M-potentials,

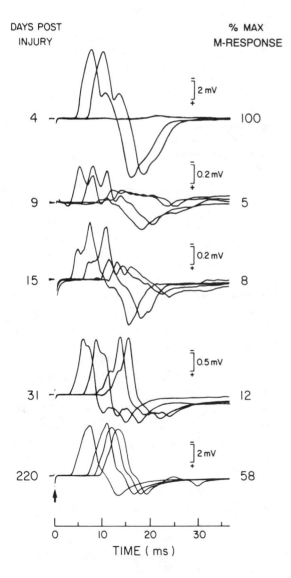

elicited by stimulation at the wrist, relative to the maximum M-potential at four days are shown as percentages of the latter value, on the right. Points here include:

1. The maximum HT M-potential on the affected side elicited by stimulation at the wrist at four days was only one-half of the corresponding potential in the other arm on the same day. This suggested that already a substantial proportion of the HT motor axon population on the injured site were no longer contributing their MUPs to the compound HT M-potential, probably because degeneration of their axons had at this point proceeded too far for the fibers to be excitable any longer or even if excitable opposite the cathode, to be able to transmit their impulses without interruption through to the muscle.

2. More of the population of HT motor axons became inexcitable between four and nine days as indicated by the further drop in the HT M-potential elicited by stimulation at the wrist. After nine days there was further decline in the size of the distally evoked M-potential; indeed, there was some increase in size, perhaps reflecting collateral reinnervation of some of the denervated muscle fibers by axons that survived the original injury. Fibrillation ultimately appeared in the hypothenar muscle by 15 days and was frequent at 31 days.

3. Between 15 and 220 days there was a progressive increase in the size of the HT M-potential, but even at 220 days the potential amplitude was still only about half of the 2-SD lower limit in healthy subjects. By 220 days the fibrillation activity was much reduced.

4. Initially, at four days, transmission across the injured elbow segment was completely blocked (the very low-amplitude positive potential seen, probably being volume-conducted from the forearm muscles). At 9 and 15 days, transmission of some impulses across the elbow was restored. By 31 days there was no indication of conduction block across the elbow.

5. By 220 days the maximum conduction velocity across the elbow segment was within the normal range and equivalent to the velocities both proximal and distal to the elbow segment.

PERONEAL NERVE

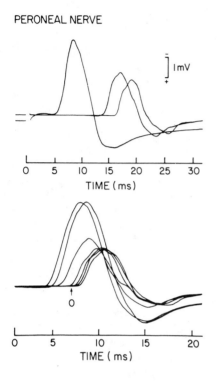

FIGURE 2.21. Acute peroneal neuropathy examined 10 days following onset. Shown are the maximum extensor digitorum brevis (EDB) M-potentials elicited by supramaximal stimulation of the common peroneal nerve.

(Top) The common peroneal nerve was stimulated at the ankle, just distal to the fibular head and proximal to the fibular head. The substantial difference in the amplitudes and areas of the maximum EDB M-potentials between the fibular head and ankle suggested that impulse transmission was blocked in a substantial proportion of the EDB motor axons between the ankle and fibular head.

(Bottom) To better establish the site of the conduction block, the nerve was stimulated percutaneously at 20 mm intervals both distally and proximally to the midpoint of the fibular head (O). This technique revealed that the site of the conduction block and associated conduction slowing was centered over a 40 mm segment adjacent to the distal fibula. Moderate numbers of fibrillation potentials developed subsequently in EDB and other muscles supplied by the common peroneal nerve.

This peroneal neuropathy developed following a period of more than one hour in which the subject squatted down to pick low-lying fresh fruit. The peroneal neuropathy fully resolved over the next 2 months.

1981) (Figure 2.22). These disproportionate local conduction abnormalities at the border zones of the tourniquet no doubt indicate local mechanical injuries to the nerve at these sites. This view is supported by the much more persistent local conduction abnormalities localized to the border zones in a case of persistent tourniquet paralysis in man (Bolton and McFarlane, 1978) (Figure 2.23). The primary cause of the persistent conduction block

and wallerian degeneration in tourniquet paralysis is local compression, even though the physiological consequences of ischemia may dominate at the time of tourniquet inflation (Yates, Hurst, and Brown, 1981).

What is the nature of the local conduction abnormalities at the borders of the tourniquet? One of the most important contributions to this subject in recent years has been the demonstration of specific structural

FIGURE 2.22. Changes in the maximum hypothenar (HT) compound potential are elicited by stimulation of the ulnar nerve at the wrist just distal to the tourniquet, and two stimulation points 30 mm apart, beneath and just proximal to the tourniquet. The interelectrode distance across the border zones of the tourniquet was 50 mm. Testing was carried out prior to tourniquet inflation, at intervals throughout the period of inflation, and through the subsequent 60 minutes after removal of the tourniquet. Note:

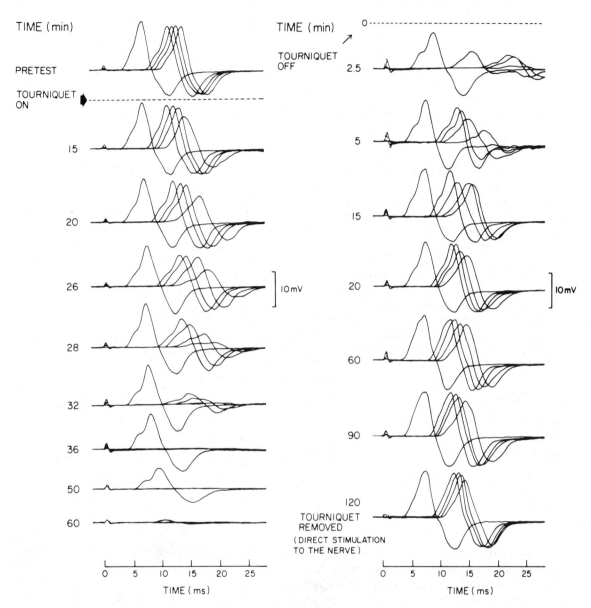

1. The earliest conduction block was evident across the proximal border zone (15 minutes)
2. The early disproportionate conduction delay across the distal tourniquet border zone in relation to the subtourniquet segment (15 minutes)
3. The overall proximal to distal cascade in the degree of conduction block
4. On release of the tourniquet, the disproportionate conduction delay across the distal tourniquet border zone at 2.5 minutes, the persistent conduction block across this segment at 15 minutes, and eventual recovery by 60 minutes

From Yates, Hurst, and Brown (1981, figure 3).

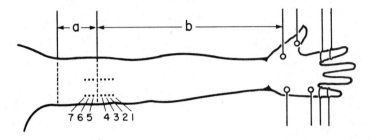

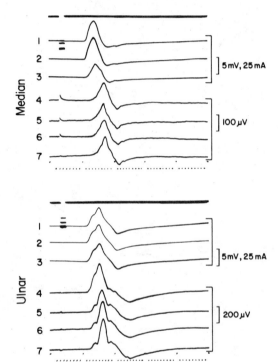

FIGURE 2.23. Five weeks prior to this study, a pneumatic tourniquet was applied to upper arm for just over two hours at a pressure exceeding the systolic blood pressure. Complete paralysis of all forearm and hand muscles resulted.

(Top) Location of the stimulating and recording sites for the motor and sensory studies. The broken vertical lines indicate the presumed location of the tourniquet. The conduction block was located at the presumed former site of the distal margin of the tourniquet. The median and ulnar nerves were stimulated proximal and distal to the tourniquet (1–7).

(Right) The maximum thenar and hypothenar M-potentials evoked by stimulation at points 1 through 7. Their maximum amplitudes proximal to 3 were only about 5 percent of the amplitudes evoked by stimulation just distal to 3, the presumed distal border of the tourniquet. The time pulses are at 1-ms intervals.

From Bolton and McFarlane (1978, figures 1 and 3).

changes in the nerve at these regions of experimental tourniquet compressions (Ochoa, Danta, Fowler, and Gilliatt, 1971; Ochoa, Fowler, and Gilliatt, 1972; Gilliatt, 1980a) (Figure 2.24). This very important work has clearly shown that the severity of the compressive injuries was related to the magnitudes of pressure in the tourniquet and the compression times. When the inflation pressure was 250 mm Hg and the compression time two hours, no persistent abnormalities were observed. Local demyelination and conduc-

tion block developed in all experiments, however, when the pressure was 1,000 mm Hg over an equivalent time. Pressures in between caused lesser degrees of demyelination and conduction block.

The most characteristic structural abnormalities were located beneath the borders of the tourniquet. Intussusceptions of nodal regions into adjacent internode segments were seen, but there was little damage to the nerve beneath the center of the tourniquet (Figures 2.24 and 2.25). The intussusceptions were

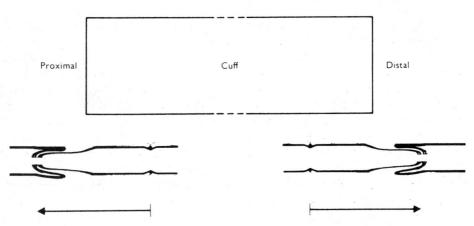

FIGURE 2.24.   Illustration of the intussusceptions of the nodes of Ranvier into their adjacent internode segments, and the polarity and location of such changes in relation to the overlying pneumatic tourniquet. In normal nerve fibers the attachment of the myelin lamellae in the region of the node of Ranvier is so strong that despite the sometimes extensive intussusceptions, the lamellae do not lose their attachments in such acute high-compression injuries as occurred in these experimental studies in the baboon.
Adapted from Ochoa, Fowler, and Gilliatt (1972), and reprinted with permission of the publisher, Cambridge University Press.

FIGURE 2.25.   The percentage of larger myelinated nerve fibers seen in transverse sections at various levels in relation to the pneumatic cuff, which appeared abnormal four days following compression of the medial popliteal fossa by the cuff inflated to 1,000 mm Hg for 90 minutes.
From Ochoa, Fowler, and Gilliatt (1972, figure 7), and reprinted with permission of the publisher, Cambridge University Press.

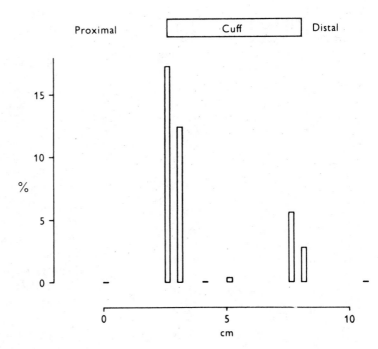

pointed away from the tourniquet. This suggested that the displacements were produced by pressure gradients acting across the border zones of the tourniquet. The locations of the structural abnormalities correlated with the locations of the predominant conduction delays and conduction blocks following tourniquet compression (Gilliatt, 1980a). These characteristic nodal displacements were seen in the early lesions. The lesions later evolved into regions of paranodal demyelination and still later remyelination with onset of recovery (Ochoa, Fowler, and Gilliatt, 1972). Equivalent structural abnormalities have been observed in local compressions produced by weighted nylon cords (Rudge, Ochoa, and Gilliatt, 1974).

Other important characteristics mark the above experimental compressive lesions. These include:

1. Nodal invaginations were most common in the larger-diameter myelinated nerve fibers. Why this is so is not known. Perhaps much higher intra-axonal pressures are required to force the invaginations into adjacent internodes in smaller nerve fibers. The degree of constriction of the axon at the node of Ranvier relative to the diameter of the internodal axon, however, is greater in larger- than in smaller-diameter myelinated nerve fibers and might be expected to act as a better check on intussusception, therefore, in the larger fibers.

2. Wallerian degeneration was common in lesions where there was a high degree of conduction block. Based on our own experience in human compressive and crush injuries of peripheral nerves when the conduction block exceeds 50 percent or more, wallerian degeneration is very common and no doubt contributes to the overall deficit.

The exact mechanisms by which compression produces these characteristics is not known. Peripheral nerves are not damaged even by very high pressures, provided the distribution of these pressures throughout the nerve is even (Grundfest, 1936). Peripheral nerves are, however, very susceptible to local injury where the pressure distributions are uneven (Bentley and Schlapp, 1943), an event to be expected beneath a local pressure point (Rudge, Ochoa, and Gilliatt, 1974) or at the borders of a tourniquet (Ochoa, Fowler, and Gilliatt, 1973; Griffiths and Heywood, 1973).

Physiological Abnormalities in Human Nerves Subjected to Short-term Compression Injuries

Conduction abnormalities in the human are just what would be expected based on the experimental evidence. They include:

1. Wallerian degeneration. Wallerian degeneration is common when the compression is severe or prolonged, as it may be in coma. By and large, the connective tissue framework in the nerve remains intact, but those axons interrupted at the site of injury degenerate distal to the level of the compression. Preservation of the endoneural tubes helps to ensure the best possible chance of accurate and complete subsequent regeneration.

The proportion of the whole nerve fiber population that has undergone degeneration can be estimated once enough time (five to ten days) has elapsed for these nerve fibers to become inexcitable and no longer contribute to the amplitude of the M-response or compound nerve potentials (Figure 2.20).

2. Slowing of the conduction velocity and conduction block at the level of the compression. Slowing of conduction and conduction block at the level of the compression makes it possible to localize the injury. Persistent and disproportionate slowing of conduction velocities and conduction block at the borders of an earlier tourniquet placement can last several weeks before recovery in the tourniquet lesion (Bolton and McFarlane, 1978) (Figure 2.23). The abnormalities noted in the re-

ported patient are the equivalent of the local conduction abnormalities noted in experimental tourniquet lesions. Sweating was also impaired in their patient, which suggests that smaller-diameter nerve fibers were also damaged, and not just the larger-diameter fibers. Similar local conduction abnormalities are common in the so-called Saturday-night radial nerve palsies, acute peroneal compression palsies, and other acute focal neuropathies (Figure 2.26).

Chronic Repeated Nerve Compression

In this group are most of the very common peripheral nerve entrapments such as the median nerve in the carpal tunnel, the ulnar nerve in the retroepicondylar and cubital tunnel sites, and some of the cervical and lumbosacral root entrapments. The majority of root entrapments are caused by bony encroachment in the intervertebral root canals or compression of the roots by herniations of nearby disk material. Fixation and compression of nerves by tough connective tissue bands or injury of the nerves in fibrous or fibro-osseous tunnels tends to dominate current thinking about the cause of the more peripheral entrapments in man. These nerves are often thinned and flattened out at the site of compression, and may be enlarged proximal and sometimes distal to the compression as seen at operation (Brown, Ferguson, Jones, and Yates, 1976). The precise pathogenesis of these lesions is uncertain, but probably depends on the location of the nerve with respect to the local tissues, the nature of those tissues (bony, disk, and connective tissues), whether or not traction and angulation as well as compression are involved, and whether or not ischemia is also present through compression and obstruction of the microcirculation of the nerve (Lundborg, 1970; Sunderland, 1976, 1978; Gilliatt, 1980a).

In the siliconized rubber tube model of chronic compression, nerve fibers were normal proximal and distal to the compression.

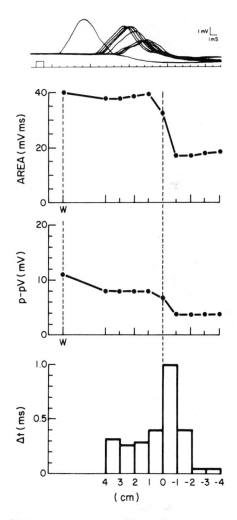

FIGURE 2.26. Alcoholic subject whose symptoms of paresthesias and weakness in the ulnar distribution were of short duration. Shown are changes in the negative peak area in millivolts and milliseconds and the peak-to-peak amplitude in millivolts [p-pV (-mV)] of the maximum hypothenar M-potentials as recorded with surface electrodes and elicited by direct stimulation of the ulnar nerve at 1-cm intervals proximal (−) and distal to the tip of the medial epicondyle as well as at the wrist. The real potentials are shown at the top; the time intervals in milliseconds over the successive 1-cm intervals at the elbow are at the bottom. Note that the major reductions in amplitude and area as well as increase in conduction time were centered about the tip of the medial epicondyle.

At the level of the compression, however, there was demyelination. This was maximum in the outermost and largest-diameter nerve fibers (Aguayo, Nair, and Midgley, 1971). Unlike the above model where no changes were apparent in the diameters of the myelinated nerve fibers distal to the compression, Baba, Fowler, Jacobs, and Gilliatt (1982) recently showed that a chronically applied ligature constricting a peripheral nerve can reduce axonal diameters distal to the constriction. These authors speculated that such reductions in axonal diameters could well help to explain the reductions in the maximum conduction velocities observed distal to the constriction. In another model of chronic compression, guinea pig median nerves compressed beneath their cartilaginous bars at the wrist (Fullerton and Gilliatt, 1967a, 1967b), local demyelination, remyelination, and wallerian degeneration were all observed. In these nerves, local conduction delays at the sites of the compression were present as well as some-

times very prolonged motor terminal latencies.

In chronic compression neuropathies, the most characteristic lesions are displacements of the myelin away from the site of compression (Figure 2.27). At those ends of the internodes nearest to the site of compression, the terminal myelin loops become detached and the myelin retracts away from the node. Toward the opposite ends of the internode the myelin becomes buckled and heaped up. The mechanisms responsible for these changes are not known, but could involve longitudinal stretching of nerves fixed at their entrapment sites and perhaps intermittent intra-axonal pressure waves moving out from the site of the compression. The above polar lesions combine with local demyelination and remyelination and regeneration clusters consisting of thinly myelinated immature regenerating nerve fibers, thus completing the pathology of chronic nerve compression in experimental and human chronic entrapment neuropathies

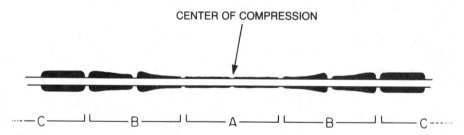

FIGURE 2.27.   Diagrammatic illustration of the effects of chronic or repeated compression of a peripheral nerve fiber. Opposite to and immediately adjacent to the site of compression (A), many fibers are demyelinated or thinly remyelinated. Internodes more removed both proximal and distal to the site of compression show strikingly polarized morphological changes (B). These consist of loss of the attachment of the myelin lamellae at the ends of internodes facing the site of compression and progressive slippage of the myelin sheath, which becomes heaped up toward the opposite end of the internode. The slippage and subsequent breakdown of the myelin sheath in the paranodal region produces paranodal demyelination. Further removed from the site of compression, these changes become less pronounced and the paranodal and internodal regions correspondingly more normal (C). Perineural thickening and endoneural edema as well as clusters of regenerated and remyelinated fibers are also common findings (see Neary and Eames, 1975).

(Neary and Eames, 1975; Neary, Ochoa, and Gilliatt, 1975; Ochoa and Marotte, 1973; Gilliatt, 1980b).

Physiological Abnormalities in Chronic Nerve Compression

Chronic nerve compression may result in the following abnormalities (Figures 2.28 and 2.29):

1. Local slowing of conduction velocities
2. Local conduction block
3. Continuous conduction
4. Wallerian degeneration
5. Ectopic impulse generation
6. Changes in nerve conduction proximal to the compression
7. Changes in nerve conduction distal to the compression

For reasons outlined earlier, partial or complete loss of the myelin sheath slows conduction velocities and may lead to conduction block at the site of entrapment. In entrapment lesions of the median nerve, the conduction velocities in single motor axons are sometimes less than one meter per second (Figure 2.30). These very low velocities are in the range of what would be expected were continuous conduction to be present. Whether or not continuous conduction develops in human entrapment neuropathies is not known. The observation that conduction block can last for many months in these conditions raises questions about just what are the necessary stimuli or impediments to reorganization of ion channel densities and their distribution in order to overcome established blocks.

Wallerian degeneration in some of the motor and sensory fibers of the entrapped nerve is common. Because of the slow progression of these injuries, however, it is possible that muscle fibers are reinnervated at rates that are able to keep pace with rates of their denervation as their parent axons degenerate. The true extent of motor axon loss is then

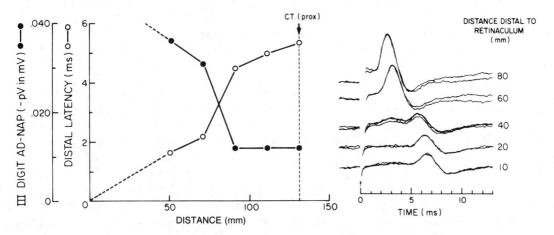

FIGURE 2.28.   Example of a focal conduction delay and block in median sensory fibers toward the distal end of the carpal tunnel. Shown are the antidromic digital sensory nerve action potentials recorded by a pair of ring electrodes about the third digit. They were elicited by percutaneous stimulation of the median nerve at 20-mm intervals, beginning in this case at the proximal border of the carpal tunnel. Note the increase in size, area, and amplitude of the potential between 40 and 60 mm distal to the proximal border of the flexor retinaculum. This patient reported intermittent paresthesias and numbness waking her at night for several months; there was some persistent numbness in the median distribution as well.

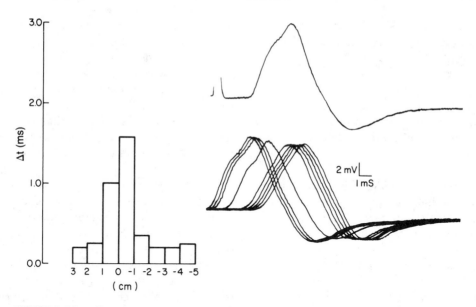

FIGURE 2.29.   Chronic ulnar neuropathy. The traces illustrate the maximum hypothenar (HT) M-potentials elicited by ulnar nerve stimulation at the level of the wrist (top) and proximal and distal to the tip of the medial epicondyle. The histogram illustrates conduction times in milliseconds over successive 10-mm segments proximal (−) and distal to the medial epicondyle (0). Note that the most abnormal increases in conduction time were observed across the 20 mm centered on the tip of the medial epicondyle. Over the worst of these two successive 10-mm segments, the maximum conduction velocity was 6.6 m/s, whereas the maximum conduction velocities across the cubital tunnel segment and proximal to the retroepicondylar regions were over 40 m/s. From Brown, Ferguson, Jones, and Yates (1976, figure 10).

masked by collateral reinnervation. Few motor units need be present to maintain normal or near-normal forces and M-response amplitudes (McComas, Sica, Campbell, and Upton, 1971; Brown, 1973).

The losses of motor units may be estimated by various methods outlined in Chapter 6. Wallerian degeneration in sensory nerve fibers is betrayed by reductions in the amplitudes of the compound sensory nerve action potential (see Chapter 3). Conduction block and wallerian degeneration may reduce both the amplitudes of nerve and muscle action potentials. It may be difficult to assess the relative contributions of these two mechanisms in entrapment or compressive neuropathies.

Some degree of loss of nerve fibers, however, is suggested when, for example, the amplitude of the muscle compound action potential as elicited by an electrical stimulus delivered to the nerve distal to the site of the injury is reduced, compared to normal values for that muscle, provided account is also taken of the possible effects of temporal dispersion on the amplitude of the potential.

Assessment of conduction block at the site of the injury requires, in the case of motor studies, that stimulation be carried out both proximal and distal to the injury site and comparison of the sizes the maximum M-potential elicited by the stimulation proximal to the injury with that elicited by the stimulation distal

FIGURE 2.30. Histogram illustrating the motor conduction time (Δt) over the most abnormal 0.5-cm segment in each of 23 median carpal tunnel neuropathies where the nerve was studied at operation by direct stimulation proximal to and through the region of the carpal tunnel. The conduction times in milliseconds (ms) are shown below and the corresponding conduction velocities above. Note that in 10 of the 23 median nerves investigated, the maximum motor conduction velocity over the most abnormal segment was below 5 m/s and in two instances it was less than 1 m/s. The last suggests the possibility of continuous conduction over these most abnormal segments.

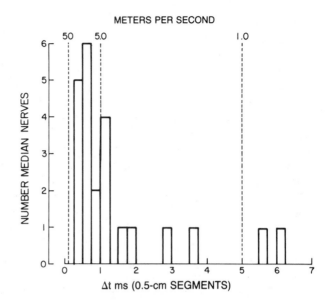

to the injury (Figures 2.28 and 2.29). Normally, over the short distance involved (50 to 100 mm) there is little appreciable difference in the shapes or sizes of the two potentials.

A major reduction in the amplitude and area of the proximally elicited M-potential with respect to the distally evoked M-potential, (provided there is no accompanying increase in the duration of the proximal stimulus-evoked M-potential as to suggest an increase in temporal dispersion) is strong evidence that transmission in a significant proportion of the axons has been blocked at or close to the injury site.

Conduction velocities may be reduced proximal to a nerve transection or crush (Cragg and Thomas, 1961; Aitkin and Thomas, 1962; Kuno, Miyata, and Muñoz-Martinez, 1974a, 1974b; Stohr, Schumm, and Reill, 1977; McComas, Sica, and Banerjee, 1978; Miller and Stein, 1981; Dyck, Lais, Karnes, Sparks, Hunder, Low, and Windeback, 1981). In chronic compressive neuropathies the evidence of this is more uncertain. While it is true that the maximum conduction velocities proximal to a nerve entrapment may well be

below normal values (Thomas, 1960), selective degeneration or conduction block of the largest-diameter nerve fibers at the site of entrapment could explain proximal slowing of conduction. To exclude the latter possibility, the examiner must measure the conduction velocity proximal to the injury in such a way that it is independent of transmission across or distal to the entrapment. To date this has not been the practice in clinical laboratories. Therefore it remains uncertain whether the slowing of conduction velocities seen proximal to the site of entrapment in humans is more apparent than real. There is some evidence to the contrary (Buchthal and Rosenfalck, 1971; Buchthal, Rosenfalck, and Trojaborg, 1974).

The proximal location of root lesions makes direct assessment of conduction across the site of the lesions impossible except by using invasive techniques. The F-response and evoked potential techniques share the same major limitation; they both force the electromyographer to include a long segment of normal or relatively normal conducting nerve distal to the root with the much shorter root segment in the overall measure of latency. Clearly, unless the root lesion is extensive and the resulting conduction slowing very pronounced, there may be no significant alteration in the overall proximal conduction time (or velocity) as assessed by these techniques.

This limitation is present to a lesser extent in lesions affecting the brachial and lumbosacral plexuses. Unless such lesions in the plexuses are extensive or wallerian degeneration has taken place, no abnormalities may be detected using presently available electrophysiological techniques.

Reduced conduction velocities in digital sensory nerve fibers distal to the site of entrapments of the median nerve in the carpal tunnel may well be explained by axonal atrophy distal to the compression such as has been described following constriction of a nerve by a ligature in experimental animals (Baba, Fowler, Jacobs, and Gilliatt, 1982). Conduction block can last several months following brief compressive injuries (Fowler, Danta, and Gilliatt, 1972; Rudge, 1974; Trojaborg, 1977) and persist for very long periods in chronic compressive nerve injuries as well. These long-lasting neuropraxic lesions are probably not responsible for the fibrillation potentials seen in such cases. A more likely explanation is wallerian degeneration in some of the motor nerve fibers (Gilliatt, Westgaard, and Williams, 1978), although this question has not been completely resolved (Gilliatt, 1980b).

TRACTION INJURIES

Peripheral nerves may also be injured by stretching. Normally, nerve fibers are protected against such stretch or traction injuries by the elastic properties of the perineurium (Sunderland, 1978). Once the rather generous elastic limits of the connective tissue framework are reached and exceeded, however, these tissues may rupture and split. Nerve fibers, now stretched beyond their limit, break and degenerate beyond the site of rupture.

Breaks and ruptures also develop in blood vessels. Nerve fibers herniate out through their perineural sheath, which leads to their subsequent degeneration. In addition to these obvious mechanical effects, traction may produce ischemic damage to the nerve by narrowing the cross-sectional areas of the funiculi, thereby increasing intrafunicular pressures enough to occlude the intrafunicular blood supply to the nerve.

Between the spinal cord and the distal extremities of the main peripheral nerve trunks, the most vulnerable site for traction injuries to take place is the junction between the spinal cord and the spinal roots. The connective tissue support is weakest at this level, the roots themselves being protected somewhat by extension of part of the perineurium into the roots, the other part becoming continuous with the pia arachnoid (Low, 1976; Sunderland, 1978). Avulsions of the roots from the spine in brachial plexus injuries are therefore common.

Clinically, it is important to establish whether the injuries are proximal or distal to the dorsal root ganglia (DRG). When they are proximal to the DRG, degeneration will not develop in the peripheral processes of the DRG cells, and tests directed toward these processes, such as recording peripheral sensory nerve action potentials, should be normal. In such lesions the central processes of the intact dorsal root ganglion cells are unable to regenerate into the central nervous system, at least in numbers and with the necessary appropriate central connections to be of any value. When the dorsal root ganglion cells themselves are destroyed, the peripheral as well as central processes of the dorsal root ganglion cells undergo degeneration, with the result that the related sensory nerve fibers lose their excitability and there is a corresponding reduction in the amplitudes of the sensory nerve action potentials recorded in the periphery. In such cases, regeneration of both the central and peripheral processes of the

DRG cells is impossible because of the loss of parent cell bodies. When the interruption of axonal continuity is distal to the DRG, the peripheral processes are able to regenerate, provided the injury is not too close to the cell body. Injuries to the spinal cord and meninges are commonly associated with lesions involving the roots.

The presence of Horner's syndrome is an indication of possible avulsion of the lower cervical and T1 roots. A normal flare response to intradermal histamine is further evidence that the peripheral sensory processes and dorsal root ganglion cells themselves are intact (Sunderland, 1978). Similarly, preserved sensory nerve action potentials in regions where clinical testing reveals impaired large fiber sensation have equivalent meaning, although it may take anywhere from one to seven days for the peripheral processes of the DRG cells to degenerate and become inexcitable once the parent cell bodies have been destroyed. It is also common for traction injuries to the brachial plexus to extend both proximal and distal to the intervertebral foramina as well as throughout the plexus, although such a broad distribution of the lesions may not be at all apparent even when the plexus is inspected directly.

The actual site of a peripheral nerve injury may not correspond to the most obvious site. For example, because of severe angulation as well as traction, it is not uncommon for the site of the nerve injury to be well proximal or distal to a displaced fracture, even though the most obvious mechanism of injury might appear to be direct trauma at the site of the bony displacement and trauma.

ISCHEMIA AND PERIPHERAL NERVES

Ischemia is not a common cause of damage to peripheral nerve and muscle, but can occur in occlusive peripheral vascular disease as well as in the compartment syndromes (Schaumburg, Spencer, and Thomas, 1982; Parry, 1983). The problems that sometimes attend use of the pneumatic tourniquet are the result of mechanical injuries to the underlying compressed nerve at the borders of the tourniquet and not the result of ischemia (Bolton and McFarlane, 1978).

Physiological Abnormalities

The physiological consequences of ischemia and hypoxia include progressive reductions in the amplitudes of compound nerve action potentials, progressive inability to generate impulses, proximal to distal progression of conduction abnormalities, progressive neuromuscular transmission failure reduction in accommodation, and ectopic generation of impulses.

Progressive Reductions in the Amplitudes of Compound Nerve Action Potentials

In multifiber preparations there is a progressive reduction in the amplitude of compound nerve potentials. This reduction could be the result of reductions in the amplitudes of individual impulses, progressive conduction block, and an increase in the temporal dispersion among the component impulses. The last is in turn the result of the progressively slower conduction velocities of the component nerve impulses.

Progressive Inability To Generate Impulses

In a hypoxic environment, generation of the impulse begins to block at nodes of Ranvier in single rat myelinated nerve fibers by about 20 minutes. Prior to the block there is progressive reduction in the amplitude of the impulses. The block is reversible at the outset by increasing the extracellular calcium ion concentration, an observation that, according to Mauhashi and Wright (1967), suggested that the binding of calcium ions to sodium channels was energy dependent. Hence in the absence of oxygen, calcium binding to the channels was reduced and the sodium channels became inoperable (Mauhashi and Wright, 1967).

Proximal-Distal Progression of the Conduction Abnormalities

Lewis, Pickering, and Rothschild (1931) observed that when a pneumatic tourniquet was inflated to above systolic blood pressure, a progressive advance in the paralysis and sensory loss followed, beginning at the periphery and advancing toward the tourniquet. This centripetal progression was thought to result from a progressive block beginning in the proximal part of the nerve and advancing toward the periphery. Others claimed this general centripetal spread in paralysis and sensory impairment was not the same in all peripheral nerves in the ischemic territory, but that some peripheral nerves appeared to be involved before others. For example, the order of involvement in the upper limb was claimed to be median, ulnar medial, and lateral cutaneous nerves of the forearm (Sinclair, 1948). This apparent relative susceptibility among the major nerves in the upper limb has been seen by ourselves as well, but the explanation is not obvious (Figure 2.31). Whatever the relative susceptibilities among the various nerves to ischemia, the central observation holds true that there is progression in the appearance and severity of conduction abnormalities toward the periphery.

Progressive increases in which the thresholds to direct electrical stimulation of the nerve trunk as well as conduction block progress in a distal direction in ischemic cat nerves (Groat and Koenig, 1946). Similarly, Kugelberg (1944) observed that the characteristic reduction in accommodation of ischemic nerve began in the proximal portions of ischemic nerve. Nielsen and Kardel (1974, 1981) and later we ourselves (Yates, Hurst, and Brown, 1981) documented progressive reduction in maxi-

mum conduction velocities and amplitudes of the maximum compound nerve trunk potential or M-response that began near the tourniquet and advanced distally in the ischemic zone distal to the tourniquet (Figure 2.21).

This proximal to distal progression has not been explained at the present time. Possible explanations include the following:

1. Even if the chance of conduction block were the same at all sites along the length of nerve, the proportion of nerve fiber population whose impulses are blocked, and hence the amplitudes of the compound nerve trunk potential or M-response, will fall as the distance over which conduction is measured increases (Figure 2.32). This could explain the apparent increases in threshold measured at more proximal sites, where the accumulative effects of the conduction block between sites of the recording and stimulating electrodes could act to remove most, if not all, of the lower-threshold nerve fibers from those still able to conduct impulses uninterruptedly between the sites. The effect would be to remove more and more of the lower-threshold nerve fibers from the test population as the distance increased between the stimulating and recording electrodes.

2. In a like manner, the proportion of nerve fiber population whose impulses are blocked increases as the length of the nerve increases over which conduction is measured. This fact could explain the apparent progressive centrifugal reduction in maximum conduction velocities because more and more of the faster-conducting nerve fibers would be blocked as the site of stimulation moved in a proximal direction. This does not imply selective block of the faster-conducting fibers. The larger the proportion of the whole population of nerve fibers whose impulses are blocked, however, the greater the chance that some of the faster-conducting fibers will be included among them.

3. One other possible explanation is that

FIGURE 2.31. Relative susceptibility of the ulnar and median nerves to ischemia. The nerves were stimulated by surface electrodes positioned over them just proximal and distal to the tourniquet and at the level of the wrist, and recordings were made over the thenar and hypothenar muscles. Pretourniquet values are shown at the top.

In the selected traces, note that at 20 minutes the earliest appearance of conduction block was in the median nerve across the tourniquet segment. Thereafter the proximal-to-distal cascade in the declines of respective M-potentials was greater in the median nerve until at 30 minutes, only the distal stimulus-evoked thenar M-potential remained. A hypothenar M-potential that was about one-half the size of that evoked at the wrist could be elicited by stimulation of the ulnar nerve just distal to the tourniquet. Finally, at 55 minutes, only the distal stimulus-elicited hypothenar potential remained.

Following release of the tourniquet, the recovery of the median nerve as seen at 2.5 minutes was considerably slower than that of the ulnar nerve.

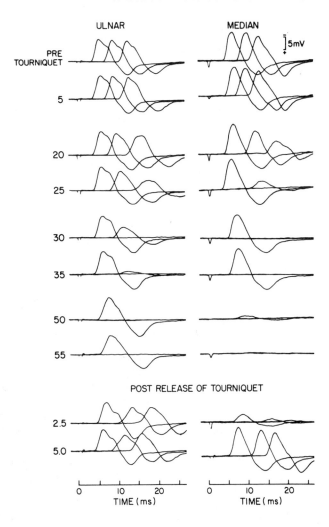

as the degree of temporal dispersion increases in response to the ischemia, the initial positive peak to which the "least" latencies are measured in the orthodromic nerve action potential technique (Buchthal and Rosenfalck, 1966) may become less and less representative of the fastest-conducting fibers as the distance away from the site of stimulation increases. Nielsen and Kardel (1974, 1981) have advanced arguments as to why their results and similar observations by others are not explicable by temporal dispersion or the selective block of conduction in faster-conducting nerve fibers.

4. There is no reason to think that one region is more ischemic than another distal to the tourniquet. Temperature gradients would be expected to reduce conduction velocities more distally than proximally.

5. Based on our present knowledge, there is no reason to suppose that oxygen use, sodium channel kinetics or densities, or the safety factor for impulse transmission are not similar along the length of peripheral nerves

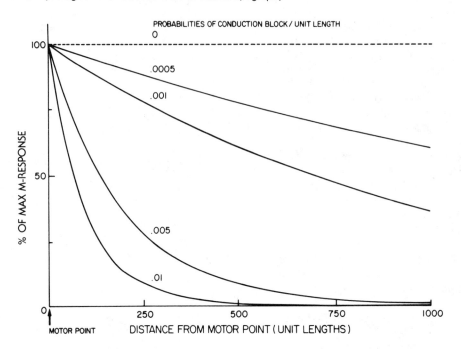

FIGURE 2.32.   Plots of the changes expected in the M-potential, here shown as a percentage of the M-potential elicited by stimulation at the motor point, as the site of the supramaximal stimulation of the motor nerve is moved progressively proximalward. In this model, the sizes of the muscle potentials elicited by all the individual motor axons is assumed to be identical. The size of the M-potential in this model is assumed to be directly proportional to the numbers of contributing MUPs and therefore, motor axons whose impulses are able to conduct without interruption from the site of stimulation to the muscle. No account is taken of any alterations in the size of the M-potentials elicited by motor nerve stimulation at various distances between the motor point and the site of stimulation, which might reflect differences among the conduction velocities of the motor axons.

Distance in the model is expressed in multiples of a unit length of the nerve, perhaps corresponding to a single internode. Note that the steepest absolute declines in the size of the M-potentials occur within the immediate vicinity of the motor point; although the percentage reduction in size of the M-potential for equivalent conduction distances remains the same. Even probabilities of conduction block per internode as low as 0.005 and 0.01 produce steep declines in the size of the M-potential. The maximum M-potential amplitude at any distance n number of unit lengths away from the motor point equals

$$y \times (1-p)^n \times V,$$

where p = the probability of the conduction
              block in each nerve fiber per unit
              length,
      y = the number of nerve fibers, and
      n = the number of unit lengths
              (or internodes) in the nerve.
From Yates, Hurst, and Brown (1981, figure 9).

except perhaps at their distal extremities. Our own observations suggest that reductions in amplitudes of nerve trunk potentials and increases in their latencies are the same for equivalent lengths of nerve irrespective of their proximal or distal location. Thus proximal regions are possibly no more susceptible than are more distal regions to the effects of ischemia. The whole question about proximal to distal progression of conduction abnormalities in ischemic nerve needs reinvestigation.

Neuromuscular Transmission

Neuromuscular transmission failures occur prior to the appearance of conduction block in the main nerve trunk. This is possibly a result of progressive depolarization of the membranes and thence reductions in the amplitudes of impulses in the presynaptic terminals (Hubbard and Loyning, 1966).

Reduction in Accommodation

Brief subthreshold stimulus pulses reduce the threshold levels at which impulses are initiated, whereas long-duration stimulus pulses can increase these levels. In the latter case the membrane accommodates because of the inactivation of sodium channels. In ischemia the capacity of nerves to accommodate to long-duration stimuli is reduced, single pulses often triggering trains of impulses (Kugelberg, 1946).

Ectopic Generation of Impulses

In the early ischemic and postischemic periods, paresthesias are experienced (Kugelberg, 1944; Nathan, 1958; Ochoa and Torebjork, 1980; Culp, Ochoa, and Torebjork, 1982).

Ischemic Injury of Peripheral Nerves

Longitudinal and regional vessels supply blood to peripheral nerve. The importance of the longitudinal blood supply is clear because healthy peripheral nerves may be dissected free from nearby tissues over surprisingly long distances without apparent hazard to the nerve (Sunderland, 1978; Schaumburg, Spencer, and Thomas, 1983). The same procedure is, however, much more risky when the longitudinal blood supply is interrupted for any reason. In such cases the nerve trunk becomes much more dependent on regional or segmental blood supplies and when the longitudinal arterial supply is compromised as by a local compressive lesion, the nerve trunk may become much more susceptible to ischemic damage when extensive mobilization procedures interrupt the segmental supply on which it is now dependent.

Because peripheral nerves have an abundant blood supply, it is difficult to produce pure ischemic injuries in them. The pneumatic tourniquet is a poor model because of the mechanical pressure injuries at the level of the tourniquet. To produce ischemic injury, all the major blood supply to a nerve must be occluded. This means, for example, that in the rabbit it is necessary to occlude both the external and internal iliac arteries or the common and internal iliac arteries (Hess, Eames, Darveniza, and Gilliatt, 1979). In this excellent ischemic model, true *coagulation necrosis* of the muscle and intramuscular nerve fibers developed with no cell survivors. In nerve trunks within the ischemic territory, wallerian degeneration developed but the Schwann cells and fibroblasts survived. Because the Schwann cells survived, regeneration was possible in the nerve trunk. In this model the intramuscular nerve fibers were clearly more vulnerable to ischemia than was the parent nerve trunk. In addition, muscle suffered before the nerve. Degeneration developed in both the myelinated and unmyelinated nerve fiber populations, there being no selective involvement of the large-diameter nerve fibers. Lesions in the peripheral nerves were concentrated in the central regions of the fascicles. Demyelination was not a prominent feature, degeneration of nerve fibers being the more characteristic abnormality. Not unexpectedly, therefore, conduction block was uncommon (Fowler and Gilliatt, 1981).

Important points to remember about ischemic injuries of peripheral nerves include the following:

1. It is difficult to produce infarction of peripheral nerves because of the dual longitudinal and segmental blood supply. Nerves must be deprived of their blood supply above, below, and at segmental levels. This can occur were occlusion of major proximal vessels to develop, for example, in the aorta or common iliac arteries in the lower limb or the axillary artery in the upper limb. Where vascular occlusions are more distal, these must involve at least two or more of the major peripheral arteries.
2. Muscle and the intramuscular nerve fibers are more susceptible to ischemic damage than are the main nerve trunks. Exceptions to this include arteriovenous shunts in limbs (Bolton, Driedger, and Lindsay, 1979).
3. Because of the loss of the connective tissue framework in the nerve, regeneration of the nerve is not possible where there is coagulation necrosis.
4. In the larger nerves, degeneration of nerve fibers is more characteristic of these lesions than is primary demyelination, and in keeping with this is the finding of reduced M-potential amplitudes in the absence of any indications of conduction block or conduction slowing in human ischemic neuropathies (Wilbourn, Furlan, Hulley, and Ruschhaupt, 1983).

COMPARTMENT SYNDROMES

The compartment syndromes are unique disorders in which trauma or spontaneous hemorrhage within compartment spaces bound by bone and the relatively inelastic fascia can lead to a substantial increase in intracompartmental pressure (see review by Mubarak and Hargens, 1981). If this pressure exceeds the perfusion pressure of the tissues, necrosis of muscle and intramuscular nerve branches within the compartment can develop, as can damage to nerves that transit through the compartment. Examples include the anterior tibial and forearm flexor compartment syndromes (Matsen and Krugmire, 1978; Rorabeck and MacNab, 1975; Rorabeck and Clarke, 1978).

The increases in intracompartmental pressure, although probably not sufficient to occlude the larger arteries, are no doubt able to occlude the smaller intramuscular and intraneural vessels. Conduction in nerves that pass through the compartment progressively fails in that the conduction velocity progressively slows (Rorabeck and Clarke, 1978) and this is accompanied by progressive increases in the completeness of the conduction block in the nerve. The rate of onset and completeness of such conduction failures is related to the compartmental pressure, conduction failures being speedier to onset and more complete the higher the intracompartmental pressure. It is not clear from the reported studies, however, whether such progressive conduction failures are caused by ischemia alone or if angulation and compression at the sites of entry of the nerves into and from the compartment may also play a role in the pathogenesis of the nerve injury. The higher the intracompartmental pressure and the longer this is maintained, the slower and less complete the recovery of function in the nerve.

In the few posttraumatic compartment syndromes we have seen in the lower limb, three or more weeks following the injury and fasciotomy, large areas of the muscle were electrically silent and inexcitable to direct or indirect stimulation. Such areas probably represented areas of muscle infarction, while other areas in the muscle, where viable muscle fibers remained, were signaled by abundant fibrillation activity, probably a result of the loss of their motor innervation. In all cases, nerves such as the anterior tibial or superficial peroneal, in the cases of the anterior and lateral compartment syndromes respectively, became inexcitable; in the case of the anterior tibial nerve, the extensor digitorum brevis muscle became completely denervated. Changes such as the above indicate infarction not only of large parts of the muscle tissue within the compartment, but as alluded to above, ischemia and possibly compression angulation injury of nerves entering and leaving the compartment.

It is hoped that further experimental studies of these syndromes will cast more light on the nature of the functional and structural changes in nerves terminating in or passing through the compartment as well as the precise sequences of the functional failures in the muscle fibers, intramuscular axons, neuromuscular junctions, and larger nerve trunks themselves.

COLD INJURY OF PERIPHERAL NERVES

Nerves can be injured by exposure to excessive or prolonged cold. Nerve impulses in myelinated nerve fibers block between 5 and 10°C, and at even higher temperatures if the nerve is abnormal for some reason (Paintal, 1965; Schauf and Davis, 1974; Davis, Schauf, Reed, and Kesler, 1975).

There is some evidence that the small myelinated nerve fibers are more susceptible to conduction block produced by cold than are larger myelinated nerve fibers (Byck, Goldfarb, Schaumburg, and Sharpless, 1972), although others have not been able to demonstrate this (Paintal, 1965). Sometimes even though the conduction block reverses with rewarming and no structural abnormalities are observed at the time, degenerative changes develop in the nerve over the next several hours (Basbaum, 1973). If the cold injury is

severe enough, wallerian degeneration may develop, the axons and myelin being more susceptible to the cold than are perineural and epineural connective tissues. The basic pathogenesis of cold injury has not been established. There is recent evidence, however, that alterations in vascular permeability and damage to the vasa nervorum may lead to increases in endoneural edema and pressure and subsequent wallerian degeneration in compressed and perhaps ischemic nerve fibers (Myers, Powell, Heckman, Costello, and Katz, 1981). Preservation of the basement membranes helps to ensure that nerve regeneration is possible.

References

Aguayo A, Nair CPV, Midgley R. Experimental progressive compression neuropathy in the rabbit. Arch Neurol 1971;24:358–64.

Aitkin JT, Thomas PK. Retrograde changes in fiber size following nerve section. J Anat 1962;96:121–29.

Allt G. Pathology of the peripheral nerve. In: Landon DN, ed. The peripheral nerve. New York: John Wiley & Sons, 1976:666–739.

Asbury AK, Arnason BG, Adams RD. The inflammatory lesion in idiopathic polyneuritis. Medicine 1969;48:173–215.

Asbury AK, Johnson PC. Pathology of peripheral nerve. In: Bennington JL, ed. Major problems in pathology. Philadelphia: W B Saunders, 1978.

Baba M, Fowler CJ, Jacobs JM, Gilliatt RW. Changes in peripheral nerve fibers distal to a constriction. J Neurol Sci 1982;54:197–208.

Ballantyne JP, Campbell MJ. Electrophysiological study after surgical repair of sectioned peripheral nerves. J Neurol Neurosurg Psychiatry 1973;36:797–805.

Basbaum CB. Induced hypothermia in peripheral nerve: electron microscopic and electrophysiological observations. J Neurocytol 1973;2:171–87.

Behse F, Buchthal F. Alcoholic neuropathy: clinical, electrophysiological and biopsy findings. Ann Neurol 1977;2:95–110.

Bentley FH, Schlapp W. The effects of pressure

on conduction in peripheral nerve. J Physiol 1943;102:72–82.

Berry CM, Grundfest H, Hinsey JC. The electrical activity of regenerating nerves of the cat. J Neurophysiol 1944;7:103–15.

Berry CM, Hinsey JC. The recovery of diameter and impulse conduction in regenerating nerve fibers. Ann NY Acad Sci 1947;47:559–72.

Bolton CF, Driedger AA, Lindsay RM. Ischemic neuropathy in uremic patients caused by bovine arteriovenous shunt. J Neurol Neurosurg Psychiatry 1979;42:810–14.

Bolton CF, McFarlane RM. Human pneumatic tourniquet paralysis. Neurology (Minneap) 1978;28:787–93.

Bostock H, Rasminsky M. Potassium channel distribution in spinal root axons of dystrophic mice. J Physiol 1983;340:145–56.

Bostock H, Sears TA. The internodal axon membrane: electrical excitability and continuous conduction in segmental demyelination. J Physiol 1978;280:273–301.

Bostock H, Sears TA, Sherratt RM. The effects of 4-aminopyridine and tetraethylammonium ions on normal and demyelinated mammalian nerve fibers. J Physiol 1981;313:301–15.

Bostock H, Sherratt RM, Sears TA. Overcoming conduction failure in demyelinated nerve fibers by prolonging action potentials. Nature 1978;274:385–87.

Brown WF. Functional compensation of human motor units in health and disease. J Neurol Sci 1973;20:199–209.

Brown WF, Feasby TE. Conduction block and denervation in Guillain-Barré polyneuropathy. Brain 1984;107:219–239.

Brown, WF, Ferguson GG, Jones MW, Yates SK. The location of conduction abnormalities in human entrapment neuropathies. Can J Neurol Sci 1976;3:111–22.

Brown WF, Hurst LN, Routhier, C. Regeneration following nerve experimental transection and microneural repair. Fifth International Congress on Neuromuscular Disease, Marseille, France, September 1982.

Brown WF, Yates SK. Percutaneous localization of conduction abnormalities in human entrapment neuropathies. Can J Neurol Sci 1982;9:391–400.

Buchthal F, Kühl V. Nerve conduction, tactile sensibility and the electromyogram after suture or compression of peripheral nerve: a longitudinal study in man. J Neurol Neurosurg Psychiatry 1979;42:436–51.

Buchthal F, Rosenfalck A. Evoked action potentials and conduction velocity in human sensory nerves. Brain 1966;3:1–122.

Buchthal F, Rosenfalck A. Sensory conduction from digit to palm and from palm to wrist in the carpal tunnel syndrome. J Neurol Neurosurg Psychiatry 1971;34:243–52.

Buchthal F, Rosenfalck A, Trojaborg W. Electrophysiological findings in entrapment of the median nerve at the wrist and elbow. J Neurol Neurosurg Psychiatry 1974;37:340–60.

Burchiel KJ. Abnormal impulse generation in focally demyelinated trigeminal roots. J Neurosurg 1980;53:674–83.

Burke RE. Motor units in mammalian muscle. In: Sumner AJ, ed. The physiology of peripheral nerve disease. Philadelphia: WB Saunders, 1980:133–94.

Byck R, Goldfarb J, Schaumburg HH, Sharpless SK. Reversible differential block of saphenous nerve by cold. J Physiol 1972;222:17–26.

Casey EB, LeQuesne PM. Evidence for a distal lesion in alcoholic neuropathy. J Neurol Neurosurg Psychiatry 1972;35:624–30.

Cavanagh JB. The significance of the "dying-back" process in experimental and human neurological disease. Int Rev Exp Pathol 1964;3:219–67.

Chiu SY, Ritchie JM. Evidence for the presence of potassium channels in the paranodal region of acutely demyelinated mammalian single nerve fibers. J Physiol 1981;313:415–37.

Collins WF, O'Leary JC, Hunt WE, Schwartz HG. An electrophysiological study of nerve regeneration in the cat. J Neurosurg 1955;12:39–45.

Cragg BG, Thomas PK. Changes in conduction velocity and fiber size proximal to peripheral nerve lesions. J Physiol 1961;157:315–27.

Cragg BG, Thomas PK. The conduction velocity of regenerated peripheral nerve fibers. J Physiol 1964;171:164–75.

Culp WJ, Ochoa J. Abnormal nerves and muscles as impulse generators. Oxford: Oxford University Press, 1982:3–250.

Culp WJ, Ochoa J, Torebjork E. Ectopic impulse

generation in myelinated sensory fibers in man. In: Culp WJ, Ochoa J, eds. Abnormal nerves and muscles as impulse generators. Oxford: Oxford University Press, 1982:490–512.

Davis FA, Schauf CL, Reed BJ, Kesler RL. Experimental studies of the effects of extrinsic factors on conduction in normal and demyelinated nerve. I. Temperature. J Neurol Neurosurg Psychiatry 1975;39:442–48.

Dayan AD. Peripheral neuropathy of metachromatic leukodystrophy: observations on segmental demyelination and remyelination and the intracellular distribution of sulphatide. J Neurol Neurosurg Psychiatry 1967;30:311–18.

Denny-Brown D, Brenner C. Paralysis of nerve induced by direct pressure and by tourniquet. Arch Neurol Psychiatry 1944;51:1–26.

Devor M, Bernstein JJ. Abnormal impulse generation in neurones: electrophysiology and ultrastructure. In: Culp WJ, Ochoa J, eds. Abnormal nerves and muscles as impulse generators. Oxford: Oxford University Press, 1982:363–80.

Devor MV, Govrin-Lippmann R. Maturation of axonal sprouts after nerve crush. Exp Neurol 1979;64:260–70.

Donoso RS, Ballantyne JP, Hansen S. Regeneration of sutured human peripheral nerve: an electrophyisological study. J Neurol Neurosurg Psychiatry 1979;42:97–106.

Dyck PJ. Pathological alterations of the peripheral nervous system of man. In: Dyck PJ, Thomas PK, Lambert EH, eds. Peripheral neuropathy. Philadelphia: WB Saunders, 1975.

Dyck PJ, Lais AC, Karnes JL, Sparks M, Hunder H, Low PA, Windebank AJ. Permanent axotomy, a model of axonal atrophy and secondary demyelination and remyelination. Ann Neurol 1981;9:575–83.

Dyck PJ, Thomas PK, Lambert EH. Peripheral neuropathy. Philadelphia: WB Saunders, 1975.

Dyck PJ, Thomas PK, Lambert EH, Bunge R. Peripheral neuropathy. Vols. I, II. 2nd Edition. Philadelphia: WB Saunders, 1984.

Eccles JC, Libet B, Young RR. The behaviour of chromatolysed motoneurones studied by intracellular recording. J Physiol 1958;143:11–40.

Eisen A, Humphreys P. The Guillain-Barré syndrome: a clinical and electrodiagnostic study of 25 cases. Arch Neurol 1974;30:438–43.

Erlanger J, Schoepfle GM. A study of nerve degeneration and regeneration. J Physiol 1946;147:550–81.

Feasby TE, Bostock H, Sears TA. Conduction in regenerating dorsal root fibers. J Neurol Sci 1981;49:439–54.

Feasby TE, Hahn AF, Gilbert JJ. Passive transfer studies in Guillain-Barré polyneuropathy. Neurology 1980;32:1159–67.

Feasby TE, Pullen AH, Sears TA. A quantitative ultrastructural study of dorsal root regeneration. J Neurol Sci 1981;49:363–86.

Fisher CM, Adams RD. Diphtheritic polyneuritis—a pathological study. J Neuropathol Exp Neurol 1956;15:243–68.

Fowler CJ, Gilliatt RW. Conduction velocity and conduction block after experimental ischemic nerve injury. J Neurol Sci 1981;52:221–38.

Fowler CJ, Danta G, Gilliatt RW. Recovery of nerve conduction after a pneumatic tourniquet. Observation on the hind limb of the baboon. J Neurol Neurosurg Psychiatry 1972;35:638–47.

Fullerton PM, Gilliatt RW. Pressure neuropathy in the hind foot of the guinea pig. J Neurol Neurosurg Psychiatry 1967a;30:18–25.

Fullerton PM, Gilliatt RW. Median and ulnar neuropathy in the guinea pig. J Neurol Neurosurg Psychiatry 1967b;30:393–402.

Gilliatt, RW. Recent advances in the pathophysiology of nerve conduction. In Desmedt JE, ed. New developments in electromyography and clinical neurophysiology. Basel: Karger, 1973:2–18.

Gilliatt RW. Peripheral nerve compression and entrapment. Proceedings of the Eleventh Symposium on Advanced Medicine. Belmont, Calif.: Pitman, 1975:144–63.

Gilliatt RW. Acute compression block. In: Sumner AJ, ed. The physiology of peripheral nerve disease. Philadelphia: WB Saunders, 1980a;287–315.

Gilliatt RW. Chronic nerve compression and entrapment. In: Sumner AJ, ed. The physiology of peripheral nerve disease. Philadelphia: WB Saunders, 1980b:316–39.

Gilliatt RW, Hjorth RJ. Nerve conduction during

wallerian degeneration in the baboon. J Neurol Neurosurg Psychiatry 1972;35:335–41.

Gilliatt RW, Westgaard RH, Williams IR. Extra-junctional acetylcholine sensitivity on inactive muscle fibers in the baboon during prolonged nerve pressure block. J Physiol 1978;280:499–514.

Greenfield JC. The spinocerebellar degeneration. Oxford: Blackwell, 1954.

Griffiths JC, Heywood OB. Bio-mechanical aspects of the tourniquet. Hand 1973;5:113–18.

Groat RA, Koenig H. Centrifugal deterioration of asphyxiated peripheral nerve. J Neurophysiol 1946;9:275–84.

Grundfest H. Effects of hydrostatic pressure upon the excitability, the recovery and potential sequence of frog nerve. Cold Spring Harbor Symp Quant Biol 1936;4:179–87.

Harrison MJG. Pressure palsy of the ulnar nerve with prolonged conduction block. J Neurol Neurosurg Psychiatry 1976;39:96–99.

Haymaker W, Kernohan, JW. The Landry-Guillain-Barré syndrome. Medicine 1949;28:59–141.

Hess K, Eames RA, Darveniza P, Gilliatt RW. Acute ischemic neuropathy in the rabbit. J Neurol Sci 1979;44:19–43.

Hodes R, Larrabee MG, German W. The human electromyogram in response to nerve stimulation and the conduction velocity of motor axons. Arch Neurol Psychiatry 1948;60:340–65.

Hodgkin AL, Katz B. The effect of temperature on the electrical activity of the giant axon of the squid. J Physiol 1949;109:240–49.

Hopkins AP, Gilliatt RW. Motor and sensory nerve conduction velocity in the baboon: normal values and changes during acrylamide neuropathy. J Neurol Neurosurg Psychiatry 1971;34:415–26.

Hubbard JC, Loyning Y. The effects of hypoxia on neuromuscular transmission in a mammalian preparation. J Physiol 1966;185:205–23.

Hudson AJ. Amyotrophic lateral sclerosis and its association with dementia, parkinsonism and other neurological disorders: a review. Brain 1981;104:217–47.

Jacobson S, Guth L. An electrophysiological study of the early stages of peripheral nerve regeneration. Exp Neurol 1965;11:48–60.

Jasper H, Penfield W. The rate of reinnervation of muscle following nerve injuries in man as determined by the electromyogram. Trans R Soc Can 1946;5:81–91.

Joseph BS. Somatofugal events in wallerian degeneration: a conceptual overview. Brain Res 1973;59:1–18.

Koles ZJ, Rasminsky M. A computer simulation of conduction in demyelinated nerve fibers. J Physiol 1972;227:351–64.

Kugelberg E. Accommodation in human nerves and the significance for symptoms in circulating disturbances and tetany. Acta Physiol Scand 1944;8(suppl)24:1–105.

Kugelberg E. "Injury activity" and "trigger zones" in human nerves. Brain 1946;69:310–24.

Kugelberg E. Properties of the rat hind-limb motor units. In: Desmedt JE, ed. New developments of electromyography and clinical neurophysiology. Basel: Karger, 1973:2–13.

Kugelberg E, Edström L, Abbruzzese M. Mapping of motor units in experimentally reinnervated rat muscle. J Neurol Neurosurg Psychiatry 1970;33:319–29.

Kuno M, Linás R. Enhancement of synaptic transmission by dendritic potentials in chromatolysed motoneurones of the cat. J Physiol 1970;210:807–21.

Kuno M, Miyata Y, Muñoz-Martinez EJ. Properties of fast and slow alpha motoneurones following motor reinnervation. J Physiol 1974a;242:273–88.

Kuno M, Miyata Y, Muñoz-Martinez EJ. Differential reaction of fast and slow alpha motorneurones to axotomy. J Physiol 1974b;240:725–39.

Kurdi A, Abdul-Kader M. Clinical and electrophysiological studies of diphtheritic neuritis in Jordan. J Neurol Sci 1979;42:243–50.

Lafontaine S, Rasminsky M, Saida T, Sumner AJ. Conduction block in rat myelinated fibers following acute exposure to anti-galactocerebroside serum. J Physiol 1982;323:287–306.

Lewis T, Pickering GW, Rothschild P. Centripetal paralysis arising out of arrested blood flow to the limb, including notes on a form of tingling. Heart 1931;16:1–32.

Lieberman AR. The axon reaction: a review of the principal features of perikaryal responses to axon injury. Int Rev Neurobiol 1971;14:49–124.

Lieberman AR. Some factors affecting retrograde neuronal responses to axonal lesions. In: Bellairs R, Gray EG, eds. Essays on the nervous system. Oxford: Clarendon Press, 1974:71–105.

Low FN. The perineurium and connective tissue of peripheral nerve. In: Landon DN, ed. The peripheral nerve. London: Chapman & Hall, 1976;159–67.

Lowndes HE, Baker T, Cho E, Jortner BS. Position sensitivity of de-efferented muscle spindles in experimental acrylamide neuropathy. J Pharmacol Exp Ther 1978;205:40–48.

Lowndes HE, Baker T, Michelson LP, Vincent-Ablazey M. Attenuated dynamic responses of primary endings of muscle spindles: a basis for depressed tendon responses in acrylamide neuropathy. Ann Neurol 1978;3:433–37.

Lundborg G. Ischemic nerve injury. Scand J Plast Reconstr Surg 1970;3(Suppl. 6):113.

Madrid R, Bradley WG. The pathology of neuropathies with focal thickening of the myelin sheath (tomaculous neuropathy): studies on the formation of the abnormal myelin sheath. J Neurol Sci 1975;25:415–48.

Matsen FA, Krugmire RB Jr. Compartmental syndromes. Surg Gynecol Obstet 1978;147:943–49.

Mauhashi J, Wright EB. Effect of oxygen lack on the single isolated mammalian (rat) nerve fiber. J Neurophysiol 1967;30:434–52.

McComas AJ, Sica RE, Banerjee S. Long-term effects of partial limb amputation in man. J Neurol Neurosurg Psychiatry 1978;41:425–32.

McComas AJ, Sica REP, Campbell MJ, Upton AR. Functional compensation in partially denervated muscles. J Neurol Neurosurg Psychiatry 1971;34:453–60.

McDonald WI. The effects of experimental demyelination on conduction in peripheral nerve: a histological and electrophysiological study. II. Electrophysiological observations. Brain 1963;86:501–24.

McDonald WI. Pathophysiology in multiple sclerosis. Brain 1974;97:179–96.

McDonald WI. Clinical consequences of conduction defects produced by demyelination. In: Culp WJ, Ochoa J, eds. Abnormal nerves and muscles as impulse generators. Oxford: Oxford University Press, 1982.

McIntyre AK, Bradley K, Brock LG. Responses of motoneurones undergoing chromatolysis. J Gen Physiol 1959;42:931–58.

McLeod JG, Walsh JC, Prineas JW, Pollard JP. Acute idiopathic polyneuritis. J Neurol Sci 1976;27:145–62.

Mendell LM, Munson JB, Scott JG. Alterations of synapses on axotomized motoneurones. J Physiol 1976;255:67–79.

Mendell LM, Scott JG. The effects of peripheral nerve cross union on connections of single 1A to motoneurones. Exp Brain Res 1975;22:221–34.

Miledi R, Slater CR. On the degeneration of rat neuromuscular junctions after nerve section. J Physiol 1970;207:507–28.

Miller TE, Stein RB. The effects of axotomy on the conduction of action potentials in peripheral sensory and motor nerve fibers. J Neurol Neurosurg Psychiatry 1981;44:485–96.

Milner-Brown HS, Stein RB, Lee RG. Pattern of recruiting human motor units in neuropathies and motor neuron disease. J Neurol Neurosurg Psychiatry 1974;37:665–69.

Mubarak SJ, Hargens AR. Compartment syndromes and Volkmann's contracture. Philadelphia: WB Saunders, 1981.

Myers RR, Powell HC, Heckman HM, Costello ML, Katz J. Biophysical and pathological effects of cryogenic nerve lesion. Ann Neurol 1981;10:478–85.

Nathan PW. Ischemic and post-ischemic numbness and paraesthesia. J Neurol Neurosurg Psychiatry 1958;21:12–123.

Neary D, Eames RW. The pathology of ulnar nerve compression in man. Neuropathol Appl Neurobiol 1975;1:69–88.

Neary D, Ochoa J, Gilliatt RW. Subclinical entrapment neuropathy in man. J Neurol Sci 1975;24:283–98.

Nielsen VK, Kardel T. Decremental conduction in normal human nerves subjected to ischemia. Acta Physiol Scand 1974;92:249–62.

Nielsen VK, Kardel T. Temporospatial effects on orthodromic sensory potential propagation during ischemia. Ann Neurol 1981;9:597–604.

Ochoa J, Danta G, Fowler TJ, Gilliatt RW. Nature of the nerve lesion caused by the pneumatic tourniquet. Nature 1971;233:265–67.

Ochoa J, Fowler TJ, Gilliatt RW. Anatomical changes in peripheral nerves compressed by a pneumatic tourniquet. J Anat 1972;113:433–55.

Ochoa J, Fowler TJ, Gilliatt RW. Changes produced by a pneumatic tourniquet. In: Desmedt JE, ed. New developments in electromyography and clinical neurophysiology. Basel: Karger, 1973:174–80.

Ochoa J, Marotte L. The nature of the nerve lesion caused by chronic entrapment in the guinea pig. J Neurol Sci 1973;19:491–95.

Ochoa JL, Torebjork HE. Paraesthesiae from ectopic impulse generation in human sensory nerves. Brain 1980;103:835–53.

Paintal AS. Effects of temperature on conduction in single vagal and saphenous myelinated nerve fibers of the cat. J Physiol 1965;180:20–49.

Parry G. Conduction changes associated with vascular lesions of nerves. In: The newer pathologic basis of nerve conduction abnormalities. Sixth Annual Continuing Education Course, Toronto, September 29–October 1, 1983. Rochester, Minn.: American Association of Electromyography and Electrodiagnosis, 1983:43–47.

Rasminsky M. The effects of temperature on conduction in demyelinated single nerve fibers. Arch Neurol 1973;28:287–92.

Rasminsky, M. Ectopic generation of impulses and cross talk in spinal nerve roots of "dystrophic mice." Ann Neurol 1978;3:351–57.

Rasminsky M. Dystrophic mouse spinal root acts as a pathological amplifier of nerve impulse activity. Neurology (Minneap) 1979;29:581.

Rasminsky M. Ephaptic transmission between single nerve fibers in the spinal roots of dystrophic mice. J Physiol 1980;305:151–69.

Rasminsky M. Ectopic excitation, ephaptic excitation and auto excitation in peripheral nerve fibers of mutant mice. In: Culp WJ, Ochoa J, eds. Abnormal nerves and muscles as impulse generators. Oxford: Oxford University Press, 1982:344–62.

Rasminsky M. Ectopic impulse generation in pathological nerve fibers. Trends Neurosci 1983; 6:38–90.

Rasminsky M, Kearney RE. Continuous conduction in demyelinated single nerve fibers. Arch Neurol Psychiatry 1976;28:287–92.

Rasminsky M, Kearney RE, Aguayo AJ, Bray GM. Conduction of nervous impulses in spinal roots and peripheral nerves of dystrophic mice. Brain Res 1978;143:71–85.

Rasminsky M, Sears TA. Internodal conduction in undissected demyelinated nerve fibers. J Physiol 1972;227:323–50.

Richardson PM, Thomas PK. Percussive injury to peripheral nerve in rats. J Neurosurg 1979; 51:178–87.

Rorabeck CH, MacNab I. The pathophysiology of the anterior tibial compartmental syndrome. Clin Orthop 1975;113:52–57.

Rorabeck CH, Clarke KM. The pathophysiology of the anterior tibial compartment syndrome: an experimental investigation. J Trauma 1978;18:299–304.

Rudge P. Tourniquet paralysis with prolonged conduction block. An electrophysiological study. J Bone Joint Surg 1974;56B:716–20.

Rudge P, Ochoa J, Gilliatt RW. Acute peripheral nerve compression in the baboon. J Neurol Sci 1974;23:403–20.

Saida G, Saida K, Saida T, Asbury AK. Axonal lesions in acute experimental demyelination: a sequential teased nerve fiber study. Neurology 1981;31:413–21.

Saida K, Saida T, Brown MJ, Silberberg DH. In vivo demyelination induced by intraneural injection of anti-galactocerebroside serum. Am J Pathol 1979;95:99–116.

Saida K, Sumner AJ, Saida T, Brown MJ, Silberberg DH. Anti-serum-mediated demyelination: relationships between remyelination and functional recovery. Ann Neurol 1979;8:12–24.

Sanders FK, Whitteridge D. Conduction velocity and myelin thickness in regenerating nerve fibers. J Physiol 1946;105:152–74.

Schauf CL, Davis FA. Impulse conduction in multiple sclerosis: a theoretical basis for modification by temperature and pharmacological agents. J Neurol Neurosurg Psychiatry 1974;37:152–61.

Schaumburg HH, Spencer PS. Toxic neuropathies. Neurology 1979;29:429–31.

Schaumburg HH, Spencer PS, Thomas PK. Disorders of peripheral nerves. Philadelphia: FA Davis, 1983.

Schaumburg HH, Wisniewski HM, Spencer PS. Ultrastructural studies of the dying-back process. Neuropathol Exp Neurol 1974;33:260–84.

Selzer M. Regeneration of peripheral nerve. In: Sumner AJ, ed. The physiology of peripheral nerve disease. Philadelphia: WB Saunders, 1980:358–431.

Sharma AK, Thomas PK. Peripheral nerve structure and function in experimental diabetes. J Neurol Sci 1974;23:1–15.

Sinclair DC. Observations on sensory paralysis prolonged by compression of a human limb. J Neurophysiol 1948;11:75–92.

Smith KJ, Hall SM. Nerve conduction during peripheral demyelination and remyelination. J Neurol Sci 1980;48:201–19.

Spencer PS, Sabri MI, Schaumburg HH, Moore CL. Does a defect of energy metabolism in the nerve fiber underlie axonal degeneration in polyneuropathies? Ann Neurol 1978;5:501–7.

Spencer PS, Schaumburg H. Central-peripheral distal axonopathy—the pathology of dying-back polyneuropathies. In: Zimmerman HM, ed. Progress in Neuropathology. New York: Grune & Stratton, 1976:253–95.

Spencer PS, Schaumburg HH. Experimental and clinical neurotoxicology. Baltimore: Williams & Wilkins, 1980.

Stålberg E, Ekstedt J. Single-fiber EMG and microphysiology of the motor unit in normal and diseased human muscle. In: Desmedt JE, ed. New developments of electromyography and clinical neurophysiology. Basel: Karger, 1973:113–29.

Stålberg E, Trontelj JV. Single-fiber electromyography. Surrey, England: Mirville Press: 1979.

Stöhr M, Schumm F, Reill P. Retrograde changes in motor and sensory conduction velocity after nerve injury. J Neurol 1977;214:281–87.

Struppler A, Huckauf H. Propagation velocity in regenerated motor nerve fibers. Electroencephalogr Clin Neurophysiol (Suppl) 1962; 22:58–60.

Sumner AJ. The physiology of peripheral nerve disease. Philadelphia: WB Saunders, 1980:340–57.

Sumner AJ, Asbury AK. Physiological studies of the dying-back phenomenon. Brain 1975;98:91–100.

Sumner AJ, Saida K, Saida T, Silberberg DH, Asbury AK. Acute conduction block associated with an antiserum-induced demyelinative lesion of peripheral nerve. Ann Neurol 1982;11:469–77.

Sumner BEH. A quantitative analysis of the responses of presynaptic boutons to post-synaptic motor neuron axotomy. Exp Neurol 1975; 46:605–15.

Sumner BEH. Quantitative ultrastructural observations on the inhibited recovery of the hypoglossal nucleus from the axotomy response when regeneration of the hypoglossal nerve is prevented. Exp Brain Res 1976;26:141–150.

Sunderland S. Nerve lesion in the carpal tunnel syndrome. J Neurol Neurosurg Psychiatry 1976;39:615–26.

Sunderland S. Nerves and nerve injuries. 2nd ed. Edinburgh: Churchill Livingstone, 1978.

Sunderland S. Advances in diagnosis and treatment of root and peripheral nerve injury. In: Thompson RA, Green JR, eds. Advances in neurology. New York: Raven Press, 1979:271–305.

Sunderland S. The anatomical basis of nerve repair. In: Jewett DL, McCarroll HR Jr, eds. Nerve repair and regeneration—its clinical and experimental basis. St. Louis: CV Mosby, 1980;14–35.

Swadlow HA, Kocsis JD, Waxman SG. Modulation of impulse conduction along the axonal tree. Annu Rev Biophys Bioeng 1980;147–79.

Thesleff S. Physiological effects of denervation of muscle. Ann NY Acad Sci 1974;228:89–103.

Thomas, PK. Motor nerve conduction in the carpal tunnel syndrome. Neurology (Minneap) 1960;10:1045–50.

Thomas PK. Nerve injury. In: Bellairs, Gray EG, eds. Essays on the nervous system. Oxford: Clarendon Press, 1974:44–70.

Trojaborg W. Rate of recovery in motor and sensory fibers of the radial nerve: clinical and electrophysiological aspects. J Neurol Neurosurg Psychiatry 1970;33:625–38.

Trojaborg W. Prolonged conduction block with axonal degeneration. J Neurol Neurosurg Psychiatry 1977;40:50–57.

Urich U. Diseases of peripheral nerve. In: Blackwood W, Corsellis JAN, eds. Greenfield's Neuropathology. Chicago: Yearbook Medical Publishers, 1976:687–720.

Wall PD, Gutnick M. Properties of afferent nerve impulses originating from a neuroma. Nature 1974a;248:740–43.

Wall PD, Gutnick M. Ongoing activity in peripheral nerves: the physiology and pharmacology of impulses originating from a neuroma. Exp Neurol 1974b;45:576–89.

Waxman SG. Conduction in myelinated, unmyelinated and demyelinated fibers. Arch Neurol 1977;34:585–89.

Waxman SG. Prerequisites for conduction in demyelinated fibers. Neurology 1978;28(2):27–33.

Waxman SG. Determinants of conduction velocity in myelinated nerve fibers. Muscle Nerve 1980;3:141–50.

Weller RO, Cervos-Navarro J. Pathology of peripheral nerves. London: Butterworth's, 1977.

Wilbourn AJ. Serial conduction studies in human nerve during wallerian degeneration. Electroencephalogr Clin Neurophysiol 1977;43:616.

Wilbourn AJ, Furlan AJ, Hulley W, Ruschhaupt W. Ischemic monomelic neuropathy. Neurology (Cleve) 1983;33:447–51.

Williams IR, Jefferson D, Gilliatt RW. Acute nerve compression during limb ischemia. An experimental study. J Neurol Sci 1980;46:199–207.

Yates SK, Hurst LN, Brown WF. The pathogenesis of pneumatic tourniquet paralysis in man. J Neurol Neurosurg Psychiatry 1981;44:759–67.

3 THE RECORDING OF CONDUCTED ELECTRICAL POTENTIALS IN NERVE TRUNKS AND CONDUCTION IN HUMAN MOTOR AND SENSORY FIBERS

The primary objectives of this chapter are not to present details of methods for measuring conduction in the now wide variety of peripheral nerves open to study in man; nor is it intended to cover the pathophysiological characteristics of all the types of peripheral neuropathies altering conduction in man. For both these, excellent sources are now available (Ludin and Tackmann, 1981; Kimura, 1983). This chapter builds on the background presented in Chapters 1 and 2 and presents the general principles of stimulation and recording techniques as applied to man, the stress being on the advantages and limitations of the techniques. Attempts are made throughout to draw attention to what correlations are now possible between the recorded potentials and the nerve fiber (NF) composition of the underlying nerve trunks. Next, methods for assessing the ranges of conduction velocities in NFs are discussed, as well as

the tendon and H-reflexes, and the F-response. Last, the general clinical and electrophysiological patterns of peripheral neuropathies are covered, with emphasis on the principal abnormalities seen with electrophysiological techniques and, where possible, the relationship these bear to clinical symptoms and signs. First, however, the general organization of NFs within peripheral nerves must be reviewed.

DIVISION OF NERVE FIBERS BY FUNCTION AND SIZE

The structure of human peripheral nerves, including the connective tissue components, has been the subject of several excellent reviews (Bischoff and Thomas, 1975; Thomas and Olsson, 1975; Webster, 1974; Landon and Hall, 1976; Low, 1976; Urich, 1976; Weller and Cervos-Navarro, 1977; Asbury and Johnson, 1980).

Cutaneous and motor nerves contain a wide variety of NFs that have traditionally been classifed into subgroups based on the major subgroups in the monophasic component potential (Erlanger and Gasser, 1937; Boyd and Davey, 1968), a system still used in respect to human cutaneous nerves (Lambert and Dyck, 1975) (Table 3.1). The subdivisions in Erlanger and Gasser's proposed system have been applied to motor NFs as well, the latter being divided into A alpha (α), beta (β), and gamma (γ) groups. Boyd and Davey (1968) have even proposed subdivision of the gamma group based on their anatomic and physiologic studies in the cat. In 1943 Lloyd proposed a subdivision of peripheral NFs by diameter (Table 3.2).

The above two classifications have been used interchangeably by many authors, the A alpha group corresponding to Lloyd's groups I and II, the A delta group to Lloyd's group III, and group IV to the C fibers. In the cat, the most rapidly conducting and largest-diameter afferents are the Golgi tendon and primary spindle (Ia) afferents. In the human, the thickest myelinated NFs in the median nerve at the wrist can reach 20 μ (Buchthal and Rosenfalck, 1966). Although there is no direct

TABLE 3.1.   Classification of Human Cutaneous Nerve Fibers

Fiber Group	Diameters (μ)	Conduction Velocities (m/s)	Relative Electrical Threshold	Types of Receptors				Physiological Characteristics of Receptors
A — Alpha	5–13[2]	30–65[3]	1X	Mechanoreceptors	Cutaneous receptors	Glabrous skin	Meissner's corpuscles	RA, S
							Merkel's disks	SA, S
							Pacinian corpuscles	RA, L
							Ruffini endings	SA, L
					Joint receptors	Hairy skin	+ Hair follicles	RA, S
A — Delta	1–5[2]	4–30[3]	5–10X	Cold receptors; Pain receptors	Pricking pain			
C	0.3–1.7[2]	0.4–1.8[3]	15–20X	Pain receptors (Polymodal nociceptors); Warm receptors; Sympathetic C units	Pain receptors; Delayed/burning/smarting pain			

1. Matthews (1972).
2. Lambert and Dyck (1975).
3. Vallbo, Hagbarth, Torebjork, and Wallin (1979).
RA = rapidly adapting.
SA = slowly adapting.
S = small receptive field.
L = large receptive field.

TABLE 3.2. Classification of Nerve Fibers in Motor Nerves (Afferents Only)

Group	Fiber Diameter (μ)	Physiological Type of Receptor
I	12–20	Spindle primaries Golgi tendon organs ?Free endings in muscle
II	6–12	Spindle secondaries Pacinian corpuscles Joint receptors Some free endings
III	1–6	Free endings, some nociceptors
IV	0.5–1.5	Autonomic fibers Nociceptors

See Lloyd (1943); critical discussion by Matthews (1972).

evidence of this, these are probably muscle and tendon afferents originating in intrinsic hand muscles and tendons innervated by the median nerve. The thickest NFs in the digital branches of the same nerve, which contain only cutaneous and joint afferents, reach only about 12 to 13 μ.

The proportions of larger and smaller myelinated NFs vary somewhat depending on the type of nerve, group III or A delta NFs being relatively much more common with respect to the larger myelinated NFs in cutaneous com-pared to motor nerves. While about 40 to 50 percent of the larger myelinated NFs (> 6 to 7 μ) in a motor nerve are probably motor (alpha motor axons) in the cat, this proportion may vary somewhat depending on the motor nerve (Boyd and Davey, 1968). In man, the proportion that are alpha motor axons has not been established, and so estimates of the pro-portion of the larger myelinated nerve fibers that are alpha motor axons in biopsied nerves, such as fascicles taken from the anterior tibial nerve just proximal to the ankle, are estimates only. Indeed, the biopsied fascicle may con-tain no motor axons at all, unless the precau-tion is taken to identify the motor fascicle to the extensor digitorum brevis muscle by direct stimulation at the time of surgery.

Figure 3.1 illustrates the relative propor-tions of NFs of various diameters in the hu-man deep peroneal nerve, a motor nerve. This nerve, unlike cutaneous or digital nerves in the hand, contains muscle and tendon affer-ents, although cutaneous nerves may contain some joint afferents. Cutaneous nerves sup-plying glabrous skin contain large numbers of cutaneous and subcutaneous mechanorecep-tor afferents as well as other afferents. The last have been the subject of intensive study in recent years using microneuronographic techniques (see the review by Vallbo, Hag-barth, Torebjork, and Wallin, 1979).

FIGURE 3.1. Fiber size distribution of myeli-nated nerve fibers in the human deep peroneal nerve. Note the large numbers of the smaller-diameter nerve fibers relative to the larger-diameter myelinated nerve fibers. (Courtesy Dr. A. Hahu).

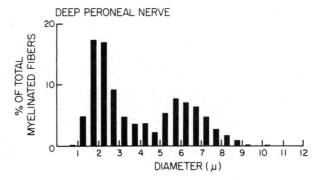

ELECTROPHYSIOLOGICAL ASSESSMENT OF CONDUCTION IN PERIPHERAL NERVE

The assessment of conduction is technically much easier in motor than in sensory NFs. For example, conduction in motor nerves may be readily assessed by recording the evoked post-synaptic muscle potentials and stimulating the motor nerve at various sites proximal to the end-plate. Each motor axon innervates a number of muscle fibers (MFs), in some cases up to several hundred. The end-plate potentials (EPPs) exceed by two to five times the thresholds needed to generate postsynaptic action potentials in the MFs. Thus each natural or stimulus-evoked impulse in the motor axon is accompanied by action potentials in the whole complement of MFs innervated by the motor axon. The amplitude of the resultant compound potential is not only much larger, it lasts two to five times longer than do the action potentials of even the largest myelinated nerve fibers when recorded extracellularly. Indeed, single motor unit potentials (MUPs) may be detected appreciable distances away from the source, whereas only when semimicroneedle or microneedle electrode recordings are made directly within the nerve trunk are the spikes of single NFs of any significant size (Figure 3.2).

The point of the above is that, although the activities of single motor axons may be readily recorded through their corresponding MUPs, the activities of single NFs are not so easily detected except with the use of near-nerve needle electrodes and electronic averaging techniques. It is also true that single NF potentials are relatively brief and usually triphasic because they are recorded extracellularly in a volume conductor. These two facts mean that the amplitude and shape of any compound nerve action potential recorded from a nerve trunk critically depend not only on the type of recording (monopolar vs bipolar), the choice of electrodes (size, shape,

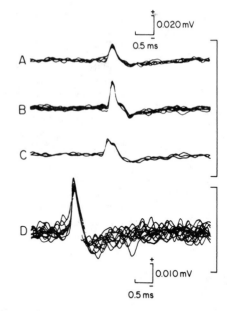

FIGURE 3.2.   Action potentials of single human nerve fibers recorded with a tungsten microelectrode (tip diameter 1 to 15 µ) from large muscle afferents within a fascicle of the median nerve of the author. The bandwidth of the recording was 200 to 5,000 Hz (3 db down), which somewhat reduces the durations of the potentials. The potentials are often diphasic, the initial and main deflection being positive, indicating that the tip of the electrode is probably within the fiber. The two peaks in the main positive deflection (B and C) may originate in two adjacent nodes, although if so, the internodal conduction time is 10 or more times normal, suggesting damage to the nerve fiber.

and electrical characteristics), and the proximities of these electrodes to the nerve trunk but on the relative conduction velocities of all the impulses in the nerve trunk and the distance between the site of origin of the impulses and the recording site. The latter two factors govern the pattern of temporal summation of single fiber potentials and hence the degree of phase cancellation between opposite phases of the component single fiber potentials. The situation is complicated further because, as was pointed out in Chapter 1, the spatial distributions and spike amplitudes of single fiber potentials are related to the conduction velocities and diameters of the NFs.

The best correspondences between the shape of the recorded compound nerve trunk potential and the NF composition in a nerve trunk are obtained through monophasic recordings. Because of the principles involved and because there is such good agreement between such recordings in vitro and quantitative morphometric data on the same nerve, it is worthwhile discussing the technique in some detail.

MONOPHASIC RECORDING OF NERVE TRUNK POTENTIALS

In nerve trunks, where there is a broad range in the diameters and hence conduction velocities of the component NFs, one of the best ways to record the conducted potentials is by the monophasic technique. This minimizes the distortions produced through phase cancellations between overlapping but out-of-phase

potentials as well as other artifacts to be discussed later.

A fascicle of the nerve or the whole nerve trunk is carefully removed and freed by microdissection of as much of its surrounding loose connective tissue as possible. Following this, the nerve is suspended on an array of stimulating and recording electrodes in air (kept moist by bubbling the air through water to avoid drying out the nerve) or sometimes in an oil medium. The air or oil serves as a nonconductive medium to prevent extension of the external longitudinal currents outside the nerve trunk and reduce their extension along the outside surface of the nerve trunk itself. The result is that the external longitudinal currents accompanying conduction of the nerve impulses are confined to the interior of the nerve trunk itself and do not as a consequence extend much ahead of the active regions. The potentials therefore tend to be monophasic (negative) and preceded by very little, if any, positive component (Figure 3.3).

To help ensure a monophasic character to the recorded potentials, the nerve may be cut or crushed beneath the positive grid 2 (G_2)

FIGURE 3.3. Monophasic recording technique. The nerve is mounted on a pair of electrodes and crushed or cut opposite the G_2 electrode to create a steady demarcation potential (G_1 positive with respect to G_2). Carrying out the recordings in air (kept moist) or oil helps to reduce the external leakage resistance (R_{ext}) between G_1 and G_2, but of course cannot alter the internal leakage resistance (R_{int}) through the nerve trunk itself. Direct impulse transmission between G_1 and G_2 is prevented by a second crush or local anesthetic block between the two electrodes. The nerve trunk is stimulated a variable distance proximal to G_2 (20 to 60 mm, usually) in human studies of nerve biopsy material.

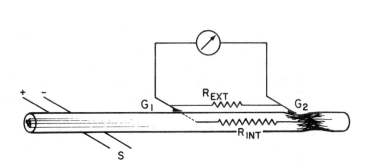

electrode. This brings the G_2 electrode in contact with the intracellular spaces of the axons by creating breaks in their underlying axolemmal membranes and produces a *demarcation potential,* G_2 becoming electronegative with respect to the negative grid 1 (G_1) electrode. The magnitude of this demarcation potential depends largely on the external longitudinal leakage resistances both just outside and within the nerve trunk between the G_1 and G_2 electrodes. The higher the value of the external longitudinal resistances, the less current is able to shunt in the extracellular space between G_1 and G_2 and the closer the demarcation potential approximates the transmembrane potential. The leakage currents outside the nerve trunk can, of course, be reduced by carrying out the recordings in air or oil, but extracellular leakage currents within the nerve trunk cannot be avoided. For this reason the demarcation potential does not reach the value of the transmembrane potential. To prevent the impulses from directly conducting through to G_2, their transmission must be blocked either by a crush or by the application of local anesthetic to the nerve between the G_1 and G_2 electrodes. Volume conduction to the G_2 electrode is of course greatly reduced, as pointed out earlier, by carrying out the recordings in oil or air, which prevents extension of the external longitudinal currents ahead of the impulse through the medium outside the nerve trunk.

Passage of the conducted impulses past G_1 is then marked by transient reductions in the steady demarcation potentials, which match the time courses of the changes in the underlying transmembrane potentials. Of course, these amplitudes are somewhat reduced because of internal leakage currents within the nerve trunk between G_1 and G_2.

The amplitudes of the monophasic compound potentials are not, however, directly related to the absolute numbers of NFs present in the nerve trunk. For example, compound nerve action potentials recorded from a fascicle may be as large as those recorded from the whole nerve trunk. In general, the larger the nerve trunk diameter, the larger the number of NFs. This increases the number of spike generators. At the same time, however, the larger volume contained by the larger nerve trunk increases the available extracellular space within the nerve trunk through which the external longitudinal currents may spread. This has the effect of increasing the internal leakage currents between G_1 and G_2 and reducing the amplitudes of individual spikes, canceling out whatever increases in the compound nerve trunk potential were derived from the larger number of NFs in the whole nerve trunk.

The amplitude of the compound nerve action potential is related more to the density of the NFs (or the number of nerve fibers per unit cross-sectional area of the nerve) than the absolute numbers of nerve fibers in the nerve trunk.

The shape of the compound nerve trunk potential is directly related to:

1. The conduction distance between the site of origin of the impulses and the G_1 electrode
2. Conduction velocities and relative numbers of various NFs within the nerve trunk
3. The relative amplitudes of the spike-generated NFs with different conduction velocities

The larger the diameters of the NFs, the larger their extracellularly recorded spikes when recorded equivalent transverse distances away from the source. This accounts for the observation that much larger numbers of unmyelinated NFs produce relatively much lower-amplitude compound potentials than do the smaller numbers of large-diameter myelinated NFs. The amplitude of the potential recorded at G_1 at any one time following onset of the volley in the nerve is thus equal to the numbers of impulses opposite G_1 at that time and the amplitudes of their respective spikes. Hence, based on reasonable assumptions about the relationships between the diameters of NFs and their conduction velocities and relative spike amplitudes, it should be possible to construct a compound nerve potential based on knowledge of the fiber size composition of a nerve trunk, which would be in reasonable agreement with potentials actually recorded

from the nerve (Figure 3.4). Such correlations turn out to be surprisingly close. The excellence of the match depends somewhat on the choice of conversion factors for fiber diameter to conduction velocity (see Chapter 1), the proportionality constant chosen for the relationship between spike amplitude and fiber diameter, and what adjustments are made for stimulus lead (Gasser, 1960).

The relationship between NF diameters and spike amplitude was dealt with briefly in

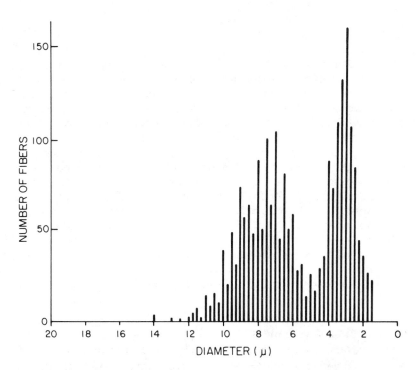

FIGURE 3.4. The correspondence between the monophasic compound action potential whose construction was based on the relative numbers of nerve fibers of different diameters within the nerve trunk and the potential actually recorded from the same nerve trunks.
(Above) Fiber size distribution for the cat saphenous nerve (myelinated nerve fibers only included).
(Next Page) The monophasic compound nerve action potential actually recorded (solid line) and reconstructed potential where it differed from the actual potential (interrupted line).
The reconstructed potential in this case was based on assumptions that

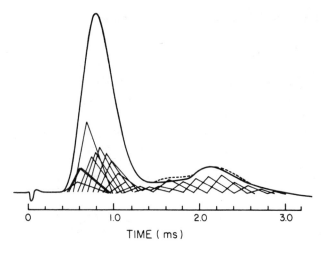

FIGURE 3.4.   *(continued)*
conduction speed and spike amplitude were both proportional to axon diameter. From knowledge of the numbers of nerve fibers of different diameters within the nerve trunk, conduction velocities and spike amplitudes were assigned to fibers of various sizes. The conduction times to the recording electrode were derived from knowledge of conduction velocity and conduction distance. Triangles with shapes simulating that of a single fiber but of a height proportional to the numbers and spike amplitudes of the fibers whose impulses reached the recording electrode at successive time intervals were then drawn above the baseline, with their leading edges corresponding to the calculated conduction time for those fibers. Such triangles were constructed for each group of fibers to reach the recording electrode in turn, and the triangles summed to produce the smooth compound potential shown.

Note the excellent agreement between the reconstructed and actual records.

From Gasser and Grundfest (1939, figures 5 and 6).

Chapter 1. Spike amplitudes were initially assumed to be proportional to the cross-sectional area of NFs (Erlanger and Gasser, 1937). This was later changed to direct proportionality between NF diameter and spike amplitude (Gasser and Grundfest, 1939) and more recently, to being proportional to the square of the diameter, especially for the smaller-diameter NFs (Gasser, 1941; Landau, Clare, and Bishop, 1968).

Progressive increases in the distance between G_1 and the site of origin of the impulses opposite the cathode are accompanied by progressive temporal dispersion of the compound nerve trunk potential. In a monophasic recording, however, the area under the potential curve remains constant because there are no phase cancellations between the component single NF potentials.

The general characteristics of monophasic recordings are summarized in Table 3.3. Such recordings do provide the most faithful correlations between the recorded potential and the fiber size composition of the nerve, and

TABLE 3.3.   Characteristics of
Monophasic Recordings

Time courses and relative amplitudes of component potentials are not distorted.

The area beneath the compound potential remains constant irrespective of the distance between the origin of the impulses and the recording site.

The technique is applicable to in vitro studies only and as such can only be applied to nerve biopsy material (Lambert and Dyck, 1975).

---

these have been very good in various human peripheral neuropathies (Lambert and Dyck, 1975).

VOLUME CONDUCTION OF CONDUCTED POTENTIALS

Human recordings of conducted potentials in nerves are not carried out in air or oil to prevent extension of the accompanying external longitudinal currents outside the nerve trunk itself. Except in the case of in vitro monophasic recordings applicable only to nerve biopsies, all recordings in vivo are necessarily carried out within the volume conduction presented by the body tissues that surround the nerve trunks (Figures 3.5 and 3.6). Under such circumstances, the external longitudinal currents can and do extend widely throughout the extracellular space outside the nerve trunks themselves.

There are two important consequences of such volume conduction of the accompanying currents into the surrounding medium. First, the currents may extend widely throughout the accompanying external tissues surrounding the nerve trunk to reach the G_1 and possibly G_2 electrode, sometimes well ahead of the arrival of the impulses themselves at the electrode. Second, the same currents are responsible for the classic *triphasic* $(+ - +)$ nature of extracellularly recorded action potentials. The *initial positive* phase indicates the approach of the conducted potentials, the subsequent *negative* phase, the arrival of impulses opposite the recording electrode, and the following *late positive* phase movement of the potentials beyond the electrode. Positive potentials are registered in regions of the extracellular field that act as *current sources,* while negative potentials are registered in regions acting as *current sinks.* In the case of the extracellular field surrounding cable conductors such as NFs or MFs, the positive potentials are recorded opposite regions where currents (electrotonic or active) are leaving the fiber, and negative potentials are recorded opposite membrane regions where currents such as the sodium current enter the fiber (Figure 3.7).

The correspondence between membrane events and the extracellular potential is closest when the recording electrode is situated just outside the fiber. The initial positive peak (or onset of the negative spike) then corresponds directly to onset of the inward sodium current, which subsequently reaches its peak just shortly before the peak of the negative spike. As the transverse (or radial) distance increases between the fiber and the recording electrode, however, not only is there a steep decline in the amplitude of the extracellularly recorded potential, but the peaks of the latter become progressively displaced both with respect to one another as well as in relation to the underlying membrane events in the fiber. Despite such distortions in the phase relationships of the recorded extracellular potentials, certain points in the potential continue to bear a constant relationship to the underlying membrane events. For example, the onset and termination times of the intracellularly and extracellularly recorded potentials continue to be the same, provided, of course, that these can be resolved in the extracellular recording. In addition, however, the zero potential crossing times of both the intracellular and extracellular potentials continue to correspond pre-

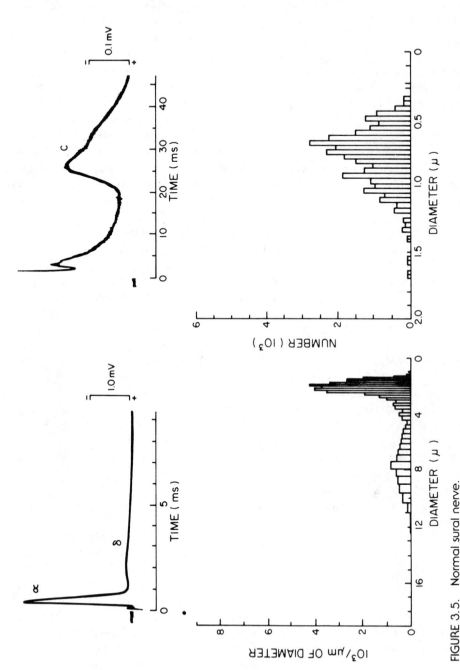

FIGURE 3.5. Normal sural nerve.

(Left) Monophasic compound nerve action potential recorded from a normal nerve. The leading edge of the A alpha peak corresponded to a conduction velocity at just over 61 m/s, the peak of the delta component at 19 m/s, and the peak of the C potential (right) at 1.1 m/s.

(Right) Fiber size distribution for the above nerve. There are many more smaller myelinated nerve fibers (A delta, 1 to 5 μ, 20 to 2 m/s) than larger ones, yet the latter are responsible for the relatively much larger amplitude of the alpha component (20 to 60 m/s or 5 to 12 μ).

From Lambert and Dyck (1975, figure 2.1).

FIGURE 3.6. Hereditary amyloidosis (dominant inheritance). (Top) Monophasic compound nerve action potential from the sural nerve. (Bottom) The corresponding fiber size distribution for this sural nerve.

Note the partial loss of myelinated and complete loss of unmyelinated nerve fibers and the correspondingly absent C potential as well as the much reduced A alpha and delta components of the compound nerve action potentials.
From Lambert and Dyck (1975, figure 20.3).

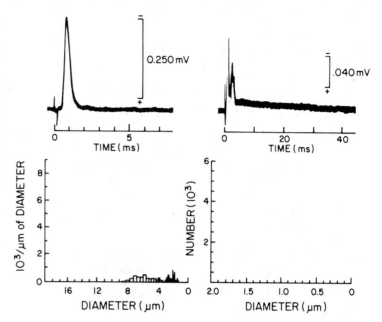

cisely irrespective of the position of the recording electrode outside the fiber. These characteristics of extracellular action potentials recorded in a volume conductor are summarized in Table 3.4 (see also Rosenfalck, 1969).

The whole subject of volume conduction is complex, although the basics at an intuitive level are not hard to grasp, and in practice the main working points that need to be kept in mind are outlined in Table 3.4. One of the clearest reviews of this subject is by Patton (1965).

One approach has been to approximate the membrane as a series of dipoles oriented perpendicular to the membrane, then to derive the potential at points in the extracellular space by analysis of the solid angles presented by the near and opposite active membrane surfaces at various times as the impulse conducts toward and passes the recording site in the

TABLE 3.4. Characteristics of Action Potentials Recorded in Volume

Potentials are triphasic.
    Biphasic potentials may be recorded near their origin or where the potentials do not conduct past the recording electrode.
There is a steep decline in amplitude as the distance between the generator(s) and the recording electrode(s) increases.
Even so, extracellular currents extend widely in volume, and the potentials may be recorded at sites remote from the current origins.
Increasing the transverse distance between the origin of the potentials and the recording electrodes results in progressive displacement of the peaks of the triphasic potentials.
Despite this, baseline (zero potential) crossings correspond in extracellular and transmembrane potential recordings irrespective of the extracellular recording site.
The duration of intracellularly and extracellularly recorded action potentials correspond.

FIGURE 3.7.   Single muscle fiber (top) shown with site of stimulating electrodes (right), intracellular and extracellular electrodes positioned at the same distance from the site of stimulation, and (middle) simulation of the corresponding intracellularly and extracellularly recorded action potentials, the latter recorded just outside the fiber.

Note:

1.   The precise correspondence between the two potentials in their times of onset as well as the termination and zero baseline crossings (vertical interrupted lines).
2.   The much larger size of the transmembrane recorded potential.
3.   The triphasic nature of the extracellularly recorded potential. The initial positive peak corresponds to the beginning of the inward sodium current opposite the recording electrode. The negative peak of the extracellular potential does not correspond to the peak of the extracellularly recorded potential.

Redrawn and adapted from Rosenfalck (1969).

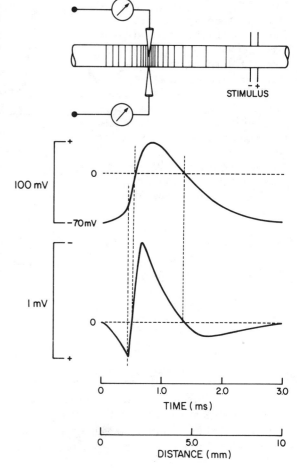

extracellular space (see Patton, 1965). This is complex and hard to grasp for many students. A simpler model is to treat the action potential as a longitudinal dipole (or perhaps tripole) in which the region of outward membrane current preceding the action potential is approximated by the leading positive (+) pole, and the region where the extracellular current is inward (sink) as the negative pole (Figure 3.8).

In this simple model, the potential recorded at a point (E) in the extracellular space in relation to a remote recording site at zero potential is related to:

1.   The absolute distances r1 and r2 between E and the respective C+ and C− poles
2.   The difference (r1 − r2), because the potential at E is the sum of the opposite potential fields exerted by the C+ and C− poles at E

Thus when r1 and r2 are equal, the opposite potentials exerted by the two poles at E are equal, and their sum therefore is zero. This happens, for example, when E is midway between C+ and C−. If the position of the dipole is kept constant and E is moved inward

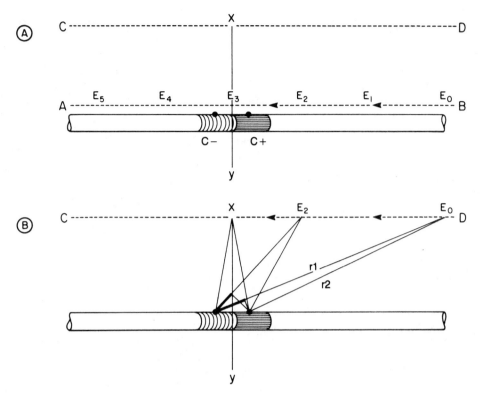

FIGURE 3.8.   Intuitive explanation for the displacement of the peaks of extracellularly recorded potentials as the transverse distance between the fiber and the recording electrode increases. Illustrated is a longitudinal dipole model for consideration of how volume conduction alters the extracellularly recorded action potential. Shown is a fiber in which the action potential has been reduced for purposes of simplification to two charges, a leading positive ($+1$) and an equal following negative (-1) charge. The longitudinal dipole here is thought of as stationary and the exploring electrode (E) as moving toward and past the dipole.

(A) The exploring electrode (E) is moved along a line (A-B) close to and parallel to the fiber.

(B) The exploring electrode is moved along the line (D-C) parallel to the fiber but at an appreciable transverse distance away. Thus as it approaches C$-$ and C$+$ the difference between r1 and r2 (r1-r2) diminishes prior to E reaching a point opposite C$+$. The result is that the difference potential between the opposite potential exerted by C$+$ and C$-$ at E reaches its maximum at some point ahead of C$+$ rather than opposite C$+$, as it would if E was much closer to the fiber. In the latter case the angle subtended by r1 and r2 would be so small that there would be no appreciable reduction in r1-r2 until E was opposite C$+$.

toward the dipole along the line A–B just outside the surface of the membrane, r1 and r2 progressively shorten and the summation potential at E progressively increases. Polarity is determined by the polarity of the nearest charge, here C$+$. The maximum positive potential is registered directly opposite C+. This happens because at this point, E is closest to C+ and there has been no change in the difference r1 − r2. Between this point directly opposite C+ and the intersect (X,Y) midway between the C+ and C− poles, the amplitude falls toward zero because the difference, r1 − r2, approaches and finally reaches zero. Once E is past the midpoint (X,Y) the polarity reverses to negative. The maximum negative potential is registered directly opposite C−. The amplitude then progressively falls off toward zero potential as E moves beyond the C− pole.

In this example, the recording site E is just outside the membrane surface and the r1 − r2 difference remains constant except when E lies between the C+ and C− poles. If, however, the electrode at E is repositioned an appreciable transverse distance away from the membrane and is once more moved toward the dipole along the line C–D parallel to the membrane, the maximum positivities and negativities are not registered directly opposite but rather ahead and behind their respective poles.

Hence, even though the potential fields exerted by C+ and C− independently at E increase as E approaches the dipole, the actual difference between these two fields at E begins to fall off at some point ahead of C+ because this difference depends on the difference r1 − r2, and the latter progressively diminishes as E approaches C+. The resultant displacements of the maximum positive and negative potentials to points in the extracellular space ahead of and behind their respective poles increase as the transverse distance between E and the dipole increases. Therefore, except when E is very close to the dipole, the maximum positive and negative potentials do not correspond to points in the extracellular field directly opposite their respective outward and inward membrane currents.

Extracellularly conducted potentials are even better approximated by a tripole of successive outward (+), inward (−), and outward (+) membrane currents. Of course the real situation is even more complicated because the spatial extents of the inward and outward membrane currents overlap to some extent and the lengths of membrane occupied by the three phases and the magnitudes of these membrane currents are not equal. The longitudinal dipole model presented here is intended simply to explain the relationships between peak latencies of the recorded potentials and the underlying membrane currents.

In human electrophysiological studies, recordings of conducted potentials are complicated because of the necessity of carrying them out in a volume conductor. The potentials so recorded of single NFs or MFs are, as pointed out, triphasic. Were all such potentials to reach the recording electrode at the same time and their wavelengths to be identical, no distortions would occur except when the recording is bipolar (see later discussion). The conduction velocities and wavelengths of NF potentials within a nerve trunk are not all the same, however, and their impulses therefore do not all reach the recording electrode at the same time. Any dispersion of their arrival times at the recording electrode such that the opposite phases of the component potentials overlap will produce phase cancellations at the electrode that records the sum of all potentials at that point. Such phase cancellations distort the later phases of the more rapidly conducting and earlier phases of the relatively slower-conducting potentials. Increasing the conduction distance by increasing the dispersion in arrival times of impulses at the recording electrode should increase the degree of phase cancellation between increasingly desynchronized potentials reaching the recording electrode. The result is that the area under the recorded potential will not remain constant as the conduction distance increases, but will decrease. This renders any assessment of conduction block hazardous in recordings of nerve action potentials unless the conduction distance over which the assessment is made is very short and the recordings are made in equivalent proximity to the nerve trunk at all recording sites.

Bipolar Recordings

The situation is complicated even further when a bipolar recording electrode arrangement is used. Unless the interelectrode distance is wide, the conducted potentials, especially those of the larger nerve fibers whose wavelengths can be appreciable (50 to 60 mm in the larger NFs), may span both electrodes

(Figure 3.9). Also, the dispersed nature of the compound potential itself (in which faster conducting impulses may reach the G_1 electrode while slower impulses are reaching G_2) may further distort the recorded potential, especially as the distance between the origin of the impulses and the recording site is increased. The effect of changing the interelectrode distance on the amplitude of the compound nerve action potential is illustrated by Figure 3.9.

Monopolar Recordings

In an attempt to avoid the added distortions of bipolar recordings, some have advocated a *monopolar (unipolar) technique* in which the reference electrode is positioned 20 to 30 mm

FIGURE 3.9. Complex interactions in bipolar recordings.

(A) Single triphasic action potential moving from left to right. Note that if the interelectrode distance is shorter than the wavelength of the potential, distortion of the latter phases of the potential as seen at G_1 may be produced because the preceding earlier components of the potential will have reached G_2. This could result in an increase or decrease of the difference potential recorded, depending on which components of the potential are seen at the two electrodes at the same time.

(B) and (C) Triphasic action potentials in two fibers whose relative conduction velocities are such that at this conduction distance the faster of the two potentials arrives opposite G_2 at a time when the slower potential is opposite G_1. Because the recorded potential is the difference between the potentials seen at the G_1 and G_2 electrodes, the potentials may interact in such a way as to distort the later phases of the earlier impulse as well as the slower of the two potentials.

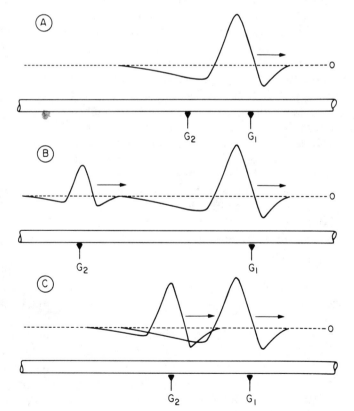

lateral to the recording electrode (Buchthal and Rosenfalck, 1966; Ludin and Tackmann, 1981). This technique helps to avoid bipolar distortions but degrades the amplitude of the recorded potentials somewhat because the reference electrode also sees the conducted potentials in volume. Especially when both G_1 and G_2 are surface electrodes, there may be an appreciable reduction in amplitude. The use of near-nerve recording electrodes reduces the problem because the potential recorded by the G_1 electrode is then so much larger than that seen by the remote G_2 electrode.

Table 3.5 summarizes the main characteristics and distortions of compound nerve action potential recordings as carried out with monopolar and bipolar recording electrode arrangements. That table makes it clear that bipolar recordings in particular distort the later phases of the recorded potentials. Even appreciably increasing the interelectrode distance (in excess of 50 to 60 mm) may not prevent the complex interaction between more rapidly and slowly conducting potentials, especially as conduction distance increases. An increase in distance would tend to enhance the problems produced through increasing temporal dispersion among the component potentials in the volley. Because of these distortions, bipolar recordings are suitable only for assessing conduction in the fastest NFs over relatively short conduction distances. In all other respects the monopolar recording arrangement is preferable.

CORRELATIONS BETWEEN COMPOUND NERVE ACTIONS

Potentials as Recorded in a Volume Conductor with the Fiber Size Composition of the Underlying Nerve

Earlier it was pointed out just how excellent was the agreement between the monophasic

TABLE 3.5.   Characteristics of Compound Nerve Action Potentials Recorded in a Volume Conductor

Monopolar Recordings

Summation at G_1 of temporally dispersed triphasic potentials is such that the later phases of more rapidly conducting potentials at G_1 may sum with the earlier phases of more slowly conducting potentials.

There is some reduction in the amplitude of the recorded potential to the extent that the G_2 (indifferent) electrode sees the potential too.

Least distortions of the later (slower) components of the compound nerve action potential occur.

Bipolar Recordings

Summations as in monopolar recordings at G_1, but here occurring at both G_1 and G_2.

Complex interactions between G_1 and G_2 because:

Longer wavelength potentials (30–60 mm) may span both electrodes at the same time.

Faster potentials reaching G_2 may sum with slower conducting potentials at G_1.

Because of these two factors, there may be serious distortions particularly of the later (slower) components of the compound nerve action potential, especially when the interelectrode distance is too short or there are appreciable differences between the conduction velocities of the component NFs the distance is increased between the site of origin of the volley and the recording sites.

The amplitudes of the potentials tend to be larger.

compound nerve action potential derived from knowledge of the fiber size, composition of the nerve, and the fiber diameter to conduction velocity on the one hand, and spike amplitude and the actual recorded potential on the other. Compound nerve action potentials recorded extracellularly in a volume conductor are distorted, however, as pointed out in the preceding discussions, by complex interactions between the temporally dispersed and triphasic component potentials even in monopolar recordings. Nonetheless, Buchthal and Rosenfalck (1966, 1971) have been able to derive from anatomical data on the median nerve, compound nerve action potentials as they would be recorded in volume that are in reasonable agreement with actually recorded potentials (Figure 3.10).

There have also been several studies relating the shape of the in vivo recorded compound nerve action potential to the results of quantitative morphometric studies of biopsy tissues taken from the same nerve (Buchthal and Rosenfalck, 1971; Buchthal, Rosenfalck, and Behse, 1975; Tackmann, Minkenberg, and Strenge, 1977; Behse and Buchthal, 1978; Ludin and Tackmann, 1981) (Figures 3.11 and 3.12).

The preceding correlative studies depend on near-nerve needle electrode recordings and the use of electronic averaging techniques to ensure identification of the earliest and slower components in the compound nerve action potentials. More is said on these correlations at the end of this chapter.

Comparison of such nerve action potential recordings with the corresponding fiber size histogram for the same nerve makes it apparent that the main potential is generated by the faster-conducting NFs (25 to 60 m/s) because of the larger amplitudes of their spikes despite the fact that they are outnumbered by the smaller-diameter NFs. The latter hardly make any contribution to the main potential but are responsible for some of the later, very low-amplitude components whose clear demonstration depends on the use of near-nerve recording and electronic averaging techniques (Buchthal and Rosenfalck, 1966; Ludin and Tackmann, 1981).

Recently there have also been attempts to derive information about the conduction velocity distribution of human nerves based on analysis of the compound nerve action potential as recorded in situ (Stegeman, 1981; Cummins, Perkel, and Dorfman, 1979; Cummins, Dorfman, and Perkel, 1979, 1981; Cummins and Dorfman, 1981). Such derivations incorporate a number of assumptions that may turn out to be incorrect in diseased nerve (Dorfman, Cummins, Reaven, Ceranski, Greenfield, and Doberne, 1983).

Interactions between Nerve Fibers

External currents accompanying the conduction of impulses in nerve and muscle fibers may cross the membranes of adjoining fibers and alter their excitabilities. Such interactions may speed up or slow down the conduction velocities of the neighboring fibers (Katz and Schmitt, 1940; Arvanitaki, 1942; Granit, Leksell, and Skoglund, 1944). In normal nerve, the importance of such interactions is probably marginal. In abnormal NFs, however, such interactions may produce ephaptic transmission among adjoining NFs (Granit, Leksell, and Skoglund, 1944; Skoglund, 1949; see also Chapter 9).

ELECTRICAL STIMULATION OF PERIPHERAL NERVE

The principles of electrical stimulation of peripheral nerve are presented in Chapter 1. In summary, the outward flow of current through the nodal regions of the NFs beneath or opposite the cathode depolarizes these regions beyond threshold and triggers the generation of impulses in these NFs. Opposite the anode, the electrical current passing through the NF membranes hyperpolarizes the membrane and may produce anodal block. In vitro, NFs are excited in order of their sizes, those of the largest diameter having the lowest thresholds, while higher-threshold NFs in general have smaller diameters and correspondingly slower conduction velocities (and longer latencies). The position of NFs within the nerve trunk with respect to the stimulating electrode is probably important, those nearest the cath-

FIGURE 3.10.   (Top) The orthodromic sensory nerve action potential as recorded in a healthy subject by the method of photographic superimposition. The conduction distance was similar to that for the reconstructed potential. The corresponding latencies and conduction velocities of the various components are shown at the bottom.

(Bottom) Reconstruction of the compound sensory nerve action from the median nerve as it would appear if recorded at the wrist in response to stimulation of the first digit based on knowledge of the relative numbers of different size myelinated nerve fibers in the nerve, the conduction distance and certain assumptions about the relationships between fiber diameter and conduction velocity and between fiber diameter and spike amplitude (see text). The shape and duration of the individual spikes were considered to be similar to those in the insert. The triangles were derived in a manner similar to that for Figure 3.4, and the compound potential by the sum of the triangles.

    Note:

1.   The close correspondence between the reconstructed and actual potentials in the normal
2.   That the main potential corresponds to activity in fibers conducting between 30 and 60 m/s and the main positive-negative spike to velocities between 40 and 60 m/s
3.   That a few fibers reach the recording electrode before the initial positive peak

s = stimulus. Time scales are shown in milliseconds. Also shown are the corresponding conduction velocities in meters per second for the various components in the potentials.

From Rosenfalck (1971).

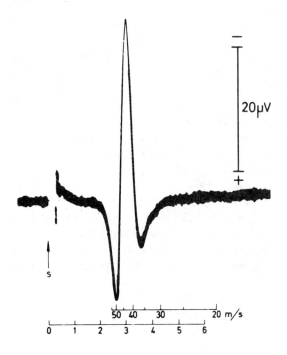

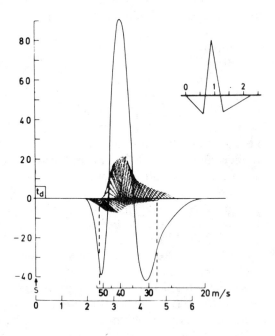

FIGURE 3.11.   Normal sural nerve.

Compound nerve action potential as recorded with near-nerve needle electrodes 50 (top) and 15 (middle) cm proximal to the site of stimulation at the level of the lateral malleolus. For each recording, 200 traces were electronically averaged. The fiber size distribution of the nerve is shown (bottom) as well as the probable correspondences among fiber diameter, conduction velocity, and the various components of the nerve action potential.

Note:

1. That the main potential as recorded 15 cm away corresponds to nerve fibers with diameters 7μ and over, and conduction velocities between 33 and 62 m/s.
2. Some slower components are apparent in the recordings, especially in the recording at the popliteal fossa.

From Buchthal, Rosenfalck, and Behse (1975, figure 21.2).

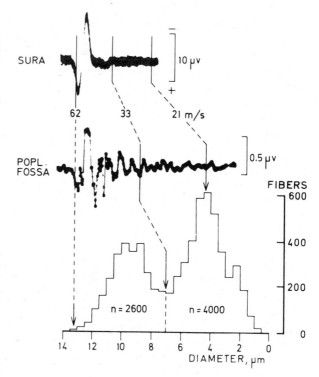

FIGURE 3.12.   Axonal type of polyneuropathy. Fiber size distribution of the sural nerve is outlined by the heavy line shown for comparison to the normal histogram (shaded). There was a severe and preferential loss of the larger- and faster-conducting myelinated nerve fibers with preservation of slow-conducting and smaller-diameter fibers. The insert shows the corresponding sensory nerve action potential as recorded 15 cm proximal to the site of stimulation at the medial malleolus. The maximum conduction velocity was somewhat reduced (40 m/s) at 36°C, and the amplitude of the potential reduced by 90 percent compared to controls.
From Buchthal, Rosenfalck, and Behse (1975, figure 21.3).

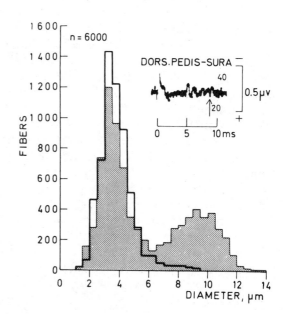

ode being excited at lower stimulus intensities than more distant NFs.

In human in vivo studies, the ranking of threshold by NF size and latency (or conduction velocity) is often not so clearly apparent as it is in vitro. Indeed, in motor axons at least, the rank order of excitability sometimes appears to be opposite the expected. Those apparent exceptions may be related to the precise method of stimulation, whether percutaneous or near-nerve, the relative positions of NFs within the nerve trunk as alluded to earlier, and possible pathological changes in some NFs (see Chapter 6 for more comment).

To make measurement of conduction velocities as accurate as possible, the stimulus must be: (1) kept as short as possible and (2) supramaximal. The briefer the stimulus, the less uncertainty there is about the time of initiation of impulses opposite the cathode. On the other hand, appreciable errors in the measurement of latencies and calculations of conduction velocities may result when, to stimulate the nerve, long-lasting, just maximal stimulus pulses are used. Such stimuli may trigger impulses in the nearby nerve only toward the end of the stimulus pulse, while the latencies are measured with respect to onset of stimulus. The resultant error may be appreciable when the stimulus duration is an appreciable fraction of the anticipated total conduction time between the sites of stimulation and recording. Brief stimuli are thought also to be less uncomfortable than longer-lasting stimuli because in the case of percutaneous stimulating electrodes, the briefer pulses may be less likely to excite smaller pain fibers in the skin opposite the electrodes.

Longer-lasting stimuli (0.2 ms and more) are sometimes necessary especially when using surface-stimulating electrodes to study conduction in chronic demyelinating neuropathies, some instances of uremic or diabetic neuropathies, hereditary hypertrophic neu-

ropathy, or recently regenerated peripheral nerve fibers where sometimes the thresholds of the NFs are exceedingly high. In these situations, longer stimulus pulses (up to 0.5 ms) may be required because of the maximum output currents of some commercial stimulators (90 to 100 mA) may be insufficient to excite the nerve fully. The need for longer stimuli may be circumvented sometimes by the use of near-nerve needle stimulating electrodes or, in the case of percutaneous stimulating electrodes, by prior careful preparation of the skin to reduce the impedance it presents to the stimulus current. To this end the skin should be abraded lightly and a little electrode paste rubbed in, after which the excess is wiped away.

The stimulus intensity should exceed threshold for all the NFs in the group under study. In the case of assessment of motor conduction, the intensity should be adjusted to be 10 to 20 percent above that necessary to excite all the motor axons in the nerve to evoke the maximum compound muscle (M) potential. This ensures that all the motor axons have indeed been activated and that this is true at all levels of stimulation of the motor nerve trunk. It is important that the stimulus intensity be no higher; this is to avoid any appreciable stimulus lead and thence excitation of the nerve ahead of the cathode, which would result in misleadingly short latencies.

Supramaximal motor stimulation as outlined above may indeed result in some stimulus lead because, especially in some pathological states where the thresholds of some motor axons may be much higher than those of other motor axons, stimulus intensities necessary to excite all the motor axons may result in some stimulus lead in the lower-threshold NFs. In these situations it is sometimes better to use submaximal stimuli, provided it can be shown that these stimuli excite the same shortest-latency NFs or groups of NFs at all levels of stimulation.

In sensory nerves the situation is complicated by the fact that these nerves contain a wider range of thresholds and diameters of NFs, and stimuli that are necessary to recruit the slower components (<25 m/s) may exceed by two to five times those necessary to excite the lowest-threshold NFs. The latter higher-intensity stimuli could result in artifactually lower latencies for the lower-threshold NFs through stimulus lead (Gasser, 1960). Therefore, the measurement of the fastest conduction velocities in sensory nerve, the stimulus intensity should be adjusted to be just supramaximal for the main initial positive to negative peak potential. If the stimulus intensity has been increased to be supramaximal for all myelinated NFs, including the higher-threshold groups, conduction velocities should be measured between successive recording sites where the latency shifts produced through stimulus lead will be the same at all recording sites. In the latter situation, the conduction velocity should not be measured between the stimulus site and the nearest recording site unless this is well distant, the longer distance serving to reduce the impact of the stimulus lead error on the overall latency.

Constant-Current versus Constant-Voltage Stimulation

Most commercial stimulators provide constant voltage stimulus pulses; that is, the voltage remains constant in successive stimuli provided no adjustments are made by the operator. Such stimuli are adequate for most purposes but may be unsatisfactory where the impedances of the stimulating electrodes or the skin, in the case of surface stimulation, change. In such situations, constant-current stimulators will, within limits, continue to deliver constant-current pulses irrespective of modest changes in the impedance. A third option is the use of a constant-voltage stimulator

while at the same time monitoring the stimulus currents delivered, changes in the latter informing the operator of changes in the electrode or skin impedance that may require correction or adjustment.

Choice of Stimulating Electrodes

The two main types of electrodes used to stimulate human peripheral nerves in situ are needle electrodes inserted near the nerve and surface electrodes. Their relative values and limitations are outlined in Table 3.6.

The usual practice with needle stimulating electrodes is to insert the cathodal needle as close to the nerve as possible in such a manner that the least stimulus intensities are needed to evoke the maximum response, for example, in the case of a mixed or motor nerve. The anode may be a second needle electrode with a larger bared surface inserted 2 to 4 cm lateral to the cathodal electrode and the nerve. In this manner, both electrodes may serve as recording electrodes (unipolar recording) as well, and the prior localization, by finding the depth and position at which stimuli evoke the maximum response with the least current, assures that the recordings will be carried out very close (near-nerve) to the nerve.

This method of positioning the needle for both stimulation and subsequent recording makes it very likely that at least on some occasions, the needle may be inserted directly into the nerve trunk. Indications of such an event probably include:

1. Shocklike sensations and paresthesia experienced in the peripheral cutaneous distribution of the nerve
2. Deep aching sensation in muscle peripherally supplied by the nerve
3. Fasciculation in the above
4. The recording of a deeply positive potential at the needle electrode site following

TABLE 3.6.   Relative Values and Limitations of Needle and Surface-Stimulating Electrodes

Percutaneous	Near-Nerve (Needle)
Advantages	
Demands less time	Can be more certain about precise origin of impulses in relation to electrodes.
No need to insert needles	Requires lower stimulus intensities; therefore less stimulus artifact and in some cases less distress to patient.
	Once in place, may be used to record, with precision, conducted potentials in the nerve trunk itself.
	Better able to reach inaccessible nerves for stimulation.
Disadvantages	
Less certain about origin of impulses in relation to overlying stimulating electrodes, especially when the nerve is deep or the size of the electrode is appreciable.	Distress caused by needle insertions.
	Insertion possible into or through the nerve trunk.
Higher stimulus intensities are often required.	May take appreciably more time.
Often the stimuli are more uncomfortable than in the case of near-nerve stimulation.	

a peripheral stimulus to the nerve; this suggests arrest of conduction in many of the NFs at the recording electrode (the killed end response)

5.   Very low thresholds to electrical stimulation through the electrode (less than 1 mA)

Despite the likelihood of such direct penetration of the nerve trunk, lasting sequelae are very rare indeed.

Needle electrodes should be kept sharp, and if the same electrodes are used to record, the impedance of the leading-off surface must be kept to a minimum both to reduce the electrode noise and to improve the frequency response of the recordings.

Surface stimulating electrodes are more convenient to use because they do not require insertion of needles and subsequent adjustment to obtain the optimal position. While

sparing the patient the discomfort of actual needle insertion and adjustments, however, surface stimuli may actually be more distressing, especially if higher stimulus intensities are required either because the nerve lies deep or the thresholds of underlying NFs are higher than usual because of a disease process.

With surface stimulating electrodes the optimal site for stimulating the underlying nerve trunk may be arrived at by adjusting the position of the electrode on the surface to where the least stimulus intensity is needed to evoke the maximum muscle (M) or nerve potential. A large size of such electrodes (3 to 5 mm) is necessary to reduce current densities through the skin so as to keep the pain experienced by the patient to a minimum. Because of this plus the short interelectrode distances (often 20 to 30 mm) and the sometimes unequal depth of the nerve with respect to the cathode and anode, the site of initiation of the volley in the nerve may not correspond to the leading edge or center of the overlying cathode.

This is especially likely to occur where the nerve lies deep beneath the cathode, as it may during an attempt to stimulate the ulnar nerve just distal to the cubital tunnel or the common peroneal nerve just beyond the fibular head, or in abnormal states where for some reason the nerve is more easily excited either proximal or distal to the cathode because of local pathological changes in the nerve beneath the cathode. Surface stimulation, however, is a quick, convenient way of locating major nerve trunks, and errors arising out of any uncertainty about the precise site of initiation of impulses in relation to the cathode become less important where the distances over which conduction is assessed are relatively long.

Stimulus Artifact

Stimulus currents, like those that accompany action potentials, spread widely throughout the tissues and can be detected in some instances a long way away. The presence of such currents is indicated, for example, in the stimulus artifact seen in recordings taken from the head, where electrical stimuli have been applied to the distal extremities. Indeed, some stimulus artifact is helpful because it indicates the onset of the stimulus pulse.

The Origins of Stimulus Artifact

Stimulus currents flow through the tissues to the recording sites both during the course of the stimulus pulse itself and for a short period following the pulse (Ranck, 1981; McGill, Cummins, Dorfman, Berlizot, Leutkemeyer, Nishimura, and Widrow, 1982). The latter currents are capacitive in origin and occur in several ways. Even though stimulus pulses are isolated with respect to ground, it is impossible to avoid stray capacitance between the stimulus leads and ground. More-

over, these stray capacitances must be charged and discharged at the onset and termination of the stimulus pulse, and should the stray capacitances and impedances of the two stimulating electrodes not be perfectly balanced, a current, the escape current, will flow to ground adding to the artifact seen following the stimulus pulse.

Capacitive coupling between the stimulating and recording leads is another potent source of artifact and depends on the proximity of the leads and the magnitude of the imbalance between the impedance of the two stimulating electrodes.

Electrolytic and current density dependent polarization capacitances exist at the interface between the metal electrode and the electrolyte, as well as at the junction between the electrolyte and the skin. The various charges on these capacitors will discharge backward through the tissues to the stimulator provided the latter has, as in the case of constant-voltage stimulators, a low enough output impedance in relation to the skin and electrode resistances. Such return currents spread through the tissues to reach the recording electrodes and produce an overshoot artifact, which lasts a variable time depending on the magnitude of the current and the low pass setting of the amplifier. Constant current stimulators, because of their higher output impedances, act to prevent current flowing backward through the tissues and therefore reduce the current flowing through the body to reach the recording electrodes. Rather, such capacitance discharge currents, as exist at the skin, tend to discharge through the resistance of the skin itself.

The AC-coupled amplifiers act as additional sources of artifacts following the stimulus pulse. Thus, even when the stimulus pulse is turned off, and even when the potential at the recording electrode is zero, the output of the amplifier will show an overshoot whose amplitude and decay time are a function by the time constant of the amplifier. The higher the value of the time constant, the higher the amplitude of the overshoot and the shorter its decay time. Sometimes, however, if the signal follows shortly after the stimulus, it is preferable to accept a longer-lasting decay time to reduce the amplitude of the overshoot in the stimulus artifact.

The AC coupling does effectively eliminate low-frequency noise generated by half-cell potentials at the electrolyte metal and electrolyte skin interfaces, as well as the galvanic potential produced through ionic processes in the skin.

Yet another source of stimulus artifact may be produced through differences in the impedance of the two recording electrodes. Such artifact may be reduced through using an amplifier with high common-mode rejection characteristics in order to reduce the common-mode voltage at the recording site. The latter is proportional in amplitude to the magnitude of the stimulus artifact.

The impact of stimulus artifact may be to overload the amplifier if the size of the artifact is too great, or seriously to distort wanted signals from muscle or nerve. Overshoot, in particular, may seriously distort recordings making it difficult or sometimes impossible to recognize the onset of the potentials or measure their size. Knowledge of the measures to reduce stimulus artifact are therefore an essential part of the practice of electromyography.

Methods for reducing stimulus artifacts include:

1. Reducing stray capacitances between the stimulating electrodes and ground
   a. Keep the impedance of the electrodes as low and as nearly equal to one another as possible.
   b. Keep the leads as short as is feasible.
   c. Use a large-ground electrode.
2. Reducing capacitance coupling between the recording and stimulating leads
   a. Keep both sets of leads as short as possible.
   b. Keep the electrode impedances low.
   c. Keep the stimulating and recording leads away from one another.
3. Reducing the effect of the metal-electrolyte and electrolyte-skin capacitances
   a. The metal surfaces of the stimulating electrodes should be free of dirt and corrosion to reduce the impedances presented by the metal surfaces themselves.
   b. The impedance of the skin should be reduced by gently abrading (reddening) it and rubbing a little electrolyte paste into the surface.
   c. The position of recording electrodes should be adjusted in such a way as to place them as close to the same isopotential line(s) for the stimulus currents as possible. Use a constant current rather than a constant voltage mode of stimulation to reduce the flow of current back through the stimulator following the stimulus pulse.
4. Optimizing the distortions produced by AC coupling in the recording amplifier
   a. Reduce the size of the overshoot by reducing the lower limit of the high-pass filter as much as possible.
5. Using as low an intensity of stimulus as possible to elicit the desired response
   a. Adjusting the position of the cathode to be as close to the nerve as possible.
   b. Where stimulus artifact is very troublesome, needle electrodes inserted nearby the nerve may be necessary.
6. Increasing the distance between the stimulating and recording electrodes as much as possible
7. Keeping the skin dry between the stimulating electrodes, ground, and recording electrodes
8. Using special techniques to reduce the stimulus artifact. These include:

a. In the case where electronic averaging is used, alternating the polarity of successive stimulus pulses as one way of reducing the stimulus artifact.

b. Recording and instantaneously injecting into the first stage of the recording amplifier, a current equal and opposite to the overshoot current.

9. Placing the ground between the stimulating and recording electrodes

In summary, the reduction of stimulus artifact requires careful attention to the condition of both the stimulating and recording electrodes, keeping their impedances as low as possible, as well as paying attention to the relative positions of these electrodes with respect to one another and the ground, as well as the filter settings of the recording amplifier. Seldom are extraordinary methods required, such as special circuits for artifact suppression; indeed, such devices sometimes distort the recorded signal and encourage sloppy stimulating and recording techniques, which, if more attention was paid to the methods of recording and stimulating, would obviate the need for most extraordinary artifact suppression techniques.

Extension of Stimulus Currents to Nearby Nerves or Muscles

Stimuli designed to excite one nerve may extend to excite other nerves and sometimes muscle in the same region, and the potentials so generated may distort the intended recordings. These unwanted effects are most likely to happen when stimulus intensities are excessive or the stimulating electrodes are positioned too close to these other nerve(s) or muscles(s). For example, the thresholds of recently regenerated and as yet very immature nerve fibers are often so high that it is difficult to avoid spread of the high-intensity stimuli required to excite such abnormal nerve fibers

to other lower-threshold nerves and muscles in the region. Excitation of these other nerves and muscles distorts the intended recordings, but may cause confusion and misinterpretation of the results unless the cause is recognized (Figure 3.13). In such situations, needle electrodes may be preferable for stimulation because they can be positioned more optimally with respect to the desired nerve. At the same time, they can be kept away from other nerves and muscles and in the process, reduce the magnitude of the stimulus currents required.

ASSESSMENT OF MOTOR CONDUCTION IN MAN

Measurement of Motor Conduction Velocities

Techniques for measuring maximum motor conduction velocities and motor terminal latencies are now well established in clinical electromyography (EMG) laboratories. Such measurements are made by recording the postsynaptic muscle (M) potential in the muscle and stimulating the motor nerve at various sites proximal to the motor point. Latency differences between the onsets of the muscle potentials elicited by electrical stimulation of the motor nerve at successively more proximal sites along the course of the nerve are used to calculate conduction velocities between successive stimulation sites (Figure 3.14). The latency between the delivery of the stimulus at the most distal site of stimulation and the M-potential is the motor terminal latency. Just proximal to the muscle and especially within the muscle, the motor axons are accompanied by progressive thinning of successive branches and slowing of the impulses in the branches. Finally, the motor axons terminate as presynaptic terminals at the neuromuscular junctions. The collective delay in conduction through the intramuscular motor axon branches and at the neuromuscular junctions is spoken of as *residual latency*.

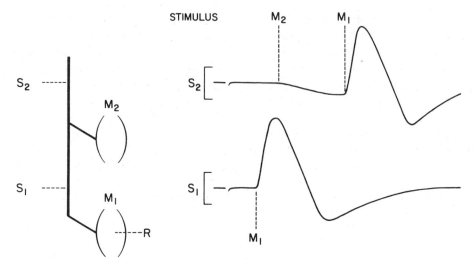

FIGURE 3.13.   Artifact from proximally innervated muscle (M_2). Note that when the stimulus is applied at the proximal site (S_2), volume-conducted activity is generated by the proximal muscles (M_2), which may result in a positive potential that precedes the main M_1-potential recorded by the distal recording electrode (R).

The residual latency may be gauged as illustrated in Figure 3.15 or by measuring the interval (about 1.5 to 2 ms) between the intramuscularly recorded motor nerve action potential recorded best near the motor point, onset of postsynaptic electrical response of the muscle (Figure 3.16). An estimate of the residual latency may also be arrived at by noting the latency difference between the antidromic sensory nerve action potential as sometimes fortuitously seen in recordings with surface electrodes over the end-plate zone, and the M-potential when a mixed nerve such as the median nerve at the wrist is stimulated (Figure 3.17).

Proper measurement of the maximum motor conduction velocity (MMCV) requires that at each site of stimulation, the stimulus intensity exceed by 10 to 20 percent that necessary to evoke a maximum M-potential. This ensures that all the alpha motor axons have been excited and that the stimulus lead will be similar at all levels of stimulation, thereby minimizing its effects on the measurement of conduction velocities among successive sites of stimulation. Latencies are measured to the initial onset of the M-potential in the muscle, which, when the recording electrode is in or over the innervation zone, is signaled by an initial negative deflection.

Choice of Electrodes for Motor Conduction Studies

Except in special circumstances, intramuscular needle electrodes are not the best electrodes for assessing motor conduction. The muscle potentials in such recordings are biased toward the electrical activities of those MFs in the immediate vicinity of the electrodes. Moreover, the muscle twitches evoked by the motor nerve stimuli may cause the position of the electrode within the muscle to change, in so doing altering the shape and size of the M-potential to successive stimuli.

Larger electrodes on the skin that span the innervation zone make better choices because

FIGURE 3.14.   General method for measuring motor conduction in man. Shown are several commonly assessed nerves: median, ulnar, radial, posterior tibial, and peroneal. In each case the maximum M-potential is recorded by surface electrodes, the stigmatic electrode of which is positioned over the innervation zones of the respective muscles or muscle groups. The nerve may be stimulated at successively more proximal sites by either percutaneous (cathode distal) or near nerve-needle electrodes (anode 2 to 4 cm laterally). The most proximal readily accessible stimulus sites are at the sciatic notch and at Erb's point respectively, although invasive techniques may be used to stimulate the roots in the cervical or lumbosacral regions.
Abbreviations:
Nerves—M = median, U = ulnar, R = radial, P = peroneal (also applied to its division in the sciatic nerve at the buttock), PT = posterior tibial.
Muscles—T = thenar, HT = hypothenar, EDC = extensor digitorum communis, EDB = extensor digitorum brevis, PL = plantar foot muscles.
S = stimulus.

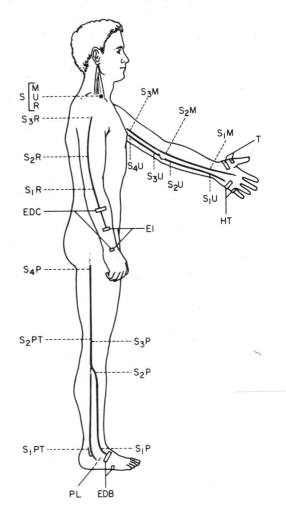

the potentials so recorded more accurately reflect the electrical activities of all the MFs and motor units contributing to the M-potential. Of course, the recorded potentials are still somewhat weighted to those MFs or motor units nearest to the overlying electrode.

The Importance of Recording in the Region of the End-plate Zone

The conduction velocities of muscle fibers are much slower (<5 m/s) than those of the parent motor axons. One consequence of this is that

when the recording electrode is positioned too far away to see, in volume, the initial onset of the muscle action potential in the region of the end-plate zone, the motor terminal latency as measured to the onset of the muscle potential will exceed the true motor terminal latency because of the time required for the muscle fiber action potentials to reach the pickup territory of the recording electrode. This error in measuring motor terminal latency may be avoided by positioning the intramuscular or surface recording electrode as close to the innervation zone as possible. At this site the surface recorded M-potential has

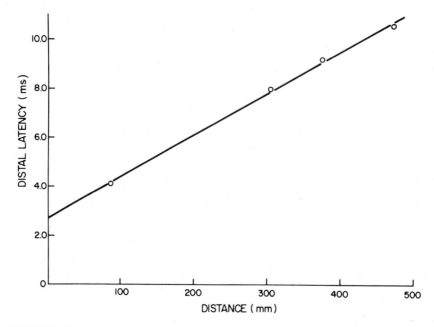

FIGURE 3.15.   Method of measuring residual latency (RL). The ulnar nerve in this case is stimulated at the levels of the wrist below and above the elbow and proximal upper arm. The intersect point with the Y axis of a line connecting the above points gives the RL. Except for preterminal and terminal slowing in the intramuscular motor axon branches and the neuromuscular delay, the intersect point would pass through the zero latency point.

an initial negative deflection and characteristically, the shortest rise time and maximum negative peak amplitude.

Range of Conduction Velocities in Alpha Motor Axons

Based on the results of a variety of techniques, it is apparent that there is about a 30 to 50 percent range in the conduction velocities of alpha motor axons innervating any individual muscle (Tables 3.7 and 3.8). Moreover, indirect evidence based on fiber size distributions of alpha motor axons in deafferented nerves and the relative numbers of MUPs of various amplitudes suggests that the fastest-conducting and largest-diameter MUPs

constitute but a small minority of the whole population of alpha motor axons within a motor nerve; the bulk of the motor axons being smaller in diameter and conducting more slowly.

Preliminary evidence based on computer simulation and patient studies in our laboratory suggests that the negative peak and peak-to-peak amplitude as well as the area of the surface-recorded maximum M-potential is dominated by the relatively much larger-sized MUP contribution generated by the few most rapidly conducting motor axons. One important result of this is the conduction block affecting impulse transmission in the fastest-conducting motor axons should have a much larger impact on the size of the maximum M-potential than conduction block affecting rel-

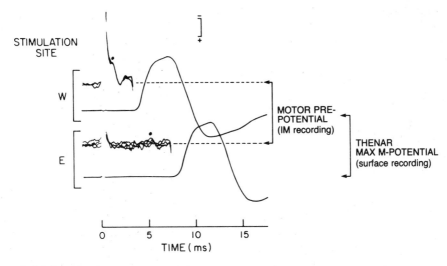

FIGURE 3.16.   Motor prepotential.

Supramaximal percutaneous stimulation of the median nerve at the wrist and elbow with recordings by surface electrodes (stigmatic over the end-plate zone) of the maximum M-potential (calculated 5 mV) and the motor nerve action potential, the latter by a concentric needle electrode inserted into the muscle near the entry point of the recurrent thenar motor branch (calculated 0.020 mV).

The motor prepotential is not seen outside the motor point or innervation zone, and while it may appear below motor threshold (antidromic potential in muscle afferents), it reaches its maximum amplitude in conjunction with the muscle (M) compound action potential.

FIGURE 3.17.   Sensory prepotential as recorded with a surface electrode positioned over the thenar eminence median nerve supramaximally stimulated at the wrist (W), elbow (E), and proximal arm (PA).

Note the prepotential precedes the much larger afterfollowing motor potential by 3.3 ms. Such sensory potentials are often as large as 0.010 to 0.050 mV (peak-to-peak amplitude) but well less than $\frac{1}{100}$ of the size of the maximum M-potential. Moreover, unlike the motor prepotential, the sensory prepotential is characteristically detectable below motor threshold and reaches its maximum amplitude at stimulus intensities at which amplitude of the maximum M-potential is but 10 to 20 percent of its maximum size.

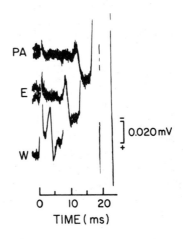

TABLE 3.7.   Diameters and Ranges in Conduction Velocities of Alpha Motor Axons in the Cat and Primate

Animal	Muscle	Nerve Fiber Diameter (μ)	% Range Nerve Fiber Diameters	Range in Conduction Velocities (m/s)	% Range Conduction Velocities
Cat	Gastrocnemius	10–18	44	57–100	47
	Soleus[1,2]	8–14	43	51–81	31
Baboon	Extensor digitorum communis[3]			49–84	42
	Abductor digiti minimi[4]			40–78	49
	Extensor digitorum brevis[4]			40–70	43

[1]Eccles and Sherrington (1930).
[2]Wuerker, McPhedran, and Henneman (1965).
[3]Eccles, Phillips, and Chien-Ping (1968).
[4]Gilliatt, Hopf, Rudge, and Baraitser (1976).

atively much larger numbers of slower-conducting motor axons whose motor unit potentials summing together make much less a contribution to the size of the M-potential.

Increasing the distance between the site of stimulation of the motor nerve and the recording site over the end-plate zone results in a progressive decline in amplitude and increase in duration of the compound M-potential (Figure 3.18). These changes result from differences between conduction velocities of motor axons whose MUPs add up to produce

TABLE 3.8.   Range in Conduction Velocities of Alpha Motor Axons in Man Expressed as a Percentage of Maximum Conduction Velocity

Technique	Muscle(s)	% of Maximum MCV (or Shortest Latency)	Source
Collision			Thomas, Sears, and Gilliatt (1959), Hopf (1962)
Abductor digiti minimi		35–40	
Extensor digitorum brevis		28	
Single motor units			
F-response	Hypothenar	30	Yates and Brown (1979)
Direct M-response	Thenar	to 53	Bergmans (1970)

See also Bergmans (1970, 1973); Kaeser (1970); Gilliatt, Hopf, Rudge, and Baraitser (1976).

TABLE 3.9. Changes in Amplitude and Duration of the
Maximum M-Potential with Increasing Distance Between
Motor Point and Site of Stimulation

Ulnar Nerve

Hypothenar	Site of Stimulation				
	W	*BE*	*AE*	*UA*	Erb's Point
p-pV (mV)	23.1	22.5	22.2	21.3	20.0
± 1 SD	4.8	4.4	4.3	4.2	4.6
p-pD (ms)	8.4	8.4	8.4	8.3	8.7
± 1 SD	1.5	1.6	1.6	1.5	1.4
Distance (mm)	74	286	385	497	703
± 1 SD	8	33	34	42	55

Peroneal Nerve

Extensor Digitorum Brevis	Site of Stimulation		
	A	*FH*	*PF*
p-pV (mV)	13.4	12.1	11.7
± 1 SD	4.6	4.1	3.9
p-pD (ms)	3.7	3.8	3.9
± 1 SD	0.6	0.5	0.5
Distance (mm)	72	372	472
± 1 SD	7	23	32

W = wrist, BE = below elbow, AE = above elbow, UA = upper arm, A = ankle, FH = fibular head, PF = popliteal fossa.

the compound M-potential. The greater the distance the motor axon impulses must travel, the greater the differences among their arrival times at the muscle and the greater the degree of desynchronization apparent in the sum of their MUPs.

If all the component MUPs were of the same phase, however, the area of the M-potential would remain constant irrespective of the distance between the site of stimulation and the innervation zone. Unfortunately, however, the potentials associated with the activities of single MUs as recorded in a volume conductor are not monophasic but biphasic (− +) when recorded in the region of the end-plate or, worse, triphasic (+ − +) when recorded outside the end-plate zone. The result is that any appreciable temporal disper-

sion among component MUPs sufficient to result in the overlapping of opposite phases of the temporally dispersed MUPs at the recording electrode will reduce the area of the summation compound M-potential through phase cancellations. The latter effect on the amplitude (p-p) or area (negative peak) of the M-potential, at least in normal human motor nerves, is minimal even over long conduction distances such as that between Erb's point and the hypothenar muscles where the reduction in negative peak area of the maximum M-potential is less than 1 percent per 100 mm between the end-plate zone and the site of stimulation (Figure 3.18).

Clearly, any tendency toward an increase in temporal dispersion among the impulses in motor axons could increase the degree of

FIGURE 3.18.   Changes in the peak-to-peak voltage (p-pV) in millivolts (mV) −2 SD (top) and peak-to-peak duration (p-pD) in milliseconds (ms) +2 SD (bottom) of the maximum hypothenar M-potential. Recording was with surface electrodes (stigmatic over the end-plate zone) and elicited by just supramaximal stimulation at the wrist (W), just distal to the cubital tunnel (BE), just proximal to the elbow (AE), the proximal arm (PA), and Erb's point.

The values are taken from 30 control subjects aged 18 to 50 years; the distances from the hypothenar innervation zone represent values for the controls.

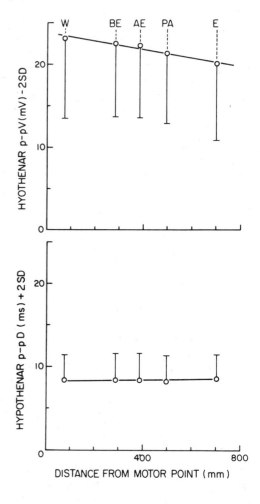

phase cancellations between MUPs making up the M-potential. The resultant reductions in M-potential amplitude and area must not therefore be taken as indications of conduction block in some of the motor axons.

The Place of Intramuscular Needle Electrodes in Measuring Motor Conduction

It was pointed out earlier that although surface electrodes are preferable for measuring motor conduction in most instances, some-times intramuscular electrodes are a better choice. For example, volume pickup of motor activity from other muscles innervated by the same or other nerves may so distort the size and waveform of the surface-recorded muscle potentials as to make it impossible to measure the latency of the desired potential properly. Use of an intramuscular electrode to record the desired muscle activity combined with filtering out of low-frequency components below 500 Hz often helps considerably by greatly attenuating more remotely generated potentials except those generated in the immediate vicinity of the electrode (Figure 3.19).

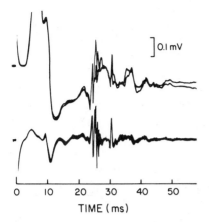

]0.1 mV

TIME (ms)

FIGURE 3.19.   Value of filtering out the lower-frequency components from a recording of the maximum M-potential.

(Top) Intramuscular concentric recording from the infraspinatus muscle in a patient with a suprascapular neuropathy. The bandwidth in the top record was 2 to 5,000 Hz (3 db down).

(Bottom) Changing the high-pass filter to 500 Hz hardly altered the late spike components originating within the supraspinatus muscle itself, but severely attenuated the volume-conducted potential from the deltoid muscle whose motor supply was also excited by the stimulus delivered at Erb's point.

METHODS OF MEASURING THE RANGE OF CONDUCTION VELOCITIES IN ALPHA MOTOR AXONS IN MAN

There is a very real possibility that some diseases may preferentially affect the more slowly conducting and smaller-diameter alpha motor axons while at the same time the faster-conducting motor axons are relatively spared. This highlights the importance not only of developing methods for assessing the range limits of conduction velocities of motor axons, but of learning something of the relative numbers of fibers conducting at different velocities in selected motor nerves. Several methods have been developed for measuring the range

of conduction velocities, all with various defects. All thus far depend on the use of the collision technique and are worth exploring in some detail because of their theoretical interest and practical limitations.

Collision Techniques

In the first method to be discussed (Thomas, Sears, and Gilliatt, 1959) the nerve is stimulated at two points, S1 and S2, a fixed distance apart (Figure 3.20). The stimulus intensity at S2 is set to be supramaximal for evoking a maximum M-potential. The S1 stimulus is then so timed with respect to the S2 stimulus that antidromic impulses in motor axons initiated at S1 collide with impulses in the same fibers originating at S2 and conducting orthodromically toward the muscle. In this model, the lowest-threshold motor axons are assumed to be those with the fastest conduction velocities. This being so, S1 stimuli just exceeding motor threshold may be expected preferentially to excite the fastest-conducting NFs.

The antidromic impulses of these NFs, on colliding with impulses in the same fibers originating at S2, would block the subsequent orthodromic conduction of the latter impulses to the muscle while at the same time leaving unblocked orthodromic impulses in the remaining higher-threshold, slower-conducting NFs.

Further increments in the intensity of the S1 stimulus would, in this model, be expected to excite progressively higher- and higher-threshold, slower-conducting motor axons until at the limit, once the S1 stimulus becomes surpamaximal for all the motor axons, all impulses initiated at S2 become blocked by collision between S1 and S2, including the slowest-conducting impulses. The range in the conduction velocities may then be calculated as follows:

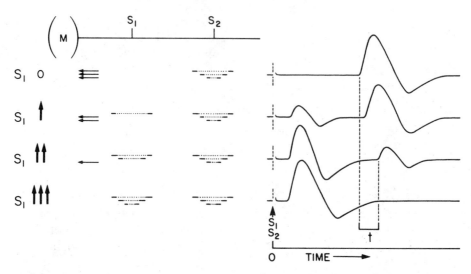

FIGURE 3.20.   This figure illustrates the principle of the method of Thomas, Sears, and Gilliatt (1959). The nerve is stimulated at two levels, S1 and S2, and the muscle potentials recorded by surface electrodes. The S2 stimulus is kept supramaximal. So long as the S1 stimulus is subthreshold for the motor fibers, all the impulses originating at S2, here reduced for simplification to three impulses, are able to reach the muscle.

It is assumed that motor axons are excited in order of their conduction velocities beginning with the fastest-conducting motor axons. Hence the first impulses originating at S2 to be antidromically blocked by weak motor stimuli at S1 are assumed to be the fastest-conducting impulses. The last to be blocked as the S1 stimulus reaches supramaximal intensity would be the slowest-conducting impulses because of their higher thresholds. The difference in latency (t) between the M-potentials elicited by S2 when S1 is just below motor threshold and when S1 is almost supramaximal provides a measure of the range of latencies of the motor axons in the motor nerve. Horizontal arrows denote impulses originating at S2 that are able to pass S1 without collision to reach the muscle (M). Vertical arrows indicate the changes in the intensity of the S1 stimulus.

$$\text{Fastest conduction velocity} = \frac{d_1}{t_1} \quad \text{and}$$

$$\text{Slowest conduction velocity} = \frac{d_1}{t_2}.$$

The method is not without its problems. For example, except where the S2 stimulus is supramaximal and all impulses originating at this site are able to reach the muscle without interruption, or where the S1 stimulus itself is supramaximal, latencies to the M1 and M2 potentials are not generated by the same motor axons. This is because impulses in those NFs that generate the M1 block orthodromically conducted impulses in the same NFs, beginning at S2. The result is that latency differences between M1 and M2 cannot be used to calculate conduction velocities for the slowest-conducting NFs with this method.

Furthermore, even when the range of conduction velocities is expressed not in actual conduction velocities but as relative latencies, for example:

$$\text{Relative latencies} = \frac{\text{longest latency to onset M2}}{\text{shortest latency to M2}},$$

the inherent assumption that the residual latencies of all the MUs are the same in such a calculation may not be true.

The preceding method has been modified to allow more direct measurement of the conduction velocities of the motor axons (Gilliatt, Hopf, Rudge, and Baraitser, 1976). In this modification, the nerve is stimulated at three sites, S1, S2, and S3 (Figure 3.21). The stimulus at S1 is increased in increments, and at each of several increments between motor threshold and reaching supramaximal intensity, the latency difference between the onsets

of the S2 and S3 stimulus-evoked M-potentials is measured. This latency difference represents the fastest conduction velocities of those motor axon impulses that are yet able to pass unblocked beyond S1 to reach the muscle. As the intensity of the stimulus at S1 increases, progressively fewer of the faster-conducting impulses beginning at S2 or S3 will be able to pass S1 without colliding with antidromic impulses in the same fibers originating at S1, until only the slowest-conducting impulses remain unblocked. Finally, even these are blocked once the stimulus at S1 becomes supramaximal.

This modification was an improvement over the original proposed by Thomas, Sears, and

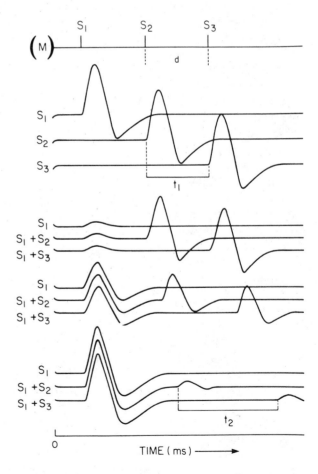

FIGURE 3.21. Diagrammatic representation of the method of Gilliatt, Hopf, Rudge, and Baraitser (1976), essentially a modification of the original method by Thomas, Sears, and Gilliatt (1959), uses an extra stimulus site S3 to measure more directly the maximum and minimum conduction velocities between S2 and S3:

$$\text{Maximum conduction velocity} = \frac{d \, (mm)}{t_1 \, (ms)}$$

$$\text{Minimum conduction velocity} = \frac{d \, (mm)}{t_2 \, (ms)}.$$

The principles behind the changes in latency of the S2 and S3 M-potentials as the intensity of the S1 stimulus is increased are as outlined for Figure 3.19; see text also.

Gilliatt (1959) in that the maximum conduction velocities of the remaining unblocked motor axons between S2 and S3 can be directly calculated. The method also has serious flaws. For example, the question remains whether submaximal stimuli at S1 are able to excite all the fastest-conducting motor axons. If not, the blockade of the fastest-conducting impulses starting out at either S2 or S3 would be incomplete. Such incomplete blockade of impulses in the fastest-conducting motor axons would tend to mask disclosure of impulses conducting in slower fibers at higher stimulus intensities. This problem is more than theoretical because there is some indication that weak stimuli may not selectively activate the fastest-conducting motor axons alone (Juul-Jensen and Mayer, 1966; Gilliatt, Hopf, Rudge, and Baraitser, 1976).

Hopf (1962) proposed yet another method for measuring the range in conduction velocities of motor axons (Figure 3.22). In this method the nerve is stimulated supramaximally at two sites. The time intervals between these stimuli at S1 and S2 are then adjusted over a range of latencies. At the outset, the S1 (distal) stimulus is timed to precede the S2 (proximal) stimulus by an interval just long enough to allow the fastest-conducting impulses originating at S1 to reach and pass the S2 site before the stimulus at S2 is delivered. This interval is so short, however, that the remaining slower-conducting impulses also beginning at S1 are unable to reach and pass S1 before orthodromic impulses in the same fibers are set off by the supramaximal stimulus delivered a short time later at S2. The result is that both volleys collide and block somewhere between the S1 and S2 sites. Hence at this interval, only impulses in the faster-conducting fibers beginning at S2 are able to reach the muscle. These evoke a low-amplitude M-response. The latency to this M-response depends on the distance between the S2 site and the motor point, the residual latencies of these motor axons, the conduction

velocities of the fibers, and the degree to which their velocities have been altered by the preceding orthodromic impulses in the same axons originating at S1.

As the interval between the S1 and S2 stimuli is increased, more and more of the slower-conducting impulses originating at S1 are able to reach and pass the S2 site prior to delivery of the S2 stimulus. The result is that more and more of the slower-conducting impulses beginning at S2 are able to conduct uninterruptedly to the muscle. Finally, at the limit, all impulses, including those in the slowest-conducting nerve fibers and beginning at S1, are able to pass S2 prior to the latter stimulus. Thus all impulses from the slowest to the fastest originating at S2 are able to reach the muscle and evoke the maximum M-potential. The range in conduction velocities of the motor axons may then be expressed in two ways:

1. As the ratio of the fastest- to slowest-conducting motor axons, namely:

$$\text{Ratio} \frac{\text{fastest } t_1}{\text{slowest } t_2}$$

where t_1 = least time interval at which S2 evokes the minimal M-potential and
t_2 = time interval at which S2 evokes the maximum M-potential.

2. In a plot of the changes in the amplitude of the M-potential against changes in the interstimulus interval. The slope of such a plot is a product both of the amplitudes of the component MUPs as well as their relative conduction velocities and numbers. These plots are an attempt to provide some indication of the quantitative distribution of motor axons of various conduction velocities in the whole population of motor axons. Such indications are, however, invalid to the degree to which there is wide range in amplitudes of component MUPs. This error is reflected by the fact that the range of conduction velocities

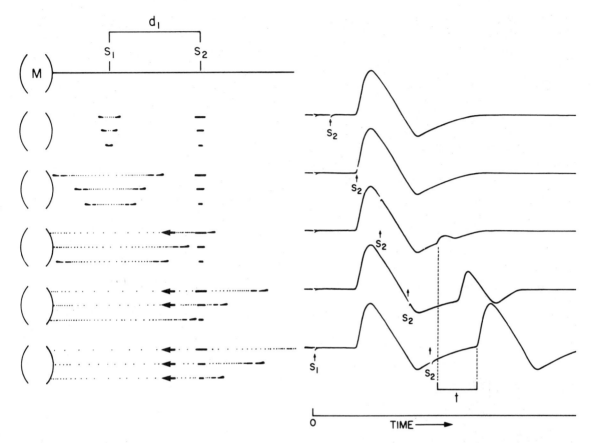

FIGURE 3.22.   In the method of Hopf (1962) the nerve is stimulated at two sites, S1 and S2. The S2 stimulus is delayed progressively with respect to the S1 stimulus so as to allow impulses in successively slower-conducting fibers which began at S1 to reach and pass S2 prior to delivery of the S2 shock. The more S1 impulses that are able to reach and pass the S2 site prior to the shock at S2, the fewer the number of S2-originating impulses will be blocked in their distal transmission to the muscle. As a consequence, the larger will be the S2 stimulus-elicited M-potential. The (t) represents the time difference between the interval at which the S2-evoked M-potential first appears and the interval at which S2 elicits the maximum M-potential. Thus (t) provides a measure of the range of the motor conduction velocities in the nerve (see text).

in human motor nerves obtained by this method is about 20 to 30 percent, an estimate about 10 to 20 percent less than those obtained by other methods and investigators.

Each of the preceding collision methods has important theoretical limitations and potential technical errors. What other methods are available to estimates of the ranges in conduction velocities in human motor nerves?

Methods for Measuring Relative Latencies of Single Motor Axons

Unfortunately, except in those instances when only a few motor axons remain, it is not often possible to excite the same axon in isolation at two or more separate sites along a motor nerve. This is because there is little chance that the same motor axon will have the lowest threshold at two or more sites, given changes in the relative positions of motor axons within the nerve trunk with respect to one another and the stimulating electrodes at the various levels of stimulation and large numbers of axons in normal motor nerves. At any one stimulus site, however, it is usually possible to excite a single motor axon in an all-or-nothing manner by surface electrical stimulation provided care is taken to adjust the stimulus intensity to avoid excitation of other motor axons.

The latencies of several such single MUPs evoked by near-threshold stimulation at sites various distances away from the motor point may be adjusted to a standard distance (Figure 3.23) provided the critical assumption is made that the residual latencies of all such single motor axons will be similar and more or less the same as the residual latency as determined for the maximum M-potentials (see Figure 3.20). The latencies of all those single MUPs obtained through stimulation at various levels may be adjusted to a standard dis-

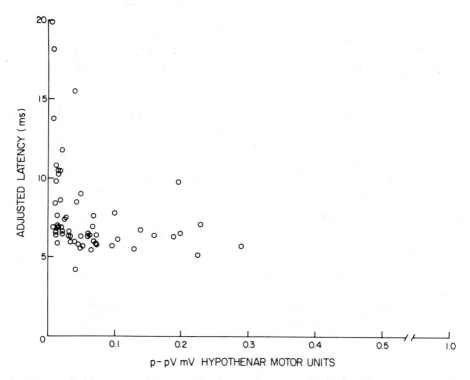

FIGURE 3.23.   Plot of the peak-to-peak voltage (p-pV) in millivolts (mV) of hypothenar MUPs as recorded with surface electrodes against the corresponding latencies adjusted to a standard distance of 200 mm from the motor point. Note the wide range of the latencies among the various motor unit action potentials. The largest-amplitude potentials generally had shorter latencies, although there was a considerable range among the relative latencies of the lowest-amplitude motor unit action potentials. From Kadrie and Brown (1978, figure 7).

tance Y millimeters from the motor point by:

$$\frac{\text{Adjusted}}{\text{latency}} = \text{latency to MUP} - \text{RL}$$

$$\times \frac{\text{distance to}}{\frac{\text{motor point}}{\text{standard}}} + \text{RL}$$
$$\text{distance Y}$$

where RL = residual latency of maximum M-potential (in ms) and

MUP = motor unit potential

Such adjusted latencies can be converted to conduction velocities for the motor axons (Figure 3.24) by:

$$\frac{\text{Conduction}}{\text{velocity}} = \frac{\text{adjusted latency} - \text{RL}}{\text{standard distance (in mm)}}.$$
$$\text{(in m/s)} = \frac{\text{(in ms)}}{\text{to which all latencies}}$$
$$\text{have been adjusted}$$

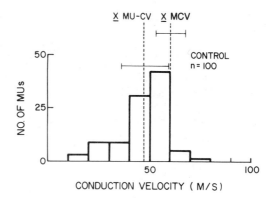

FIGURE 3.24.   Range in the conduction velocities of single median motor axons as derived from their adjusted latencies (see text). Shown also are the mean (± 1 SD) of the maximum motor conduction velocities (MCV) in this nerve as well as the mean (± 1 SD) conduction velocity of all the calculated single motor axon velocity of all the calculated single motor axon velocities (X MU-CV).

The spread in conduction velocities is misleadingly wide, probably because of the error of assuming that the residual latencies of all single motor axons are the same and equal to the residual latency for the whole M-potential.

From Kadrie and Brown (1978, figure 8).

Assessment of Conduction in Peripheral Sensory Fibers

Conduction in peripheral sensory fibers is the subject of an excellent earlier monograph by Buchthal and Rosenfalck (1966) and a more recent work by Ludin and Tackmann (1981). The assessment of sensory conduction, like that of motor conduction in vivo, depends on recording the conducted potentials in a volume conductor. Unlike motor conduction where each motor axon innervates sometimes several hundred muscle fibers and the resultant MUPs are appreciable in size and therefore readily detectable, there is no amplification device on the sensory side (except see SEP discussion, Chapter 4). Single nerve fiber potentials are not only very small even when recorded with needle electrode but they are relatively brief (spike <3 ms usually). The latter and the biphasic or, more often, triphasic

nature of the potentials makes phase cancellation between component single fiber potentials in the compound nerve action potentials a very important factor governing the shape and size of the compound potential. Sensory conduction studies in man are generally confined to the larger myelinated NFs within mixed, motor, or cutaneous nerves.

The types of afferents studied by clinical tests of sensory conduction in man and their relationship to common clinical tests of sensation are presented in Table 3.10. The major components of the nerve action potential, as recorded with surface electrodes, are generated by nerve fibers with conduction velocities between 40 and 65 m/s, although slower con-

TABLE 3.10.   Types of Larger Myelinated Nerve Fibers and their Related Sensory Functions as Tested Clinically

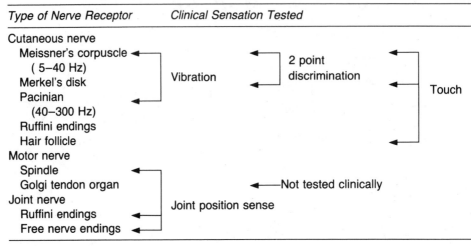

See Vallbo, Hagbarth, Torebjork, and Wallin (1979).

ducting components as low as 15 m/s may be detected when near-nerve and electronic averaging techniques are employed. This means that, as usually studied, activity in A delta (or group III) or C (group IV) nerve fibers is not assessed, nor would the recorded nerve action potential be expected to correlate with sensory functions such as temperature (warm or cold) or nociception (pinprick and tickle) subserved by these fibers.

The origin of joint position sense at the present time is a subject of some controversy because the present roles of the joint or joint capsule receptors, cutaneous receptors, and muscle stretch receptors to the overall subjective assessment of joint angle or movement have not yet been adequately defined in man or lower animals (see Horch, Clark, and Burgess, 1975; Clark, 1975; Clark and Burgess, 1975; Gandevia and McCloskey, 1976; Grigg and Greenspan, 1977; McCoskey, 1978; Ferrell, 1980; Moberg, 1983; McCloskey, Cross, Honner, and Potter, 1983).

METHODS FOR MEASURING SENSORY CONDUCTION IN MAN

Figure 3.25 illustrates the two basic ways sensory conduction may be assessed in man. In the most commonly employed method, the sensory nerve fibers are electrically stimulated in the periphery and the orthodromically conducted volley is recorded at one or more sites along the path of the volley on its way to the spinal cord or brainstem. For example, in the upper limb the stimuli may be delivered to the digits through a pair of ring electrodes (cathode proximal) and the resulting orthodromic volley recorded over the respective peripheral nerves at the wrist, elbow, proximal arm, and even Erb's point. The segmental and peripheral nerve innervation of the digits varies (Table 3.11). Digital nerves include cutaneous, joint, and possibly tendon afferents but no muscle afferents, whereas at a more proximal level, the related mixed nerves such as the median and ulnar nerves at the wrist con-

FIGURE 3.25.   Illustration of sensory recording techniques in selected nerves. The orthodromic technique is shown for the ulnar, radial, and superficial peroneal nerves. In the case of the ulnar nerve, the fifth digit may be stimulated through a pair of ring electrodes (cathode proximal) and the resultant orthodromically conducted volley recorded at the levels of the wrist, and below and above the elbow and proximal arm by near-nerve needle electrodes or surface electrodes. The reference electrodes are situated 30 to 50 mm lateral to the recording electrodes. Similar arrangements are made for recording the orthodromically conducted volleys in the radial and superficial peroneal nerves. In these two instances, the peripheral branches of the respective cutaneous nerves are often visible and, in most instances, palpable. In such situations the stimulating electrodes can be accurately positioned over the nerve (surface) or in the immediate vicinity of the nerve in the case of needle electrodes.

The inset shows an example of the antidromic recording technique. Here the antidromic sensory nerve action potential is recorded by a pair of ring recording electrodes about the third digit, and the median nerve is stimulated at various sites proximally S_1M-S_2M.

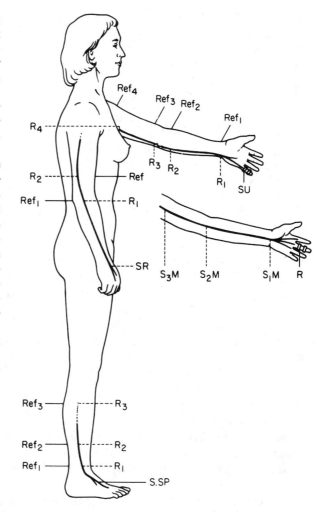

tain not only joint and cutaneous afferents but muscle afferents and motor axons as well. These points must be kept in mind when stimulating such mixed nerves in the periphery because nerve action potentials recorded proximal to the electrical stimulation of such mixed nerves may include antidromic motor impulses also in the compound nerve trunk potential. Generally speaking, however, because the latter conduct more slowly than the fastest af-

TABLE 3.11.   Segmental and Peripheral Nerve Sensory Supply of the Digits in the Hand

Digit	Segmental Innervation	Peripheral Nerve
I (thumb)	C6	Radial and median
II	C6–7	Median
III	C7	Median
IV	C7–8	Median-ulnar
V	C8	Ulnar

ferents in a mixed nerve, they make little or no contribution to the maximum conduction velocity, in normal subjects at least.

The other common option is to stimulate electrically the peripheral branches of cutaneous nerves such as the radial in the upper limb, saphenous, superficial peroneal, or sural in the lower limb, and as in digital stimulation in the upper limb, record the orthodromically conducted potential at two or more progressively proximal sites.

The maximum conduction velocities are measured between successively recorded initial positive peaks. The stimulus intensities for both digital and cutaneous branch stimulation are adjusted to be supramaximal for evoking the maximum amplitude (initial positive to negative spike peak). Because any artifacts produced through stimulus lead ahead of the cathode will be repeated at each recording, the conduction velocities measured between successive recording sites should be unaffected by the stimulus lead.

The initial positive peaks of such compound nerve action potentials do not always indicate the arrival of the fastest-conducting impulses at the recording electrode. Not uncommonly, a few poorly defined spikes are seen in the rising initial positive phase. Nonetheless, the initial positive peaks so recorded do represent the most consistently identifiable points in the compound nerve action potential to correlate with the arrival of the majority of the fastest-conducting impulses at the recording electrode, especially in orthodromic and near-nerve recordings.

The amplitude and shape of the recorded compound nerve action potential are dependent on the nearness of the recording electrode to the nerve trunk. In the case of some cutaneous nerves, such as some portions of the radial or the superficial peroneal nerve, the peripheral nerve trunk is readily palpable and sometimes seen. This makes placement of the recording electrode much easier. Sim-

ilarly, in the case of orthodromic recordings from mixed nerves such as the median or ulnar nerve, prior motor conduction studies help to locate the underlying nerve more precisely. Needle stimulating electrodes that have been inserted previously for stimulation of the nerves may serve as ideal recording electrodes as well, because of their close proximity to the nerve trunk achieved through prior stimulation and adjustment in the position of the electrode to the depth at which the maximum motor response is elicited for the least stimulus intensities.

Alternatively, surface electrodes may be used to record the nerve action potential. They provide better reproducibility of the shape and amplitude of the potentials in serial studies, but often the initial positive peak and the later components are less well defined. Near-nerve electrodes, on the other hand, although they take more time because of the need to optimize their position, provide much better resolution of the slower components, especially when combined with electronic averaging. In such recordings at high gain, it is not unusual to resolve the spikes of single NFs. As pointed out in the section on electrical stimulation, however, such electrodes must penetrate the nerve trunk from time to time, although lasting sequelae are very rare. The relative virtues of the two types of recording electrodes are summarized in Table 3.12.

To ensure the best resolution of nerve action potentials, impedance of the electrodes must be kept as low as possible. This not only reduces the noise but optimizes the frequency response of the recorded potentials. To this end, disposable electrodes may be used (they are expensive) or the leading-off surface of the electrodes may be etched by passing a small DC current through the electrode in saline as advocated by Buchthal and Rosenfalck (1966). In the case of surface electrodes, the impedance of both the electrode and the skin should be kept as low as possible. The skin

TABLE 3.12. Near-Nerve (Needle) versus Surface Electrodes for Recording Nerve Action Potentials

Needle Electrodes	Surface Electrodes
Advantages	
Better definition of early positive peak	Convenience
Early positive peak better corresponds to arrival time of most of the fastest-conducting impulses opposite the electrode (G_1)	Amplitudes are more reproducible in serial examinations because the distance between the recording electrode and underlying nerve is more constant
Better resolution of later components	
Amplitudes of potentials are larger	
Disadvantages	
Less convenient	Poor resolution of later components
More distressing for patients	The initial positive peak may be absent or poorly defined

may be prepared, for example, by removing surface oils with acetone followed by light abrasion with sandpaper or a suitable alternative, then rubbing a little electrode paste into the skin, being careful to wipe off the excess before application of the electrode. Such skin electrodes should have impedances of less than 5,000 and in most cases 2,000 ohms between 100 and 2,000 Hz.

Unipolar versus Bipolar Recording

For both surface and near-nerve recording electrodes, unipolar (or monopolar) recordings are preferable to bipolar arrangements. Distortions of later components of the nerve action potentials occur with bipolar arrangements (see earlier discussion).

Antidromic Recording of Sensory Conduction Velocities

One alternative method of assessing sensory conduction is to record the antidromic volley at some distant site on the nerve and stimulate the nerve then at one or more sites successively proximal to the recording electrode. For example, in the upper limb the antidromic volley may be recorded by a pair of ring electrodes about the digit and, in the case of the median nerve, the nerve may be stimulated at the wrist, elbow, and upper arm.

Such potentials have one particularly serious flaw, namely, distortion of the potential by the sometimes unavoidable volume conduction of proximally innervated muscle potentials. Other flaws include possible differences in the stimulus lead artifact at successive stimulus sites and the sometimes poorly defined onset of the potentials. Such potentials have no initial positive deflection, possibly because of the small volume of the digit in the face of the approaching volley, and as a consequence, latencies must be measured to the initial negative deflection.

The amplitude of antidromic nerve action potentials recorded with ring electrodes about the digit have been shown to depend on the circumference of the digit; the smaller the digit, the larger the amplitude of the recorded potential (Bolton and Carter, 1980).

Antidromically recorded nerve action potentials recorded from the nerves themselves do have initial positive deflections and well-defined positive peaks, as Figure 3.26 illustrates.

As pointed out earlier, sometimes when surface recordings are made for the purpose of recording the M-potential, a small prepotential may be detected. That this potential is generated by an antidromic volley in a nearby cutaneous nerve is supported by the twin observation that the potential develops at stimulus intensities below motor threshold and as

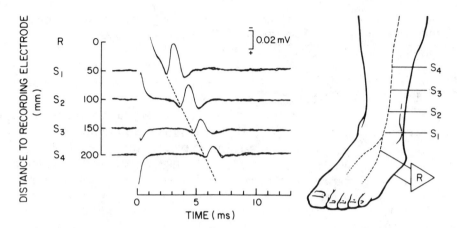

FIGURE 3.26.   Antidromic recording of sensory nerve action potential from the superficial peroneal nerve. The recording needle electrode was inserted in the immediate vicinity of the readily visible and palpable nerve and the reference needle electrode was inserted 30 mm laterally. The nerve was stimulated percutaneously at progressively proximal 50-mm intervals. The records shown are from a patient with a mild diabetic neuropathy (temperature near the nerve was 32°C). The maximum sensory conduction velocity (S_1-S_4) was 45.2 m/s.

the site stimulation is moved proximally, the latency difference between the prepotential and the M-potential increases. The latter indicates that not only does the volley generating the prepotential have a faster conduction velocity compared to the motor axons, but that the former have lower thresholds to electrical stimulation.

Comparative Excitabilities of Sensory and Motor Axons

Normally, the largest sensory fibers have appreciably lower thresholds than the lowest-threshold motor axons. This can be shown by comparing the onset and relative amplitudes as percentages of their maximum of the antidromic sensory nerve action potential and the M-potential when the median nerve is stimulated at the wrist (Figure 3.27). It is also shown in the earlier appearance of the cortical somatosensory evoked potential before the M-

potential when the median or ulnar nerves are stimulated (see Chapter 4 and Figure 4.6), the relative excitabilities of motor and sensory fibers may vary somewhat in any one individual if the position of the stimulating electrode is varied. This suggests that relative proximity to the cathode is also important.

Dependence of Conduction Velocities in Motor and Sensory Fibers on Age of Subject and Environmental Temperature

Influence of Age

Conduction velocities are very dependent on the age of the subject. In utero, myelination begins at about four months of gestation (Ochoa and Mair, 1971) and becomes complete by about five years of age (Gutrecht and Dyck, 1970), by which time the diameters of the nerve fibers will have reached adult values. In term babies, the maximum impulse velocities are about one-half of the corre-

FIGURE 3.27. Comparative excitabilities of motor and sensory fibers in the median nerve. Above illustrates the percentage of the maximum amplitude of the negative peak ($-p$), antidromic sensory nerve action (AP), and peak-to-peak voltage (p-pV) of the thenar M action potential as elicited by changes in the stimulus intensity (in milliamperes—mA) delivered to the median nerve by percutaneous electrodes at the wrist. In this person, the sensory action potential reached its maximum value while the M-potential was less than 20 percent of maximum.

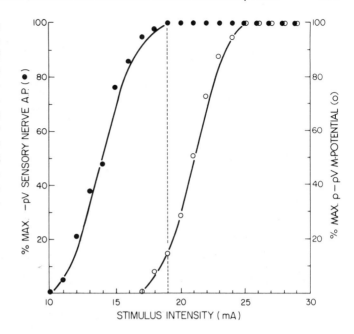

sponding values in adults (Gamstrop, 1963; Gamstrop and Shelburne, 1965; Desmedt, Noel, Debecker, and Namèche, 1973), subsequently reaching adult velocities somewhere between 5 and 8 years of age (Gamstrop, 1963; Buchthal, Rosenfalck, and Behse, 1975). Others have suggested that the attainment of adult velocities is reached somewhat earlier (Desmedt, Noel, Debecker, and Namèche, 1973). The above changes in the maximum impulse velocities are illustrated by Figure 3.28.

Later in life there are progressive declines in the maximum conduction velocities of both motor and sensory fibers (Buchthal, Rosenfalck, and Behse, 1975; Desmedt and Cheron, 1980; Norris, Shock, and Wagman, 1953) proceeding at a rate of about 1 m/s per decade between 20 and 55 years of age. Beyond 55 to 60 years of age the decline is more rapid (3 m/s per decade). These declines in conduction velocities are accompanied by reductions in amplitudes and increases in the durations of nerve action potentials (Buchthal, Rosen-

falck, and Behse, 1975; Lehmann, Muche, and Schutt, 1977).

Later life is also accompanied by progressive losses of myelinated nerve fibers (Swallow, 1966; O'Sullivan and Swallow, 1968) and increasing evidence of segmental demyelination as well as irregularities in internode length (Lascelles and Thomas, 1966). It is not known to what extent the reductions in conduction velocities can be correlated with these changes in diameters of nerve fibers, defects in myelination, losses of nerve fibers, or possibly even changes in the properties, distributions, and numbers of ion channels in the axolemmal membranes.

Influence of Environmental Temperature

The cooler the nerve, the slower are the time courses of the transmembrane ionic currents accompanying the impulse. This not only slows conduction of the impulse but prolongs the duration of the potential and tends to increase the amplitude of the action potential (Hodgkin and Katz, 1949). Such changes not

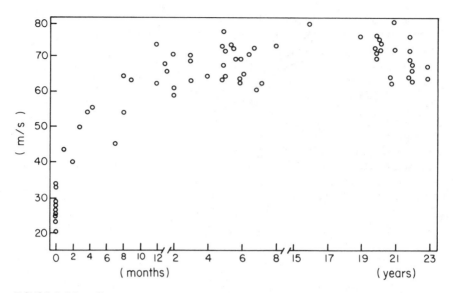

FIGURE 3.28.   Changes in maximum peripheral sensory conduction velocity as a function of age. Above are pooled data from subjects of various ages from birth to early adulthood. Note that normal velocities are reached as early as two years of age.
Redrawn from Desmedt, Noel, Debecker, and Namèche (1973, figure 2).

only explain the progressive slowing of conduction velocities, about 1.5 to 2.5 m/s per degree Celsius (Buchthal and Rosenfalck, 1966; Lowitzsch, Hopf, and Galland, 1977; Luden and Beyelar, 1977) seen as human nerves are progressively cooled, but the alterations in amplitude and prolonged durations of compound nerve action potentials (Hulley, Wilbourne, and McGinty, 1977; Bolton, Sawa, and Carter, 1981; see also review by Denys, 1980).

Proximal Conduction in Peripheral Nerves

In human peripheral nerves maximum motor and sensory conduction velocities tend to be more rapid when measured over intermediate as compared to more distal segments in the peripheral nerves (Table 3.13). To what extent these gradients in conduction velocity reflect progressive cooling of the nerve toward the distal extremities of the limb or pro-

gressive tapering of axonal diameters and myelin thickness has not been entirely resolved in man. There are obvious difficulties in such morphological studies because of the inability to be certain the diameters and myelin thicknesses are being measured in the same fibers at all levels of study. Similarly, warming the limb and even monitoring the temperature near the nerve trunk at one or more sites does not ensure that the temperature of the nerve is uniform throughout its entire length.

Even less is known about conduction velocities across the most proximal segments of the peripheral nervous system because the distances in vivo cannot be measured accurately. Nor, except with invasive techniques, can conduction be measured directly across the roots or plexuses.

Assessments of proximal conduction using indirect methods such as the F-response or H-reflexes all suffer from the inherent weak-

TABLE 3.13.   Maximum Orthodromic Sensory Conduction Velocities

Nerve	Age	n	W	E	E	AX
Median	18–25	66	64.8 ± 5.2		68.7 ±	7.2
	48–64	11	55.5 ± 2.6		67.6 ±	10.2
	70–88	24	53.5 ± 4.7		60.9 ±	7.8
			A	PF	PF	B
Sciatic	18–25	6	52.6 ± 5.2		55.1 ±	6.3

From Buchthal and Rosenfalck (1966).
W—wrist.
E—elbow.
AX—axilla.
A—ankle.
PF—popliteal fossa.
B—buttock.

nesses of being unable to measure proximal distances accurately or being certain that the respective late responses are truly representative of the fastest-conducting fibers (see later discussion of F- and H-potentials). Therefore although the above techniques have a place in assessing proximal conduction times and making relative comparisons between normal and abnormal subjects or between affected and unaffected nerves in the same subject, they have little value as direct indicators of the true conduction velocities across the roots or plexuses.

Conduction velocities across the proximal segments of the peripheral nervous system have, however, been directly measured in the baboon (Clough, Kernell, and Phillips, 1968). In this study the relevant distances could all be measured directly and the temperature of the nerves properly maintained throughout their length. The peripheral nerves were stimulated at progressively more proximal levels and recordings made of the respective volleys in the dorsal and ventral roots. Also, the antidromic action potentials of the motoneurons were recorded by means of intracellular electrodes. This technique makes it possible to assess conduction in single motor axons in addition to assessments of whole nerve volleys as recorded by root electrodes.

Clough and others (1968) conclusively showed, at least in the baboon, that the maximum conduction velocities in both motor and sensory fibers were slower across the brachial plexus and roots than in the more distal segments of the peripheral nervous system (Figure 3.29), a difference not explicable by temperature differences between the regions. Whether similar slowing of conduction in proximal segments of the peripheral nervous system occurs in man is unknown. Based on the smaller diameters of the central compared to the peripheral processes of dorsal root ganglion cells, one would anticipate proximal slowing of conduction at least over the sensory roots, which in the lumbosacral region have very appreciable lengths.

Errors in Assessment of Latency and Conduction Velocity

Accurate measurement of latency and conduction velocity depends on a number of factors (Table 3.14). Sources of error with re-

FIGURE 3.29.   The relationship between the proximal (proximal upper arm-spinal cord) and distal (proximal forearm-distal forearm) conduction velocities in motor axons innervating forearm and hand muscles in the baboon. Conduction velocities in single motor axons were measured by recording the antidromic spikes in the motoneurons as recorded with intracellular electrodes and elicited by stimulation at the peripheral sites mentioned above. The motoneurons were pooled into four groups based on their peripheral conduction velocities (<55 m/s, 55 to 64 m/s, 65 to 74 m/s, and >75 m/s). For each group the mean values and standard errors of the mean are shown. Note the slower conduction velocities over the proximal portion of the peripheral nervous system in relation to the peripheral velocities in all four groups.
From Clough, Kernell, and Phillips (1968, figure 2).

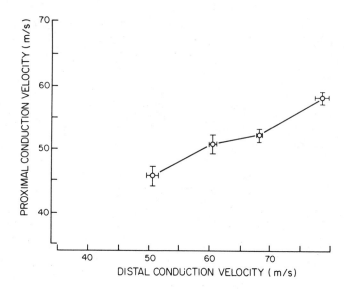

spect to stimulation and recording have been covered in earlier discussions. Just as common, perhaps, in clinical practice are those errors produced through improper measurement of distance and time.

Time Measurement

Because analog oscilloscopes and related hard-copy printout devices are likely to develop inaccuracies in their calibrated time bases, these must be rechecked and recalibrated at regular intervals. Even so, provision for a precise time marker, such as is provided by a crystal clock generator, is vital to the accurate measurement of latencies. Such time markers should be capable of providing pulse indicators at 0.1-ms intervals.

Even more common are the simple errors of recognizing the true onsets of potentials, especially when these are distorted by stimulus- or volume-conducted muscle artifacts, or are hard to discern because the trace width is too broad because the beam is out of focus or

is too intense. Displays should take advantage of the full width of the recording screen or printout device and not be crowded to one side if resolutions of the potentials and accurate measurements of latency are to be enhanced (Figure 3.27). Distortions of onset times may also be produced through the filtering out of various frequency components in the initial onset of the signal.

Digital recording devices are inherently much more accurate than are analog instruments with respect to time.

Distance Measurement

Accurate measurements of conduction velocity depend on precise assessment of both latency and the distances between the recording and stimulation sites. Such distances are measured over the surface of the limb. To a surprising degree, such surface measurements do correlate very well with the corresponding distances as measured more directly in cadavers or on the exposed nerves at operations, at

TABLE 3.14.   Sources of Error in the Measurement of Sensory and Motor Conduction

Motor Conduction	Sensory Conduction
Stimulus	
Uncertainty about precise time of onset of impulses in the nerve in relation to stimulus pulse (especially when stimulus duration is too long)	Same
Uncertainties about just where impulses in underlying nerve begin in relation to position of the cathode	Same
Submaximal stimulation	Same
Stimulus lead	Same
Recording	
Volume-conducted potentials from other muscles innervated by the same or other motor nerves or which have been activated directly at the stimulus site	Same
Movement artifact in relation to the above muscles	Inability to resolve the faster conducting components in the compound nerve action potential because, for example, initial positive peak is poorly defined
Recording so far away from the end-plate zone that earliest postsynaptic activity at end-plate zone is not seen	Distortion of nerve action potentials by excessive noise because of excessive electrode impedance
Distance measurements	
Errors in measurement of distance between stimulating and recording sites or between successive recording sites	Same
Time measurements	
Errors in manual reading of latencies	Same

least in the intermediate and distal segments of the peripheral nervous system.

More uncertain, however, are distances across more proximal segments of the peripheral nervous system; for example, between Erb's point and the spinal cord, or sciatic notch and lumbosacral roots or sacral cord. Such distances should be measured with calipers, but even here the degree of accuracy is unknown. Unfortunately, x-rays including computed tomographic pictures are unable to provide any more accurate gauges of distance.

Also, even with the use of needle electrodes positioned near the nerve, distances on the surface as measured between sites where the needles penetrate the skin may not correspond to the actual site of stimulation when needles are not inserted perpendicular to the skin.

The Tendon Reflex

Tapping a muscle tendon abruptly lengthens the muscle. This stimulus excites the spindle stretch receptors within the muscle whose primaries monosynaptically excite and may cause to fire some of the motoneurons supplying the stretched muscle, so evoking a reflex contraction of the muscle. For the purposes of this discussion, other more complex central interactions are excluded. The latency of the tendon reflex (TR) is a product of:

1. The time interval between the tendon tap and onset of the primary spindle afferent discharge. This interval depends in part on the passive viscoelastic properties of the muscle and tendon, the velocity of the stretch imparted to the muscle, and the sensitivities of the spindles to stretch. The last, in turn, is influenced by the level of background gamma motoneuronal activity and the resting lengths of the muscle and spindles.

2. Conduction velocities of the spindle primaries and distances between the receptors and the spinal cord. In long muscles such as the rectus femoris, there may be substantial differences in this distance depending on the positions of the receptors within the muscle. The arrival times of impulses in different spindle afferents at the spinal cord may therefore differ somewhat between receptors.

3. Central delays. These include the time taken up in conduction through the central processes and terminal branches of the spindle primaries, the respective monosynaptic synaptic delays, and the subsequent intervals between onset of the excitatory postsynaptic potentials (EPSPs) and the motoneuronal discharges that follow once the EPSPs exceed the firing thresholds for the motoneurons.

4. Conduction velocities and terminal conduction times of the motor axons.

5. Neuromuscular delays.

6. Length of the reflex arc.

7. Nearness of the recording electrode to the innervation zone. If the recording electrode is too far away from the innervation zone, the earliest detected potentials may not correspond to the earliest postsynaptic activity in the muscle, but to some subsequent time required for the conducted potentials in the muscle to approach near enough to the recording electrode to be detected as an approaching positive wave.

The overall latency is then the sum of the reflex time plus the time necessary to bring the muscle potentials to within the detection zone of the recording electrode. This problem can be especially troublesome in larger muscles such as the quadriceps group, gastrocnemius, or soleus muscles when the recording electrode is situated well away from the innervation zone and especially when needle electrodes with very restricted pickup territories are used.

It is clear from the above that the latencies of tendon reflex depend on more than simply the conduction velocities of the respective motor and sensory fibers. Thus, even though tendon reflexes are useful ways of testing the segmental stretch reflex arc in the neurological examination, they are perhaps a little less valuable as means of measuring conduction over the proximal segments of the peripheral nervous system. Moreover, unfortunately, they are often absent just in the very situations where it would be of greatest value to measure their latencies. For example, the tendon reflexes are often absent in peripheral neuropathies either because of the loss of too many peripheral afferents or efferents or because of excessive temporal dispersion in the afferent sensory volley. Tendon reflexes may also be reduced or even lost where the central excitabilities of the motoneurons are depressed for some reason. On the other hand, EMG recording of the jaw jerk is a useful adjunct to assessment of the trigeminal nerve (see Chapter 2), and tendon reflex latencies may be prolonged in cervical or lumbosacral root entrapments (Table 3.15).

The H-Reflex

One way of assessing proximal conduction in the peripheral nervous system that bypasses the spindle end-organs in the muscle is through

TABLE 3.15.   Tendon Reflex Latencies Prolonged
in Root Entrapments

Tendon Reflex	Primary Root Involved
Biceps	C6
Triceps	C7
Finger flexor	C8
Quadriceps	L3–L4
Achilles tendon reflex	S1

the H-reflex (Figure 3.30). In the human, one of the most accessible sites from which to elicit both a tendon jerk and H-reflex is the soleus muscle (Desmedt, 1973). The tendon jerk may be evoked by tapping the Achilles tendon and the H-reflex by electrically stimulating the posterior tibial nerve just posterior to the knee in the popliteal fossa. In most subjects, as the stimulus intensity to this nerve is gradually increased, an EMG potential at a latency of

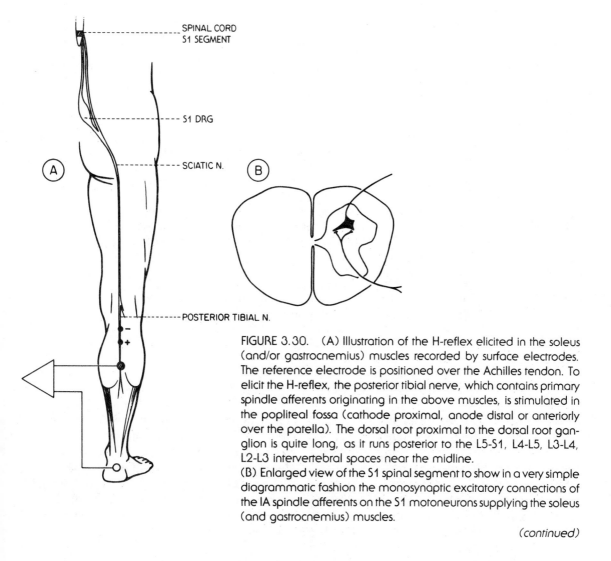

FIGURE 3.30.   (A) Illustration of the H-reflex elicited in the soleus (and/or gastrocnemius) muscles recorded by surface electrodes. The reference electrode is positioned over the Achilles tendon. To elicit the H-reflex, the posterior tibial nerve, which contains primary spindle afferents originating in the above muscles, is stimulated in the popliteal fossa (cathode proximal, anode distal or anteriorly over the patella). The dorsal root proximal to the dorsal root ganglion is quite long, as it runs posterior to the L5-S1, L4-L5, L3-L4, L2-L3 intervertebral spaces near the midline.

(B) Enlarged view of the S1 spinal segment to show in a very simple diagrammatic fashion the monosynaptic excitatory connections of the IA spindle afferents on the S1 motoneurons supplying the soleus (and gastrocnemius) muscles.

(continued)

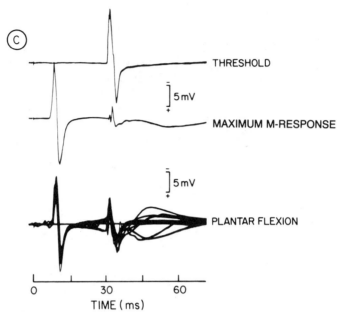

FIGURE 3.30.   *(continued)*
(C) Actual recordings of an H-reflex. Here stimulus intensities yet submaximal for the direct M-response were able to elicit an H-reflex from the soleus (and/or gastrocnemius) muscle, which in its amplitude almost matched that of the maximum M-potential elicited with supramaximal stimulation of the posterior tibial nerve (middle). Note that at the later intensity, the late response was much reduced but usually not absent. The remaining late potentials are probably due to the reflection of impulses from the motoneurons themselves when antidromically invaded (the F-response). In the bottom, the subject was instructed to plantar flex the foot strongly. While there was some potentiation of the late response, this was small. The participation of most or all of the available motoneuron population in the H-reflex as shown in the top record and the reduced capacity to potentiate the H-reflex as shown in the bottom record are common in disorders of the upper motoneuron. These recordings were made on the side of a hemiparesis caused by a contralateral cerebral infarction.

about 30 ms will appear prior to the appearance of the much shorter-latency direct M-potential. Continued increases in stimulus intensity are accompanied by increases in the amplitude of the late potential. Once the stimulus intensity exceeds threshold for soleus motor axons, however, a shorter-latency (about 5 ms) M-potential appears. Further increases in the stimulus intensity are accompanied by a progressive increase in the M-potential amplitude, while at the same time the amplitude of the late potential begins to decline. Once the stimulus intensity becomes supramaximal for the direct M-potential, only a small low-amplitude late response usually remains (Figure 3.30).

The usual interpretation of the above classic sequence is that some, at least, of the soleus primary spindle afferents have lower thresholds than do any of the soleus motor axons. Therefore stimuli that are below motor threshold but that excite some of the primary spindle afferents evoke an orthodromic volley in the latter, which monosynaptically excite and may discharge some of the soleus motoneurons. Impulses in the later axons then centrifugally conduct to the muscle to activate their respective complements of muscle fibers and produce the late M-potential at about 30 ms. The amplitude of the later H-potential continues to grow as increasing numbers of spindle primaries are excited. Once above motor threshold, however, more and more of the resultant reflex volley is blocked by antidromically conducting impulses in more and more soleus motor axons. When the stimulus intensity is increased to the point at which all motor axons in the underlying nerve are excited, all reflex volleys in the motor axons are blocked through collision. What remains of the late potential at supramaximal motor intensities must be F-potentials, although throughout the stimulus intensity range from motor threshold to supramaximal motor stimulation, a variable number of F-potentials is undoubtedly mixed in with H-reflex potentials.

Sometimes it is difficult even in healthy subjects to demonstrate a late potential at stimulus intensities below motor threshold. In such instances the initial disproportionate growth of the late potential compared to the direct M-potential establishes the H-reflex identity of the late potential.

In healthy subjects the latency of the H-reflex is determined by:

1. The very brief time required for the electrical stimulus to activate the primary spindle afferents when short-duration stimulus pulses are used (< 0.2 ms)

2. Conduction velocities of the primary spindle afferents

3. The central delay (see discussion on tendon reflex central delay)

4. Conduction velocities and terminal conduction times of the motor axons

5. Neuromuscular delay

6. The distance between the site of stimulation and the spinal cord

7. Whatever time is required for the muscle potentials to be detected by the recording electrode

Normally, the H-reflexes are difficult to elicit in the upper limb. Indeed, when they are seen in the intrinsic hand muscles, there may be an upper motor neuron disorder affecting the limb, although occasionally such H-reflexes are seen in healthy subjects. They are most regularly seen in the soleus and quadriceps muscles, but not in the plantar or extensor digitorum brevis muscles or the common peroneal group of muscles (tibialis anterior, extensor hallucis longus, extensor digitorum longus, or peroneus muscles).

The H-reflex latencies may be increased for many of the same reasons that tendon reflexes are lost or their latencies increased. There are, however, important distinctions between tendon and H-reflexes (Table 3.16).

As might be expected based on the known wide range in conduction velocities of motor axons, the latencies of individual MUPs participating in the H-reflex may differ substantially. These differences could also reflect differences in the central activation times of their respective motoneurons, and possibly even some among conduction velocities of spindle afferents eliciting the responses.

Even in some healthy persons H-reflexes are not always obtainable, and their latencies may be difficult to interpret because of differences among healthy subjects. Normative data on the relationship between latencies of the H-reflex and body height help in this respect.

TABLE 3.16.   Principal Distinctions Between Tendon and H-Reflexes

	Tendon Reflex	H-Reflex
Stimulus	Muscle stretch and subsequent direct activation of stretch receptors within the muscle	Direct electrical excitation of primary spindle afferents (bypassing receptor end organs)
Sensory volley	Characteristically repetitive discharges in primary spindle afferents The resultant afferent volleys are often very synchronous. Also differences in the distances between the spinal cord and the peripheral locations of the receptors in the muscle may be substantial	Because of the above, the latency is independent of whatever differences there may be in the distances between the receptors in the muscle and the spinal cord. Hence the afferent volley is much more synchronous, and there are no repetitive discharges in primary spindle afferents as a rule
Central delays	This could be substantial because of the wide temporal dispersion of the arrival times of the impulses in the Ia afferents at the spinal cord and subsequent onsets of their excitatory postsynaptic potentials in their target motoneurons	Central delays might be expected to be shorter because of better synchronization of the afferent volley and more optimal summation of the Ia excitatory postsynaptic potentials in the motoneurons
Efferent output	The numbers of motoneurons activated and the resultant size of the M-potential and twitch reflect the above factors	

The H-reflex has an important place in electrophysiological assessment of S1 root lesions. Unilateral absence of the soleus H-reflex or a significantly prolonged latency on the affected side is support for a lesion affecting the S1 root and can be an early indication of such, prior to the appearance of any denervation activity in muscles supplied by the S1 root. Very discrete lesions of the root, however, may produce little significant alteration of the overall latency because, as in the case of the soleus H-reflex, such latencies incorporate conduction times in much longer lengths of presumably much more normally conducting segments of the reflex pathway.

The F-Response

Electrical stimuli exceeding motor threshold trigger impulses in motor axons opposite the cathode, which then proceed to conduct both peripherally toward the muscle, where they evoke a direct M-response, and centrally toward the parent motoneurons. The latter centripedally conducting impulses in motor axons may be blocked at the first node of Ranvier or the initial segment because of the impedance mismatch presented by the greatly expanded and unmyelinated membrane of the cell body itself (Figure 3.31). The result is that the internal longitudinal currents preceding the

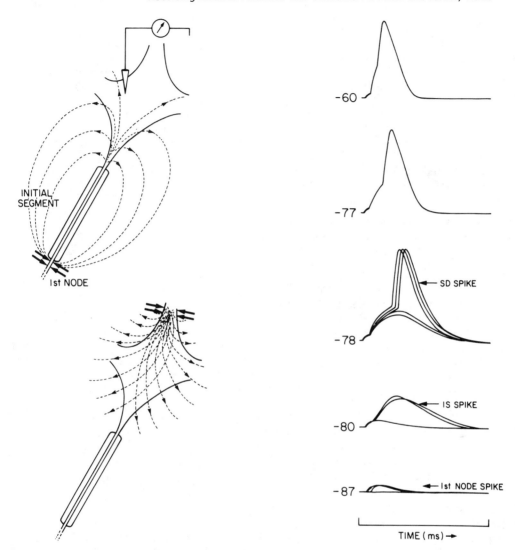

FIGURE 3.31.   (Top left) Antidromic invasion of the motoneuron initial segment and soma by the internal longitudinal currents preceding the inward action currents *(arrows)* at the first, second, or even third node of Ranvier. Should such outward somal membrane currents depolarize the membrane to threshold, a somal dendritic (SD) spike may result (right). Whether or not this happens is probably actually dependent on the transmembrane potential of the soma, hyperpolarization tending to block the impulse at the initial segment or even first node (right), leaving the initial segment (IS) node or 1st node (1st NODE) spike.

Continuation of the somal spike into the proximal dendritic tree may produce sufficient electrotonic depolarization of the membrane at the initial segment to regenerate the action potential at the initial segment or perhaps even first node of Ranvier. Such a reflected impulse could then conduct toward the periphery to activate the whole complement of muscle fibers innervated by the motoneuron.
Based on Eccles (1955).

impulse may be unable to depolarize the membrane of the initial segment or adjacent soma beyond the level necessary to generate an action potential.

If, however, the internal longitudinal currents preceding the antidromic impulse are able to overcome the impedance mismatch presented by the junction of the myelinated portion of the axon with the cell body, a somal spike may be generated that may then conduct into the proximal dendritic tree. In these circumstances the membrane of the initial segment or first node may be reactivated by the electrotonically conducted depolarizing potentials generated by the action potential in the proximal dendritic tree, provided the membranes of the initial segment or first node have had sufficient time to recover from their absolute refractory periods. Any factors that would prolong the absolute refractory period in the latter membrane regions or speed conduction of the somal spike into dendritic network would tend to prevent regeneration of the impulse at the initial segment or first node. Conversely, factors slowing conduction of the somal spike into the dendritic regions, such as would be expected if the motoneuron was hyperpolarized, or shortening the absolute refractory period would tend to increase the chance of reflection of the impulse (Eccles, 1955). The absolute refractory period at the initial segment is of the order of 0.9 to 1.2 ms. Whether or not regeneration of the impulse takes place therefore depends to a critical degree on the membrane potential of the motoneuron.

In humans, it turns out that only about one-half of the MUs generate F-responses. Furthermore, the chance of an F-response (Figure 3.32) occurring in any MU is normally less than about 1 in 10 peripheral stimuli.

The latency of the F-response in health is determined by:

1. The conduction velocities of the MUs (axons) generating the F-response. The fact

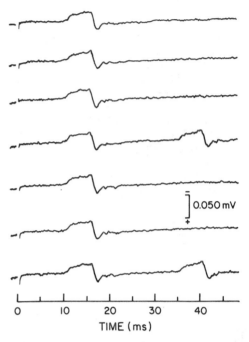

FIGURE 3.32.   The F-response in a single hypothenar MUP (surface-recorded) whose axon at the wrist was stimulated percutaneously with intensities that just exceeded threshold for the axon most but not all the time (note the absent direct response in one trace). In three of the six traces a second late potential was seen whose shape and size was identical to that in the direct response, and which was never seen except in the presence of the latter.

that F-responses are not seen in all motor units (potentials) suggests the possibility that in some instances the latency of the F-response may not reflect participation of the fastest-conducting motor axons in the F-response. That this is not a serious problem in normal subjects is suggested by the fact that the maximum conduction velocities as measured between two successive sites of stimulation of a motor nerve correspond very closely whether measured between the direct M-potentials or between the corresponding F-potentials at the two levels of stimulation. To increase the chance of including some of the faster-conducting axons in the F-response, the minimum number of stimuli that should be used is ten. Even more may be preferable to avoid missing on chance alone the shortest-latency potentials in the F-responses.

2. The distance between the site of stimulation and the spinal cord and between the latter and the muscle. The closer the site of stimulation is to the motoneuron, the shorter the antidromic conduction time. The orthodromic conduction time, of course, is not altered by changing the site of stimulation and is proportional to the distance between the motoneuron and the target muscle.

3. Following in the wake of the peripherally conducted impulses in the motor axon originating at the site of stimulation, the excitability of the nerve fiber may be altered for a variable period lasting up to several hundred milliseconds (Bergmans, 1970, 1973; also see Chapter 1). Such altered excitability states may speed up or slow down the reflected F-impulse to follow depending on the interval between the impulses. Similarly, the antidromic impulse preceding the reflected impulse alters the excitability of the axon proximal to the site of stimulation.

4. The residual latencies of the motor units (potentials) generating the F-response.

5. The turnabout time at the level of the motoneuron. This is thought to be somewhere between 0.5 and 1.5 ms, although it has never been directly measured in single motoneurons and may well be different in different motoneurons. In any one motoneuron, however, the turnabout time must be quite constant because fluctuations in latency of single MUPs in the F-response are little more than those of single MUPs in the direct M-response (Stålberg and Trontelj, 1979) (Table 3.17). The apparent great variability in amplitude and latency of the F-response as seen in the usual clinical recordings of the responses to successive stimuli is the result of changes in the participating MUPs whose absolute latencies may differ substantially, even though the latency

TABLE 3.17. Variations in Latency of Single Motor Units in M-, F-, and H-Responses

Response	Variation in Latency (μsec)	Source
M	10–30	Trontelj (1973a, 1973b)
F	40 ± 10	Schiller and Stålberg (1978)
H	150	

fluctuation for any one MUP in successive responses is quite constant.

The range of latencies of single MUPs in the F-response simply reflects the broad range in conduction velocities of motor axons (see Tables 3.7 and 3.8; Figure 3.33). In some peripheral neuropathies, especially those with prominent demyelination and remyelination, the range of F-latencies may be much broader, reflecting in this case the greater slowing of conduction in some motor axons than in others. Moreover, such temporal dispersion may be especially evident in the F-response because of the very long conduction distance over which such impulses travel (antidromic ± orthodromic), especially with distal sites of stimulation.

Factors Altering the Latency
of the F-Response in Disease

In various diseases the latency of the F-response may be altered for a number of reasons, including:

1. Slowing of motor axonal conduction velocities
2. Increases in residual latency values of MUPs in the F-response

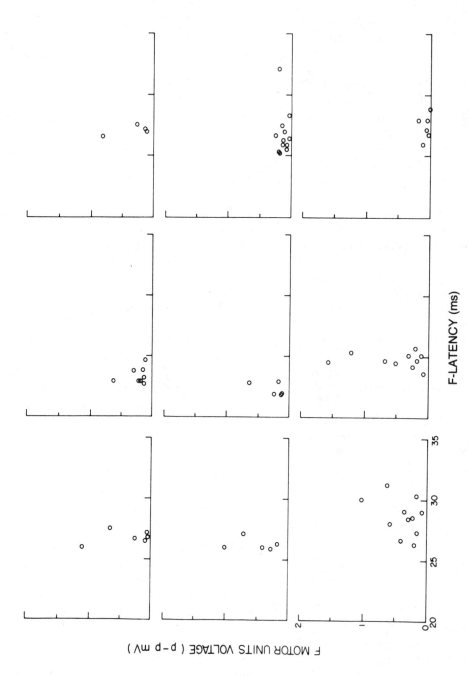

F-LATENCY (ms)

F MOTOR UNITS VOLTAGE (p-p mV)

FIGURE 3.33.   Range in latencies of single MUPs in the F-response as recorded from the thenar or hypothenar muscle groups in response to percutaneous stimulation at the wrist of the respective median and ulnar nerves in 9 subjects. The surface-recorded peak-to-peak voltages (p-pV) of the MUPs in millivolts (mV) are also shown. The range in latencies varied between 2.5 and 7 ms, indicating a possible range in the conduction velocities of the motor axons of 10 to 30 percent with these methods.

3. Conduction block in some of the antidromically conducted impulses in the motor axon
4. Possible changes in turnabout time because of alterations in central excitability of the motoneuron
5. Changes in the chance of reflection of impulses because of changes in central excitabilities of motoneurons

Slowing of motor conduction is the most obvious reason for delaying the F-response. Such slowing may be throughout the length of the motor axon or may, as in many axonopathies, be most pronounced in the distal positions of the axon. Alternatively, the slowing may be proximally located, perhaps in a root or plexus. Not proved is whether minimum latencies of the potentials in the F-response are as representative of the fastest-conducting motor axons in all the above diseases as is true in health. In certain diseases the antidromic impulses in some motor axons may be blocked between the site of stimulation and the spinal cord or the excitabilities of the motoneurons changed so as to alter the chances of reflection of the impulse; here the shortest-latency F-potentials may be representative of conduction in the fastest motor axons.

For example, conduction block among the fastest motor axons proximal to the stimulus site may result in an apparently slowed proximal conduction velocity. The longer latencies of the F-response in this case, however, may simply reflect only the F-responses of normally slower-conducting motor axons whose antidromic impulses were not blocked proximally. Such selective block of the faster-conducting myelinated NFs is a feature of nerve compression.

Recent evidence, however, suggests the opposite, namely, selective block of the more slowly conducting, smaller myelinated NFs in experimental allergic neuritis (Sumner, 1980; Lafontaine, Rasminsky, Saida, and Sumner,

1982) and perhaps also in human Guillain-Barré polyneuropathy. The point to be remembered is that one must be cautious in interpreting the F-latencies as measurements of proximal conduction where conduction block may coexist.

As was also mentioned, the chance of reflection of the antidromic impulse may change in various diseases. For example, even though in healthy subjects the chance of an F-response in any one motoneuron is somewhat less than $1:10$ antidromic impulses, our experience has been that in some peripheral neuropathies this is sometimes increased dramatically, to as high as $1:2$ antidromic impulses or higher. Thus even though large numbers of motoneurons (or their axons) may have been lost, a greater proportion of the remaining motoneurons is able to generate reflected impulses.

Other Late Responses

Not all late responses are the reflected impulses of motoneurons. Other possible late potentials include H-reflexes, proximal axon reflexes, and possible recurrent direct excitation.

1. H-reflexes (see earlier discussion). The latency fluctuations of MUPs in the H-response exceed 0.1 ms, values well in excess of comparable latency fluctuations of single MUPs in the F-response (Table 3.17). The absolute latencies of H-potentials are sometimes 1 to 2 ms shorter than those of F-potentials, possibly because the afferent limb of the H-reflex may conduct faster than do the motor axons themselves.

The H-potentials, of course, are most characteristically identified when they appear below threshold for the direct M-response. Continuing to increase the stimulus intensity beyond motor threshold does eventually cause a progressive reduction in amplitude of not only the H-reflex (see earlier discussion), but the F-potential as well (Yates and Brown, 1979).

The H- and F-potentials can and do probably combine to produce the late response at stimulus intensities above motor threshold, but it is difficult to distinguish between them. Assessing the fluctuations in latency of single MUPs using single-fiber EMG techniques is one way to do this. Experimentally, they may be readily separated by sectioning the dorsal roots, the remaining late potentials being reflected impulses in motor axons only (Gassel and Wiesendanger, 1965; McLeod and Wray, 1966; Mayer and Feldman, 1967).

2. Proximal axon reflexes. There is no evidence as yet in normal subjects of motor axon branching in the plexuses or roots. Such proximal axon branching could, however, develop following injuries to the roots or plexuses or, in the case of other diseases, where regeneration of motor axons begins at very proximal levels. Such hypothetical axon reflexes could be expected to share the characteristics of axon reflexes seen elsewhere and, as such, to disappear once the stimulus intensity is increased to a level at which all peripheral branches are excited directly by the stimulus.

3. Possible recurrent direct excitation (transsynaptic) by collaterals belonging to nearby motoneurons (Cullheim, Kellerth, and Conradi, 1977; see related discussion in Yates and Brown, 1979).

Methods for Eliciting and Studying the F-Response

The simplest way to elicit the F-response for clinical study, for example, in the ulnar nerve, is to stimulate the nerve at the wrist and record the direct M- and F-response latencies from the hypothenar muscles. The F-latency in such a case is the sum of: the antidromic conduction time between the site of stimulation and the motoneuron plus turnabout time (about 1 ms) plus the time for the reflected impulse to conduct from its site of origin to the muscle. When the site of stimulation is so distal, the F-potentials are distorted the least by the preceding stimulus and direct M-potential artifacts.

In peripheral neuropathies where conduction velocities in the motor axons are slowed, the latencies of the F-response will be correspondingly prolonged unless there is some very disproportionately greater delay over the most proximal segments. In this case the F-latency should be increased out of proportion to any peripheral slowing.

To assess proximal conduction in motor axons more directly, the F-response may be elicited by stimulation of the motor nerve at a more proximal level and calculating the proximal conduction time between the site of stimulation and the spinal cord by:

$$\text{Proximal conduction time (ms)} = \frac{\left(\begin{array}{cc} & \text{direct M} \\ \text{F-latency} & \text{latency} \\ \text{(in ms)} & -\text{ (in ms)} \end{array} \right)}{2} - 1$$

One millisecond is subtracted because part of the F-latency is accounted for by the turnabout time here considered to be 1 ms. Technically, however, in such recordings the F-response is severely distorted by the direct M-potential. The latter may be removed by delivery of a second supramaximal stimulus distally, so timed that the resulting antidromic impulses collide with and block all the distally conducting impulses in the same fibers that began their course at the proximal site of stimulation (Kimura, 1974; Kimura, Bosch, and Lindsay, 1975; Kimura and Butzer, 1975; Kimura, 1977, 1978) (Figure 3.34).

The preceding modification through the use of the two stimulus sites makes it possible to measure:

FIGURE 3.34. The F-response collision technique. (Top) Shown is a representative single motoneuron, its axon and postsynaptic complement of muscle fibers. A stimulus (S1) delivered distally along the path of the axon and of sufficient intensity to generate an action potential in the axon will result in both a centripetally and centrifugally conducted impulse. The latter generates the M-potential in the muscle.

Should a second stimulus (S2) be delivered more proximally to the same axon and be so timed in its delivery with respect to the S1 stimulus that the centripetal impulse originating at S1 collides with the centrifugally conducted impulse from S2, the M-potential the latter would otherwise have produced will be abolished. Such an M-potential would, because of its latency, have severely distorted the F-response produced by the S2 stimulus.

(Bottom) The use of this technique in whole motor nerves is illustrated below, where it can be seen that the M-potential distorts the F-potential when the proximal S2 stimulus is delivered alone (S2). However, when supramaximal stimuli are delivered both at S2 and distally (S1) and these stimuli are so timed with respect to one another that the direct M-potential elicited by the stimulus at S2 is abolished by collision with centripetally conducted impulses originating at S1, the way is cleared for a relatively distortion free presentation of the S2 elicited F-potentials (S1 + S2) and for the electromyographer to identify more reliably the onset of the proximal stimulus elicited F-potentials.

Note that the difference in latency (t2) between the shortest latency F motor unit potentials (F2 bottom trace) and longer latency F motor unit potentials (F1 top trace) is usually equal to the latency difference (t1) between the respective maximum M-potentials (M1 and M2). This indicates that equivalently fast conducting fibers are responsible for the earliest components of both the F- and M-potentials.

F-RESPONSE + COLLISION

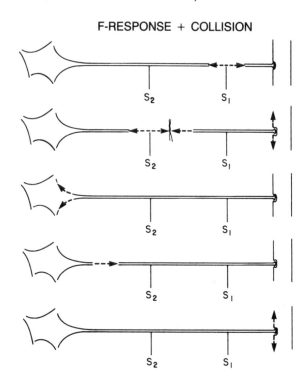

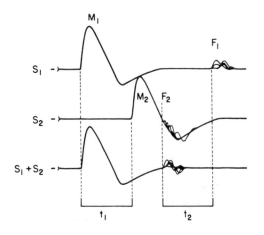

1. The maximum conduction velocity between these two sites of stimulation both with respect to the direct M- and the F-potentials
2. The motor terminal latency
3. The proximal conduction time

Thus it combines in one study several useful measures of motor conduction.

Measurement of the maximum motor conduction velocity between two or more sites of stimulation using the F-responses has the added advantage of proving whether or not the F-responses have been generated by the fastest-conducting fibers. There is no point in converting proximal conduction times measured with the F-response to conduction velocities because the distances to the spinal cord cannot be measured accurately (Young and Shahani, 1978).

One method proposed for comparing proximal and distal conduction times is to calculate the so-called F-ratio; namely, the ratio of the F-latency central to the point of stimulation to the direct M-latency measured distal to the point of stimulation.

$$\text{Central F-latency (ms)} = \frac{\text{F-latency (ms)} - \text{Direct M-latency (ms)}}{2} - 1$$

$$\text{F-ratio} = \frac{\text{Central F-latency (ms)}}{\text{Direct M-latency (ms)}}$$

$$\text{or} = \frac{\left(\dfrac{\text{F-latency (ms)} - \text{Direct M-latency (ms)}}{2}\right) - 1}{\text{Direct M-latency (ms)}}$$

Clearly, as the point of stimulation is moved proximally, the latency of the direct M-potentials will increase and that of the F-potential decrease. This changes the ratios, and so normal values and ranges of these ratios must be established for each level of stimulation because their values depend on the site of stimulation. Normative values have been established for this ratio.

Value of the F-Response in Clinical EMG

The primary value of the F-response technique is its use as an adjunct to other electrophysiological procedures for assessing conduction in motor axons in various disorders of the peripheral nervous system (see discussions by Kimura, 1978; Young and Shahani, 1978; Lachman, Shahani, and Young, 1980). Five examples follow.

Demonstration of Proximal Conduction Delays in Root Lesions

Despite reports by others (Eisen, Schomer, and Melmed, 1977a, 1977b), the author has not found that the F-response technique has much value in the assessment of the common root entrapments (C6 and C7) in the upper limb. The easiest motor nerves to test in the arm, namely, the median and ulnar nerves, include motor axons of multisegmental origin; namely, C7–T1 for the median and C8–T1 in the ulnar nerve. Even though the C7 root does make some contribution to the innervation of intrinsic muscles in the hand, this contribution is minor in relation to the C8 and T1 contributions. Also, the C6 contribution to the median nerve at the wrist is sensory, not motor. For muscles whose motor innervation is multisegmental, normal conduction in the preserved segment may well mask any apparent conduction delays of F-responses transmitted through the abnormal root segment.

The technique may be more valuable in the lower limb where the two most common root entrapments, namely, the L5 and S1 roots, may be tested in relative isolation by stimulating either the common peroneal or posterior tibial nerve, L5 being the dominant root contribution to peroneal muscles and S1 the main root innervation of the gastrocnemius and soleus muscles (see Eisen, Schomer, and Melmed, 1977b). The author has yet, however, to detect a delay in the F-response or combined H- and F-responses in the latter muscle where there were not already strong clinical indications of such root lesions.

Demonstration of Conduction Delays in Brachial and Lumbosacral Plexus Lesions

The F-response techniques are more valuable in brachial and lumbosacral plexus lesions because these lesions are more extensive than root lesions, and motor axons of multiple segmental origin are involved. Therefore F-latencies tend to be more prolonged in plexus than in single root lesions.

Demonstration of Slower Proximal Conduction in Guillain-Barré Polyneuropathy

Several authors have reported prolonged latencies of the F-response across proximal segments of the peripheral nervous system in Guillain-Barré polyneuropathy (Kimura and Butzer, 1975; Kimura, 1977; King and Ashby, 1976). Disproportionate increases in proximal conduction times in relation to more distal conduction were thought to suggest more severe involvement of the proximal segments (plexus and roots). While this interpretation may be correct, proximal conduction block in the fastest-conducting motor axons could also account for the same apparent slowing as pointed out earlier. Moreover, it is not uncommon for the F-response in Guillain-Barré polyneuropathy to be composed of very few MUPs. The latter raises questions about how representative the remaining MUPs in the F-response are of the fastest-conducting motor axons. Moreover, the F-response is all too often absent in Guillain-Barré polyneuropathy in the early course of the disease, possibly because of conduction block in most or all of the motor axons that would normally be capable of reflected impulses.

Demonstration of Conduction Abnormalities in other Peripheral Neuropathies and Motoneuron Diseases

Conduction abnormalites may be shown by the F-response technique in peripheral neuropathies and amyotrophic lateral sclerosis at stages when more conventional measures of motor conduction may be less abnormal or indeed, their values in the normal range. Examples include Charcot-Marie-Tooth disease (Kimura, 1974), amyotrophic lateral sclerosis (Argyropoulos, Panayiotopoulos, and Scar-palezos, 1978), and other peripheral neuropathies (Lachman, Shahani, and Young, 1980).

Assessment of the Excitabilities of Motoneurons

The F-technique is one way of measuring the excitabilities of motoneurons in central disorders (Fisher, Shahani, and Young, 1978; Schiller and Stålberg, 1978).

In summary, the F-technique is of some value for assessing conduction in peripheral neuropathies. Critical uncertainties remain, however, about how representative the MUPs participating in the F-response are of the fastest-conducting motor axons, especially where conduction block may be present or the number of MUPs is very reduced.

CLINICAL ASSESSMENT OF PERIPHERAL NEUROPATHIES

The objectives of clinical and electrophysiological examinations are to establish the basic distribution and functional characteristics of the peripheral neuropathy. When taken together with the history and other laboratory evidence, these data provide information about the probable cause, severity of the neuropathy, and, in some instances, direction as to its appropriate treatment. Clinical examination should provide an indication as to the general distribution of the abnormalities in the peripheral nervous system based on an assessment of the pattern of weakness (and wasting, if present) and the sensory examination. The two most common patterns of neuropathies seen in practice are the mononeuropathies and distal, symmetrical, peripheral neuropathies (see review by Schaumberg, Spencer, and Thomas, 1983).

The most common *mononeuropathies* are the root and peripheral nerve entrapment syndromes. In many of these entrapments the best evidence as to localization is the patient's description of the distribution of *paresthesias* referred to the peripheral cutaneous distribution of the root or nerve, and the *pain*. Pain, commonly of a deep quality, is often more widespread and perhaps referred to deeper structures such as muscles, interosseous membranes, joints, and other tissues innervated by the affected nerve. These paresthesias and perhaps pain are probably explained by the generation of ectopic impulses and possibly multiplication of the same by ephaptic transmission to nearby fibers at the injury site (see recent review by Culp and Ochoa, 1982; see also Chapter 9). Such abnormal trigger zones in nerves may sometimes be brought out by tapping the nerve (Tinel's phenomenon). In the early stages of such neuropathies, the neurological examination is often normal and electrophysiological studies may be normal as well, either because the functional disturbances are truly intermittent with full restoration of normal impulse transmission and membrane excitability between times of injury; or the injury is so discrete or mild as to make detection of any local and persisting conduction abnormalities impossible. Of course, in entrapment or other injuries involving pure motor nerves such as the suprascapular, long thoracic, and posterior and anterior interosseous nerves, there are no cutaneous phenomena. Therefore recognition must await the development of weakness, which may signal conduction block, axonal degeneration, or some combination of the two in the distribution of the nerve. Only later in the evolution of the mononeuropathy when persisting conduction abnormalities are extensive or severe enough to be detected and possibly wallerian degeneration develops, is the electromyographer able to detect and localize the site of the lesion.

The contrary problem occurs also; that is, local conduction abnormalities may be demonstrable in a peripheral nerve at a common site of entrapment or compression such as the median nerve in the carpal tunnel, and the patient may report either no symptoms or only occasional symptoms in respect to the nerve in question. Provided the electrophysiological studies have been properly chosen, executed, and interpreted, there is little reason to question the validity of the findings. Such apparently subclinical abnormalities do raise the important point that clinical symptoms and demonstrable conduction abnormalities do not always coincide. The proper course is to note the electrophysiological findings but proceed to manage the patient on the basis of the primary complaints except where subclinical abnormalities shed new light on the diagnosis.

The other common neuropathy pattern is that of the distal, symmetrical, sensorimotor neuropathy. In such neuropathies, weakness (with or without wasting) and sensory loss often make their earliest appearance in the distal lower limb and advance centripedally. By the time the sensory loss reaches or passes the ankle, sensory signs appear in the tips of the fingers. Further proximal advance of sensory impairment to the thigh and forearm may be accompanied by the appearance of sensory impairment over the ventral abdomen and still later, the central face. The whole pattern suggests that sensory fibers are affected in order of their length, although not necessarily in order of their diameters. Proximal advance of the motor signs may also be apparent.

In such neuropathies, electrophysiological abnormalities tend to parallel the distribution and severity of clinical findings in that conduction and evidence of nerve fiber degeneration (if present) are often more severe in the lower limbs and toward the distal extremities of the limbs. Often, however, conduction abnormalities and sometimes denervation are apparent well before the appearance of clinically apparent alterations in sensation.

It should also be pointed out here that in many such generally distributed peripheral neuropathies, abnormalities in conduction at common entrapment sites (carpal tunnel, cubital tunnel or tansepicondylar segments in the ulnar nerve, fibular head in the peroneal nerve, etc.) exceed those present proximal or distal to the compression site. These localized and disproportionate conduction abnormalities suggest that they have been caused by local trauma to which such patients may be disposed because they are prevented by paralysis, sensory loss, or mental disturbance from avoiding the compression or traction of these nerves. In any cases, such local injuries and conduction abnormalities are very common, for example, in chronic neuropathies such as the symmetrical sensorimotor or acute Guillain-Barré polyneuropathy. There may be special liability to injury of these nerves because of the general neuropathic changes as has been suggested in experimental diphtheritic neuritis (Hopkins and Morgan-Hughes, 1968).

Less common patterns in peripheral neuropathies include pure motor or sensory neuropathies or those involving plexuses and multiple peripheral nerves in an asymmetrical pattern (often called mononeuritis multiplex). Electromyographical studies in the last may be valuable because they help to define the localization of the clinically apparent neuropathies, they may unmask some that are not clinically apparent, and they provide informative data about the severity of the nerve fiber loss, both motor and sensory.

Correlations between Motor and Sensory Abnormalities Based on Clinical Examination and Electrophysiological Changes

The objective of clinically examining the motor system is to work out the pattern and semiquantitate the degree of weakness as well as wasting, if the latter is present. In most cases, it should be possible to localize, some-

times precisely while at other times more approximately, the distribution of the neuropathy from the clinical examination.

The critical motor findings of weakness and wasting need some comment. Weakness is produced through one of two basic mechanisms in peripheral neuropathies: degeneration of motor axons (and possibly the parent motoneurons) or conduction block somewhere between the motoneuron and the axon terminals or, as in some cases, a combination of the two. Neuromuscular block is probably not an important source of weakness except in rapidly progressive motoneuronal or axonal degeneration where failures are common in neuromuscular transmission at junctions undergoing degeneration or in immature, recently established end-plates. Excessive temporal dispersion alone of impulses in motor axons is a most unlikely cause of any weakness because MUs in most cases are asynchronously recruited. In any case, twitch durations are so long in relation to conduction times in the motor axons that even substantial temporal disarray in the arrival times of impulses in motor axons at the muscles probably produces very little if any noticeable motor disability.

Wasting, the other cardinal motor sign, is most commonly an indication of the presence of substantial axonal degeneration. Wasting may, however, take from three to five weeks or more to become apparent in acute neuropathies such as acute compression injuries, neuralgic amyotrophy, or axonopathies. Conversely, in chronic, very slowly progressive neuropathies, it may not be apparent at all because of ongoing reinnervation despite substantial losses of motor axons.

Wasting may also not be detected in some muscles such as the iliacus, psoas, subscapularis, deep jaw, extraocular, or lid muscles, because they are either inaccessible by palpation or inspection, or loss of muscle mass may be masked by overlying thick subcutaneous tissue, as in the case of the thigh and hip girdle muscles, even in otherwise lean individuals. In some such instances computed tomography or nuclear magnetic resonance scanning may more fully reveal the full extent of wasting.

Of course, wasting may also be caused by disuse. Here EMG recordings may be invaluable in providing clear indications of denervated muscle fibers, collateral reinnervation, and other evidence of reconstituted MUs (see Chapter 8).

To what extent motor conduction velocities and maximum M-amplitudes appear to correlate with the clinical picture and severity of the neuropathy depends on the selection of muscles, nerves, and functions to be studied. For example, within the first 1 to 2 weeks following onset of paralysis in acute Guillain-Barré neuropathy, the maximum motor and sensory conduction velocities, as commonly studied, are often within the normal range, becoming abnormally slowed only later, when the patients are often recovering clinically. This apparent discrepancy is clarified somewhat by the realization that the paralysis correlates much better with the presence of demonstrable conduction block in the nerves and that one of the reasons that the peripheral conduction velocities remain so normal may be because of preferential involvement of the more slowly conducting motor axons (Lafontaine, Rasminsky, Saida, and Sumner, 1982).

Good correlations have been shown between nerve fiber densities in nerve biopsies and the size of the maximum M-potential (Bolton, Gilbert, Girvin, and Hahn, 1979) in chronic neuropathies. Of course, this would not be expected in neuropathies where conduction block is present to any degree.

Motor conduction studies are also done most commonly using distal muscles (foot and hand) as the recording site. Such a selection works out best where the primary objective in the electrophysiological study is early detection of a motor abnormality in, for example, a dying-back neuropathy that becomes manifest earliest and most severely in the distal extremities. The choice of distal muscles may be less useful for correlating electrophysiological abnormalities with clinical status unless the clinical examination makes specific reference to the functions of the distal muscles tested electrophysiologically. Disability measures such as walking, sitting up, rolling over, or using the arms correlate much better with changes in the proximal limb and trunk muscles than they do with distal extremity muscles. In the case of the foot muscles, they may be so severely affected as to be completely denervated in patients who have very little overall functional disability. In those who are moderately to severely affected, the maximum motor conduction velocities to such distal muscles may be based on fewer than five fibers; not a very representative number in a nerve such as the anterior tibial nerve branch to the extensor digitorum brevis muscle that normally contains 100 or more motor axons (see Chapter 6).

Better correlations between clinical disability and electrophysiological studies are possible when the latter also include more proximally innervated and often less severely affected muscles and nerves in assessment of the neuropathies.

Fasciculation and *neuromyotonia* are usually readily recognized clinically and indicate ectopic spontaneous activity at various sites in the motor axons (see Chapter 9).

Sensory Examination

It was pointed out earlier in this chapter that the main spike components of the sensory nerve action potential are generated by the larger and faster-conducting (30 to 65 m/s) myelinated sensory fibers. Therefore alteration in maximum sensory conduction velocity and the size and shape of the sensory nerve action potential should correlate best with clinical sensory functions served by the larger sensory afferents. These include vibration sense, two-point discrimination, and touch localization as well as the tendon reflex, rather than abnormalities in the smaller myelinated and unmyelinated fibers serving nociceptive temperature and autonomic functions. While this generally holds true, there are exceptions.

For example, lesions central to the dorsal root ganglia involving the dorsal roots or ascending sensory tracts may be associated with clinical sensory disturbances attributable to the activities of the larger peripheral afferents and their receptors, and sensory conduction assessed peripheral to the dorsal root ganglia will, as expected, be normal. Conduction block confined to the proximal portion of the larger afferents may also be associated with normal peripheral sensory conduction, provided no appreciable number of the larger sensory fibers has undergone degeneration distal to the lesion.

Where neuronopathies affect the dorsal root ganglion cells, the resulting degeneration of the central as well as peripheral processes of these cells, sometimes advancing in a centripetal fashion toward the cell body, may be apparent in peripheral and central (dorsal column) sensory conduction studies. Such a pattern of combined peripheral and central degeneration, for example, may be seen in vitamin B_{12} deficiency.

It sometimes happens too, that even though clinical sensory testing reveals abnormalities in large fiber functions, sensory conduction in the same nerve is normal. This could, for example, happen in an axonopathy affecting the receptor end-organs first, and which subsequently progresses centripetally. Conventional sensory conduction studies bypass the receptor end-organs and indeed, in most instances, begin as much as 30 to 100 mm proximal to the end-organs. Experimental acry-

lamide neuropathy (see Chapter 2) is one such example in which degeneration begins in the distal extremity of the sensory axon, interrupts receptor function first, and then advances centripedally toward the CNS (see review by Sumner, 1980). In such cases it may be useful to devise a means of testing sensory function through methods designed to stimulate the receptor end-organs themselves rather than by stimulating the afferents proximally, thereby effectively bypassing the receptors themselves. Such natural stimulus-evoked nerve action potentials are often difficult to detect, however, because of the usually very asynchronous nature of the afferent volley.

Unlike the motor side where abnormal spontaneous impulse activity in axons or the muscle is readily betrayed in some instances by simple inspection or palpation (fasciculation, neuromyotonia) or by recording from the muscle, similar activity in sensory fibers is not so easily detected. The reason is that the signals, nerve fiber action potentials, are much smaller and more difficult to record, requiring intraneural recordings with microelectrodes.

Abnormal spontaneous activity in sensory fibers is apparent, however, to the patient who reports sensations such as tingling, prickling, or pain. Careful attention to the distribution of such symptoms, as mentioned in the discussion on mononeuropathies, often provides the earliest evidence of a neuropathy and very helpful information about the localization of the responsible lesions.

Finally, it is worth pointing out the extent to which the clinical examination can indicate something of the nature of the morphological and physiological changes in the underlying nerves. Clearly, any substantial degree of wasting strongly suggests the presence of degeneration of motor axons, and the absence of such in the face of much weakness in an established neuropathy probably indicates the presence of a significant degree of conduction block. Conduction block in turn is a strong indicator of the probable presence of demyelination.

Other suggestive evidence of demyelination (and possibly remyelination) as the predominant morphological change in the peripheral nerves are the early or disproportionate loss of tendon reflexes and vibration, both functions that probably depend on a high degree of temporal coincidence in the transmission of their respective afferent impulses. Nerve hypertrophy, often accompanied by increased firmness of the nerve and especially when seen or felt outside of common entrapment sites where thickenings of the epineurium of peripheral nerve are common, is usually an indication of onion bulb formation and repeated demyelination and remyelination in the underlying nerve.

The preceding discussion is intended simply to indicate the limits of the correlations possible between the neurological and EMG examinations. The two are entirely complimentary and an adequate EMG examination cannot be practiced or its results interpreted properly without reference to the knowledge derived from the clinical examination. Both are enriched by selected studies of nerve and muscle biopsies.

The Place of Nerve Biopsies and the Correlation Between Electrophysiological and Morphological Studies

Nerve biopsy has become an important tool in the investigation of peripheral neuropathies in selected cases (Stevens, Lofgren, and Dyck, 1973; Weller and Cervos-Navarro, 1977; Asbury and Johnson, 1980; Buchthal and Behse, 1978). Morphological changes revealed by such biopsies do correlate closely with electrophysiological changes in monophasic action potentials recorded in vitro and the clinical study of conduction in the same or nearby nerves, as well as studies of muscles in the innervation territory of the nerve (i.e., motor) (Table 3.18).

Biopsy examination of peripheral nerve tissues should provide quantitative morphological data on:

1. The density of nerve fibers per unit cross-sectional area
2. Fiber size (diameter) distribution of the nerve, including myelinated and unmyelinated nerve fiber populations
3. Morphologic changes in the nerve fiber including, most important, evidence of axonal/wallerian degeneration, axonal regeneration (with regeneration clusters), and demyelination (paranodal and internodal) and remyelination

The frequency and distribution of the changes noted in point 3 are best appreciated by quantitative analysis of teased fibers.

Complete study of nerve tissue should also include examination of the connective tissue and vesicular components, especially where there is reason to suspect abnormalities in these structures and where their study may provide an indication of the specific cause of the neuropathy.

Biopsy specimens studied in the above manner provide an appreciation of the fiber sizes predominantly affected and the nature of the fundamental process, namely, if the disorder is one predominately affecting the axons or the Schwann cells and myelin sheath.

This appreciation is helpfully supplemented by obtaining biopsy tissue from a nearby muscle, study of which may provide important evidence of denervation, reinnervation, vasculitis, or other specific changes of value in the appreciation of the neuropathies. There are, however, certain limitations in the value of nerve biopsies.

First, of course, biopsies are not indicated in all patients with generalized neuropathies, only those where such information as it may provide may help to make a specific diagnosis possible. Second, the biopsy is necessarily a one-time study and therefore cannot be used

TABLE 3.18.   Correlation of Nerve Biopsy and Electrophysiological and Clinical Tests

Morphological Features in the Biopsy	Electrophysiological Correlates	Clinical Correlates	
		Motor	Sensory
Loss of nerve fibers			
Larger myelinated	↓ Amplitudes sensory nerve action	Weakness	↓ 2 point discrimination
	↓ Amplitudes M-potentials	± Wasting	↓ Vibration
	↓ Motor unit recruitment patterns		
	EMG evidence of denervated muscle fibers and neurogenic MUPs	± Fasciculation	↓ Touch
Smaller myelinated	No changes	—	
Unmyelinated			
Demyelination (± remyelination)	↓ Maximum sensory and motor sensory conduction velocities	—	↓ Pinprick sensation
			↓ Temperature sensation
	↑ Temporal dispersion of nerve action potentials and maximum M-potentials		↓ Tickle appreciation
			↓ Tendon reflex
			↓ Vibration sense
	± Conduction block	Weakness ± Neurogenic tremor	

to follow the progress of a disease, unlike clinical and EMG examinations that lend themselves admirably to serial studies. Third, the biopsy represents but a short length of nerve at a very distal location and may not be representative, quantitatively at least and possibly qualitatively, of changes in the peripheral nerves at more proximal levels.

In some neuropathies the biopsy is able to provide more direct clues to the specific etiology of the neuropathy, examples being, metachromatic leukodystrophy, amyoloidosis, leprosy, the inflammatory polyneuritides, and the neuropathies seen in association with the various vasculities.

Unlike the EMG studies, however, biopsies provide critical information about smaller myelinated and unmyelinated nerve fibers; information that can be better appreciated by clinical examination when attention is paid to testing nociception, temperature appreciation, and autonomic function.

All three—the clinical examination, EMG studies, and nerve biopsy in selected cases—play mutually supporting roles in establishing the clinical diagnosis and in appreciating the physiological disturbances caused by the neuropathies.

References

Argyropoulos C, Panayiotopoulos CP, Scarpalezos S. F- and M-wave conduction velocity in amyotrophic lateral sclerosis. Muscle Nerve 1978;1:479–85.

Arvanitaki A. Effects evoked in an axon by the activity of a contiguous one. J Neurophysiol 1942;5:89–108.

Asbury AK, Johnson PC. Pathology of peripheral

nerve. In: Bennington JL, ed. Major problems in pathology. Vol. 9. Philadelphia: WB Saunders, 1980.

Behse F, Buchthal F. Sensory action potentials and biopsy of the sural nerve in neuropathy. Brain 1978;101:437–93.

Bergmans J. The physiology of single human nerve fibers. Louvain, Belgium, Vander, 1970.

Bergmans J. Physiological observations on single human nerve fibers. In: Desmedt JE, ed. New developments in electromyography and clinical neurophysiology. Basel: Karger, 1973:89–127.

Bischoff D, Thomas PK. Microscopic anatomy of myelinated nerve fibers. In: Dyck PJ, Thomas PK, Lambert EH, eds. Peripheral neuropathy. Philadelphia: WB Saunders, 1975:104–30.

Bolton CF, Carter K. Human sensory nerve compound action potential amplitude. Variation with sex and finger circumference. J Neurol Neurosurg Psychiatry 1980;43:925–28.

Bolton CF, Gilbert JJ, Girvin JP, Hahn A. Nerve and muscle biopsy: electrophysiology and morphology in polyneuropathy. Neurology (Minneap) 1979;29:354–62.

Bolton CF, Sawa GM, Carter K. The effects of temperature on human compound action potentials. J Neurol Neurosurg Psychiatry 1981; 44:407–13.

Boyd IA, Davey MR. Composition of peripheral nerves. Edinburgh: Livingstone, 1968.

Buchthal F, Behse F. Sensory action potentials and biopsy of the sural nerve in neuropathy. In: Canal N, Pozza G, eds. Peripheral neuropathies. Amsterdam: Elsevier North-Holland, 1978.

Buchthal F, Rosenfalck A. Evoked action potentials and conduction velocity in human sensory nerves. Brain Res 1966;3:1–122.

Buchthal F, Rosenfalck A. Sensory potentials in polyneuropathy. Brain 1971;94:241–62.

Buchthal F, Rosenfalck A, Behse F. Sensory potentials of normal and diseased nerve. In: Dyck PJ, Thomas PK, Lambert EH, eds. Peripheral neuropathy. Philadelphia: WB Saunders, 1975:442–64.

Clark FJ. Information signaled by sensory fibers in medial articular nerve. J Neurophysiol 1975;38:1466–72.

Clark FJ, Burgess PR. Slowly adapting receptors in cat knee joint: can they signal joint angle. J Neurophysiol 1975;38:1448–63.

Clough JFM, Kernell D, Phillips CG. Conduction velocity in proximal and distal portions of forelimb axons in the baboon. J Physiol 1968; 198:167–78.

Cullheim S, Kellerth JO, Conradi S. Evidence for direct synaptic inter-connections between cat spinal alpha-motoneurons via the recurrent axon collaterals: a morphological study using intracellular injection of horseradish peroxidase. Brain Res 1977;132:1–10.

Culp WJ, Ochoa J. Abnormal nerves and muscles as impulse generators. Oxford: Oxford University Press, 1982.

Cummins KL, Dorfman LJ. Nerve fiber conduction velocity distributions: studies of normal and diabetic human nerves. Ann Neurol 1981;9:67–74.

Cummins KL, Dorfman LJ, Perkel DH. Nerve fiber conduction velocity distributions. II. Estimation based on two compound action potentials. Electroencephalogr Clin Neurophysiol 1979;46:647–58.

Cummins KL, Dorfman LJ, Perkel DH. Nerve conduction velocity distributions: a method for estimation based upon two compound action potentials. In: Dorfman LJ, ed. Conduction velocity distributions: a population approach to electrophysiology of nerve. New York: Alan R. Liss, 1981:181–231.

Cummins KL, Perkel DH, Dorfman LJ. Nerve fiber conduction velocity distributions. I. Estimation based on the single fiber and compound action potentials. Electroencephalogr Clin Neurophysiol 1979;46:634–46.

Denys EH. The role of temperature in electromyography. Minimonograph 14. Rochester, Minn.: American Association of Electromyography and Electrodiagnosis, 1980:1–22.

Desmedt JE. A discussion of the methodology of the triceps surae T- and H-reflexes. In: Desmedt JE, ed. New developments in electromyography and clinical electromyography and neurophysiology. Basel: Karger, 1973:773–80.

Desmedt JE, Cheron G. Somatosensory evoked potentials to finger stimulation in healthy octogenarians and in young adults: wave forms, scalp topography and transit times of parietal and frontal components. Electroencephalogr Clin Neurophysiol 1980;50:404–25.

Desmedt JE, Noel P, Debecker J, Namèche J. Maturation of afferent conduction velocity as studied by sensory nerve potentials and by cerebral evoked potentials. In: Desmedt JE, ed. New developments in clinical electromyography and neurophysiology. Basel: Karger, 1973:52–63.

Dorfman LJ, Cummins KL, Reaven GM, Ceranski J, Greenfield MS, Doberne L. Studies of diabetic polyneuropathy using conduction velocity distribution (DCV) analysis. Neurology 1983;33:773–79.

Eccles, JC. The central action of antidromic impulses in motor nerve fibres. Pfluegers Arch 1955;260:385–415.

Eccles JC, Sherrington CS. Numbers and contraction values of individual motor units examined in some muscles of the limb. Proc R Soc Biol 1930;106:326–57.

Eccles RM, Phillips CG, Chien-Ping W. Motor innervation, motor unit organization and afferent innervation of M. extensor digitorum communis of the baboon's forearm. J Physiol 1968;198:179–92.

Eisen A, Schomer D, Melmed C. The application of F-wave measurements in the differentiation of proximal and distal upper limb entrapments. Neurology (Minneap) 1977a;27:662–68.

Eisen A, Schomer D, Melmed C. An electrophysiological method for examining lumbosacral root compression. Can J Neurol Sci 1977b;4:117–23.

Erlanger J, Gasser HS. Electrical signs of nervous activity. Philadelphia: University of Pennsylvania Press, 1937.

Ferrell WR. The adequacy of stretch receptors in the cat knee joint for signalling joint ankle throughout a full range of movement. J Physiol 1980;299:85–99.

Fisher MA, Shahani BT, Young RR. Assessing segmental excitability after acute rostral lesions. I. The F-response. Neurology 1978;28:1265–71.

Gamstrop I. Normal conduction velocity of ulnar, median and peroneal nerves in infancy, childhood and adolescence. Acta Paediatr Scand [Suppl] 1963;146:68–76.

Gamstrop I, Shelburne SA. Peripheral sensory conduction in ulnar and median nerves of nor-mal infants, children and adolescents. Acta Paediatr Scand 1965;54:309–13.

Gandevia SC, McCloskey DI. Joint sense, muscle sense, and their combination as position sense, measured at the distal interphalangeal joint of the middle finger. J Physiol 1976;260:387–407.

Gassel MM, Wiesendanger M. Recurrent and reflex discharges in plantar muscles of the cat. Acta Physiol Scand 1965;65:138–42.

Gasser HS. The classification of nerve fibers. Ohio J Sci 1941;41:145–59.

Gasser HS. Effect of the method of leading on the recording of the nerve fiber spectrum. J Gen Physiol 1960;43:927–40.

Gasser HS, Grundfest H. Axon diameters in relation to the spike dimensions and the conduction velocity in mammalian fibers. Am J Physiol 1939;127:393–414.

Gilliatt RW, Hopf HC, Rudge P, Baraitser M. Axonal velocities of motor units in the hand and foot muscles of the baboon. J Neurol Sci 1976;29:249–58.

Granit R, Leksell L, Skoglund CR. Fibre interaction in injured or compressed region of nerve. Brain 1944;67:125–40.

Grigg P, Greenspan BJ. Response of primate joint afferent neurons to mechanical stimulation of knee joint. J Neurophysiol 1977;40:1–8.

Gutrecht JA, Dyck PJ. Quantitative teased-fibre and histologic studies of human sural nerve during postnatal development. J Comp Neurol 1970;138:117–30.

Hodgkin AL, Katz B. The effect of sodium ions on the electrical activity of the giant axon of the squid. J Physiol 1949;108:37–77.

Hopf HC. Untersuchungen uber die unterschiede in der leitgeschwindegkeit motorischer nervenfasern. Dtsch Z Nervenheilkd 1962;183:579–88.

Hopkins AP, Morgan-Hughes JA. The effect of local pressure in diphtheritic neuropathy. Electroencephalogr Clin Neurophysiol 1968;25:399.

Horch KW, Clark FJ, Burgess PR. Awareness of knee joint angle under static conditions. J Neurophysiol 1975;38:1436–47.

Hulley WC, Wilbourn AJ, McGinty K. Sensory nerve action potential amplitudes; alterations with temperature. Abstract in twenty-fourth Annual Meeting American Association of Electromyography and Electrodiagnosis, Salt Lake City, September 30–October 1 1977.

Juul-Jensen P, Mayer RF. Threshold stimulation for nerve conduction studies in man. Arch Neurol (Chicago) 1966;15:410–19.

Kadrie H, Brown WF. Neuromuscular transmission in human single motor units. J Neurol Neurosurg Psychiatry 1978;41:193–204.

Kaeser HE. Nerve conduction velocity measurements. In: Vinken PJ, Bruyn GW, eds. Handbook of clinical neurology. Amsterdam: Elsevier North-Holland, 1970:116–94.

Katz B, Schmitt OH. Electric interaction between two adjacent nerve fibers. J Physiol 1940;97:471–88.

Kimura J. F-wave velocity in the central segment of the median and ulnar nerves: a study in normal subjects and in patients with Charcot-Marie-Tooth disease. Neurology 1974;24:539–46.

Kimura J. Proximal versus distal slowing of motor nerve conduction velocity in the Guillain-Barré syndrome. Ann Neurol 1977;3:344–50.

Kimura J. Clinical value and limitations of F-wave determination. A comment. Letter to the editor. Muscle Nerve 1978;1:350–51.

Kimura J. Electrodiagnosis in diseases of nerve and muscle. Philadelphia: FA Davis, 1983.

Kimura J, Bosch P, Lindsay G. F-wave conduction velocity in the central segment of the peroneal and tibial nerves. Arch Phys Med Rehabil 1975;56:492–97.

Kimura J, Butzer JF. F-wave conduction velocity in Guillain-Barré syndrome. Assessment of nerve segment between axilla and spinal cord. Arch Neurol 1975;32:524–29.

King D, Ashby P. Conduction velocity in the proximal segments of a motor nerve in the Guillain-Barré syndrome. J Neurol Neurosurg Psychiatry 1976;39:538–44.

Lachman T, Shahani BT, Young RR. Late responses as aids to diagnosis in peripheral neuropathy. J Neurol Neurosurg Psychiatry 1980; 3:156–62.

Lafontaine S, Rasminsky M, Saida T, Sumner AJ. Conduction block in rat myelinated fibers following acute exposure to antigalactocerebroside serum. J Physiol 1982;323:287–306.

Lambert EH, Dyck PJ. Compound action potentials of sural nerve in vitro in peripheral neuropathy. In: Dyck PJ, Thomas PK, Lambert EH, eds. Peripheral neuropathy. Philadelphia: WB Saunders, 1975:427–41.

Landau WM, Clare MH, Bishop GH. Reconstruction of myelinated nerve tract action potentials. An arithmetic method. Exp Neurol 1968;22:480–90.

Landon DN, Hall S. The myelinated nerve fiber. In: Landon DN, ed. The peripheral nerve. London: Chapman & Hall, 1976:1–105.

Lascelles RG, Thomas PK. Changes due to age in internodal length in the sural nerve in man. J Neurol Neurosurg Psychiatry 1966;29:40–44.

Lehmann HJ, Muche H, Schutt P. Refractory period of human sural nerve action potential related to age in healthy probands. Eur Neurol 1977;15:85–93.

Lloyd DPC. Neuron patterns controlling transmission of ipsilateral hindlimb reflexes in cat. J Neurophysiol 1943;6:293–315.

Low FN. The perineurium and connective tissue of peripheral nerve. In: Landon DN, ed. The peripheral nerve. London: Chapman & Hall, 1976:159–87.

Lowitzsch K, Hopf HC, Galland J. Changes of sensory conduction velocity and refractory periods with decreasing tissue temperature in man. J Neurol 1977;216:181–88.

Ludin HP, Beyelar F. Temperature dependence of normal sensory nerve action potentials. J Neurol 1977;216:173–80.

Ludin HP, Tackmann W. Sensory neuropathy. New York: Thieme-Stratton Incorporated, 1981.

Matthews PBC. Mammalian muscle receptors and their central action. London: Edward Arnold, 1972.

Mayer RF, Feldman RG. Observations on the nature of the F-wave in man. Neurology (Minneap) 1967;17:147–56.

McCloskey DI. Kinesthetic sensibility. Physiol Rev 1978;58:763–820.

McCloskey DI, Cross MJ, Honner R, Potter E. Sensory effects of pulling or vibrating exposed tendons in man. Brain 1983;106:21–38.

McGill KC, Cummins KL, Dorfman LJ, Berlizot BB, Luetkemeyer K, Nishimura DG, Widrow B. On the nature and elimination of stimulus artifact in nerve signals evoked and recorded using surface electrodes. IEEE Trans Biomed Eng 1982;BME29:129–36.

McLeod JG, Wray SH. An experimental study of the F-wave in the baboon. J Neurol Neurosurg Psychiatry 1966;29:196–200.

Moberg E. The role of cutaneous afferents in position sense, kinaesthesia and motor function of the hand. Brain 1983;106:1–20.

Norris AH, Shock NW, Wagman JH. Age changes in the maximum conduction velocity of motor fibers of human ulnar nerves. J Appl Physiol 1953;5:589–93.

Ochoa J, Mair WGP. The normal sural nerve in man: changes in axons and Schwann cells due to aging. Acta Neuropathol (Berl) 1971;13:217–39.

O'Sullivan DJ, Swallow M. The fiber size and content of the radial and sural nerves. J Neurol Neurosurg Psychiatry 1968;31:464–470.

Patton HD. Special properties of nerve trunks and tracts. In: Ruch TC, Patton HD, Woodbury JW, Towe AL, eds. Neurophysiology. Philadelphia: WB Saunders, 1965:73–94.

Ranck JB Jr. Extracellular stimulation. In: Patterson MM, Kesner RP, eds. Electrical stimulation research techniques. New York: Academic Press, 1981.

Rosenfalck A. Peripheral nerve. In: Cobb WA, ed. Handbook of electroencephalography and clinical neurophysiology. Amsterdam: Elsevier North-Holland, 1971:22–32.

Rosenfalck P. Intra- and extracellular potential fields of active nerve and muscle fibers. Acta Physiol Scand 1969;75(Suppl)321:1–168.

Schaumburg HH, Spencer PS, Thomas PK. Disorders of peripheral nerves. In: Plum F, ed. Contemporary neurology series. Philadelphia: FA Davis, 1983.

Schiller HH, Stålberg E. F responses studied with single fibre EMG in normal subjects and spastic patients. J Neurol Neurosurg Psychiatry 1978; 41:45–53.

Skoglund CR. Transsynaptic and direct stimulation of post fibers in the artificial synapse formed by severed mammalian nerve. J Neurophysiol 1949;8:365–76.

Stålberg E, Trontelj JV. Single-fibre electromyography. Surrey, England: Mirvalle Press, 1979.

Stegeman D. Compound nerve action potentials, an electrophysiological model study of human peripheral nerves in situ. Krips Repro Meppel, 1981.

Stevens JC, Lofgren EP, Dyck PJ. Histometric evaluation of branches of peroneal nerve: technique for combined biopsy of muscle nerve and cutaneous nerve. Brain Res 1973;52:37–59.

Sumner AJ. The physiological basis for symptoms in Guillain-Barré syndrome. Ann Neurol 1980;9(suppl):28–30.

Swallow M. Fiber size and content of the anterior tibial nerve of the foot. J Neurol Neurosurg Psychiatry 1966;29:205–13.

Tackmann W, Minkenberg R, Strenge H. Correlation of electrophysiological and quantitative histological findings in the sural nerve of man, studies on alcoholic neuropathy. J Neurol 1977;216:289–99.

Thomas PK, Olsson Y. Microscopic anatomy and function of the connective tissue components of peripheral nerve. In: Dyck PJ, Thomas PK, Lambert EH, eds. Peripheral neuropathy. Philadelphia: WB Saunders, 1975:168–89.

Thomas PK, Sears TA, Gilliatt RW. The range of conduction velocity in normal motor nerve fibers to the small muscles of the hand and foot. J Neurol Neurosurg Psychiatry 1959;22:175–81.

Trontelj JV. A study of the F-responses by single-fibre electromyography. In: Desmedt JE, ed. New developments in electromyography and clinical neurophysiology. Basel: Karger, 1973a:318–22.

Trontelj JV. A study of the H-reflex by single-fiber EMG. J Neurol Neurosurg Psychiatry 1973b;36:951–59.

Urich H. Diseases of peripheral nerves. In: Blackwood W, Corsellis JAN, eds. Greenfield's neuropathology. Chicago: Year Book Medical Publishers, 1976:688–770.

Vallbo AB, Hagbarth KE, Torebjork HE, Wallin BG. Somatosensory, proprioceptive and sympathetic activity in human peripheral nerves. Physiol Rev 1979;59:919–57.

Webster HdeF. Peripheral nerve structure. In:

Hubbard JI, ed. The peripheral nervous system. New York: Plenum Press, 1974:3–26.

Weller RO, Cervos-Navarro J. Pathology of peripheral nerves. London: Butterworth's, 1977.

Wuerker RB, McPhedran AM, Henneman E. Properties of motor units in a heterogeneous pale muscle (M. gastrocnemius of the cat). J Neurophysiol 1965;28:85–99.

Yates SK, Brown WF. Characteristics of the F-response: a single motor unit study. J Neurol Neurosurg Psychiatry 1979;42:161–70.

Young RR, Shahani BT. Clinical value and limitations of F-wave determination. Letter to the editor. Muscle Nerve 1978;1:248–49.

4 EVOKED POTENTIALS

Evoked potential techniques have been useful electrophysiological tools with which to investigate the projection of the skin surface onto the cerebral cortex in lower animals. Plots of the amplitude distributions of these potentials formed the basis of the now famous cartoon-like homunculi shown superimposed on the surface of the sensorimotor cortex. The sizes of the various body parts in such homunculi were approximately proportional to the areas of underlying cortex devoted to those parts. These potentials were evoked by mechanical taps delivered to the skin surface or through stimulation of the hair, and were carried out under deep barbiturate anesthesia. Electronic averaging techniques were not needed because of the large amplitudes of these potentials when recorded directly from the cortical surface (Woolsey and Erickson, 1950; Woolsey, 1952, 1964).

The techniques have been used to plot, in a more approximate manner, the localization of sensory function in the human cortex (Woolsey, Erickson, and Gilson, 1979). For the most part, these investigations were limited to the exposed cortical surface; little or no attempt was made to explore buried cortex.

Evoked potential techniques have been used also to locate and estimate quantitatively the level of electrical activity generated by large populations of neurons or neural elements. They are especially valuable when combined with single unit recordings to provide a picture of the background activities of large populations of neural elements against the activity of single units (Nicholson, 1979).

The detection of electrical stimulus and tendon jerk-evoked cortical potentials preceded the development of the earliest electronic averager (Dawson, 1947). Photographic superimposition and the good fortune that the first patient investigated had myoclonic epilepsy, in which disorder the amplitudes of the somatosensory evoked potentials are sometimes much enhanced, helped to ensure early success. Development of the electronic averager, however, was critical to the evolution and present success of these techniques and their application to the investigations of neurological disease.

Basic electrophysiological investigations have established the character of potentials recorded near the nerve roots or spinal cord in response to peripheral nerve stimulation in lower animals (see review by Willis, 1980); equivalent records being obtained by near root and cord recordings in man (Magladery, Porter, Park, and Teasdall, 1951). Much of the early work on the cortical evoked potentials in man concentrated on the effects of anesthesia, changes in the rates of stimulation on the potentials, and preliminary surveys of the changes in these potentials in various diseases (Halliday and Wakefield, 1963; Giblin, 1964; Domino, Matsuoka, Waltz, and Cooper, 1965; Desmedt, 1971). The shortest-latency components in the scalp-recorded potentials that could be reliably detected with the techniques then available were in the case of stimulation of the median nerve at the wrist, the negative potential at 20 to 22 ms, and sometimes a preceding positive potential at 15 ms (Broughton, 1969).

In recent years there has been renewed interest in evoked potential techniques in general because of technical improvements in electronic averagers and other components of the recording systems. In addition, the techniques have repeatedly demonstrated their value as detectors of subclinical lesions in multiple sclerosis and as aids to the localization of lesions in other central and peripheral nervous diseases. This chapter is devoted solely to the techniques of recording evoked potentials and their electrogenesis, with only brief comment on their value in diseases of the spinal cord and peripheral nerves.

GENERAL PATTERN OF THE SOMATOSENSORY EVOKED POTENTIAL EVOKED BY STIMULATION IN THE UPPER LIMB

Figures 4.1 and 4.2 illustrate the methods employed for the median nerve stimulus-evoked somatosensory evoked potential (SEP). In the median nerve and other peripheral nerves two basic methods may be employed: *far field recording* (FFR) and, for lack of a better term, *near field recording* (NFR) (Figure 4.3). Except when the recording electrode is immediately adjacent to or in the neural structure that generates the potential(s), all electrode recording sites are remote to some extent from the origins of the various potentials. In FFR,

however, no attempt is made to place the recording electrodes near the generators. These recordings take advantage of the fact that in the largely homogeneous conductor of the body, all recording sites are active to some extent and see the potentials. In FFRs, then, the reference (positive grid 2, or G_2) electrode is positioned at the most remote site possible; for example, the opposite hand or foot in the case of median nerve stimulation, or opposite leg in the case of posterior tibial nerve stimulation, the negative grid 1 (or G_1) being located on the scalp. In such recordings there is a series of *subcortical* (or precortical) positive waves that correspond to potentials generated in various neural structures in the peripheral and central nervous systems in the ascending sensory pathway.

In an attempt to increase the sizes and definition of the various subcortical potentials, NFR techniques may be used in which the G_1 electrode is placed as close to the probable generator(s) as possible; for example, over the peripheral nerve trunk at various levels, the spinal cord entry zone (cervical or lumbosacral), and various levels of the ascending pathway in the spinal cord (thoracic or cervical) in the case of lower limb stimulus sites. Even here, however, the distances between the neural generators and G_1 electrode may be appreciable (30 to 50 mm).

In the case of trigeminal evoked potentials, similar subcortical potentials can be detected. Here, however, NFR cannot be done because the peripheral and brainstem generators are obviously not accessible to a near-electrode recording.

In this chapter, the techniques employed to record somatosensory evoked potentials are discussed, including the technical aspects of these tests as well as the probable electrogenic origins of the various potentials. An outline of the practical uses of these tests is presented at the end of the chapter.

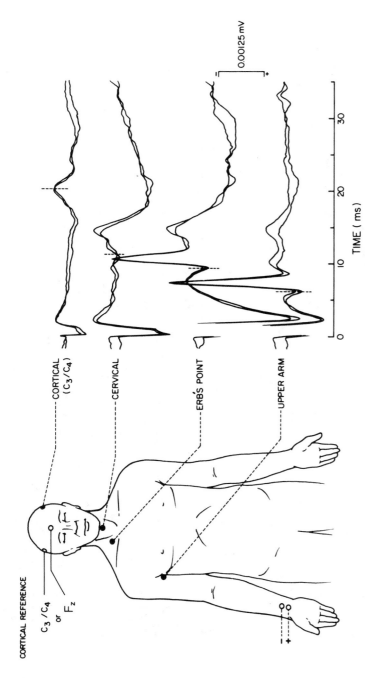

FIGURE 4.1.   Method for eliciting somatosensory evoked potentials in the upper limb. Here the median nerve is stimulated at the wrist (cathode proximal) and the orthodromic compound nerve action potentials at the levels of the proximal upper arm and Erb's point are recorded by surface electrodes over these sites. The cervical potential is recorded by a surface electrode over the C_6 spinous process and the contralateral cortical evoked potential by a needle electrode over C_3 or C_4. Suitable reference sites for all recording electrodes may be F_z; we prefer the ipsilateral C_3 or C_4 as the case may be.

The corresponding averaged potentials are shown on the right. The latencies (*interrupted vertical lines*) to the upper arm and Erb's point potentials are measured to the initial positive peak and to the cervical potential and cortical potentials to the onset and N20 peaks respectively. For each recording site two averages of 256 traces are shown.

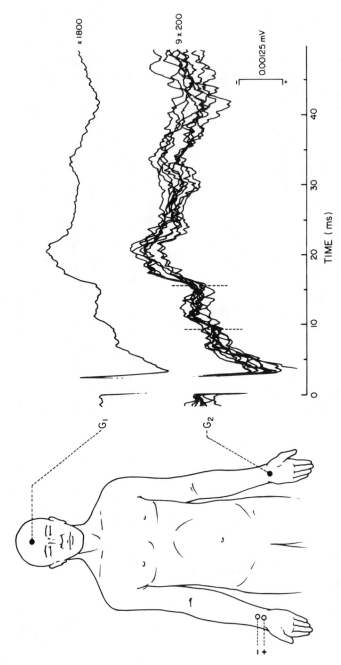

FIGURE 4.2.   Far field recording of somatosensory evoked potentials in response to median nerve stimulation at the wrist in the same subject as Figure 4.1. The G_1 electrode is positioned in this case at F_z and G_2 over the opposite hand. The top tracing is the electronic average of 1,800 responses; while below are superimposed electronic averages of successive groups of 200 responses in the above 1,800 to show variations among them.

The positive peak of the far field potential at 8 to 9 ms (*vertical interrupted line*) approximately corresponds with the potential recorded at Erb's point in Figure 4.1, although usually the latter occurs a little later, suggesting that the far field potential at 7 to 8 ms has a more distal origin in the brachial plexus than the Erb's point potential. The P15 potential in the far field recording (*vertical interrupted line*), although corresponding roughly in latency to the cervical potential, may well originate in the medial lemniscus. The negative potential at 20 ms corresponds closely to the $N_{20.9}$ potential in the cortical recording trace in Figure 4.1.

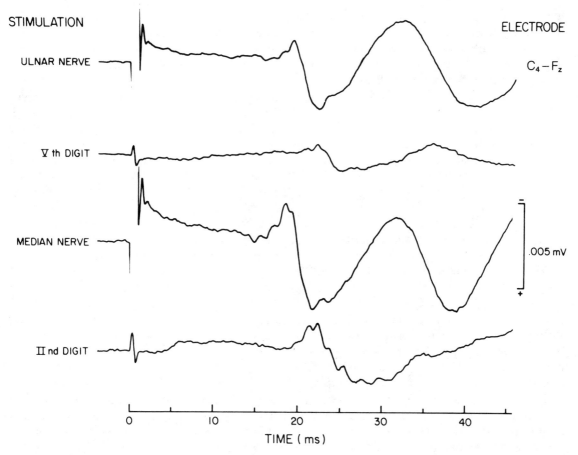

FIGURE 4.3. Comparison of cortical evoked potentials elicited by stimulation of mixed motor nerves such as the ulnar (top) and median nerves (bottom) at the wrist and the cortical potentials evoked by stimulation of the fifth and second digits. The recording electrode in this case was situated at C_4 and the reference electrode at F_z.

Note the longer latencies of the cortical potentials evoked by digit stimulation because of the longer peripheral conduction distances. The configurations of the potentials are basically very similar despite the fact that muscle afferents probably contribute to the cortical potentials elicited by mixed nerve stimulation, while such afferents are absent in digital nerves.

NOMENCLATURE

One important block to communication between laboratories has been the thorny problem of just how to name the potentials (see review by Donchin, Callaway, Cooper, Desmedt, Goff, Hillyard, and Sutton, 1977). The most practical and easiest method in the author's view is to designate the potentials by their latency and polarity, because it does not imply electrogenic sources. Such naming also accommodates any alterations in shape and latency because of differences in technique. This method that represents the best compromise is not without its problems, however, especially because the latencies of the peripherally and centrally generated potentials are dependent on the subject's height and limb length and may be characteristically changed in diseases of the peripheral and central nervous systems.

One important problem introduced by labeling potentials by their polarity is that sometimes G_1 is not the more active electrode and therefore one cannot make automatic assumptions about the polarity of a potential or its origin. Only when it is known which electrode (G_1 or G_2) is the more active can conclusions be drawn about the polarity of the potential. Thus the convention that upward deflections as seen at G_1 indicate a negative potential at G_1 may be correct only if G_1 is the more active electrode. The same upward deflection at G_1 could be produced if there were positivity at G_2, in which case G_1 would be negative only with respect to the greater positivity at G_2. The true polarity of the potential in the latter case is positive, not negative. Indeed, if G_1 and G_2 are both positive but the greater positivity is at G_2, there will be an upward deflection at G_1 because G_1 is less positive compared to G_2. The preceding illustrates the hazards of assuming polarity from any source of the potential based on the direction of the polarity shift at G_1 alone.

Therefore before drawing any conclusions about the sources of various potentials, it is important to establish the polarity and size of the potentials as seen at both G_1 and G_2. This can be accomplished by recording at each site against a remote reference; for example, an opposite limb at which sites are generally much less active in relation to a cervical or scalp electrode. The problem of the potentials as seen at G_2, especially when they are unappreciated, has led to interpretive problems in assessing the electrogenic origins of some of the subcortical and cortical potentials, particularly when comparing potentials of similar po-

larity as recorded in different laboratories with different electrode configurations.

To avoid the misinterpretations sometimes presented by labeling potentials as N (negative) or P (positive), others have suggested labeling components, for example, the cervical potential, by letters (A, B). This avoids implications about the likely electrogenic sources or which electrode is the more active (Chiappa, Choi, and Young, 1980); there has been no general acceptance of this system, nor has it been extended to later potentials in the SEP. Clearly too, such a system becomes cumbersome in the face of the wide variety of SEPs now recorded, including those in the trigeminal and lower limb distributions. Also, even in the upper limb, potentials at similar latencies, for example, those between 13 and 15 ms evoked by median nerve stimulation at the wrist may have quite different electrogenic origins, intracranial or spinal, depending on the electrode recording sites.

Overall therefore, despite the unhappy compromises inherent in designating potentials by latency and deflection at the G_1 electrode, this system is probably the most adaptable to the SEP techniques applicable, and so long as the investigator keeps clearly in mind that G_2 may be active, indeed more active than G_1, misinterpretations of the sources of potentials are less likely to happen.

In practice, the convention of labeling the major components of the SEP by polarity and latency works reasonably well. Even where the latencies vary because of differences in limb length or temperature or the potentials are delayed because of peripheral or central lesions, the configurations of the potentials are usually distinctive enough to allow for their confident identification.

Finally, it must be stressed that the convention of identifying various components by their peaks should not be taken to imply that electrical activity at some particular site or level begins or even reaches its peak at that time. This is especially true of the central components. Thus the identification of the N11 and N13–14 peaks in the cervical potential with the ascending volley in the dorsal column and the cord dorsum potential respectively (see later section) should not be taken to mean that these peaks necessarily correspond to the onset or peak activity times of these potentials.

In the peripheral nervous system the initial positive peak or onset of the negative spike does correspond more or less to the arrival of the nerve trunk potential beneath the leading recording electrode (see Chapter 3). Such a convention has little meaning with respect to the central nervous system, however, because here potentials at multiple levels often overlap and there are likely to be complex polarity and latency interactions between the various neural generators. For example, the posterior cervical-recorded cord dorsum potential, which is a broad potential lasting several ms and begins within 1 to 2 ms of the entry of the afferent volley into the cord, must clearly overlap with ascending volleys in the dorsal columns, spinocervical tract, and medial lemniscus, and perhaps even the earliest activity in the thalamocortical pathway to cortex. Since both electrodes are often active, especially in the case of cephalic references such as F_z, complex interactions between these spatially distributed but temporally coincident potentials are not only possible but likely.

ELECTRONIC REQUIREMENTS

Bandwidth Requirements

Somatosensory potentials do not contain the high-frequency (HF) components of motor unit potentials (MUPs) and it is not necessary therefore to use as wide a bandwidth in the recording system to record them. The main objective of the system is to record the poten-

tials as faithfully as possible to avoid displacements of peak latencies (Desmedt, Brunko, Debecker, and Carmeliet, 1974), while at the same time using as narrow a bandwidth as is compatible with this objective to reduce unwanted noise, primarily electroencephalographic (EEG) and electromyographic (EMG) potentials. The upper limit of the bandwidth of some of the subcortical potentials extends to about 1,000 c/s (3 db down), but that of the slower cortical potentials is lower (about 300 c/s) (Figure 4.4). The high-pass filter settings can be usefully set as high as 30 c/s in the case of cortical potentials, and in the case of spinal potentials as high as 100 c/s without serious distortions of the potentials being introduced. The higher high-pass filter setting for the spinal potentials helps to exclude 60 Hz of noise, which can be particularly troublesome in the operating room or intensive care unit. These bandwidth requirements may be maintained throughout the recording system, including tape recordings and electronic averaging systems.

The input impedances of the amplifiers should exceed by 1,000 times (less than 0.1 percent phase and amplitude distortion) the impedance of the electrodes used to record the evoked potentials. Because noise levels are a function of the impedance of the electrodes, these impedances should be kept as low as possible.

Electronic Averaging

Over a broad range of frequencies, noise reduction is proportional to the square root of the number of trials ($\sqrt{n}$) (Figure 4.5). The actually observed reductions in noise may be somewhat less when the amplitude of the noise greatly exceeds the size of the signal, especially when the noise is sinusoidal or includes electromyographical (EMG) potentials, when noise or artifact is time locked in some way to

FIGURE 4.4. Illustration to show the effect of changing the low-pass filter on the shapes and latencies of the nerve trunk potential recorded at the upper arm and the cortical potential recorded over the opposite hand region of the postcentral region in response to stimulation of the median nerve at the wrist. Individual traces are the electronic average of the 500 responses recorded previously on magnetic tape and subsequently replayed through a precision filtering device (Krohn-Nite Model 3700R Filter) at 10 to 2,000 Hz, 10 to 500 Hz, and 10 to 200 Hz (all 12 db down).

Note the reductions in amplitude, especially of the highest-frequency components (the spike component in the upper arm potential) relative to the slower components of the potentials as well as changes in the interpeak latencies of some of the components. For example: N19.1 to N21 (difference 1.9 ms), N27.9 to N31.7 (difference 3.8 ms), and P39.2 to P41.9 (difference 2.7 ms). There is an apparent shift in latencies with respect to onset of the stimulus, although not with respect to the peak of the stimulus artifact itself.

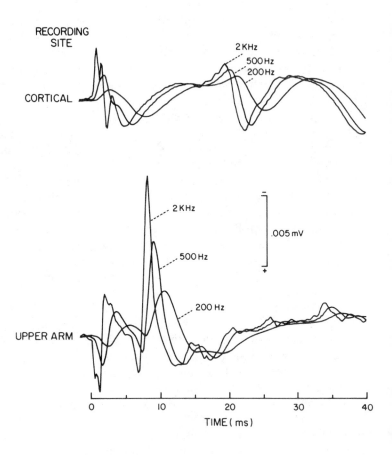

the stimulus, or when weighted averaging techniques are used. The sampling rate per channel should exceed by at least two times—or, better, four times—the upper limit of the bandwidth of the signals to be recorded. This corresponds to a bin width of no more than 250 μsec, and better 25 μsec (for 1,000 c/s upper frequency limit in a single-channel recording).

The vertical resolution should be 10 to 12 bits, or for a full-scale vertical deflection, the number of possible amplitude increments should be between 1,024 and 4,096. This is especially important if the amplitude of the event to be detected is less than 10 percent of the full-scale deflection. This degree of resolution provides 100 to 400 increments with which to resolve the recorded signals.

Most commercially available electronic averagers do not provide a true average but a

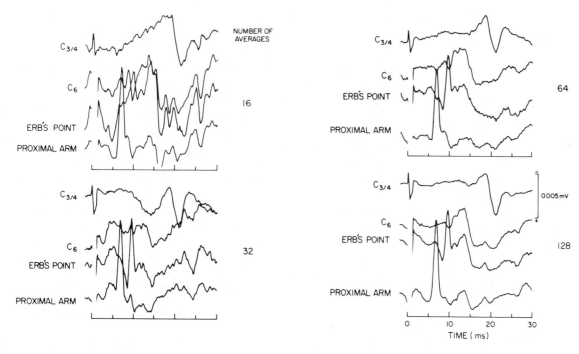

FIGURE 4.5. The progressively improved resolution of the various peripheral and central components of the somatosensory evoked potentials (same subject as Figure 4.3) as the number of averages is increased from 16 to 32 to 64 and 128 (top to bottom). Note that the general character of the potentials is defined well by 32 and not much improvement takes place between 64 and 128 in this relatively low-noise recording.

weighted average, and sometimes constantly rescale to provide a calibrated average in the course of the test in order to monitor the progress of the recording. Weighted averaging techniques, however, mean that the first few events averaged have more weight in the final average than later events.

Artifacts

The primary artifacts are listed in Table 4.1. It is not possible to exclude all artifact. It is possible in most subjects, however, to reduce the amount of *EMG activity* by taking a few moments to explain the procedure and help them to feel at ease. Sometimes excessive EMG activity makes it all but impossible to

obtain good recordings without the use of drugs to reduce anxiety and promote more complete relaxation. We prefer to use diazepam, 5 to 10 mg delivered slowly, if necessary by the intravenous route or preferably orally about one hour before the study.

The *corneoretinal potentials* accompanying ocular movement and the *EKG* artifacts may be excluded from the final average by incorporating a so-called pre-look facility in the recording. By this means any potentials occurring within the first 50 to 100 ms (exclusive of stimulus artifact) that exceed operator-adjustable preset amplitude limits in each channel can be rejected prior to their inclusion in the final average. Such devices are now incorporated in some commercial equipment and can be built at minimal expense as well. They are

TABLE 4.1.   Artifacts in Somatosensory Evoked Potentials

Origin	Prevention
EMG	Reduce anxiety, improve patient
Scalp ⎫	relaxation
Jaw ⎪	Make patient comfortable
Neck ⎬	Instruct patient in how to relax
Arm ⎪	various muscle groups
Thorax ⎭	± Diazepam
Ocular	All of the above and
Corneoretinal potential	Pre-look and rejection of large
Blink reflex—EMG	artifacts
EKG	Pre-look and rejection, or
	Trigger the stimulus after the QRS
	complex
Respiration	Pre-look and rejection
Electrode	Proper selection, preparation, and
	placement of electrodes
Electroencephalographic	Pre-look and rejection
activity	

very important because they automatically reject excessive artifact prior to inclusion in the average. Even so, it must be stressed that no electronic device can reject or average out excessive EMG activity.

THE SOMATOSENSORY SYSTEM IN RELATION TO THE SEP

Peripheral Mechanisms

Functional Types of Afferents Stimulated

Cutaneous nerves include group II and III cutaneous mechanoreceptors and sometimes joint receptors (McClosky, 1979). Mixed nerves, on the other hand, such as the median nerve, contain a broader spectrum of sensory fibers including muscle afferents and efferents (see Chapter 3). In such mixed or motor nerves, antidromically conducted potentials in motor axons would add to the compound nerve trunk potentials recorded proximal to the site of stimulation. Moreover, muscle and tendon afferents could contribute to the spinal and cortical potentials. In this last respect there is clear evidence that primary and secondary spindle afferents do project to the cortex (see review by Phillips and Porter, 1977; and Chapter 12) and cortical potentials can be recorded in man over the scalp in response to muscle stretches or tendon taps when cutaneous inputs have been excluded by local anesthetic blocks (Brown, 1980; Starr, McKeon, Skuse, and Burke, 1981).

There are about 600 myelinated nerve fibers per digit in the hand (Buchthal and Rosenfalck, 1966). These digital nerves contain both cutaneous and joint afferents. The fact that clearly defined cortical evoked potentials can be evoked by stimulation of the digits or cutaneous nerves suggests that muscle afferents, although they may contribute to the cortical potentials evoked by stimulation of a mixed nerve like the median nerve and can evoke cortical potentials on their own, are not the dominant or even essential afferents responsible for the cortical potentials.

Number of Sensory Fibers Activated

Cortical evoked potentials can be detected at or just above threshold levels at which subjects can barely detect electrical stimuli delivered to a digit (Libet, 1973; Libet, Alberts, Wright, and Feinstein, 1967). This may correspond to activation of as few as ten or fewer of the sensory nerve fibers in the digit (Buchthal and Rosenfalck, 1966). At this stimulus intensity it may not be possible to detect an orthodromic sensory nerve action potential at the level of the wrist, although the capacity to detect such a potential is a function of how near the recording electrode is positioned in respect to the nerve, the number of potentials averaged, and the degree of the amplification of the potential.

Cortical evoked potentials reach their maximum amplitudes at stimulus intensities that are clearly below those necessary to evoke the maximum orthodromic sensory nerve action potential (Dawson, 1947, 1956) (Figure 4.6). Their latencies also progressively decrease as the stimulus intensity is increased to the point

FIGURE 4.6. The effect of increasing the stimulus current delivered to the median nerve at the wrist (top) or first digit (bottom) on the respective amplitude (onset to negative peak) of the antidromic first digit nerve action potential (recorded by a pair of ring electrodes) and the amplitude (initial positive to negative peak) of the orthodromically recorded median nerve action potential (NAP) at the wrist (surface electrodes, monopolar configuration). These are plotted in comparison to the amplitude (N20 to P23–25) of the corresponding cortical evoked potentials, all expressed as percentages of their maximum values.

In both cases the cortical potential increases its amplitude and reaches maximum value earlier than does the corresponding, peripherally recorded nerve action potentials.

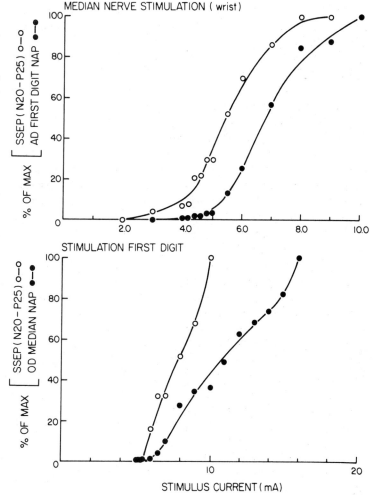

at which the amplitude of the cortical potential reaches its maximum, beyond which the latencies become more or less constant (Figure 4.7).

Stimulus Frequency

Short trains of stimuli at frequencies as high as 100 to 300 impulses per second produce no change in peripheral compound nerve action potentials or dorsal root potentials. The same frequencies, however, cause a substantial fall-off in the amplitude of cervical and cortical evoked potentials (Figure 4.8). The declines in amplitudes of the latter at the higher frequencies of stimulation no doubt reflect failures of synaptic transmission as well as possible failures in presynaptic action potentials to invade the axon terminals (Desmedt and Noel, 1973; Shimoji, Matsuki, Ito, Masuko, Maruyama, Iwane, and Aida, 1976; El-Negamy and Sedgwick, 1978; Maruyama, Shimoji, Shimizu, Kuribayashi, and Fujioka, 1982). The more synapses between the sites of stimulation and recording, the lower the safety factor for transmission through the chain. This is reflected in the fact that the cervical potential is relatively more resistant to higher-frequency stimulation than the cor-

tical potential. Even at stimulation frequencies of 20 to 50 Hz, the amplitudes of the cervical and cortical potentials may fall off. Stimulation frequencies therefore should not exceed 10 Hz if distortions of the central potentials are to be avoided.

Mechanical or Electrical Stimulation?

Electrical stimulation of digits or underlying cutaneous or motor nerves is the most common type of stimulation used in clinical laboratories. It has the obvious advantage that the orthodromic (and antidromic) nerve impulses originate beneath the cathode at more or less the same time, and the evoked potentials are therefore time locked in a precise manner to the onset of the stimulus. This type of stimulation, however, is not "natural," and selects afferents more on the basis of their relative electrical thresholds and position in the nerve relative to the cathode than by the functional types of afferents.

There have been numerous attempts to use more natural stimuli such as cutaneous taps or muscle stretch to activate cutaneous, joint, or muscle mechanoreceptors. These have met with variable success. As pointed out earlier,

FIGURE 4.7.   Changes in the latencies of the N21 and P24 components of the cortical evoked sensory potentials as well as latency to onset of the initial negative deflection of the antidromic first digit nerve action potential (NAP). The median nerve was stimulated at the wrist (in mA). Note the initial reductions in the latencies to all three potentials, but with no significant further increases in latency beyond 10 mA.

The plot emphasizes the importance of being certain that the stimulus intensity is sufficiently high to record the shortest latencies. Note also the absence of stimulus lead between 10 and 18 mA.

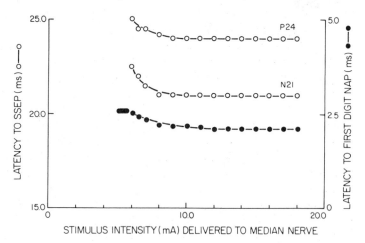

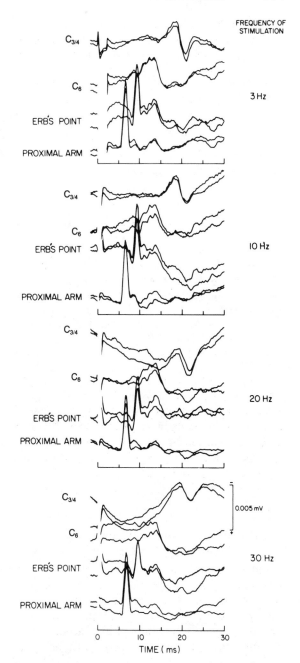

FIGURE 4.8. The effect of changing the frequency of stimulation on the latencies and shapes of the peripheral and centrally generated somatosensory evoked potentials.

Stimulation of the median nerve at the wrist at 3, 10, 20, and 30 Hz. The evoked potentials are recorded at the proximal upper arm, Erb's point, C6 spinous process, and contralateral receiving area of the primary sensory cortex (reference, the corresponding region of the ipsilateral hemisphere).

In this subject there were no changes in latencies of the proximal arm or Erb's point potentials at 10, 20, or 30 Hz compared to the latencies at 3 Hz.

Similarly, there were no changes in the onset (9.7 ms) or various negative peak components (N11.0, N12.3, and N13.4 ms) of the cervical or cortical potentials at 10 Hz compared to 3 Hz.

At 20 Hz and at 30 Hz, there was a 0.3-ms increase in latency to onset of the cervical potential (now 10 ms) and its 11 ms component (now 11.3 ms), a greater increase (0.7 ms) in the latency to the N12.3 and N13.4 components, and an even larger increase in the latency to the N18.3 and P21 cortical components (by 1.5 and 1.3 ms respectively). The greater latency shifts to the longer-latency components probably reflects increasing numbers of synapses between the primary afferents and the primary sensory cortex as the sensory volley ascends to the cortex.

cortical potentials were evoked by muscle stretches (Brown, 1980; Starr, McKeon, Skuse, and Burke, 1981), in which studies attempts were made to block inputs from cutaneous afferents.

Unless special precautions are taken, how-

FIGURE 4.9. Comparison of tendon tap and electrical stimulation-evoked cortical potentials. All traces are electronic averages of 256 potentials. (Top) Cortical potential (C_4–F_z) recorded in response to electrical stimulation of the ulnar nerve at the wrist. (Bottom) Cortical potential recorded in response to lateral tapping of second digit. Note the absence of the initial negativity (here N22) and the longer latencies of the other components.

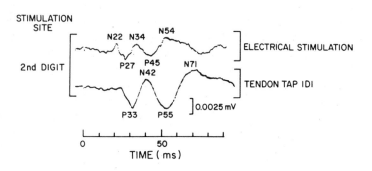

FIGURE 4.10. Deep afferent evoked cortical potential recording C_4–F_z. Lateral top of the second digit (II) following complete xylocaine block of the radial and median nerves at the wrist, rendering the second digit completely anesthetic to touch or pinprick. The block in the median nerve was proved to be complete by (D) supramaximally stimulating the median nerve proximal to the local block and eliciting no thenar potential. At the same time, supramaximal ulnar nerve stimulation at the wrist evoked normal (B) hypothenar and (C) thenar M-potentials. Complete block of cutaneous or joint afferents supplying the second digit was further proved by the absence of any cortical potential when the digit was stimulated electrically through ring electrodes.

The tendon tap-evoked cortical potential therefore must have been mediated by ulnar muscle afferents and not cutaneous or joint afferents belonging to the median or radial nerves.

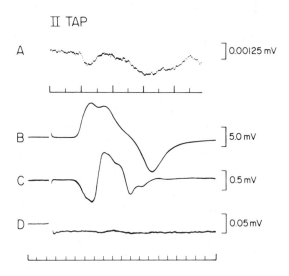

ever, light skin taps could excite deeper receptors in muscle, tendons, or even joints. Similarly, tendon taps or muscle stretches may excite receptors in the skin and other tissues, even when the skin beneath the tap is anesthetized. Even so, mechanical stimuli do have the theoretical advantage of activating the afferents through their receptors instead of at more proximal sites as in electrical stimulation. Although not yet taken advantage of, such direct receptor stimulation could provide a more sensitive means of detecting the earliest physiological abnormalities in dying-back neuropathies (see Chapter 2), and could possibly be useful in detecting root lesions where

the skin in various segmental cutaneous territories on the body surface could be tapped. Our experience with these, however, has been disappointing because of the very small amplitudes of some of the potentials as recorded on the scalp. Mechanical stimulation is also potentially less distressing than electrical stimulation of peripheral nerves, but unfortunately, as pointed out, the potentials so obtained are often much more poorly defined (Figures 4.9 and 4.10).

Cortical potentials evoked by mechanical stimuli have some important differences when compared to those evoked by electrical stimulation (Sears, 1959; Halliday and Mason,

1964; Larsson and Prevec, 1970; Pratt, Starr, Amlie, and Politoske, 1979; Pratt, Amlie, and Starr, 1979; Pratt and Starr, 1981; Starr, McKeon, Skuse, and Burke, 1981) (Table 4.2). For example, the latencies of mechanically evoked cortical potentials exceed by 3 to 5 ms the latencies of corresponding cortical potentials evoked by electrical stimulation of peripheral nerves even when the stimuli are delivered at equivalent distances from the spinal cord. Moreover, in the arm the N20–22 potential, which probably represents the onset of cortical activity, is not usually seen in most mechanically evoked cortical potentials (Figure 4.9). These unique characteristics of the latter no doubt reflect important differences between the two types of stimulation, and as a consequence, the nature of the afferent volley.

For clinical purposes therefore, mechanical stimuli are not as useful as electrical stimulation because the much better synchronized volleys in the latter make recording the compound potentials from the nerve trunks easier. Also, these potentials and those recorded over the spinal cord and scalp are much better defined. Thus assessments of peripheral conduction velocities and central conduction times are easier and more reliable when electrical rather than mechanical stimuli are used. It is much more difficult to detect the subcortical centrally originating potentials when mechanical stimuli are used, probably for the same reason, namely, higher temporal dispersion of the ascending afferent volleys (Sears, 1959; Halliday and Mason, 1964; Larsson and Prevec, 1970; Pratt, Starr, Amlie, and Politoske, 1979; Pratt, Amlie, and Starr, 1979; Pratt and Starr, 1981; Starr, McKeon, Skuse, and Burke, 1981).

Age-related Changes

Maturation of the peripheral nervous system was discussed in Chapter 3. By term, the

TABLE 4.2. Comparison of Electrical and Mechanical Stimulus Evoked Potentials

Electrical Stimulation	Mechanical Stimulation
Peripheral nerve volley	
Much easier to detect because the peripheral volley is better synchronized	Much harder to detect because the volley is very asynchronous because:
	Many receptors discharge repetitively in response to the stimulus
	The distances between various receptors excited by the stimulus and the spinal cord may differ substantially
Types of afferents stimulated	
Selection depends on:	Selection depends on:
Relative thresholds of afferents in the nerve	Site of stimulation
Positions of these afferents in the nerve trunk in relation to the stimulating electrode	Precise nature of the stimulus—taps delivered to the skin or nail, tendon tap, muscle stretches
Composition of afferents in the nerve at site of stimulus (whether the nerve contains muscle or other deep afferents)	
Characteristics (duration and shape) of the stimulus	
Cortical potential	
Latency shorter	Longer latency
± Larger amplitude	± Lower amplitude

medial lemniscus is myelinated, and by the ages of 8 to 10 years the central conduction time measured between the cervical and cortical evoked potentials reaches adult values (Desmedt, Noël, Debecker, and Namèche, 1973) whereas the peripheral motor and sensory conduction velocities reach adult values earlier (2 to 5 years).

The potential, which is the equivalent of the primary sensory cortical in the adult, is more prominent and has a longer duration in the newborn (Figure 4.11). With subsequent maturation there are progressive reductions in its latency and duration.

Little is known, unfortunately, about possible changes in the numbers and diameters of central somatosensory pathways in the later decades of life (Figure 4.12). The potential that many again associate with onset of cortical activity in the primary sensory cortex (areas 3, 2 and 1), the N20–22 potential evoked by distal stimulation in the upper limb, increases in amplitude and duration in late life for reasons that at this point are quite unknown (Desmedt and Cheron, 1980a, 1980b). The later changes are not, however, accompanied by any increase in central conduction time.

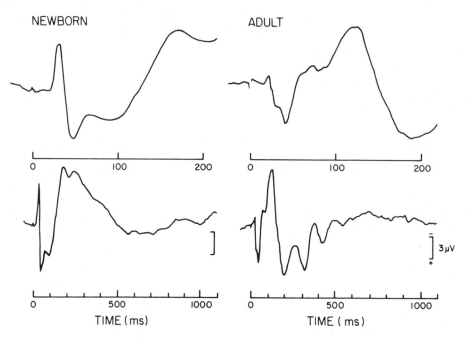

FIGURE 4.11.   Comparison of somatosensory cortical evoked potentials in the newborn (left) in REM sleep and a conscious adult (right) shown on two separate time scales (top and bottom). Despite the much smaller size of the newborn, the initial cortical negativity (here called N1) has a similar latency to the adult value, reflecting the much slower peripheral and central conduction velocities in the afferent pathway at this age. The N1 component is much broader in the infant perhaps because of a greater degree of temporal dispersion in the afferent volley and the synaptic immaturity of the cortical connections.
From Desmedt (1971, figure 5).

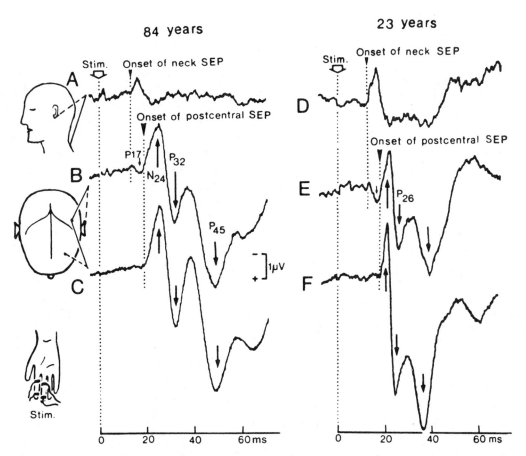

84 years

Stim. Onset of neck SEP

A

Onset of postcentral SEP

P17   P₃₂

B   N₂₄

P₄₅

C

Stim.

23 years

Stim. Onset of neck SEP

D

Onset of postcentral SEP

E   P₂₆

F

]1µV

0   20   40   60 ms

0   20   40   60 ms

FIGURE 4.12.   Comparison of cervical and cortical evoked potentials (parietal to forehead reference) as elicited by stimulation of the second and third digits in subjects 84 (left) and 23 (right) years of age. In this and other octogenarians, Desmedt and Cheron were unable to show significant increase in the conduction time of the central somatosensory pathway. There were, however, increases in the conduction time to the spinal cord, reflecting slower conduction in peripheral afferent pathways in older subjects. The number of trials averaged in both cases was 1,024. From Desmedt and Cheron (1980c, figure 2).

Limb Length

The latencies to the cervical evoked potential in adults are proportional to limb length (Small, Beauchamp, and Matthews, 1980) (Figure 4.13). Similarly, the latencies to the N20–22 component increase in relation to limb length and body weight (Desmedt and Brunko, 1980). In the lower limb, length is also an important determinant of the onset of spinal cord activity (Lastimos, Bass, Stanback, and Norvell, 1982).

Hence limb length must be taken into account when decisions are made about whether latencies to cervical or cortical potentials are normal in any one subject. One possible solution in respect to the upper limb is to measure the latencies to the cerebral and cervical potentials with reference to Erb's point. The

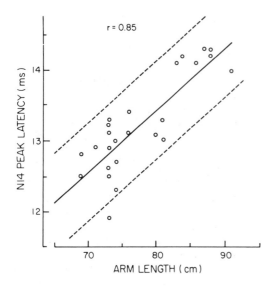

FIGURE 4.13.   Increase in latency of the cervical N14 peak latency (in ms) as a function of arm length. Note the almost linear relationship between limb length and N14 latency.

From Matthews, Beauchamp, and Small (1974, figure 2), reprinted with permission of the publisher. © 1974, Macmillan Journals Ltd.

assumption is that differences in the distances between that point and the cervical cord will show much less variation among individuals than would be apparent in differences in the lengths of their limbs. The strategy has the added advantage that the proximal peripheral and central conduction times would not be as subject to the influence of differences among subjects in limb temperature. The preceding points also emphasize the value of comparing latencies of the potentials on the two sides, especially when there is reason to think that one side is normal; the latter then serves as the normal for the abnormal side, with less need to be concerned about adjustments for differences among subjects in their limb lengths, temperatures, and ages. Of course if there is any cause to suspect that the other side may be abnormal, such comparisons between limbs are not valid.

Central Mechanisms SEP

Spinal

The observation that abnormalities in the cortical evoked potentials were associated with defects in position and vibration sense, but not thermal or pain sensation (Halliday and Wakefield, 1963; Giblin, 1964) led to the suggestion that the dorsal columns mediated the cortical evoked potentials at the level of the spinal cord. There is, however, recent evidence that the dorsal columns do not mediate vibration or position senses (Wall, 1970; Wall and Noordenbos, 1977; Ross, Kirpatrick, and Lastimos, 1979). The most constant abnormalities associated with dorsal column lesions were impairments in the manipulative actions of the hands, appreciation of the direction of movements across the skin surface, and impaired two-point discrimination (Wall, 1970).

In lower animals, evidence suggests that sensory transmission through both the dorsal columns and other ascending pathways can evoke cortical potentials. Forelimb spindle primaries in the cat and primate are known to be transmitted through the cuneate fasciculus (Webster, 1977; Brown and Gordon, 1977) (Figure 4.14). In the cat, weak stimuli that excite Ia afferents do evoke cortical potentials and these are abolished by section of the dorsal column (Oscarsson and Rosén, 1963). Similarly, in the primate, section of the dorsal columns abolishes the muscle stretch evoked input originating in the forelimb to sensorimotor cortex (Phillips, Powell, and Wiesendanger, 1971), as well as the cortical potentials in response to peripheral nerve stimulation (Cusick, Myklebust, Larson, and Sances, 1979).

In the cat, however, stronger stimulation of the same motor nerves sufficient to excite group II muscle and tendon afferents will evoke cortical potentials even in the presence of section of the dorsal columns (Oscarsson and Rosén, 1963). Moreover, in contradis-

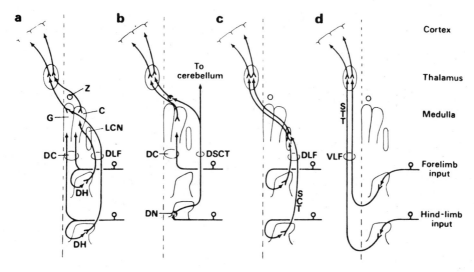

FIGURE 4.14.

(a) Dorsal column projection system for peripheral cutaneous afferents.
(b) Proprioceptive projection systems for muscle and tendon afferents from the upper and lower limbs.
(c) Spinocervical-lemniscothalamic pathways.
(d) Spinothalamic pathway.

Abbreviations: Tracts and fascicles—DC = dorsal column, DLF = dorsolateral fascicle, DSCT = dorsal spinocerebellar tract, SCT = spinocervical tract, STT = spinothalamic tract, VLF = ventrolateral fascicle.

Nuclear regions—C = cuneate nucleus, DH = dorsal horn (shown in transverse section), DN = dorsal nucleus (Clarke's column), G = gracile nucleus, LCN = lateral cervical nucleus, Z = nucleus Z.

Reprinted by permission of the publisher from Brown and Gordon (1977, figure 1).

tinction to the claims of Cusick, Myklebust, Larson, and Sances (1979), there is other evidence that cutaneous stimulus evoked cortical potentials, although reduced somewhat in amplitude, do indeed persist despite dorsal column section (Andersson, Norrsell, and Norrsell, 1972).

The importance of the above observations is that projections other than those from the dorsal column may participate in the generation of cortical potentials. Their contributions may depend on the nature and intensity of the stimulus. Other spinocortical projection systems that could contribute to the scalp evoked potentials are the spinocerebellar, dorsolat-

eral (including the spinocervical tract), and anterolateral (spinothalamic) tracts. As yet there is no evidence for or against the possibility that cerebellar cortical potentials in response to *spinocerebellar tract* inputs could contribute to the scalp-recorded potentials in man, although in lower animals the spinocerebellar tract probably makes no important contributions to the cortical evoked potential (Werner and Whitsel, 1973).

The maximum conduction velocities in the *spinothalamic tracts* are, however, too slow for cortical potentials generated by activity in this tract to contribute to the earliest components of the cortical potential. The *spinocervical tract,* in contrast, is mainly concerned with signals originating in hair follicle receptors, and impulses in this tract conduct rapidly toward the brainstem. This tract therefore could contribute to the cortical evoked potential, especially where cutaneous afferents are stimulated. In man, much remains to be worked out about which ascending spinal tracts participate in the generation of the spinal and cortical evoked potentials. There may well be important species differences in the relative importance of these spinal tracts to the cortical potentials.

Brainstem and Thalamic Mechanisms

The dorsal columns project to the gracile cuneate nuclei and related nuclei, nucleus Z, and the lateral cervical nucleus (Brodal, 1981). These in turn project by way of the medial lemniscus to the ventral posterolateral (VPL) nucleus of the thalamus. The thalamic destinations of muscle and joint receptors may, however, lie somewhere between the VPL and the ventrolateral (VL) nuclei (Brown and Gordon, 1977; Brodal, 1981; see also Wiesendanger and Miles, 1982). The various spinocortical projections are illustrated in Figure 4.15.

Lesions restricted to VPL nuclei abolish the cortical evoked potentials, whereas these persist when the lesion is limited to VL nuclei. The thalamus behaves as if it were a *closed field* in that electrical activity originating within the thalamus itself may be difficult to detect even in the immediate vicinity outside the thalamus (Hunt and O'Leary, 1952; Celesia, 1979). In the human, the earliest electrical activity recorded by an electrode in VPL nuclei in response to contralateral distal median nerve stimulation begins at 15.8 ± 0.4 ms, the maximum positive potential and multispike activity being registered between 17 and 18.7 ms. The earliest positive potential and spike activity probably originate in the medial lemniscus that terminates within the nucleus (Arezzo, Legatt, and Vaughan, 1979). This means

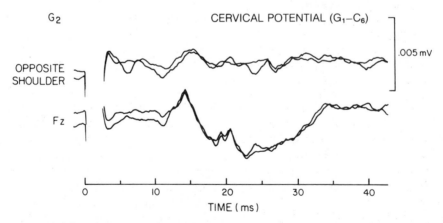

FIGURE 4.15. Comparison of the potential recorded by a surface electrode positioned over the C_6 spinous process as elicited by stimulation of the median nerve at the wrist, with the reference electrode positioned over the opposite shoulder (top) and F_z (bottom). The negative potential is larger in the latter case. This may be a result of the combination of a negativity at G_1 and an almost coincident positivity as seen at F_z, the latter possibly being produced by the ascending volley in the medial lemniscus and the former by the cord dorsum potential itself. Each potential is the electronic average of 500 traces.

that electrical potentials with latencies much below 15 ms (when evoked by a distal peripheral nerve stimulus in the arm) must originate in subthalamic structures. Other nonlemniscal and probably slower-conducting projections to the thalamus could also make important contributions, especially to the later cortical potentials.

Sensorimotor Cortex

The ventrobasal thalamic complex projects to the ipsilateral postcentral cortex inclusive of the cytoarchitectonic areas 3A, 3B, 1, 2, the precentral cortex, and the second sensory area (SII) (Jones and Powell, 1973; Powell, 1977; Brodal, 1981). The heaviest projections in subhuman primates are to areas 4, 3A, and 3B. The thalamocortical projections to areas 1 and 2 are for the most part collateral branches of thalamocortical connections to areas 3B and 3A. Direct thalamic projections to areas 1 and 2 are few and the fibers are small in diameter (Jones and Powell, 1973). The muscle stretch receptor projections to area 2 may explain in part the observation that neurons in this region register static joint angle and changes in joint angle (Rose and Mountcastle, 1959). These latter properties were earlier ascribed to receptors originating in the joints themselves when originally investigated.

The SII sensory area in the subhuman primate receives its primary projection by way of branches of ventrobasal fibers to the primary sensory area (SI) (Jones and Powell, 1973; Powell, 1977). The topographic organization is similar to that in SI but is less precise, and the neurons, although responding to cutaneous mechanoreceptor stimulation, do not respond to joint displacement. Unlike SI, ipsilateral and contralateral thalamic projections project to SII, although the latencies of evoked responses in SII are longer than to SI (Woolsey, Erickson, and Gilson, 1979). In the marginal posterior zone, neurons exist that respond to convergent somatic, auditory, and at times, visual stimuli, some even responding to nociceptive stimulation. Precise reciprocal connections exist between SI and SII.

The primary projections from SI are to SII and areas 4 and 5 (Powell, 1977). These projections are heavy and the diameters of these nerve fiber connections are large. Projections to the supplementary motor areas are much less dense. Yet a third somatosensory area (SIII) has been postulated to exist and equated with area 5, although this remains a subject of controversy. Surface cortical stimulation in this region in man does not produce any subjective sensory experiences, nor have potentials been recorded in this region in response to peripheral stimulation. Perhaps these negative observations are explained by the fact that the face and arm areas are lost in the intraparietal sulcus (Jones and Powell, 1973; Woolsey, Erickson, and Gilson, 1979). Except for the distal upper and lower limbs, there are important interhemispheric connections between areas SI and SII.

In summary, peripheral somatic stimuli can evoke activity in sensory pathways that project by lemniscal and nonlemniscal paths to the ventrobasal complex, thence to areas 4 and SI and SII. There is later extension to other cortical areas, including the parietal region and the opposite hemisphere by transcallosal connections, except in the last case for the most distal regions in the limbs. Possibly all the above tracts, nuclei, and cortical regions contribute at their appropriate times to the recorded scalp and neck potentials. The primary surface positive response (recorded under barbiturate anesthesia) is localized to the SI area, however (Woolsey, Erickson, and Gilson, 1979).

The organization of the primary sensory cortex has been investigated by evoked potential techniques, examination of physiological responses of single neurons in this region, anatomical studies, and study of the patterns of sensory localization in human subjects in whom the sensory cortex has been stimulated. In lower animals, the general pattern of sensory localization in the primary sensory cortex (see review of Werner and Whitsel, 1973) is such that the cortical representations of the dermatomes moving from medial to lateral across the postcentral cortex trace a continuous line over the surface of the body beginning in the sacral strips and successively through the lower limb, trunk, upper limb, and trigeminal areas. This pattern sometimes produces unexpected results. For example, some regions of the skin surface are represented by two or more cortical areas or nearly adjacent areas on the body surface, such as the heel and dorsum of the ankle, and may be widely separated in their cortical representations.

The cortical projections from the digits are discrete, exhibiting very little overlap between the cortical representations of other digits in both subhuman primates and man.

Neurons in the cortical area 3B and the anterior part of area 1 respond to cutaneous stimulation, whereas those more caudally located in area 1 as well as area 2 respond to muscle, joint, and other noncutaneous afferent inputs. Some neurons in 3A and the rostral part of 3B may receive convergent projections from the skin and muscle afferents, whereas other neurons in 3A receive inputs from primary spindle afferents. Vertical cell columns serving different sensory modalities but of similar segmental dorsal root origins are linked together by anteroposterior reciprocal connections.

Organization of the Human Sensorimotor Cortex

In the human, the patterns of sensory representation in the sensory cortex have been studied by evoked potentials (Woolsey and Erickson, 1950; Jasper, Lende and Rasmussen, 1960) and cortical stimulation techniques. In the latter, threshold or near-threshold faradic stimulation of the sensorimotor cortex was carried out under local anesthesia (Penfield and Boldrey, 1937; Woolsey, Erickson, and Gilson, 1979). The patterns of sensory representation obtained were based on a limited number of observations made on a large number of patients.

In these important pioneer investigations there was extensive overlap between cortical regions related to quite separate areas on the body surface. Moreover, the fact that the digits were represented by narrow bands on the precentral and postcentral cortex adjacent to the central sulcus, while other regions of the limb were much more widely represented on cortical surface, clearly suggests that projection of the digits to the primary sensory cortex is primarily to the cortex of the posterior wall of the central sulcus (Woolsey, Erickson, and Gilson, 1979).

There have been few opportunities to stimulate the buried cortex on the banks of the central sulcus because of the necessity of opening the sulcus. Moreover, conclusions about localization based on cortical stimulation must be cautiously interpreted because such stimuli can produce widespread direct and indirect excitation of cortical and subcortical structures well beyond the cortical region stimulated (see review by Phillips and Porter, 1977).

In other studies, localization in the human sensory cortex was investigated by mapping the distribution of the *primary surface positive potentials* evoked by mechanical taps or hair stimulation delivered to various points on the skin surface (Woolsey and Erickson, 1950; Woolsey, Erickson, and Gilson, 1979). Here too, no explorations were made of the banks of the central sulcus. Also, electronic averaging techniques were not used such as would be necessary to detect subcortical far field potentials. The recordings in such studies of evoked potentials over the precentral cortex were too few in number to permit any useful comment to be made about sensory projections anterior to the rolandic fissure.

VOLUME CONDUCTION AND OTHER FACTORS AS THEY AFFECT RECORDED POTENTIALS

Possible origins of SEPs in the central nervous system include conducted potentials in central ascending sensory tracts and cellular potentials in the dorsal horn, brainstem, and diencephalic nuclei, and the cerebral cortex. The sources overlap somewhat depending on the latencies and durations of their respective potentials. The durations of the conducted tract potentials depend on the range in the conduction velocities of the nerve fibers that compose the tract and the conduction distances of these fibers. The latter of these, for example, may vary substantially depending on the functional type of the fiber, in the case of thalamocortical fibers, because of their different cortical destinations, near the base or crown of the postcentral or precentral gyrus.

Because of the open nature of the fields *(open fields)* about peripheral and central tracts, the dorsal horn, and the cerebral cortex, the potentials generated by these structures are likely sources for various components of the SEP depending on their respective latencies and the locations of both the G_1 and G_2 electrodes that may variably be active, depending on their location with respect to these potentials. Less likely as sources of SEP potentials are the *closed fields,* characteristic of the thalamic and possibly gracile and cuneate nuclei. Thus even though electrical activity can be recorded from within the thalamus beginning at 15 ms (see earlier discussion), this activity cannot be readily detected outside the thalamus (Celesia, 1979; and see earlier work in the cat, Hunt and O'Leary, 1952).

Theoretically, the most likely sources for the subcortical and earliest cortical potentials include:

1. The centripedally conducted peripheral nerve volley
2. Ascending volleys in the dorsal columns and other fast-conducting ascending spinal sensory pathways such as the spinocervical tract
3. Presynaptic and postsynaptic segmented activity in the dorsal horn
4. Ascending volleys in the medial lemniscus
5. Conducted potentials in thalamocortical pathways
6. Postsynaptic potentials and afterpotentials in the postcentral and precentral cortex

For more commentary on the above the reader is encouraged to refer to the work on volume conduction by O'Leary and Goldring (1964), Landau (1967), Humphrey (1968), Schlag (1973), and Nunez (1981), and the experimental investigations of SEPs in primates by Legatt and Vaughan (1979) and Arezzo, Vaughan, and Legatt (1981).

In addition to the importance of the openness of the potential fields about the various neural generators, there are other factors to consider in the electrogenesis of the SEP. These include the distance between the generators and the recording electrodes, the orientation of the potential field in respect to those electrodes, possible changes in the impedance presented by the pathways between the potentials and the recording electrodes at certain points in the neural pathway between the site of origin of the sensory volley and the cerebral cortex, and the nature of the electrical potentials at various levels of the somatosensory pathway.

The importance of the positions of both electrodes G_1 and G_2 was alluded to earlier in this chapter. The reader is reminded that these interpretations of the origins and polarity of potentials may occur because both electrodes may be active, and especially where G_2 is the more active electrode. This, for example, is probably the case with respect to ascending propagated potentials in the medial lemniscus when G_2 is located on the scalp (F_z) and G_1 is cervical (Figure 4.15). In this case, the polarity and origin of the recorded potential may be incorrectly thought to be cervical in origin and negative in polarity (the N14) (see Desmedt and Cheron, 1980b). It may more correctly be a positive potential (P14 at G_2) originating above the foramen magnum, as pointed out in the medial lemniscus. More will be said of the origin of these and often similar latency potentials later.

The amplitude of potentials is proportional to $1/d^2$, where d is the distance between the source and the recording electrode. Ideally then, one of the electrodes should be as close to the generator as possible and the other as remote as possible. The greater the interelectrode distance, however, the greater the chances of picking up unwanted potentials such as respiration artifact, EKG, and especially, EMG activity with FFR.

Alternatively, the electrode positions can be chosen so they record the maximum opposite polarities for the desired potentials. For example, to enhance the cervical potentials, a cephalic reference may be chosen that sees the approaching peripheral and centrally conducting volleys and the cervical activity as a series of positive potentials (Figure 4.15); whereas the cervical electrode, although seeing the brachial plexus potentials as positive, sees the cervical activity as negative potentials. Because the differential amplifier registers the difference potential, the precervical potentials will be diminished in size, but potentials originating in the cervical cord will be enhanced.

Theoretically, orientation of electrodes with respect to the generator(s) of the potentials is important. For example, if both electrodes lie on the same isopotential lines, no potential difference will be recorded even though both electrodes may lie quite close to the generator. Lueders (1982) has drawn attention also to the importance of impedance changes in the path between the recording electrode(s) and the electrical generator. He suggests that changes in impedance presented by the compound nerve trunk potential as it moves from the proximal upper limb into the much larger conductor presented by the trunk accounts for the apparently standing wave recorded by far field recording and apparently originating in the distal brachial plexus. Possible changes in the composition or arrangements of nerve fiber bundles at this level may also be an important factor here.

Other possible sites of impedance change include the transitions as the conducted action potentials pass through the intervertebral canals and later the spinal canal, and again as the rostrally conducted action potentials pass through the foramen magnum to enter the skull.

The nature of the potentials is also an important determinant of whether they will be seen at any appreciable distance by a recording electrode. Longer-lasting potentials such as *postsynaptic potentials* (PSPs) and *afterpotentials* are much more likely sources of far field or cortical potentials than are spikes, except where there is a high degree of synchrony between large numbers of spike generators as in the peripheral nerve trunks in central tracts. Because there is relatively much less synchrony between the spike discharges of cortical elements, the latter are not as likely to be sources of potentials as recorded with scalp electrodes as are the slower potentials. The longer duration of PSPs and afterpotentials also makes them much less likely to be lost in the face of minor degrees of temporal dispersions among their activities. In addition, however, the higher-frequency components characteristic of spike potentials are attenuated much more rapidly with increasing distance than are the lower frequencies more characteristic of PSPs and afterpotentials (see also Chapters 3 and 7).

Postsynaptic potentials and afterpotentials are therefore the probable primary sources of the potentials originating in the dorsal horn and cerebral cortex as seen in volume in SEP recordings (Humphrey, 1968; Schlag, 1973; Nicholson, 1979; Desmedt and Brunko, 1980).

In summary, the most important determinants of whether a neural structure contributes to the SEP are:

1. The nature of the source, including
   a. The degree of synchronization in the activity of its neural elements
   b. The nature of the potentials, i.e., whether these are spikes, postsynaptic potentials, or afterpotentials
   c. Whether the field is open or closed
2. The nearness and orientation of the source with respect to the recording electrodes
3. Possible impedance changes in the path between the recording electrode and the conducted electrical activity as it propagates rostrally

With the preceding in mind and comments made earlier about the likely neural generators of the components, subcortical and cortical, of the SEP, it is time to turn our attention to present views about the actual generation of these potentials, to highlight the points of agreement and disagreement between investigators in this field, and to point out possible strategies for resolving these issues. It must be mentioned here that as of the present time there is very little direct evidence clearly establishing the generation of the components of the SEP.

ORIGIN OF SUBCORTICAL SOMATOSENSORY POTENTIALS

Upper Limb Stimulation

There is now general agreement that the positive potential P7–8 recorded in FFR originates in the distal brachial plexus (Figure 4.2). This is based on its appropriate latency and the fact that nearer brachial plexus recordings, as for example at Erb's point, record a propagated triphasic potential (the classic + − + potential recorded as the wave front approaches, reaches, and passes the recording electrode) that has the same or if anything, a little longer latency, indicating the latter originates more proximally in the brachial plexus. This brachial plexus potential, whether recorded by direct Erb's point or by far field techniques, may be used to help to localize lesions in the brachial plexus and possibly nerve roots (Figures 4.16 and 4.17) (see Siivola, Myllylä, Sulg, and Hokkanen, 1979; Jones, 1979, 1980).

The major controversies occur with the next series of potentials beginning at 9 to 10 ms in the case of median nerve stimulation at the wrist and extending through to 20 ms. The interpretations of Desmedt and Cheron (1980, 1981a, 1981b) based on their analysis of far field potentials and nearer field recordings over the posterior neck and prevertebral sites seem most consistent with our present knowledge of the physiological activities and anatomy of the somatosensory pathway. Thus I will concentrate on these initially before pointing out areas of disagreement.

First, in prevertebral recordings (esophageal electrode) against a remote reference (opposite hand), Desmedt and Cheron (1981b) recorded a large positive precervical potential (Figure 4.18). This potential had several important characteristics, namely:

FIGURE 4.16.   Patient with compression of the lower brachial plexus at the thoracic outlet on the right. Shown are recordings at the proximal arm (PA), Erb's point (E), sixth cervical spine (C6), and scalp (C4-C3)] of the potentials elicited in response to electrical stimulation of the median (M) nerve (top trace of each pair) and the ulnar (U) nerve. Each trace represents the electronic average of 250 responses.

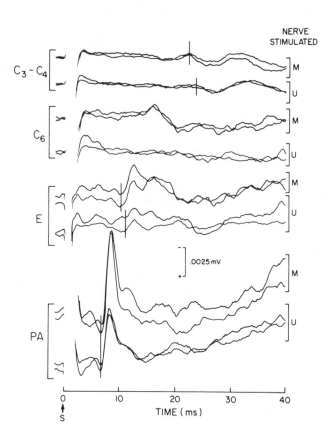

In this patient, the potentials elicited in response to median nerve stimulation were all in the normal range with respect to their shapes, sizes, and latencies. In response to ulnar nerve stimulation, the potential recorded at the proximal arm site was identical in latency to that elicited by median nerve stimulation. The ulnar stimulus elicited Erb's point potential, however, was obviously delayed; the corresponding cervical potential absent and the contralateral cortical potential were even more delayed with respect to the corresponding median stimulus evoked potentials, indicating a lesion(s) situated in the brachial plexus and primarily involving the C8-T1 contributions to the lower trunk (and possibly medial cord) of the plexus. The gain is the same for all traces. These recordings were somewhat noisy, largely because of excessive EMG activity.

1. Amplitude was maximal in the midcervical region, falling off steeply at more rostral cervical recording sites.
2. There was no detectable shift in latency from low to high at the cervical recording site.
3. The potential was positive.

Desmedt and Cheron concluded that the precervical positive potential (P13 in response to stimulation at the wrist) corresponded to the *cord dorsum potential,* a negative potential when recorded posteriorly over the cord, and which originates in presynaptic and postsynaptic activity in the dorsal horn based on an extensive body of evidence.

In the human, direct epidural recordings at the midcervical level reveal a series of distinctive potentials in response to electrical stimulation of the ulnar nerve at the elbow or wrist (Shimoji, Kano, Higashi, Morioka, and Henschel, 1972; Shimoji, Matsuki, Ito, Masuko, Maruyama, Iwane, and Aida, 1976; Shimoji, Matsuki, and Shimizu, 1977; Shimoji, Shimizu, and Maruyama, 1978; Maruyama, Shimoji, Shimizu, Kuribayashi, and Fujioka, 1982; Shimizu, Shimoji, Maruyama, Matsuki, Kuribayashi, and Fujioka, 1982).

The earliest potential is a brief spike (onset and peak latencies of about 10 and 12 ms respectively, with stimulation at the wrist) (Figure 4.19). This sometimes triphasic potential, like the peripherally conducted nerve trunk

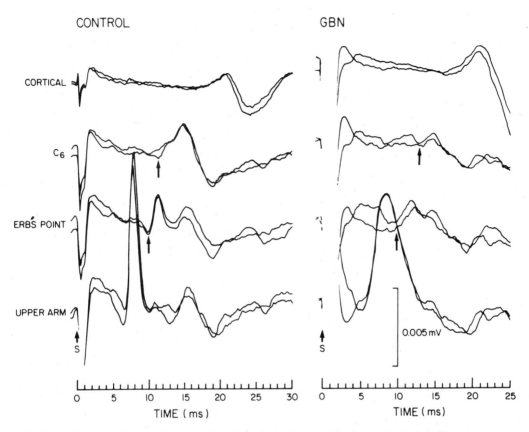

FIGURE 4.17. Conduction abnormalities in Guillain-Barré polyneuropathy (right). Comparable normal peripheral, cervical, and cortical evoked potentials are shown on the left as elicited by stimulation of the median nerve at the wrist in both cases. The most obvious abnormalities include the broader upper arm potential whose negative peak duration exceeded the 3-SD upper limits for controls and the increase in the conduction time between onset of the Erb's point and cervical potentials (here 3.1 ms; upper limit of normals 2.0 ms). The latter points to abnormal slowing of conduction across the proximal brachial plexus or roots (or both). The maximum conduction velocity between the proximal arm and wrist was within the 2-SD lower limit of controls. The broader upper arm potential suggests an increase in the degree of desynchronization among the orthodromically conducting afferent impulses (and possibly to some extent antidromically conducting afferent impulses in motor axons).

potential, is very resistant to stimulation at intervals as short as 3 to 5 ms (Shimoji, Shimizu, and Maruyama, 1978), and therefore probably represents the conducted potential in the dorsal roots as has been shown in lower animals. This spike potential is not well seen in posterior surface recordings in the neck. Conducted potentials in the roots themselves are unlikely to be readily detected in surface recordings because of their steep attenuation with distance (Inouye and Buchthal, 1977).

In posterior epidural recordings, the early spike potential is characteristically followed by a slower and longer-lasting negative-positive potential. This potential is nearly identical in its characteristics to the intermediary cord po-

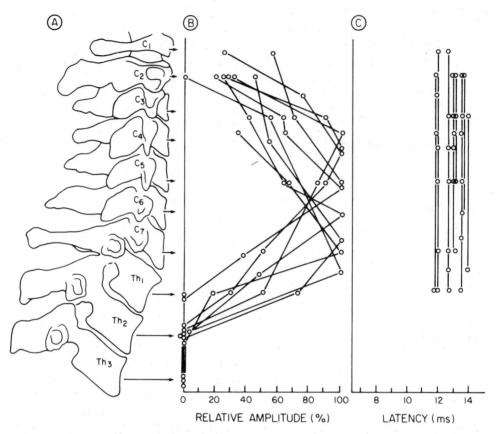

FIGURE 4.18.   Distribution of the cervical potential as recorded anterior to the cervical vertebral column (A) with esophageal electrodes. In (B) are plotted the relative amplitudes of this potential and in (C) the peak latencies in ms at various cervical levels. The location of the peak amplitude between C4 and T1 varies widely among individuals. There is also wide rostrocaudal distribution of the potential. The amplitude of the anterior cervical potential is lower at the higher cervical compared to the midcervical level, and the peak latency of the potential is constant throughout the cervical region. The latter observations strongly suggest that the anterior cervical potential corresponds to the cord dorsum potential.
From Desmedt and Cheron (1981b, figure 6).

tentials or cord dorsum potentials (see review by Willis, 1980); the negative component reflecting postsynaptic activity generated by various afferents in the dorsal horn and the later positive potential.

Primary Afferent Depolarization

In lower primates (Table 4.3), although not in man, secondary negative peaks imposed on the main negative potential have been recognized (Beall, Applebaum, Foreman, and Willis, 1977) and attributed to dorsal horn activity in response to successively higher-threshold afferents.

Similar cord dorsum potentials have also been recognized as originating in the lumbosacral cord in response to segmental inputs (Magladery, Porter, Park, and Teasdall, 1951; and see later section on spinal evoked poten-

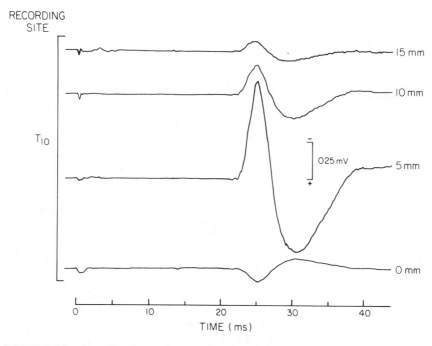

RECORDING SITE

T₁₀

0.25 mV

15 mm
10 mm
5 mm
0 mm

TIME (ms)
0   10   20   30   40

FIGURE 4.19.   Needle electrode recording at the T10-11 interspace of the cord dorsum potential from a patient rendered quadriplegic previously by a fracture dislocation at C5-6. The posterior tibial nerve was stimulated at the level of the ankle.

In this instance the intention was to insert the Teflon-coated needle electrode only as far as the epidural space, but inadvertently the electrode passed more deeply, and probably through to the anterior spinal cord (0). Note the reversal of polarity of the potential as the electrode was subsequently withdrawn 5, 10, and 15 mm posteriorly. Fortunately, there were no immediate or late ill effects from this procedure. The study was done to look for evidence of central ascending afferent transmission through the cervical injury site, but no cortical potential was elicited.

tials). Such intermediary cord potentials reverse polarity anterior to the cord (Figure 4.20), thus explaining the P13 precervical potential of Desmedt and Cheron (1981a) (see also Figure 4.18). Because they are segmentally generated they do not propagate rostrally, although simply because more rostral spinal segments may be activated slightly later, there may be some apparent increase in latency of the negative wave recorded over higher segments, as was noted by Magladery, Porter, Park, and Teasdall (1951) in the human lumbosacral cord potential.

Also, because the negative potential is postsynaptic, the potential amplitude falls off when the stimulus intervals are too short because of synaptic transmission failures (Shimoji, Shimizu, and Maruyama, 1978; Dimitrijevic, Sedgwick, Sherwood, and Soar, 1980).

Second, at the lowest precervical recording sites (C8, T1–2) an earlier negative potential was recorded whose negative onset latency occurred at about 10 ms and which reasonably must represent orthodromic conducted potentials in the dorsal roots plus possibly antidromic motor activity in the ventral roots, es-

TABLE 4.3.   Origin of Cord Dorsum Potential

Potential		Origin
Early negative		Postsynaptic activity in the dorsal horn generated by
Subcomponents	N1	Activation of lowest-threshold cutaneous afferents (A alpha, beta)
	N2	Activation of higher threshold cutaneous afferents (slower beta and faster delta)
	N3	Activation of highest-threshold cutaneous afferents (A delta)
(Superimposes on positive potential)		At these stimulus intensities, burst activity in spinothalamic tract neurons
Later positive		Primary afferent depolarization

From Beall, Applebaum, Foreman, and Willis (1977).

pecially with mixed nerve stimulation as in the case of median stimulation at the wrist. The latency of this precervically recorded potential is therefore very similar to the early spike potential in the posterior epidural recordings noted earlier.

When the median nerve is stimulated at the wrist, nerve fibers belonging to several root segments are excited, the nerve at this level containing C6–8 cutaneous and joint and C7–T1 muscle afferents. On entering the spinal cord, cutaneous afferents divide into rostral and caudal branches from which collaterals pass into the dorsal horn one or even two spinal cord segments above and below their levels of entry into the cord. This means that dorsal horn segments between C3 and T2 could be excited by median nerve stimulation at the wrist. Even stimulation of single digits could excite postsynaptic neurons in as many as two or three cervical segments.

In posterior neck recordings the same authors recorded a large negative potential, the N13 component of which corresponded to the P13 in precervical recordings. Preceding the N13 potential, however, was an earlier N11

potential, which when recorded against a hard reference site, progressively increased in latency from lower to higher cervical recording sites. This indicated that it at least was a traveling potential, and because of its latency, probably originated as a propagated wave in the dorsal columns. In precervical recordings this potential was not seen.

The origin of the N14 potential recorded with a posterior cervical G_1 electrode has been a matter of controversy, partly because of differences among investigators in the sites chosen for the reference electrode. The clear cervical origin for the N13 potential in Desmedt's (1981b) remote reference recordings is supported by the characteristics of the precervical P13 potential. The problem is compounded, however, where a cephalic reference is used because in this case, as pointed out earlier, both electrodes are active. Indeed, G_2 may be the more active because it sees the approaching volley in the medial lemniscus, which is known to reach the basal thalamus at the earliest by about 15 ms, based on direct thalamic recordings in man (Arezzo, Legatt, and Vaughan, 1979; Fukushima, Mayanagi, and

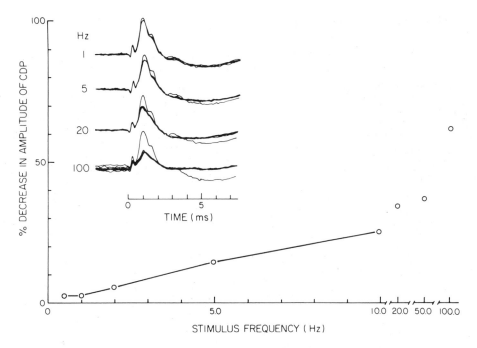

FIGURE 4.20.   Changes in the cord dorsum potential (CDP) of the cat in response to trains of stimuli delivered to the sural nerve at various frequencies, successive traces in the train are shown superimposed, the initial CDP in each train being normal in size. Even at 5 Hz there was some reduction in the size of the CDP potential. At interstimulus intervals of 50 to 10 ms these reductions were much more dramatic. They were not accompanied by any change in the size or shape of preceding dorsal root potential. Such changes in the size of the CDP indicate that this potential must be generated postsynaptically. These changes in the CDP at various stimulus frequencies are shown in the plot surrounding the insert of the actual potentials.
(From Brown, Hurst, and Routhier, unpublished observations)

Bouchard, 1976). The negativity registered by G_1 over the neck in such cephalic reference recordings therefore may not entirely reflect an underlying cervical negative potential generated in the dorsal horn, but an even more positive cephalic G_2 electrode because of the lemniscal activity. Moreover, in such cephalic reference recordings the progressive increase in latency of the N11 potential (posterior cervical G_1) is not seen, which probably explains the controversy as to whether there is any true latency shift in the cervical potential to indicate the presence of a conducted tract potential (Cracco, 1973; Cracco, Cracco, Sar-

nowski, and Vogel, 1980; Matthews, Beauchamp, and Small, 1974; Small, Beauchamp, and Matthews, 1980).

The lemniscal origin of the far field recorded P13–14 potential is supported by its persistence in the presence of thalamic lesions (Nakanishi, Shimoda, Sakuta, and Toyokura, 1978; Mauguière and Courjon, 1981). A dominant cervical contribution to the N14 potential (G_1 posterior neck and $G_2–F_z$) has been suggested because of its preservation in the face of pontine or midbrain lesions (Chiappa, Choi, and Young, 1980). It was not clear in the latter reports, however, whether or not the medial lemniscus was destroyed and if so, how complete that destruction was.

The completeness of the lesion is an important point because it apparently requires few peripheral afferents or their second-order sensory fibers to generate a nearly complete cortical SEP. This is suggested by the fact that the SEP reaches its maximum amplitude where the peripheral sensory nerve action potential is clearly submaximal, and the ability to record an SEP in the presence of severe sensory neuropathies where no peripheral sensory nerve action potentials can be recorded (Desmedt, 1971) (Figure 4.21).

It was pointed out in the section on the thalamus in this chapter, that in the human thalamus the earliest activity begins in the ventrobasal complex (posterior lateral nucleus) at 15 ms and reaches a peak at about 18 ms in response to a contralateral stimulus delivered to the median nerve at the wrist (Fukushima, Mayanagi, and Bouchard, 1976; Celesia, 1979). Celesia (1979) observed a steep decline in the amplitudes of these potentials as the electrode prod was moved even a few millimeters off this target, in keeping with the closed-field nature of thalamic activity. This last suggests that electrical potentials gener-

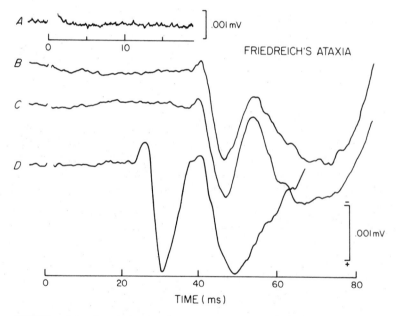

FIGURE 4.21.   Patient with Friedreich's ataxia (age 23 years).
(A) In a recording from median nerve at the wrist no nerve action potential was detectible in response to stimulation of the second and third digits. Cortical evoked potentials in response to the stimulation at the wrist (B and C repeated to show reproducibility of recordings) and median nerve in the axilla (D). The calculated maximum afferent conduction velocity between the wrist and axilla was 31.5 m/s. Despite this demonstration of very slow peripheral conduction velocity, the shape of the cortical potential was normal, indicating its central generators probably operated more or less normally once the afferent volley reached them.
From Desmedt and Noel (1973, figure 5).

ated by neuronal potentials in the thalamus probably do not contribute much if at all to the SEP.

More likely generators of SEPs are the ascending activity in the medial lemniscus, which probably accounts for the far field recorded P13–15 as outlined earlier, and thalamocortical activity projecting to the sensorimotor cortex. Indeed, such later activity could well account for the increasing negativity between 17–20–22 ms recorded with G_1 over the contralateral C_3 or C_4 position and the reference electrode (G_2) over the corresponding ipsilateral cortical regions (Figure 4.1). In such an electrode arrangement, electrical activity originating in the central neuraxis, brainstem, and perhaps even thalamus would be seen equally by both electrodes, and only above the thalamus would a different potential be seen. In view of the evidence that electrical potentials beginning at 20 to 22 ms probably originate in the sensorimotor cortex it seems

reasonable to assume that the increasing negativity (see above) preceding the N20–22 peak is thalamocortical in origin. This is a view shared by Desmedt and Cheron (1981a), who claim that the N18 component of this activity that is seen initially in contrast to the N20–22 must represent thalamocortical activity.

It must be admitted at the present time that very little is known about the conduction distances in the various function-specific thalamocortical afferents, their diameters, or conduction velocities. In view of the depth of the rolandic fissure, it seems clear that the deeper regions 3 and 1 must be activated earlier than the cortex on the crown of the postcentral gyrus. Possibly the series of negative peaks on the increasing negativity leading up to N20–22 (see Figures 4.1 and 4.3) represents different components of this thalamocortical rostrally conducting activity.

Table 4.4 summarizes present views about the origin of the subcortical potentials. It must

TABLE 4.4.   Electrogenic Origins of Various Subcortical Potentials (Median Nerve Stimulation at Wrist)

	Potential	Probable Electrogenic Source
Far Field		
G_1 Cephalic and	P8–9	Brachial plexus
G_2 Opposite hand, knee, or foot	P15	Ascending medial lemniscus
Nearer Field		
G_1 Posterior neck and	P8–9	Brachial plexus
G_2 Opposite hand	N11	Ascending dorsal column activity
	N13–14	Postsynaptic activity in dorsal horn (C3–T2)
G_1 Posterior neck and	P8–9	Brachial plexus
G_2 Cephalic (F_z)	N11	? ascending tract or postsynaptic activity in spinal cord
	N13–14	Postsynaptic activity dorsal in horn (C3–T2) +
G_1 Contralateral scalp (C3/4) and	N15–20	Ascending medial lemniscus
G_2 Ipsilateral scalp (C3/4)		Thalamocortical activity

be thought of as a tentative and, in need of more direct confirmation by direct or nearby recordings from the various neural structures, a careful analysis of discrete lesions in the somatosensory pathway whose precise localization and completeness is confirmed by pathological examination and more detailed anatomical measurements of the fiber spectra of the central tracts and their conduction distances.

SEP Potentials of Cortical Origin

For most EMG laboratories it is the earliest (20 to 22 ms from upper limb) rather than the more intermediate and later cortical potentials that are of the most interest. For this reason, this chapter focuses on the electrogenesis of the earliest cortical activity.

When the median or ulnar nerve at the wrist or their respective digits are stimulated, a N20–22 potential can be recorded posterior to the rolandic fissure at the scalp and directly on the cortical surface where its amplitude is substantially higher (Figure 4.22). As befits its origin in the distal limb dermatomal representation in the postcentral cortex, the N20–22 potential is strictly contralateral (there are no transcallosal connections for central afferent projections from the skin surface of the distal limbs). Unfortunately, this potential was not consistently or clearly recognized in earlier direct cortical investigations in man where transcortical recordings were made and the effects of ablation were studied on the cortical potentials. The positive potential that followed P20–25, however, was seen clearly and this potential not only reversed its polarity in transcortical recordings (Kelly, Goldring, and O'Leary, 1965; Stohr and Goldring, 1969) but was lost when ablation of the postcentral cortex was carried out (Stohr and Goldring, 1969; Goldring, Aras, and Weber, 1970). The reversal of polarity began just below the cortical

surface. Such reversals of phase point to the recruitment of successively more superficial neurons beginning in layer IV by the thalamocortical afferents to the primary sensory cortex (Amassian, Waller, and Macy, 1964).

The above observations indicate that not only does the N20–P25 potential originate in the postcentral cortex, but that it is almost certainly the equivalent of the primary surface positive potential. This potential in man (Woolsey and Erickson, 1950; Jasper, Lende, and Rasmussen, 1960; Woolsey, Erickson, and Gilson, 1979) and lower animals is discretely localized to the contralateral primary sensory cortex in the case of distal limb stimulation (see also review Werner and Whitsel, 1973).

Within the postcentral cortex, the potentials are probably generated predominantly by postsynaptic potentials in pyramidal neurons oriented perpendicularly to the cortical surface, though not necessarily the convexity of the brain. This is because much of the primary cortical representation for the distal portions of the limbs lies in the posterior wall of the rolandic fissure. Other postsynaptic potentials, in short interneurons and long afterpotentials, may also contribute to the primary cortical potentials.

The precise relationships between the recorded scalp potentials and the actual underlying cortical generators have not yet been established with any certainty in man. The N20–22 potential that immediately precedes the major positive-negative potential P20–N30 as recorded posterior to the rolandic fissure is not seen in lower primates, or for that matter in man, in response to mechanical stimuli. This is possibly because of the resultant poorly synchronized peripheral afferent volley and the poor resolution of the averaging techniques available in some of the earlier studies. A potential equivalent to N20–22 was detected, however, in response to taps delivered to the nail bed (Sears, 1959).

One current, and in the author's view, rea-

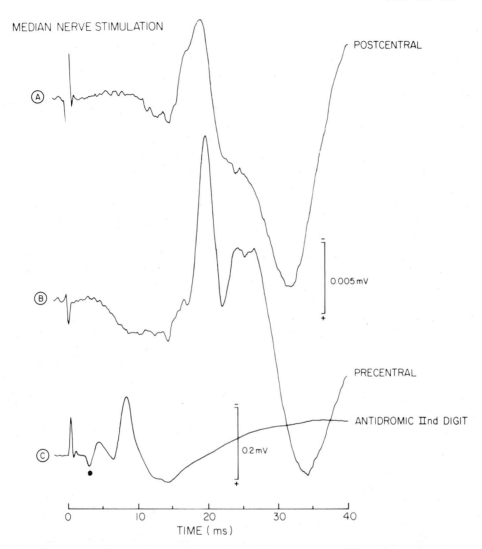

FIGURE 4.22.   Direct cortical recordings on the surface of the precentral (B) and postcentral cortex (A) of somatosensory evoked cortical potentials elicited by contralateral stimulation of the median nerve. Such potentials are usually 3 to 10 times larger than the equivalent potentials recorded from the scalp. The precentral and postcentral regions from which these potentials were recorded were also the sites at which direct stimulation elicited low-threshold thumb twitches and paresthesias in the hand respectively.

The latency of the N20 potential was about 1 ms shorter when recorded over the postcentral compared to the precentral cortex. Also, the N20 potential was clearly preceded by a series of positive waves beginning as early as 10 ms in the postcentral recording. These must be volume-conducted potentials originating in subcortical structures. The reference electrode for all recordings was attached to the electrode holder clamped onto the skull at the posterior margin of the craniectomy.

In (C) is shown the antidromic sensory nerve action recorded from the second digit (onset marked with •) followed by the volume-conducted motor response from the median innervated lumbrical and thenar muscles.

sonable hypothesis is the suggestion that the P20–N30 potential recorded anterior to the central sulcus (or the equivalent, the N20–P30 potential registered over the parietal region) originates in the postcentral gyrus and is the equivalent of the primary cortical response seen in lower animals. Indeed, two responsible generators have been postulated to be present in the postcentral gyrus (Allison, Goff, Williamson, and VanGilder, 1980; Arezzo, Vaughan, and Legatt, 1981). One compromising areas 3 and anterior area 1 receives cutaneous and muscle afferent inputs. Electrical potentials originating in this region of the cortex could account for the apparent horizontal anterior–posterior dipole and phase reversal across the central sulcus noted by several authors in scalp and direct cortical recordings (Broughton, 1969; Allison, Goff, Williamson, and VanGilder, 1980). A second generator may also exist in the crown of the postcentral gyrus, a region comprising areas 1 and 2 and which receives inputs from deep afferents. Electrical potentials originating here could explain the P25–N35 potential seen best in direct cortical recordings.

Not all investigators have been able, by direct cortical recordings, to detect a clear phase reversal across the central sulcus (Stohr and Goldring, 1969; Woolsey, Erickson, and Gilson, 1979; Celesia, 1979). The two-generator hypothesis, however, is consistent with what is known about the physiological and anatomical organization of the postcentral cortex (see review by Brodal, 1981) and cortical recordings in lower primates (Arezzo, Vaughan, and Legatt, 1981).

The latter group of authors have suggested that if the N20–P30 (or P20–N30) potentials do originate in the postcentral cortex, the earlier N20–22 potential may not be cortical in origin at all, but pre-precortical. It would therefore have to be generated by propagated potentials in thalamocortical connections. It is worthwhile recalling here that the anterior and posterior banks of the rolandic fissure have not been subjected to detailed evoked potential recordings in man.

The central sulcus is about twice as deep as the precentral or postcentral gyri are wide. In short, about two-thirds or more of the sensorimotor cortex is buried and not accessible to direct convexity recordings. This point is important because, as pointed out earlier, the posterior and anterior banks of the central sulcus are the sites of the representation of the distal limbs (Woolsey, Settlage, Meyer Spencer, Hamuy, and Travis, 1952; Werner and Whitsel, 1973; Jones and Powell, 1973; Wong, Kwan, Mackay, and Murphy, 1978; Kwan, Mackay, Murphy, and Wong, 1978; Woolsey, Erickson, and Gilson, 1979; Murphy, Kwan, Mackay, and Wong, 1980; Brodal, 1981). When the skin or the peripheral nerves in the distal parts of limbs are stimulated, as in most SEP studies, it is precisely these deeper regions, areas 3 and anterior 1, that would be excited earliest. Areas 2 and posterior area 1 would be activated later through collaterals of projections to areas 3 and anterior 1. Such activation of the postcentral gyrus could lead to an overlap of conducted potentials in the thalamocortical pathway with direct cortically originating potentials. The N20–22 potentials could therefore be generated by rostrally conducting electrical potentials in the thalamocortical pathway, as suggested recently by Chiappa, Choi, and Young (1980), or the combination of this with generators in the cortex itself, as suggested by Kritchevsky and Wiederholt (1978) and Desmedt and Brunko (1980).

The cortical potentials beyond 30 ms no doubt represent the activation of other cortical regions by cortical-cortical connections and extralemniscal projections to other cortical regions. For example, it is known that SI projects to the secondary sensory area (SII), the contralateral SI (except for distal limb regions), and the parietal region, area 5. Indeed, potentials can be detected over SII that have onset latencies between 30 and 50 ms in man (Woolsey, Erickson, and Gilson, 1979). Moreover, area 4 receives direct thalamic proprioceptive projections independent of the thalamocortical projections to the postcentral cortex, as well as cortical-cortical connections originating in areas 3 and 2. Desmedt and Cheron (1981a), in disagreeing with the earlier suggestions of a positive-negative dipole across the rolandic fissure (see earlier discussion), contend that the prerolandic positivity P22 has a little longer latency than the postrolandic negativity N20. They further state that this, plus the preservation of this P22 prerolandic potential in the presence of parietal lesions, indicates that the prerolandic P22 originates in the precentral cortex itself by thalamic projections independent of those to the postcentral gyrus. Thus the P22 is not the mirror or dipole image of the postcentral N20.

The premotor region area 6 also receives projections from areas 4 and 5 and the frontal cortex from posterior parietal cortex. These connections and others could explain the progressive activation of other cortical areas and the later cortical potentials. Table 4.5 summarizes present speculations about the origins of cortical potentials in the SEP.

Somatosensory Evoked Potentials in Response to Stimulation in the Lower Limb

Up to now the discussion has concentrated on the technical aspects and basic physiology and mechanisms using upper limb SEP studies in man to highlight the important issues and illustrate various phenomena. Clearly, however, the same techniques are applicable in the lower limb and would be a potentially valuable means to investigate peripheral conduction in the lower limbs, including the plexus and roots and central ascending conduction in

TABLE 4.5.   Electrogenic Origins of Cortical Potentials

Postcentral recordings	N20–22	Earliest activity in postcentral cortex or thalamocortical
Postcentral recordings	N20 to P30	Primary sensory cortical activity
Precentral	P22	?Precentral cortical activity

the spinal cord, as well as the more rostral conduction through to the cortical representation areas for the lower limb.

In a landmark study of immediate relevance, Magladery, Porter, Park, and Teasdall (1951) characterized the potentials recordable with wire electrodes introduced into the lumbosacral subarachnoid space in response to electrical stimulation of cutaneous and motor nerves in the lower limb. Their records are remarkably clear and even today stand as the best-documented series of such recordings in man. As these early observations inform us about the potentials now recorded with electronic averaging techniques with surface electrodes, it is worthwhile reviewing the characteristics of these potentials (Figure 4.23).

These authors, even with the use of "near" spinal cord or root electrodes, experienced problems with the pickup of EMG activity from nearby paraspinal muscles and therefore used sodium phenobarbital sedation to help relax the subjects. The electrical stimulus pulses were delivered through percutaneous electrodes to mixed (posterior tibial nerve or peroneal nerve) or cutaneous nerves (sural) and recordings made at the various lumbosacral levels. The main potentials they recognized included the dorsal root potential (DRP), ventral root potential (VRP), "intermediate" potential, and spinal potential.

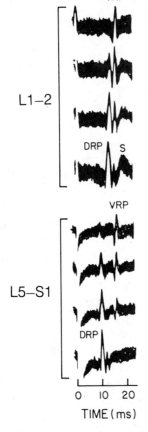

VRP

L1–2

DRP   S

VRP

L5–S1

DRP

0   10   20
TIME (ms)

FIGURE 4.23.   Spinal root recordings made with in-trathecal needle electrodes insulated except near their tips and inserted near the roots at the L1–2 and L5–S1 levels. The intensity of the electrical stimulus delivered to the posterior tibial nerve at the level of the popliteal fossa was increased from top to bottom through the four traces at the above two recording sites.
DRP = Dorsal Root Potential
VRP = Ventral Root Potential
S = Spinal (cord dorsum potential)
Adapted from Magladery JW, Park AM and Teasdall (1951, figures 4 and 6).

Dorsal Root Potential

1. The dorsal root potential (DRP, Figure 4.23) appeared at stimulus intensities (posterior tibial nerve stimulation) exceeding those necessary to evoke an H-reflex in the gastrocnemius and soleus muscles.
2. Of the various root potentials, the DRP had the shortest latencies at all levels (L1 and L5).
3. The latency of this potential progressively increased between the L5 and L1 (10 to 11ms at L5 in response to stimulation of the posterior tibial nerve in the poplite-al fossa), establishing the orthodromic na-ture of the potential.

Ventral Root Potential

1. The ventral root potential (VRP, Figure 4.23) appeared in concert with, and its amplitude increased and decreased in parallel with, the H-reflex.
2. The latency of this potential progressively increased between L1 and L5 (latency 17 ms at L5), thus establishing the fact that the potential originated in the spinal cord and conducted toward the periphery.
3. The least time interval between the DRP and VRP at L1 was 1.8 ms an interval, which suggests a monosynaptic reflex.

Intermediate Potential

1. The intermediate potential (IP) appeared only at stimulus intensities that exceeded threshold for the DRP.
2. Its amplitude paralleled changes in the amplitude of the direct M-potential in contradistinction to the behavior of the reflex VRP, whose amplitude diminished as did the H-reflex at higher stimulus in-tensities, probably because of collisions between antidromic and reflex impulses in the ventral roots.

Magladery, Porter, Park, and Teasdall (1951) suggested that this intermediate poten-tial was an antidromic VRP. Alternatively, Debecke, McComas, and Kopec (1978) sug-gested that it more likely represented anti-dromic conducted potentials in gamma motor axons.

Spinal Potential

At the lumbosacral and lower thoracic levels a slow negative-positive potential was seen sometimes preceded by a smaller sharper potential. The main characteristics of these potentials were:

1. The potential was mainly distributed between T10 and L1–2 and was not seen at middle to lower lumbar levels in their recordings.
2. Rostral to L1 the preceding spikelike root potentials were not seen.
3. Between the L1 and T9 levels the latency of this potential progressively increased, possibly through the sequential activation of the successively more rostral dorsal horn segments.
4. The latency of the onset of the negative potential was 13 to 14 ms and the duration of the whole negative potential was 17 to 20 ms (posterior tibial nerve stimulation in the popliteal fossa).
5. The succeeding positive potential lasted approximately twice as long as the preceding negative potential at the T11 level.
6. Similar potentials could be evoked by cutaneous nerve (sural) stimulation.
7. Progressive declines in the amplitudes of these slow potentials developed at interstimulus pulse intervals as short as 10 ms, suggesting the presence of at least one synapse between the site of stimulation and the generator of the potential, here postsynaptic neurons in the dorsal horn.

It was concluded by the original authors that the slow negative-positive lumbosacral cord potential in man was the equivalent of the intermediate cord or so-called cord dorsum potentials (CDP) seen in lower animals and discussed earlier in this chapter (Gasser and Graham, 1933; Bernard, 1953; Bernard and Widen, 1953; Coombs, Curtis, and Landgren, 1956; Willis, 1980). This potential is therefore the equivalent of the N13–14 segmental cervical potential.

In the monkey, the lumbosacral cord dorsum potential extends over the entire length of the lumbosacral cord, although the amplitude is maximum opposite the dorsal root that contributes the largest number of the afferents to the cord (Beall, Applebaum, Foreman, and Willis, 1977). In the cat, the amplitude of the cord dorsum potential evoked by motor nerve stimulation is relatively smaller than that produced by stimulation of cutaneous nerves (Figure 4.24). In the monkey, however, group I and II muscle afferents can evoke a large negative cord dorsum potential. This potential has a broad longitudinal distribution in the lumbrosacral cord (Foreman, Kenshalo, Schmidt, and Willis, 1979), suggesting important species differences in the connectivities of peripheral afferents to the spinal cord. In man, like the monkey, muscle or cutaneous afferents alone can generate a cord dorsum potential that has broad distributions in the lumbosacral cord.

Conducted ascending and descending tract potentials have been recorded in man by near-cord electrodes. Using these techniques, Ertekin (1976a, 1976b) estimated the maximum conduction velocity in the dorsal columns to be between 30 and 50 m/s (mean, 37 m/s). Maximum velocities in the sciatic nerve between the popliteal fossa and cord were appreciably higher, between 50 and 73 m/s (mean, 63 m/s), an observation compatible with anatomical studies that have shown that the diameters of nerve fibers in the dorsal columns (range, 1 to 7 μ) are about one-half of the diameters of the largest nerve fibers in the peripheral nerve (Onishi, O'Brien, Okazaki, and Dyck, 1976). Recently, however, much higher conduction velocities in the dorsal columns have been reported (82 ± 5.4 m/s) by Maruyama, Shimoji, Shimizu, Kuribayashi, and Fujioka (1982).

In Ertekin's (1976a, 1976b) studies the characteristics of the recorded spinal poten-

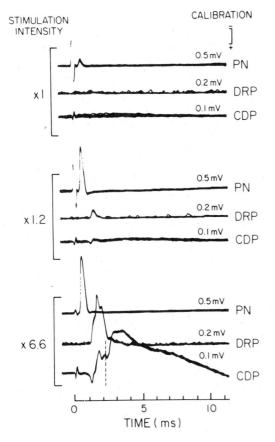

FIGURE 4.24.   Relationships between the cord dorsum potential (CDP), dorsal root potential (DRP), and the monophasic compound nerve action potential here recorded antidromically from the peroneal nerve (PN) in the cat. Stimulus currents expressed as multiples of the least current shown (top) are indicated on the left. The stimulus was delivered directly to the common peroneal nerve. Note that the CDP, which begins at the second interrupted vertical line, is preceded by a spike potential produced by the volley in the primary afferents at the root entry zone. There is about 1 ms between onset of this spike and onset of the negative CDP; this is time enough for one or possibly more synapses within the dorsal horn of the spinal cord.

cal intrathecal electrodes recorded conducted potentials in the roots, the cord dorsum potential when the electrode was more dorsolateral in position, or the dorsal column potential and possibly the cord dorsum potential when the electrode was in the middorsal position.

The sources of potentials at or near the spinal cord therefore include:

1. Dorsal and ventral root potentials, including antidromic activity in the ventral roots when motor nerves are stimulated.
2. The dorsal horn (this has been discussed earlier).
3. Conducted potentials in various central tracts, such as the dorsal, dorsolateral, and the anterolateral columns. The latencies of the tract potentials could be expected to increase the more rostral the site of the recording electrodes, as has indeed been shown in the cervical region by Desmedt and Cheron (1981a). In the case of the dorsal horn potential, although some slight progressive increases in latency through sequential activation of more rostral dorsal horn segments may be seen, these should be much less than in the case of tract potentials that conduct at much faster velocities.

In studies such as Ertekin's (1976a, 1976b) where needle electrodes are inserted near the cord, there must be concern about possible injuries to the spinal cord. The reports of paresthesia in these studies suggest that the electrodes in some instances did indeed touch or even penetrate the spinal cord. Fortunately, no lasting sequelae developed after these investigations, to the best of our knowledge.

SURFACE RECORDINGS OF LUMBOSACRAL AND ROOT POTENTIALS

There have been numerous attempts to record lumbosacral root and lower cord potentials by

tials were critically dependent on the precise position of the recording electrode. For example, in response to stimulation of peripheral nerves in the arm, laterally placed cervi-

surface electrodes (Figure 4.25). Cracco and colleagues, for example, were able to identify and characterize three main potentials recorded over the lumbosacral, thoracic, and cervical regions in response to peripheral nerve

stimulation in the lower limb (Cracco, Cracco, Sarnowski, and Vogel, 1980). Sequential bipolar electrode recordings were made between the lumbar and cervical regions and revealed:

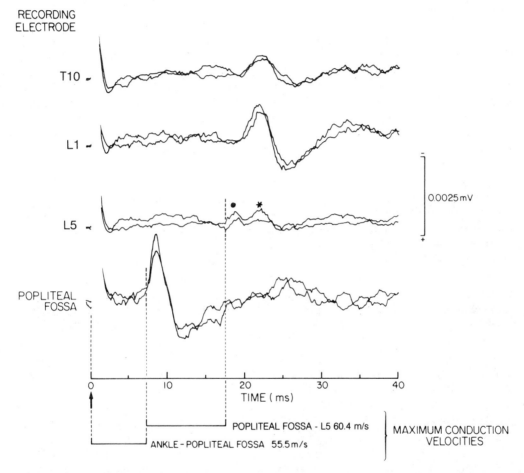

FIGURE 4.25. Lumbosacral evoked potentials recorded with surface electrodes over the L5, L1, and T10 spinous processes (reference electrode T6 in all cases) in response to stimulation of the posterior tibial nerve at the ankle. For the knee-level recording, the recording electrode was situated over the posterior tibial nerve and the reference electrode 50 mm laterally.

Note the larger cord dorsum potential (− +) at L1 compared to T10, and the two successive potentials marked by a dot (•) and an asterisk (*) over the L5 level. The first of these (•) probably represents the orthodromic traveling afferent volley in the dorsal roots, with a possible contribution from antidromic motor impulses in the ventral roots. The second of the potentials (*) could be generated by a reflex motor volley (although there was only a small and very variable late response in the plantar muscles here) or volume conduction within the spinal space of the rostrally generated cord dorsum potential.

1. A triphasic potential was recorded over the lumbar region. The latency of this potential increased between L5 and L1 and therefore this potential was in all likelihood a conducted potential in the dorsal roots.
2. A larger negative potential was recorded over the lower thoracic spine, which in some records showed an apparent increase in latency between the low thoracic and midthoracic levels. This potential probably corresponded to the cord dorsum potential and the progressive increase in latency to sequential activation of higher dorsal horn segments and the attendant conduction in intersegmental fibers. Sometimes this large negative potential was preceded by a low-amplitude, short-duration, positive-negative potential that was probably generated by conducted potentials in intraspinal branches of primary sensory afferents.
3. Between the midthoracic to cervical regions a small triphasic potential was seen in most recordings. This was postulated to be generated by a conducted potential in the dorsal columns and possibly other spinal rostral tracts.

Others have reported various modifications to the technique that better record and characterize these lumbosacral root and lower cord potentials (Dimitrijevic, Larsson, Lehmkuhl, and Sherwood, 1978; Debecke, McComas, and Kopec, 1978; Phillips and Daube, 1980). In our own laboratory we have chosen to stimulate the posterior tibial nerve at the level of the ankle and record the potentials at the levels of the popliteal fossa, L5, L1–2, and cephalic levels. The best position of the reference electrode varies a little with the subject. In general we have chosen either the opposite iliac crest or a T6 electrode.

The main problems with the surface recordings are the low amplitudes of the potentials and EKG and EMG artifact, which may make it very difficult to resolve the various potentials even in healthy subjects. If necessary, EKG can be avoided by triggering the averager off the EKG potential, although this prolongs the recording time (stimulation at about 1 per second instead of 3 or 4 per second). The EMG artifact in such recordings in our experience is much the worst villain. It sometimes helps to place one or two pillows under the patient's stomach and take other measures to promote relaxation. In some subjects, diazepam may be necessary to obtain the requisite relaxation. In the better of such recordings, several potentials can be identified, namely:

1. A large negative-positive potential whose amplitude is maximum over T10–12 and steeply declines toward the midthoracic region, but which may be seen with opposite polarity in the lower lumbar recordings (L5). This again is likely the cord dorsum potential, and as in Cracco and associates' (1980) records, this large potential may be preceded by a small positive notch on the onset of the main negative potential.
2. At the lumbosacral levels sometimes two potentials can be recognized. There is usually an early positive-negative potential that must be generated in the dorsal roots because the latency of the potential increases between the S1 and L1 levels. A second potential that has a longer latency and whose amplitude parallels the amplitude of the H-reflex in some subjects may be detectable and could originate in the ventral roots, although others, including Debecke, McComas, and Kopec (1978) and Phillips and Daube (1980), have argued that this potential was simply the cord dorsum potential seen in volume by the lumbar electrode.

Based on our recent experience, spinal evoked potentials seem to offer little as yet to the study of diseases of the roots or lumbosacral cord because of the small size of some of the potentials, especially as recorded with surface electrodes, and problems of obtaining the necessary relaxation in some subjects. The resolution of the root and cord potentials can, of course, be substantially increased by using needle electrodes, inserted into the epidural or subarachnoid space. The latter position provides a sometimes convenient means of stimulating the ventral roots and assessing proximal motor conduction as well (Figures 4.26 and 4.27).

There are other ways for assessing peripheral and central conduction from the lower limb. For example, in a manner akin to the FFR techniques used for upper limb studies, FFRs can be done for the lower limb (Yamada, Machida, and Kimura, 1982). Various components of these far field potentials correspond in timing at least, to potentials generated in the lumbosacral plexus or roots, lumbosacral cord, and perhaps ascending potentials as well as the cortical evoked potential. The author has no experience with this technique as applied to the lower limb, but if it shares the same problems of poor definition of the subcomponents even in some normal subjects and especially in patients with disorders affecting the peripheral and central sensory pathways as it does in the upper limb, it is unlikely to have much practical value; to me, nearer source recording techniques seem preferable.

The other option is to record the cortical evoked potential in response to stimulation of peripheral nerves in the lower limb at several distal to proximal sites as a way of measuring peripheral sensory conduction velocities. This technique is especially valuable when the patient has lost an appreciable number of the larger peripheral sensory afferents or the conduction velocities are slowed, and when peripheral sensory nerve action potentials are difficult to detect with surface electrodes or even in some instances, near-nerve electrodes. As pointed out in Chapter 3, however, stimulation at two or more levels may not excite the same afferents because some afferents present in the proximal nerve trunk leave the trunk proximal to the distal sites of stimulation. Moreover, there is no certainty that the afferents that evoke the SEP, especially in abnormal states, are truly the fastest-conducting afferents.

TRIGEMINAL EVOKED POTENTIALS

Recently, techniques have been described for recording the cortical potentials evoked by stimulation of trigeminal afferents (Figure 4.28). The methods of stimulation vary from mechanical stimuli such as taps delivered to the tongue (Ishiko, Hanamori, and Murayama, 1980) or face (Larsson and Prevec, 1970), to electrical stimulation of peripheral branches of the trigeminal nerve or the gums (Bennett and Jannetta, 1980; Stöhr and Petruch, 1979; Stöhr, Petruch, and Scheglmann, 1980; Drechsler, 1980; Singh, Sachdev, and Brisman, 1982; Eisen, Paty, Purves, and Hoirch, 1981). Alternating the polarity of the electrical stimulus helped to reduce the stimulus artifact. Using these techniques, abnormalities in trigeminal somatosensory central pathway have been shown in multiple sclerosis (Eisen, Paty, Purves, and Hoirch, 1981).

PRESENT VALUE OF SOMATOSENSORY EVOKED POTENTIALS

The preceding techniques have proved very useful for detecting subclinical lesions not seen with computerized tomographic scanning, the prime example being multiple sclerosis (Figure 4.29). Their value in this regard may be

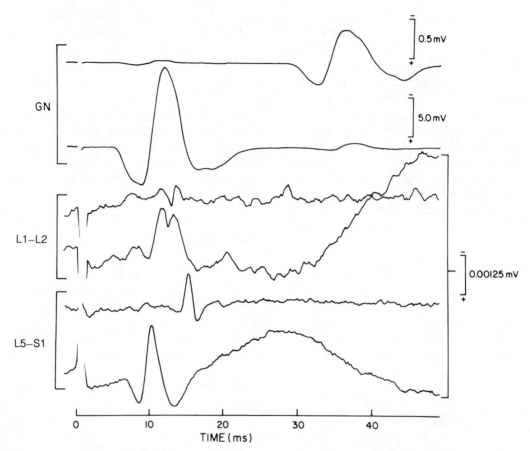

FIGURE 4.26.   Lumbosacral evoked potential study carried out using needles insulated except at their tips and inserted into the subarachnoid spaces at the L1−2 and L5−S1 levels. The posterior tibial nerve was stimulated in the popliteal fossa and the respective gastrocnemius (GN) muscle and root potentials at the L1−2 and L5−S1 levels recorded when the stimulus intensity was adjusted to be just below motor threshold and sufficient to elicit a maximum M-potential (top and bottom traces respectively, of each pair).

The weaker of the two stimuli elicited an H-reflex response in the gastrocnemius muscle and clearly defined root potentials at both the L1−2 and L5−S1 levels. The rostrocaudal increase in latency strongly suggested these root potentials were generated in the ventral roots and were the same volley which more peripherally elicited the H-reflex. This view was substantiated by the disappearance of the latter potential at L5−S1 when the stimulus was supramaximal for eliciting the maximum M-potential. The late M-potential still evident must have been generated by reflected F-impulses in motor axons whose centrifugally conducting volley must, in this case, have been too asynchronous to elicit a well-defined volley in ventral roots.

The same supramaximal stimulus evoked shorter latency potentials at both the L5−S1 and L1−2 levels, which probably originated in the dorsal roots. In keeping with the latter view, the latency of the volley increased from L5−S1 to L1−2. Superimposed on the root potential at L1−2 when the stimulus was supramaximal was the cord dorsum potential.

The above recordings from a volunteer rendered quadriplegic by a C6−7 traumatic cord lesion clearly illustrates the well defined root potential readily recordable from most subjects when subarachnoid or sometimes epidural needle electrodes are used. The reference electrodes for the L1−2 and L5−S1 electrodes were in each case a second needle electrode inserted subcutaneously in the next (rostral) interspace.

FIGURE 4.27. Same subject as in Figure 4.26. Here the ventral roots were stimulated supramaximally at the L5–S1 level and the maximum M-potentials as recorded with surface electrodes, recorded from the gastrocnemius (GN) and extensor digitorum brevis (EDB) muscles. The peroneal nerve, in the case of EDB, was stimulated supramaximally in the popliteal fossa and at the ankle and the posterior tibial nerve in the popliteal fossa in the case of the GN recording. Such a method makes it possible to measure motor conduction velocities and assess the presence or absence of conduction block across the proximal portions of the peripheral nervous system. Note that in this subject as in other subjects where peripheral conduction in motor fibers is normal, no more than a 20 percent reduction in the peak-to-peak amplitude or 40 percent increase in the duration of the negative peak of the potentials was seen.

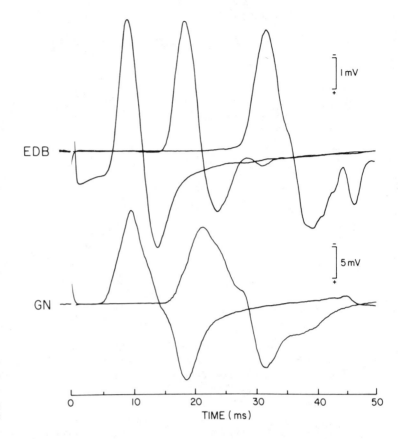

superseded by newer nuclear magnetic resonance scanning procedures, however.

In the peripheral nervous system, the main value of SEP techniques is in the assessment of conduction in the brachial or possibly lumbosacral plexuses (see Figure 4.16). In the author's view, they have had little value in evaluating cervical root lesions, especially where digit stimulation has been used, because the amplitude and resolution of the cervical and even cortical potentials have been too poor to identify any but the most affected roots (Figure 4.30). It is just such severe root entrapments that are the easiest to recognize by their clinical presentation and radiological assessments.

The SEP techniques can demonstrate proximal conduction abnormalities in Guillain-Barré polyneuropathy (see Figure 4.17) at very early stages in the evaluation of this disease at a time when more peripheral sensory as well as motor conduction velocities are normal.

Further developments are necessary in technology and clinical experience before these tests can be held to have an established value. One of the problems here, however, is that in order to improve the resolution of the potentials recorded near the cord or roots, the recording electrodes will have to be inserted nearer to the structures, and this will limit their use to the most unusual and diagnostically difficult cases. That these developments will turn out to be necessary in the face of recent advances in neuroradiological techniques is doubtful.

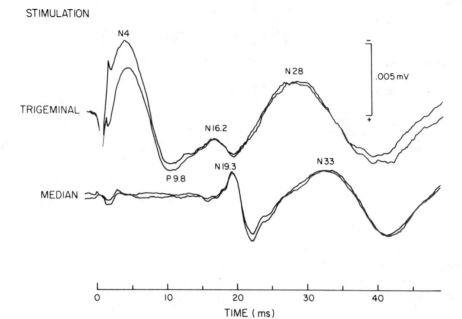

STIMULATION

N4

N 28

.005 mV

TRIGEMINAL

N16.2

N 19.3

N 33

P 9.8

MEDIAN

TIME (ms)

FIGURE 4.28.   Trigeminal somatosensory evoked potential (Top). Electrode G_1 was situated over the contralateral postcentral face area and G_2 at the vertex. The contralateral lower lip was stimulated by means of a bipolar electrode (5 mA) just sufficient to produce a small twitch in the underlying orbicularis oris muscle. The general configuration of the potential was similar to the somatosensory evoked potential elicited by contralateral distal upper limb stimulation (median nerve wrist G_1 and G_2 over the contralateral and ipsilateral C4–3 regions respectively).

(Bottom) Comparable median nerve stimulus (wrist) evoked cortical potential recorded over the hand area of the postcentral region. Note the similarity in the wave forms, N16.2 trigeminal evoked potential being equivalent to the N19.3 potential of the median stimulus-elicited cortical potential. Preceding the N16.2 potential are N4 and P9.8 potentials, which are possibly generated in the gasserian ganglion, trigeminal, nerve or brainstem (Singh, Sachdev, and Brisman, 1982). Each of the above potentials is the electronic average of 500 responses.

MULTIPLE SCLEROSIS

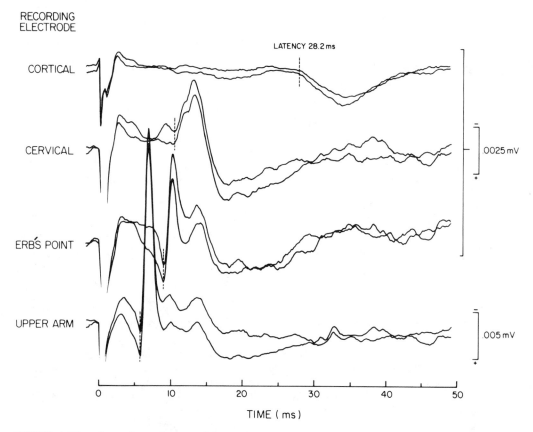

FIGURE 4.29. Central conduction delay in multiple sclerosis. Shown are the orthodromic nerve action potentials as recorded at the levels of the proximal arm and Erb's point, the cervical potential recorded over C6, and the contralateral cortical evoked potential recorded at C4 (reference electrode for all recording sites was the ipsilateral C3).

The peripheral sensory conduction velocities and latency to the onset of the cervical potential were well within the respective −2-SD and +2-SD limits for controls. Also, the cervical potential has a normal shape and size; however, the cortical potential was obviously delayed. The delay could have been caused by lesion(s) affecting the medial lemniscus and/or thalamocortical projections.

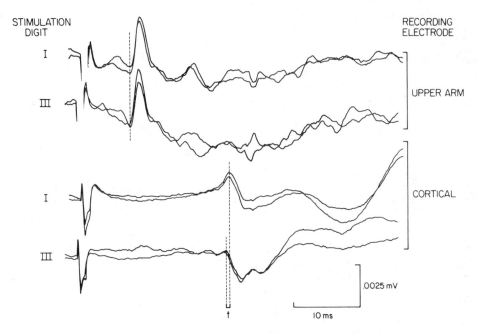

FIGURE 4.30.   Patient with C7 radiculopathy, in whom an obvious displacement of the C7 root at the C6–7 level was evident in the myelogram. In the recordings the first (C6) and third (C7) digits were stimulated to elicit the maximum orthodromic potential over the median nerve in the proximal upper arm. The recordings at the upper arm and contralateral (C4) cortical regions have been displaced with respect to one another so that onsets of the respective potentials at the upper arm coincide. Here there was a 0.6-ms delay in onset of the third digit (C7) N20 potential compared to the potential elicited by stimulation of the first digit (C6). Such a delay in a single root entrapment is unfortunately not too readily seen in many patients because the recordings are too often technically unsatisfactory.

References

Allison T, Goff WR, Williamson PD, VanGilder JC. On the neural origin of early components of the human somatosensory evoked potential. In: Desmedt JE, ed. Clinical uses of cerebral, brainstem and spinal somatosensory evoked potentials. Progress in clinical neurophysiology. Basel: Karger, 1980:51–68.

Amassian VE, Waller MJ, Macy J Jr. Neuronal mechanism of the primary somatosensory evoked potential. Ann NY Acad Sci 1964;112:5–32.

Andersson SA, Norrsell K, Norrsell U. Spinal pathways projecting to the cerebral first somatosensory area in the monkey. J Physiol (Lond) 1972;225:589–97.

Arezzo J, Legatt AD, Vaughan HG. Topography and intracranial sources of somatosensory evoked potentials in the monkey. Early components. Electroencephalogr Clin Neurophysiol 1979;46:155–72.

Arezzo JC, Vaughan HG, Legatt AD. Topography and intracranial sources of somatosensory evoked potentials in the monkey. II. Cortical components. Electroencephalogr Clin Neurophysiol 1981;51:1–8.

Beall JE, Applebaum AE, Foreman RD, Willis WD. Spinal cord potentials evoked by cutaneous afferents in the monkey. J Neurophysiol 1977;40:199–211.

Bennett MH, Jannetta PJ. Trigeminal evoked potentials in humans. Electroencephalogr Clin Neurophysiol 1980;48:517–26.

Bernard CG. The spinal cord potentials in leads from the cord dorsum in relation to peripheral source of afferent stimulation. Acta Physiol Scand 1953;106 (suppl):1–29.

Bernard CG, Widen L. On the origin of the negative and positive spinal cord potentials evoked by stimulation of low-threshold cutaneous fibers. Acta Physiol Scand 1953;106 (suppl):42–54.

Brodal A. Neurological anatomy in relation to clinical medicine. Oxford: Oxford University Press, 1981.

Broughton RJ. Average evoked potentials. In: Donchin Lindsley Washington: US Government Printing Office, NA SA SP 191 1969:79–84.

Brown AG, Gordon G. Subcortical mechanisms concerned in somatic sensation. Br Med Bull 1977;33:121–28.

Brown WF. Muscle input to human motor-sensory cortex. 1980 Meeting Society for Neuroscience Abstracts. Unpublished observations.

Buchthal F, Rosenfalck A. Evoked action potentials and conduction velocity in human sensory nerves. Brain Res 1966;3:1–122.

Celesia GG. Somatosensory evoked potentials recorded directly from human thalamus and Sm I cortical area. Arch Neurol 1979;36:399–405.

Chiappa KH, Choi S, Young RR. Short-latency somatosensory evoked potentials following median nerve stimulation in patients with neurological lesions. In: Desmedt JE, ed. Clinical uses of cerebral, brainstem and spinal somatosensory evoked potentials. Progress in clinical neurophysiology. Basel: Karger 1980:264–81.

Coombs JS, Curtis DR, Landgren S. Spinal cord potentials generated by impulses in muscle and cutaneous afferent fibers. J Neurophysiol 1956;19:452–67.

Cracco RQ. Spinal evoked response: peripheral nerve stimulation in man. Electroencephalogr Clin Neurophysiol 1973;35:379–86.

Cracco RQ, Cracco JB, Sarnowski R, Vogel HB. Spinal evoked potentials. In: Desmedt JE, ed. Clinical uses of cerebral, brainstem, and spinal somatosensory evoked potentials. Progress in clinical neurophysiology. Basel: Karger 1980:87–104.

Cusick JF, Myklebust JB, Larson SJ, Sances A Jr. Spinal cord evaluation by cortical evoked responses. Arch Neurol 1979;36:140–43.

Dawson GD. Investigations on a patient subject to myoclonic seizures after sensory stimulation. J Neurol Neurosurg Psychiatry 1947;10:141–49.

Dawson GD. The relative excitability and conduction velocity of sensory and motor nerve fibers in man. J Physiol 1956;131:436–51.

Debecke J, McComas AJ, Kopec SJ. Analysis of evoked lumbosacral potentials in man. J Neurol Neurosurg Psychiatry 1978;41:293–302.

Desmedt JE. Somatosensory cerebral evoked potentials in man. In: Remond A, ed. Handbook of EEG and clinical neurophysiology. Amsterdam: Elsevier, 1971:55–82.

Desmedt JE, Brunko E. Functional organization of far-field and cortical components of somatosensory evoked potentials in normal adults. In: Desmedt JE, ed. Clinical uses of cerebral, brainstem and spinal somatosensory evoked potentials. Progress in clinical neurophysiology. Basel: Karger, 1980:27–50.

Desmedt JE, Brunko E, Debecker J, Carmeliet J. The system bandpass required to avoid distortion of early components when averaging somatosensory evoked potentials. Electroencephalogr Clin Neurophysiol 1974;37:407–10.

Desmedt JE, Cheron G. Central somatosensory conduction in man: neural generators and interpeak latencies of the far-field components recorded from neck and right or left scalp and earlobes. Electroencephalogr Clin Neurophysiol 1980a;50:382–403.

Desmedt JE, Cheron G. Somatosensory evoked potentials to finger stimulation in health octogenarians and in young adults: waveforms, scalp topography and transit times of parietal and frontal components. Electroencephalogr Clin Neurophysiol 1980b;50:404–25.

Desmedt JE, Cheron G. Somatosensory pathway and evoked potentials in normal human aging. In: Desmedt JE, ed. Clinical uses of cerebral, brainstem and spinal somatosensory evoked potentials. Progress in clinical neurophysiology. Basel: Karger, 1980c:162–69.

Desmedt JE, Cheron G. Non-cephalic reference recording of early somatosensory potentials to finger stimulation in adult or aging normal man: differentiation of widespread N18 and contralateral N20 from the prerolandic P22 and N30 components. Electroencephalogr Clin Neurophysiol 1981a;52:553–70.

Desmedt JE, Cheron G. Prevertebral (oesophageal) recording of subcortical somatosensory evoked potentials in man: the spinal P13 component and the dual nature of the spinal generators. Electroencephalogr Clin Neurophysiol 1981b;52:257–75.

Desmedt JE, Noël P. Average cerebral evoked potentials in the evaluation of lesions of the sensory nerves and of the central somatosensory pathway. In: Desmedt JE, ed. New developments in electromyography and clinical neurophysiology. Basel: Karger, 1973:352–71.

Desmedt JE, Noël P, Debecker J, Namèche J. Maturation of afferent conduction velocity as studied by sensory nerve potentials and by cerebral evoked potentials. In: Desmedt JE, ed. New developments in electromyography and clinical neurophysiology. Basel: Karger, 1973;2:52–63.

Dimitrijevic MR, Larsson L-E, Lehmkuhl D, Sherwood A. Evoked spinal cord and nerve root potentials in humans using a non-invasive recording technique. Electroencephalogr Clin Neurophysiol 1978;45:331–40.

Dimitrijevic MR, Sedgwick EM, Sherwood A, Soar JS. A spinal cord potential in man. J Physiol 1980;303:37P.

Domino EF, Matsuoka S, Waltz J, Cooper IS. Effects of cryogenic thalamic lesions on somesthetic evoked response in man. Electroencephalogr Clin Neurophysiol 1965;19:127–38.

Donchin E, Callaway E, Cooper R, Desmedt JE, Goff WR, Hillyard SA, Sutton S. Publication criteria for studies of evoked potentials in man: report of a committee. In: Desmedt JE, ed. Attention, voluntary contraction and event-related cerebral potentials in man. Progress in clinical neurophysiology Basel: Karger, 1977:1–11.

Drechsler F. Short- and long-latency cortical potentials following trigeminal nerve stimulation in man. In: Barber C, ed. Evoked potentials. Baltimore: University Park Press, 1980.

Eisen A, Paty D, Purves S, Hoirch M. Occult fifth nerve dysfunction in multiple sclerosis. Can J Neurol Sci 1981;8:221–25.

El-Negamy E, Sedgwick EM. Properties of a spinal somatosensory evoked potential recorded in man. J Neurol Neurosurg Psychiatry 1978; 41:762–68.

Ertekin C. Studies on the human evoked electrospinogram. I. The origin of the segmental evoked potentials. Acta Neurol Scand 1976a;53:3–20.

Ertekin C. Studies on the human electrospinogram. II. The conduction velocity along the dorsal funiculus. Acta Neurol Scand 1976b;53:21–38.

Foreman RD, Kenshalo DR, Schmidt RF, Willis WD. Field potentials and excitation of primate spinothalamic neurones in response to volleys in muscle afferents. J Physiol 1979;286:197–213.

Fukushima T, Mayanagi Y, Bouchard G. Thalamic evoked potentials to somatosensory stimulation in man. Electroencephalogr Clin Neurophysiol 1976;40:481–90.

Gasser HS, Graham HT. Potentials produced in spinal cord by stimulation of dorsal roots. Am J Physiol 1933;103:303–20.

Giblin DR. Somatosensory evoked potentials in healthy subjects and in patients with lesions of the nervous system. Ann NY Acad Sci 1964;112:93–142.

Goldring S, Aras E, Weber PC. Comparative study of sensory input to motor cortex in animals and man. Electroencephalogr Clin Neurophysiol 1970;29:537–50.

Halliday AM, Mason AA. The effect of hypnotic anaesthesia on cortical responses. J Neurol Neurosurg Psychiatry 1964;27:300–12.

Halliday AM, Wakefield GS. Cerebral evoked potentials in patients with dissociated sensory loss. J Neurol Neurosurg Psychiatry 1963;26:211–19.

Humphrey DR. Re-analysis of the antidromic cortical response. II. On the contribution of cell discharge and PSPs to the evoked potentials. Electroencephalogr Clin Neurophysiol 1968;25:421–42.

Hunt WE, O'Leary JL. Form of thalamic response evoked by peripheral nerve stimulation. J Comp Neurol 1952;97:491–514.

Inouye Y, Buchthal F. Segmental sensory innervation determined by potentials recorded from cervical spinal nerves. Brain 1977;100:731–48.

Ishiko N, Hanamori T, Murayama N. Spatial distribution of somatosensory responses evoked by tapping the tongue and finger in man. Electroencephalogr Clin Neurophysiol 1980;50:1–10.

Jasper H, Lende R, Rasmussen T. Evoked potentials from the exposed somato-sensory cortex in man. J Nerv Ment Dis 1960;130:526–37.

Jones EG, Powell TPS. Anatomical organization of the somatosensory cortex. In: Iggo A, ed. Handbook of sensory physiology. II. Somatosensory system. Berlin: Springer-Verlag, 1973.

Jones SJ. Investigation of brachial plexus traction lesions by peripheral and spinal somatosensory evoked potentials. J Neurol Neurosurg Psychiatry 1979;42:107–16.

Jones SJ. Somatosensory evoked potentials in traction lesions of the brachial plexus. In: Barber C, ed. Evoked potentials. Baltimore: University Park Press, 1980:443–48.

Kelly DL, Goldring S, O'Leary JL. Averaged evoked somatosensory responses from exposed cortex of man. Arch Neurol 1965;13:1–9.

Kritchevsky M, Wiederholt WC. Short-latency somatosensory evoked potentials. Arch Neurol 1978;35:706–11.

Kwan HC, Mackay WA, Murphy JT, Wong YC. Spatial organization of precentral cortex in awake primates. II. Motor outputs. J Neurophysiol 1978;41:1120–39.

Landau WM. Evoked potentials. In: Quarton GC, Melnechuk T, Schmitt FO, eds. The neurosciences. New York: Rockefeller University Press, 1967:469–82.

Larsson L-E, Prevec TS. Somato-sensory response to mechanical stimulation as recorded in the human EEG. Electroencephalogr Clin Neurophysiol 1970;28:162–72.

Lastimos ACB, Bass NH, Stanback K, Norvell EE. Lumbar spinal cord and early cortical evoked potentials after tibial nerve stimulation: effects of stature on normative data. Electroencephalogr Clin Neurophysiol 1982;54:499–507.

Legatt AD, Vaughan HG. Topography and intracranial sources of somatosensory evoked potentials in the monkey. I. Early components. Electroencephalogr Clin Neurophysiol 1979;46:155–72.

Libet B. Electrical stimulation of cortex in human subjects and conscious sensory aspects. In: Iggo, A, ed. Handbook of sensory physiology. Berlin: Springer-Verlag, 1973:744–90.

Libet B, Alberts WW, Wright EW Jr, Feinstein B. Responses of human somatosensory cortex to stimuli below threshold for conscious sensation. Science (NY) 1967;158:1597–1600.

Lueders H. Introduction to somatosensory evoked potentials. Fifth Annual Continuing Education Course, American Association of Electromyography and Electrodiagnosis, October 1982.

Magladery JW, Porter WE, Park AM, Teasdall RD. Electrophysiological studies of nerve and reflex activity in man. IV. The two-neurone reflex and identification of certain action potentials from spinal roots and cord. Bull Johns Hopkins Hosp 1951;88:499–519.

Maruyama Y, Shimoji K, Shimizu H, Kuribayashi H, Fujioka H. Human spinal cord potentials evoked by different sources of stimulation and conduction velocities along the cord. J Neurophysiol 1982;48:1098–1120.

Matthews WB, Beauchamp M, Small DG. Cervical somatosensory evoked responses in man. Nature (Lond) 1974;52:230–32.

Mauguière F, Courjon J. The origin of short-latency somatosensory evoked potentials in man. A clinical contribution. Ann Neurol 1981;9:707–10.

McClosky DI. Kinesthetic sensibility. Physiol Rev 1979;58:763–820.

Murphy JT, Kwan HC, Mackay WA, Wong YC. Physiologic basis for focal motor seizures and the Jacksonian "march" phenomena. Can J Neurol Sci 1980;7:79–85.

Nakanishi T, Shimoda Y, Sakuta M, Toyokura Y. The initial positive component of the scalp-recorded somatosensory evoked potentials in normal subjects and in patients with neurological disorders. Electroencephalogr Clin Neurophysiol 1978;45:26–34.

Nicholson C. Generation and analysis of extracellular field potentials. In: Electrophysiological techniques. Bethesda, Md.: Society for Neuroscience, 1979:93–148.

Nunez PL. Electric fields of the brain. New York, Oxford: Oxford University Press, 1981.

O'Leary JL, Goldring S. D-C potentials of the brain. Physiol Rev 1964;44:91–125.

Onishi A, O'Brien PC, Okazaki H, Dyck PJ. Morphometry of myelinated fibers of fasciculus gracilis of man. J Neurol Sci 1976;27:163–72.

Oscarsson O, Rosén I. Projections to cerebral cortex of large muscle-spindle afferents in forelimb nerves of the cat. J Physiol 1963;169:924–45.

Penfield W, Boldrey E. Somatic motor and sensory representation in the cerebral cortex of man as studied by electrical stimulation. Brain 1937;60:389–443.

Phillips CG, Porter R. Cortico-spinal neurones. London: Academic Press, 1977.

Phillips CG, Powell TPS, Wiesendanger M. Projections from low-threshold muscle afferents of hand and forearm to area 3a of baboons cortex. J Physiol (Lond) 1971;217:419–46.

Phillips LH, Daube JR. Lumbosacral spinal evoked potentials in humans. Neurology 1980;30:1175–83.

Powell TPS. The somatic sensory cortex. Br Med Bull 1977;33:129–35.

Pratt H, Amlie RN, Starr A. Short-latency mechanically evoked somatosensory potentials in humans. Electroencephalogr Clin Neurophysiol 1979;47:524–31.

Pratt H, Starr A. Mechanically and electrically evoked somatosensory potentials in humans: scalp and neck distribution of short-latency components. Electroencephalogr Clin Neurophysiol 1981;51:138–47.

Pratt H, Starr A, Amlie RN, Politoske D. Mechanically and electrically evoked somatosensory potentials in normal humans. Neurology (NY) 1979;29:1236–44.

Rose JE, Mountcastle VB. Touch and kinesthesis. In: Field J, Magoun HW, Hall VE, eds. Handbook of physiology. I. Neurophysiology. Washington: American Physiology Society, 1959:387–429.

Ross ED, Kirpatrick JB, Lastimos AB. Position and vibration sensations: functions of the dorsal spino-cerebellar tracts. Ann Neurol 1979;5:171–76.

Schlag J. Generation of brain-evoked potentials. In: Thompson RF, Patterson MM, eds. Bioelectric recording techniques. A. Cellular processes and brain potentials. New York: Academic Press, 1973;1:273–316.

Sears TA. Action potentials evoked in digital nerves by stimulation of mechanoreceptors in the human finger. J Physiol 1959;148:30P.

Shimizu H, Shimoji K, Maruyama Y, Matsuki M, Kuribayashi H, Fujioka H. Human spinal cord potentials produced in lumbosacral enlargement by descending volleys. J Neurophysiol 1982;48:1108–1120.

Shimoji K, Kano T, Higashi H, Morioka T, Henschel EO. Evoked spinal electrograms recorded from epidural space in man. J Appl Physiol 1972;33:468–71.

Shimoji K, Matsuki M, Ito Y, Masuko K, Maruyama M, Iwane T, Aida S. Interactions of human cord dorsum potential. J Appl Physiol 1976;40:79–84.

Shimoji K, Matsuki M, Shimizu H. Waveform characteristics and spatial distribution of evoked spinal electrogram in man. J Neurosurg 1977;46:304–13.

Shimoji K, Shimizu H, Maruyama Y. Origin of somatosensory evoked responses recorded from the cervical skin surface. Neurosurgery 1978;48:980–84.

Siivola J, Myllylä VV, Sulg I, Hokkanen E. Brachial plexus and radicular neurography in relation to cortical evoked responses. J Neurol Neurosurg Psychiatry 1979;42:1151–58.

Singh N, Sachdev KK, Brisman R. Trigeminal nerve stimulation: short-latency somatosensory evoked potentials. Neurology 1982;32:97–101.

Small DG, Beauchamp M, Matthews WB. Subcortical somatosensory evoked potentials in normal man and in patients with central nervous system lesions. In: Desmedt JE, ed. Clinical uses of cerebral, brainstem and spinal somatosensory evoked potentials. Progress in clinical neurophysiology. Basel: Karger, 1980:190–204.

Starr A, McKeon B, Skuse N, Burke D. Cerebral potentials evoked by muscle stretch in man. Brain 1981;104:149–66.

Stöhr M, Petruch F. Somatosensory evoked potentials following stimulation of the trigeminal nerve in man. J Neurol (Berl) 1979;220:95–98.

Stöhr M, Petruch F, Scheglmann K. Somatosensory evoked potentials following trigeminal nerve stimulation in trigeminal neuralgia. Ann Neurol 1980;9:63–66.

Stohr PE, Goldring S. Origin of somatosensory evoked scalp responses in man. J Neurosurg 1969;13:117–27.

Wall PD. The sensory and motor role of impulses travelling in the dorsal columns towards cerebral cortex. Brain 1970;93:505–24.

Wall PD, Noordenbos W. Sensory functions which remain in man after complete transection of dorsal columns. Brain 1977;100:641–53.

Webster KE. Somaesthetic pathways. Br Med Bull 1977;33:113–20.

Werner G, Whitsel BL. Functional organization of the somatosensory cortex. In: Iggo A, ed. Handbook of sensory physiology. Berlin: Springer-Verlag, 1973:621–700.

Wiesendanger M, Miles TS. Ascending pathway of low-threshold muscle afferents to the cerebral cortex and its possible role in motor control. Physiol Rev 1982;62:1234–70.

Willis WD. Spinal cord potentials. In: Windle WF, ed. The spinal cord and its reaction to traumatic injury. New York: Marcel Dekker, 1980:159–87.

Wong YC, Kwan HC, Mackay WA, Murphy JT. Spatial organization of precentral cortex in awake primates. I. Somatosensory inputs. J Neurophysiol 1978;41:1107–20.

Woolsey CN. Patterns of localization in sensory and motor areas of the cerebral cortex. In: The biology of mental health and disease. London: Millbank Memorial Fund, 1952:193–206.

Woolsey CN. Cortical localization as defined by evoked potentials and electrical stimulation studies. In: Schaltenbrand J, Woolsey CN, eds. Cerebral localization and organization. Wisconsin: University of Wisconsin Press, 1964:17–26.

Woolsey CN, Erickson TC. Study of the postcentral gyrus of man by the evoked potential technique. Trans Am Neurol Assoc 1950;75:50–52.

Woolsey CN, Erickson TC, Gilson WE. Localization in somatic sensory and motor areas of human cerebral cortex as determined by direct recording of evoked potentials and electrical stimulation. J Neurosurg 1979;51:476–506.

Woolsey CN, Settlage PH, Meyer DR, Spencer W, Hamuy TP, Travis AM. Patterns of localization in precentral and "supplementary" motor areas and their relation to the concept of a premotor area. Res Publ Assoc Nerv Ment Dis 1952;30:238–64.

Yamada T, Machida M, Kimura J. Far-field somatosensory evoked potentials after stimulation of the tibial nerve. Neurology 1982;32:1151–58.

5 THE NORMAL MOTOR UNIT

The motor unit (MU) is composed of the motoneuron, the motor axon, and the whole population of muscle fibers innervated by that neuron (Figure 5.1). Motor units are the motor "output" of the central nervous system and are responsible for both movements and the maintenance of posture. The choice of MUs and their rates and times of discharge are made by the central nervous system on the basis of current intention and prior experience in order best to carry out a movement or sequence of movements. To this central selection, adjustments are made in response to visual, vestibular, cutaneous, muscle, and other feedback about the present situation. The resultant displacements and forces are products of the numbers and choices of MUs, their rates of discharge, and the lengths of the muscles.

The examination of MUs, their respective motor unit potentials (MUPs), and motor conduction velocities is often of enormous value to the electromyographer in establishing the nature and location of abnormalities in motoneurons or their peripheral motor axons. It is important therefore to examine in turn the location and organization of motoneurons in the spinal cord, the physiological properties of motoneurons and MUs, the organization of MU in muscle, patterns of MU recruitment, and the effects of exercise and fatigue on MUs

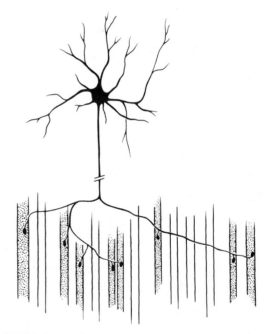

FIGURE 5.1. Major components of the motor unit, which include the motoneuron cell body and its dendritic tree, the axon, and the whole complement of muscle fibers innervated by the motoneuron.

and muscle as a whole (for detailed reviews see Buchthal and Schmalbruch, 1980; Burke, 1980, 1981; Henneman and Mendell, 1981; Freund, 1983).

ORGANIZATION OF MOTONEURONS IN THE SPINAL CORD

The ventral horn region includes lamina VII, VIII, and IX, but it is in lamina IX that most of the cell bodies of motoneurons are located (Brodal, 1981) (Figure 5.2). In man, ventral horn cells can be divided into two main groups: (1) larger motoneurons (diameters of 34 to 60 μ) that are probably alpha motoneurons and (2) more intermediate-sized neurons (diameters of 24 to 34 μ) that probably include the gamma motoneurons. Neurons of various sizes intermingle in the ventral horn, there being no apparent segregation according to size alone. The ratio of large to intermediate neurons in the ventral horn is about 3 : 1 and there is a similar ratio between large- and smaller-diameter motor nerve fibers in the ventral root. Not all neurons in lamina IX, however, are motoneurons. Some are propriospinal neurons and others are Renshaw cells. Some of the motoneurons innervate both intrafusal and extrafusal muscle fibers (MFs), the so-called beta motoneurons (Burke, 1981).

The cell bodies of motoneurons supplying

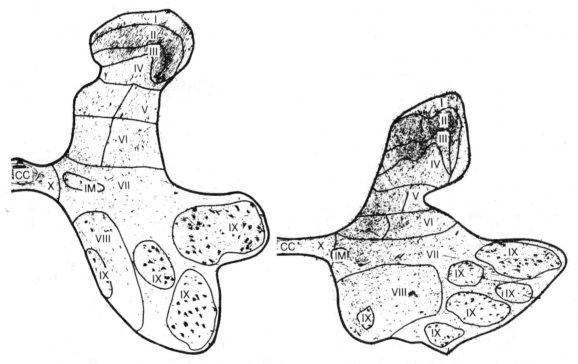

FIGURE 5.2.   Cross sections of the gray matter of the human spinal cord at the C6 (left) and L5 (right) levels to illustrate the division of the gray matter into lamina based on the various morphological features in different regions. The motoneurons (alpha, gamma, and beta) are concentrated in lamina IX. Cell columns supplying individual muscle usually extend over two or more spinal segments. The more distal the position of the muscle in the limb, the more lateral the position of its motoneurons within the ventral gray matter (see Sharrard, 1953).
CC = central canal.
IM = intermediomedial nucleus.
From Carpenter and Sutin (1983, figures 9.12 and 9.19).

individual muscles are arranged in rostrocaudal columns (Romanes, 1951) that extend over two or more segments in the spinal cord. The locations of motoneurons supplying various muscles have been worked out on experimental animals by locating those motoneurons that develop a chromatolytic reaction to peripheral motor nerve section or that stain with horseradish peroxidase following the retrograde transport of this substance from the cut end of the respective motor axons in the periphery. These techniques have been applied to the cat (Romanes, 1964; Sterling and Kuypers, 1967; Burke, Strick, Kanda, Kim, and Walmsley, 1977) as well as to the primate (Reed, 1940; Sprague, 1948). There is recent evidence to suggest that motoneurons innervating separate muscles may intermingle to some extent (Burke, Strick, Kanda, Kim, and Walmsley, 1977). There also appears to be some relationship between the location of motoneurons within the cell columns and the territories of MUs in muscle.

The relative juxtaposition of motoneuronal cell columns probably reflects complex, to this time poorly understood, functional relationships between the various groups and columns of motoneurons. Certainly at the cruder level of groups of functionally related muscles, the motoneurons are topographically organized in the ventral horn. Thus within lamina IX, axial, trunk, and neck motoneurons are ventromedial in location, flexor motoneurons are more dorsal than extensor motoneurons, and in the lumbosacral and cervical enlargements the motoneurons innervating limb muscles are the most laterally placed in the ventral horn.

In man, even less is known about the arrangement of motoneurons in the spinal cord. What evidence we have comes from the examination of the spinal cord following amputations, peripheral nerve injuries, and polio, where careful examinations of the patterns of neuronal loss and chromatolysis have been made (Elliott, 1942, 1943; Sharrard, 1955; Brodal, 1981). Even in experimental animals, including the subhuman primates, little is known about the precise locations and organization of spinal motoneurons that innervate single distal, intermediate, and proximal muscles, or even the relative positions of motoneurons acting synergistically across the same or adjacent joints or innervating antagonistic muscles.

Nonetheless, in man the general pattern holds true whereby trunk and axial motoneurons are ventromedial in the ventral horn and limb motoneurons are concentrated in the caudal cervical and lumbar enlargements in the spinal cord. Segmental innervation patterns in man have been established by the electrical stimulation of ventral roots and recording the EMG from various target muscles (Thage, 1965) (Table 5.1). All muscles are

TABLE 5.1.   Segmental Innervation Patterns in Man

Muscle	Spinal Segment					
	L2	L3	L4	L5	S1	S2
Quadriceps	+ +	+ +	+ +	+	−	−
Tibialis anterior	−	−	+ + +	+ +	+	−
Peroneus longus	−	−	−	+ +	+ +	−
Extensor digitorum brevis	−	−	−	+ +	+ +	−
Gastrocnemius	−	−	−	+ +	+ + +	+
Biceps femoris	−	−	+	+	+	−

From Thage (1965).

supplied by two or more roots just as in the distal muscles in the macaque upper limb (Wray, 1969).

Fiber Size, Distributions, and Conduction Velocities of Alpha Motor Axons

The proportion of myelinated nerve fibers in a motor nerve that are motor fibers varies. In the baboon, 57 percent of the myelinated nerve fibers in the motor nerve to gastrocnemius were alpha and gamma nerve fibers, the equivalent proportion in the recurrent motor thenar branch being 52 percent (Wray, 1969). In the cat this proportion varies somewhat with the motor nerve (Boyd and Davey, 1968).

In man, the relative proportions of sensory and motor fibers in motor nerves are not known because these determinations depend on prior destruction of the dorsal root ganglion cells, and opportunities to study this question in man are rare. Even in the experimental preparations, it is well to remember that ganglionectomies can injure ventral root fibers (Boyd and Davey, 1968). In man, probably about 50 percent of the total myelinated nerve fiber population is motor.

There is a wide range in the conduction velocities of motor nerve fibers. For example, in the baboon, these fibers can be divided into two main groups. In the group with larger diameters, the conduction velocities of single fibers range between 49 to 84 m/s and the smaller fibers between 22 and 41 m/s (Eccles, Phillips, and Wu-Chien Ping, 1968). This wide range, where the slowest motor axons have conduction velocities as low as 65 percent of the velocities in the fastest fibers and where the range of diameters was equivalently wide (alpha, 6 to 14 μ; gamma 1 to 6 μ), could complicate interpretations of conduction velocity determinations in man. For example, the observations of slower maximum conduction velocities may not indicate real reductions in the

conduction velocities of nerve fibers, but selective or even random loss of the faster-conducting motor nerve fibers.

Branching in motor nerve fibers begins about 100 mm proximal to the motor point in normal subjects (Eccles and Sherrington, 1930) (Figure 5.3). Branching at more proximal levels cannot be excluded, however, although electrophysiological evidence of this is rare in control motor nerves.

Innervation Ratios in Whole Muscles

By estimating the number of motor axons in the motor nerve supplying a particular muscle and counting the number of MFs within the muscle, Feinstein, Lindegård, Nyman, and Wohlfart (1955) were able to derive some very approximate estimates of the mean innerva-

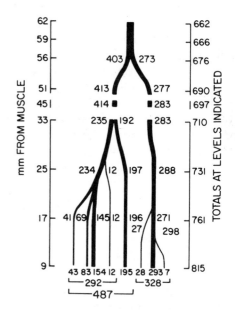

FIGURE 5.3. Branching in motor axons and consequent increase in the numbers of nerve fibers in the nerve to the medial gastrocnemius muscle of the cat as the nerve approaches the muscle.
From Eccles and Sherrington (1930, figure 1).

tion ratios for several muscles (Figure 5.4). These studies showed the extraocular muscle to have the lowest innervation ratio, or numbers of MFs per motor axon. While large muscles, such as the gastrocnemius, were supplied by fewer motor axons than an extraocular muscle, single gastrocnemius motor axons on the average innervated a far greater number of MFs than in the case of the extraocular muscle. Occupying an intermedite position are the intrinsic muscles of the hand. It is tempting to suggest that the larger numbers of motoneurons supplying the extraocular and facial muscles, in comparison to larger and bulkier muscles elsewhere, indicates that the CNS exercises a greater degree of precise control over the former than the latter.

These early studies provided, of course, no anatomical information about innervation ratios or territories occupied by single MUs with respect to the various types of MUs present in these muscles; information still lacking today.

Distribution Patterns of Muscle Fibers Belonging to Single Motor Units Within a Muscle

Knowledge of the numbers and locations of MFs within a muscle belonging to individual MUs is vital to understanding the changes in MUPs as recorded with single-fiber, concentric, and more recently, macro needle electrodes in the various diseases that affect peripheral nerves. To work out the innervation patterns of MFs in single MUs one of two methods may be used. In the first, a single filament belonging to an alpha motor axon is gently separated from other fibers in the ventral root and mounted on a pair of stimulating electrodes. The filament is then stimulated at a sufficiently high frequency for a long enough period to exhaust the glycogen content of all the MF within the innervation territory of that single motor axon. Following this program of stimulation, histochemical staining of cross sections of the muscle in question reveals the innervation pattern of the MU in the MFs de-

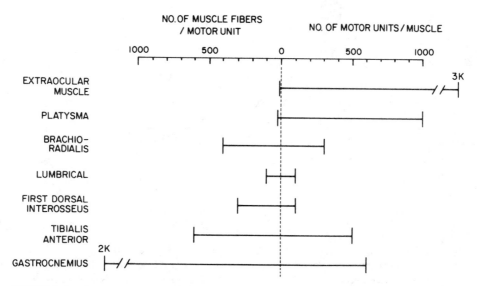

FIGURE 5.4.   Innervation ratios (number of muscle fibers per motor unit or motoneuron) and numbers of motor units (motoneurons) per muscle for various human muscles. Based on Feinstein, Lindegård, Nyman, and Wohlfart (1955).

pleted of their glycogen (Kugelberg, 1973; Brandstater and Lambert, 1973). The second method is similar in all respects except the single MU is isolated from other MUs by inserting a glass microelectrode into its cell body and stimulating the latter by passing a depo-larizing current through the electrode (Burke and Tsairis, 1973) (Figure 5.5).

The preceding methods, applied so far to the rat and cat, are the single best tools available for experimentally working out the innervation patterns and ratios of single MUs.

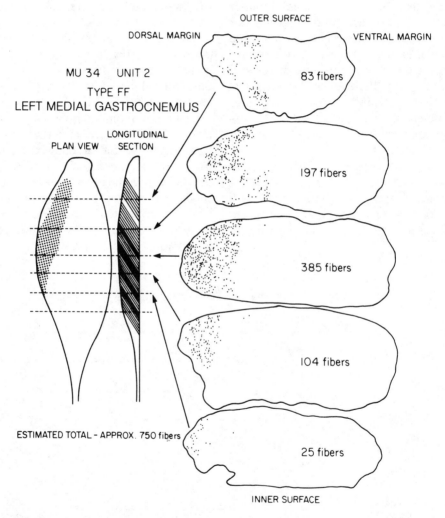

FIGURE 5.5.   Reconstruction of the distributions of the muscle fibers in a FF motor unit in the medial gastrocnemius muscle of the cat. Note that in this pennate muscle a cross section taken at any one level does not include all the muscle fibers in the motor unit. Counts of glycogen-depleted muscle fibers are indicated within the cross section panels.
From Burke and Tsairis (1973, figure 13).

The methods are not, however, without their limitations. For example, not all the MFs belonging to a single MU may be represented within any one cross section through the whole muscle. Furthermore, problems may arise in the less glycogen-dependent MUs where it may be more difficult to define which MFs have been depleted of their glycogen in sections stained for glycogen. Even in more glycogen-dependent MFs, the extent of the depletion may vary somewhat throughout the length of the MFs, with the result that in some sections some MFs belonging to the MU fail to be identified (Walsh, Burke, Rymer, and Tsairis, 1978; Buchthal and Schmalbruch, 1980; Burke, 1981).

Whatever the failings and limitations of the above histochemical techniques for studying the innervation patterns of MUs, they have clearly shown in normal muscle that MFs belonging to separate MUs freely intermingle with MFs belonging to several other MUs. Even within the cross-sectional territory of a muscle occupied by a single MU, the distribution of the MFs in the MU is such that most MF in the MU are found singly, less often in pairs and much less commonly are three or more MFs sharing the same innervation to be found adjacent to one another (Kugelberg, 1973; Brandstater and Lambert, 1973). This intermingling between the MFs of different MUs probably serves to smooth interactions between twitches in neighboring MUs. As well, such intermingling might also serve to effectively limit interactions between the action currents of MFs of the same MU and in this way might help to discourage reactivation of these MF and possible backfiring of their intramuscular terminal and preterminal motor axons.

The innervation patterns of MUs revealed by Kugelberg (1973) and Brandstater and Lambert (1973) were anticipated by earlier electrophysiological studies of the locations of MFs belonging to single MUs in the rat

diaphragm by Krnjević and Miledi in 1958 and anatomical studies of the terminal innervation patterns of motor axons within rat muscle by Feindel (1954). In keeping with all the above experimental studies is the observation that in normal muscle no more than two independent MF spike sources belonging to the same MU are usually found within the pickup territory of a single fiber needle electrode (Stålberg and Trontelj, 1970; see also Chapter 7).

In man, estimates of the transverse territories occupied by single MUs within a muscle have been arrived at by several techniques. In the earliest to be applied, the potential profile of the whole MU was studied by using a multielectrode incorporating a number of recording electrodes in the side of a carrier needle cannula (Buchthal, Guld, and Rosenfalck, 1957a, 1957b) (Figure 5.6). The linear array was so designed as to span the width of the territories of most of the MUs likely to be encountered. The multielectrode was inserted into the territory of the MU and its position adjusted so that one of the central electrodes in the array was approximately positioned in the center of the MU. Then by recording the potentials as seen by other electrodes, the transverse voltage profile of the MU could be plotted. By making certain assumptions about the proximity of MFs to the recording electrodes based on the amplitude and rise time of the potential recorded at each electrode in the array, an approximate estimate of the transverse territory occupied by single MUs in various muscles could be made.

The original studies by Buchthal, Guld, and Rosenfalck (1957a, 1957b) used a relatively large-bore carrier cannula (1-mm diameter) and the leading-off surfaces in the linear array were also large (1.5 mm in length). More recently, Stålberg, Schwartz, Thiele, and Schiller (1976) described the use of yet another multielectrode designed for the same purpose, but which used much smaller leading-off surfaces for recording electrodes in the array. The lat-

FIGURE 5.6. Multielectrode for measurement of the transverse territory occupied by single motor units within a muscle (left). In this electrode, 12 electrodes, each 1.5 mm wide, are arranged in line along the side of the cannula (interelectrode separation 0.5 mm). The electrode is inserted perpendicular to the muscle and its position adjusted so that the maximum voltage is recorded by one of the central electrodes (electrode 5 or 6) and one of the end electrodes in the array registers little or no potential. The latter is therefore able to serve as a reference electrode for the others. The amplitudes of the MUP registered at each of the remaining electrodes in the array are then recorded (right). In these recordings, peak-to-peak spike amplitudes exceeding 50 μV were assumed to indicate the presence, within 1 mm of the electrode, of one or more muscle fibers belonging to the motor unit.
From Buchthal, Erminio, and Rosenfalck (1959, figure 2).

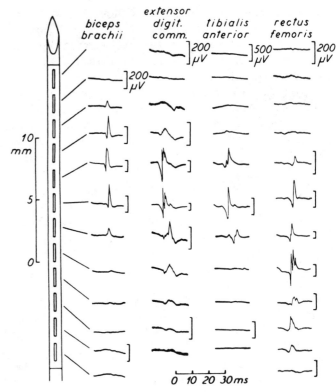

ter made it possible to work out the positions and numbers of MFs belonging to one MU along the transverse corridor through which the multielectrode was inserted (Figure 5.7).

Such recordings, however, are not without their drawbacks. The small area of the electrodes incorporated in the multielectrodes means the impedance of these electrodes may be substantial and this enhances the possibility of capacitive cross-talk between nearby leads and some degrading of the discriminative value of the electrodes.

In addition, electrophysiological studies of the spatial limits of MUs in man have, in all likelihood, been biased toward the lowest-threshold MUs to be recruited in voluntary contraction, because these studies were all done in the course of weak voluntary contractions.

These studies probably therefore, provide no information about the transverse territories of normally higher-threshold MUs; studies that would necessarily be technically more difficult because of the interfering activities of other MU potentials. Also, the multielectrode may not have been passed through the center of the MU and in the case of bipennate or multipennate muscles, the actual geometry of the MU may be much too complex to represent in a single needle tract. These limitations all combine to make estimates of MU territories by means of such multielectrode techniques very approximate.

One recent attractive way to visualize the transverse potential profile of a single MU recruited in a weak voluntary contraction is to record the potentials associated with the activity of this MU at intervals as a recording

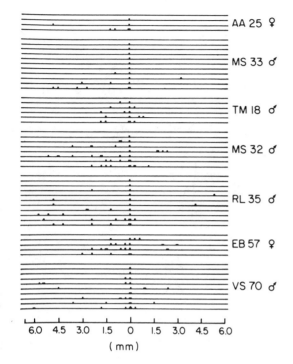

6.0 4.5 3.0 1.5 0 1.5 3.0 4.5 6.0

(mm)

FIGURE 5.7.   Locations of single muscle fibers in single motor units in successive transverse corridors of the biceps brachii in normal human subjects. These were established with the use of a multielectrode consisting of 14 electrodes, each 25 μ in diameter, arranged in a linear array along the side of a 0.6-mm-diameter needle cannula. The multielectrode was inserted perpendicular to the muscle fibers within the muscle.

When action potentials exceeded 200 μV in amplitude, their rise times were less than 300 μsec, and they were seen in consecutive discharges, time locked but jittering with respect to the reference potential, they were considered to indicate the presence of a single muscle fiber spike source within 300 μ of any of the electrode recording sites. One of the muscle fibers in the center of the motor unit served as the reference spike for all other muscle fiber spikes belonging to the same motor unit.

Note that for the most part, muscle fibers belonging to single motor units are separate from one another, although sometimes a pair of adjacent fibers are seen.

From Stålberg, Schwartz, Thiele, and Schiller (1976, figure 6).

electrode (concentric needle) is drawn transversely through the territory of the MU (Stålberg and Antoni, 1980). The potentials recorded at successive sites throughout the territory of the MU are then displayed in raster fashion time locked to a stable spike recorded with a single-fiber electrode from the same MU. Raster displays of the MUPs recorded in this fashion provide a graphic view of the transverse spatial distribution MUP as seen along a transverse corridor through the muscle.

The preceding studies in experimental animals and the electrophysiological studies in man, bearing on the territories and innervation patterns of MUs establish three main points:

1. The cross-sectional territories of MUs occupy but a small part of the whole cross-sectional area of most muscles. In the human biceps brachii muscle, for example, the transverse diameters of MUs range between 2 and 15 mm and clearly span but a small fraction of the whole cross section of the adult muscle (Buchthal, Guld, and Rosenfalck, 1957b).

2. MFs belonging to separate MUs intermingle so that the territories of from 10 to 30 MUs may overlap to some extent in any one region of the muscle.

3. Because of the intermingling of MFs belonging to separate MUs, the majority of MFs in a MU are found alone, less often a pair of MFs are found together, and still less often are groupings of three or more MFs belonging to the same MU found together in normal muscle.

The spike pickup territories of concentric needle electrodes are such that only a small fraction of the MF belonging to any particular MU can contribute to the spike component of the motor unit potential (see Chapter 7). Probably even the slower components of the MUP do not reflect the activities of all the

MFs in the MU. The shape and amplitude in particular of MUPs recorded by concentric needle electrodes are therefore critically dependent on the precise position and orientation of the recording surface with respect to the MFs in the MU. Such recordings provide no indications of the spatial limits or innervation ratios of the underlying MU, but do provide an approximate indication of the innervation density or numbers of MFs belonging to one MU within the pickup territory of the electrode. The latter can be even better appreciated by the single-fiber electrode, which allows the electromyographer to count the number of independent spike generators in the MU within the very immediate pickup territory of the electrode (about 0.6 mm in diameter).

End-plate Zone

The end-plate zone, or innervation zone, is located midway between the origin and insertion of MFs. In this region, the end-plates are arranged in narrow bands (usually single) running at right angles to the direction of the MFs. The innervation zone in a muscle may not be in the center of or run transverse to the whole muscle, however, but may have a complex distribution, depending on the orientation and distribution of MFs within the muscle (Figure 5.8). Even in the intrinsic muscles of the human hand, the innervation zones may be widely scattered or complex because of the complex patterns and arrangements of the MFs in some of these muscles (Desmedt, 1958; Christensen, 1959; Bergmans, 1970; Burke, Skuse, and Lethlean, 1974). The sartorius and iliacus muscles have numerous tendinous insertions present throughout the muscle, which consists of parallel bundles of short MFs linked together by tendinous bands. This accounts for the numerous innervation bands scattered randomly through these muscles. Several

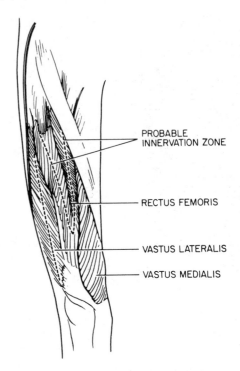

FIGURE 5.8.   The probable distribution of innervation zone of the rectus femoris and vastus lateralis muscles based on the arrangement of fibers in this muscle. The assumption is that the end-plate in any one muscle fiber is positioned roughly halfway between the origin and insertion of the muscle fiber. In electrophysiological studies in our laboratory, end-plate activity in this muscle has been found to be widely distributed throughout the proximal-distal extent of this muscle.

techniques exist for staining axon terminals and end-plates that make it possible to localize the innervation zone (see reviews by Coërs and Woolf, 1959, 1981).

Electrophysiological Localization of the End-plate Zone

In the end-plate zone the initial transmembrane currents accompanying the end-plate and subsequent action potentials are inward.

The associated potential as recorded in the extracellular space in the immediate vicinity is negative, the region being spoken of as a current sink (Figure 5.9). Outside the end-plate zone the above inward currents pass outward through the muscle fiber membrane, and in these regions an electrode situated in the extracellular space will record a positive potential, other regions being said to act as potential sources.

The electrical sign therefore, that indicates a recording electrode is situated in the region of the end-plate zone, is an initial negative deflection of the muscle compound action potential whether recorded with a surface or intramuscular electrode. Conversely, an initial positive deflection signifies that the initial postsynaptic inward current is taking place some distance away from the recording electrode, the subsequent negative deflection pointing to the arrival of the subsequently conducted action potentials of the MFs at a position opposite the recording electrode. The time between the onset of the initial positive deflection and the positive peak of the muscle action potential provides an approximate indication of the conduction time between the site of origin and the arrival at the recording electrode of the muscle fiber action potentials in surface recordings. This is so provided the onset and peak of the positive deflection are not distorted by the filter settings and the recording electrode is positioned along the longitudinal axis of the muscle fiber, and not so far away from the end-plate zone that the end-plate currents cannot be seen in volume at the recording electrode.

Electrophysiological criteria for the localization of the end-plate zone include:

1. The initial voltage deflections of MU potentials, the compound muscle action potential, as well as single MF action potentials as recorded with surface or

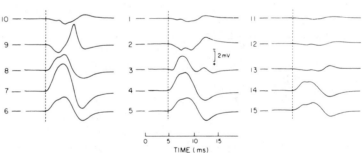

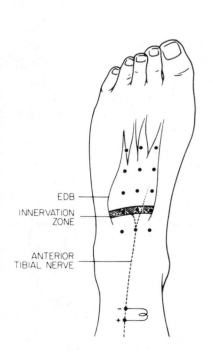

FIGURE 5.9. Surface-recorded amplitudes and shapes of the extensor digitorum brevis maximum M-potential as recorded at various sites over the dorsum of the foot. Note that the initial deflection is negative and the negative peak amplitude is maximum in the vicinity of the innervation zone. The larger amplitude recorded over the lateral innervation zone probably reflects the fact that the lateral part of this muscle is closer to the recording electrode, the tendons of the extensor digitorum longus muscle covering the middle and medial portions of the muscle. Toward the distal end of the muscle the initial deflections are positive and the amplitudes somewhat lower. Vertical interrupted lines denote onset of the negative deflection at the innervation zone.

intramuscular electrodes are negative. The reasons are outlined in the preceding discussion.

2. The rise time to the negative peak of the maximum compound action potential of the muscle as recorded with surface electrodes is usually briefest when recorded in the region of the end-plate zone. This is probably explained by the lesser degree of temporal dispersion of all the component MF action potentials whose compound sum accounts for the M-potential in the end-plate zone.

3. The amplitude of the maximum compound action potential of the muscle is maximum. The reason is undoubtedly the same as accounts for the two.

4. Intramuscular needle electrode recordings in the region readily detect miniature end-plate potentials.

All the above criteria provide reliable indicators of the position of the end-plate zone, especially in simpler and smaller muscles such as the extensor digitorum brevis, and to a lesser extent for the more complex and overlapping end-plate zones of the muscle comprising thenar and hypothenar muscle groups, respectively. In some muscle groups it is difficult and at times impossible to find a position on the surface where the initial negative response is negative. In other muscles, such as tibialis anterior, the end-plate zone simply cannot be covered by any one electrode because of its complex orientation.

PHYSIOLOGICAL, BIOCHEMICAL, AND MORPHOLOGICAL CHARACTERISTICS OF MOTOR UNITS

There is now abundant evidence that MUs in most mammalian muscles can be divided into three main groups on the basis of their physiological and biochemical characteristics. The three classifications proposed by Brooke and Kaiser (1970), Peter (1971), and Burke (see review of 1981) agree for the most part in how they subdivide the MF and MU types. Table 5.2 provides an overview of how all the various morphological, physiological, and biochemical characteristics of MUs and MFs interrelate. It must be recognized, however, that there are exceptions to such simple systems both among individual muscles and among species. Even within a particular muscle the range of conduction velocities, contraction times and tensions of any one subtype of MU can be quite broad and at the limits, overlap with MUs belonging to other subtypes.

In general, the lower the input resistance of the motoneuron, the higher the threshold for recruitment in response to peripheral and central inputs, the larger the twitch tension of the MU, and the less resistant the MU is to fatigue.

There is also a close correlation between the sizes of motoneurons and the conduction velocities of their peripheral axons, and the twitch tensions of MUs. Despite the reasonable view that the twitch tensions should correlate with the innervation ratios of the MUs, there is some recent evidence, at least in the cat gastrocnemius, that the innervation ratios of the higher-tension MUs may not exceed by much the innervation ratios of lower-tension MUs. The higher tensions must in these cases have been the product of the larger diameters of the MFs in the higher-tension MUs. This would generate larger tensions per MF because of their larger cross-sectional areas and possibly other differences in their contractile apparatus. Whether or not this holds true in man is unknown, but one would expect that larger motoneurons would support larger peripheral motor axon branching networks and hence innervate more MFs.

The longer-lasting periods of afterhyperpolarization in slow-twitch (S) MUs though effectively limiting their capacity to fire at high

TABLE 5.2.   Characteristics of MUs

Classification	I[1,2] SO (Slow-twitch, oxida- tive) S[3] (Slow)	IIA FOG (Fast-twitch, oxida- tive, glycolytic) FR (Fast fatigue-resis- tant)	IIB FG (Fast-twitch, glyco- lytic) FF (Fast fatigable)
Motoneuron			
Size	Smallest		Largest
Input resistance	Highest		Lowest
Threshold	Lowest		Highest
Duration of afterhyperpolarization	Longest		Shortest
Accommodation	Least		Maximum
Firing characteristics	Slow, steady		High-frequency bursts
Axons			
Diameter	Smallest		Largest
Conduction velocity	Lowest		Fastest
Neuromuscular transmission			
End-plates	Smallest area		Largest area
Quantal content of EPP[3]	Least		Most
Muscle fibers			
Diameters	Smallest		Largest
Myofibrillar			
ATPase (pH 9.4)	Low	High	High
Oxidative enzymes	High	Medium-high	Low
Glycogen	Low	High	High
Phosphorylase	Low	High	High
Capillary supply	Rich	Rich	Sparse
Contractile characteristics			
Contraction time	Slow	Fast	Fast
Tension	Low	Medium	High
Resistance to fatigue	High	High	Low
"Sag"	No		Yes

Based on Guth (1968), Close (1972), Buchthal and Schmalbruch (1980), Burke (1980, 1981), Henneman and Mendell (1981).
[1]Brook and Kaiser (1970, 1974).
[2]Peter (1971).
[3]Burke, Levine, Zajac, Tsairis, and Engel (1971).

frequencies, would not necessarily limit their capacity to generate their maximum tension because the twitches in S-MUs could be expected to fuse at lower firing frequencies. The higher degree of accommodation in fast-twitch (F) motoneurons, however, would restrict their capacity to fire at high frequencies for more than short bursts.

Both MFs and MUs vary in the degree to which they depend on aerobic or anaerobic metabolism to meet their energy needs. Some histochemical techniques, by making visible the enzymes (oxidative or anaerobic glycolytic) or substrates (glycogen) of the major aerobic and anaerobic energy systems, provide semiquantitative indications of the dominant energy system in MFs. These correlate for the most part, with the extent of the capillary network, the diameters of the MFs, and the use to which the MUs are put in the course of the animals' activities. These histochemical properties also correlate well with various other morphological differences in MFs (for review see Buchthal, 1980; Burke, 1981). For example, a high dependence on aerobic metabolism correlates with the presence of large numbers of mitochondria and heavy staining for mitochondrial enzymes. On the other hand, MFs and MUs that depend on glycogen for their main source of energy have relatively few and smaller mitochondria but more abundant glycogen and the related enzyme phosphorylase. The speed of muscle contraction appears to correlate best with the extent of the development of the sacroplasmic reticulum (see Dubowitz and Brooke, 1973).

The larger MFs, because of their larger volumes, have lower input resistances. This imposes an extra load on the presynaptic terminal, which, to compensate, releases larger numbers of quanta per presynaptic impulse (Kuno, Turkanis, and Weakly, 1971). The synaptic junctions also occupy larger areas in such MFs.

Cat S-MUs are particularly specialized to provide the more or less constant discharges needed to maintain posture and for the fine grading of force output. These small MUs make it possible for the central nervous system to recruit extra MUs and increase the force of contraction very gradually without producing large, abrupt step-ups in force, which would happen were the larger MUs to be recruited.

To meet the constant demands placed on

such S-MUs to maintain a steady contraction and tensions, these MUs must be resistant to fatigue. This need can best be met by aerobic metabolism, but this in turn demands a constant source of oxygen and a rich blood supply and deeper location in the muscle to prevent heat loss. Perhaps the smaller diameters of these MFs help also to facilitate the exchange of oxygen across their sacrolemmal membranes.

By contrast, the FF (fast fatigable) MUs generate the much larger forces per MU necessary for short bursts of muscle contraction and for greatly increasing the force of a muscle contraction. In the cat, these MUs could be expected, for example, to participate in jumps or sprints where brief bursts of activity in larger MUs may be necessary. Because only brief bursts are required, these MUs could be relatively oxygen independent and less dependent on a rich capillary blood supply or warmer temperature. The major energy source of these MUs is glycogen, but because the supplies are limited, the MUs are unable to maintain their contractions well.

Between the two extremes are the FR (fatigue-resistant) MUs. They combine both a capacity for anaerobic and aerobic energy production and have fast contraction times. In fact, endurance training in humans may be able to convert at least some FF-MUs to FR-MUs.

Overall, the correlations among structure, function, and chemistry are quite good, but there are important differences among species and even among various muscles within the same species. The latter should make us all more cautious about assuming too direct a correlation between the physiological and histochemical properties of MUs as revealed by studies in lower animals and MUs in various muscles in man. The matter is further complicated by the fact that as mentioned above, the properties of some MUs may be altered by changing their work histories.

CONTRACTILE CHARACTERISTICS OF HUMAN MOTOR UNITS

The contractile characteristics of MUs in man have been measured both by direct nerve stimulation and by isolating their activities from the actions of other MUs in isometric contractions by the spike-triggered averaging technique.

Studies of single MUs isolated by direct nerve stimulation have shown a wide range in contraction times. For example, in the human extensor hallucis brevis (EHB), the contraction times of MUs isolated by incremental stimulation of the anterior tibial nerve fall into two main groups: one between 35 and 74 ms and the other between 78 and 98 ms (Sica and McComas, 1971). Even though the tensions generated by these MUs ranged between 2 to 14 gm, there was no obvious correlation between the tensions and contraction times. The latter incidentally was also true of MUs in the human masseter muscle (Goldberg, and Derfler, 1977). Buchthal and Schmalbruch (1969, 1970, 1980) have also shown that there is a range in the contraction times of MUs within and between various limb muscles in man.

The twitch tensions of single MUs in the abductor digiti minimi have been measured when these have been isolated by weak incremental stimuli delivered in the region of the motor point over the surface of the muscle (Burke, Skuse, and Lethlean, 1974), or by intramuscular stimulation of the motor axons in the first dorsal interosseus muscle (Taylor and Stevens, 1976; Young and Mayer, 1981). Whether or not the tensions measured by the latter technique represent the whole MU or only part of it remains in question because of the substantial branching of motor axons within the substance of the muscle. Such intramuscular stimulation could excite only a fraction of the intramuscular branches in any one MU and it cannot be assumed that the remainder are all excited antidromically.

Sometimes, however, it was possible to show that the potentials evoked by intramuscular microstimulation were truly identical to MUPs recruited by voluntary muscle contractions. The latter suggests that, at least in some instances, microstimulation was able to excite all the MFs in the MU.

The isometric contraction method, discussed in more detail later, has also indicated a broad range in the contraction times and tensions of MUs, and at least in the first dorsal interosseus muscle there was a reasonable correlation between the tensions and contraction times.

Table 5.3 shows some human muscles and the ranges in their contraction times and twitch tensions where available of single MUs in these muscles. To date, no direct correlations have been established for human MUs among their contractile properties, the histochemical properties of their MFs, and the conduction velocities of their parent motor axons. Freund, Budingen, and Dietz (1975), however, were able to demonstrate a correlation between the threshold force levels at which MUs were recruited and their relative conduction velocities (Figure 5.10).

Few attempts have been made to examine the relative resistance of MUs to fatigue in human muscles. Stephens and Usherwood (1977) were able to demonstrate fatigue in some high-tension MUs that had short contraction times (probably analogous to the FF-MUs), but no MUs equivalent to FR-MUs were seen in the first dorsal interosseus muscle by the same authors.

MOTOR UNIT RECRUITMENT

Early Observations in Man

In the course of needle electrode recordings from human muscles, Norris and Gasteiger (1955) early observed that the amplitudes of

TABLE 5.3.   Contraction Times in Human Muscle

Muscle	Contraction Time (ms)	Tension (gm)
Masseter[1]	38–69	11–205
Masseter[2]	30–85	
Platysma[3]	30–58	
Biceps[3]	16–84	
Triceps[3]	16–60	
First dorsal interosseus[4]	30–100	0.1–10
fatigable[5]	33–57	15–26.0
nonfatigable[5]	59–146	0.18–1.9
Tibialis anterior[3]	40–80	
Gastrocnemius (lateral)[3]	56–100	
	35–74	
Extensor hallucis brevis[6]	78–98	2–14

[1]Goldberg and Derfler (1977).
[2]Yemm (1977).
[3]Buchthal and Schmalbruch (1969, 1970, 1980).
[4]Milner-Brown, Stein, and Yemm (1973a).
[5]Stevens and Usherwood (1977).
[6]Sica and McComas (1971).

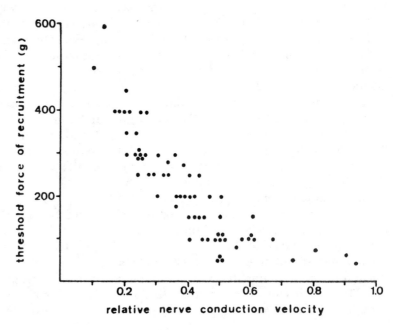

FIGURE 5.10.   Threshold isometric tension levels at which motor units in the first dorsal interosseus muscle were successively recruited as the force of the contraction was increased. Levels are shown plotted against the conduction velocities of the motor axons relative to one another (0 = fastest fibers and 1 = slowest). From Freund, Budingen, and Dietz (1975, figure 2).

MUPs recruited at lower thresholds were clearly lower than the amplitudes of those recruited in stronger contractions, although there were no obvious systemic changes in MUP duration throughout the recruitment range. The lowest-threshold MUP discharged at frequencies between 10 and 20 Hz in weak contractions, but the rates could increase to as high as 60 to 140 Hz in bursts in very strong contractions; whereas the highest-amplitude MUP recruited only in strong contractions tended to discharge at much lower frequencies. These observations pointed to a recruitment order among MUs that depended on the force of a muscle contraction. The relationships between the amplitudes of these intramuscularly recorded MUPs and the acutal sizes of the responsible MUs were not known. Thus the experiments could be criticized because of the known important dependence of the amplitudes of MUPs on the distance between MFs in the MU and the leading-off surface of the recording electrode.

Motor Unit Size

The size of MUs is most often thought of by electromyographers in terms of the amplitude and sometimes the duration of the MUP. The amplitude of MUPs as recorded by needle electrodes within the muscle bears little direct relationship to the actual innervation ratios and tensions of MUs, but more to the numbers of MFs in the immediate vicinity of the recording electrode. This brings us to a discussion of the concepts of MU size, which may be measured with respect to:

1. Number of MFs per MU (innervation ratio)
2. Forces generated per MU
3. Territories within muscles (cross-sectional areas) occupied by MUs

4. The amplitude of the MUP as recorded by surface or intramuscular needle electrodes

The above indices of MU size, although interrelated, do not reflect the same characteristics in MUs. It is possible for an MU to be large in one respect but not in another. Factors that govern the tensions of MU are listed in Table 5.4.

Even where the innervation ratios of MUs are very similar, the tensions MUs can generate can vary widely. This is probably mainly because of the larger diameters of the MFs in the higher-tension MUs, the number of contractile elements being approximately related to the cross-sectional area of the MF. The type of MF is also important because the force generated per unit cross-sectional area is higher in fast compared to slow MFs. Firing frequency is important because in slow MFs no significant change in force output occurs in a train of twitches, whereas in FF-MUs, appreciable force decrements may occur.

Similarly, the amplitudes of MUPs depend on a number of factors (Rosenfalck, 1969; Buchthal and Schmalbruch, 1980):

1. Number of MFs per MU
2. The numbers of MFs belonging to individual MUs that are nearest to the recording electrode
3. Characteristics of the electrode, including the area of the recording surfaces, loca-

TABLE 5.4. Characteristics that Govern Forces Generated by MUs

Number of MFs per MU (innervation ratio)
Diameters of MFs
Force output per unit cross-sectional area of the MF
Types of MFs
Discharge frequency of MUs
Initial length of MFs

tion of the reference electrode, and impedance of the electrode(s)

4. Orientation of the electrode(s) with respect to MFs
5. Diameters of the MFs
6. The degree of synchronization in the summation of the component single MFPs

Of the above factors, the most important is the number of MFs nearest to the leading-off surface of the recording electrode (see Chapter 7). Any tendency toward the clustering together of MFs belonging to single MUs could increase the amplitudes of MUP whether or not there has been any real increase in the numbers of MFs per motoneuron. The diameters of MFs are important because the larger the diameters of the MFs generating the potential, the larger the amplitude of the extracellularly recorded action potential. Moreover, the rise times are shorter and the amplitudes higher in extracellularly recorded action potentials generated by fast-twitch compared to slow-twitch MFs.

In healthy muscles there is a correlation between the tensions of MUs and the amplitudes of their MUPs in both experimental animals and in man. For example, in the first lumbrical muscle in the cat foot there is a clear positive correlation between twitch tension and

the amplitudes of the MUPs recorded by electrode on the surface of the muscle in MUs of various sizes (Appelberg and Emonet-Dénand, 1967; Kernell, Ducati, and Sjoholm, 1975; Kernell and Sjoholm, 1975) (Figure 5.11). The same was also true when the comparison was made between MU tensions and the amplitudes of their MUPs as recorded by intramuscular electrodes in the cat gastrocnemius (Olson, Carpenter, and Henneman, 1968).

In the human, clear correlations have been shown between the amplitudes of MUPs and the tensions of these same MUs for the first dorsal interosseus muscle (Tanji and Kato, 1973; Milner-Brown and Stein, 1975; Monster and Chan, 1977) and in the masseter muscle (Goldberg and Derfler, 1977). These correlations have held true between intramuscularly recorded MUPs and tension (Tanji and Kato, 1973; Goldberg, Louis, and Derfler 1977) and between the surface MUP amplitudes and tension (Milner-Brown and Stein, 1975) (Figures 5.12 and 5.13).

The twitch tension of MUs in the first dorsal interosseus muscle in the human increases linearly with threshold force at which the MUs are recruited, and the corresponding surface amplitudes of their MUPs increases as the square root of the tensions of the MUs.

FIGURE 5.11. Relationship between the amplitude of MUPs as recorded directly over the surface of the muscle and the maximum tetanic tension generated by the motor unit in the first deep lumbrical muscle of the cat foot (20 motor units studied in 6 cats). Shown also is the regression line (least squares method correlation coefficient was +0.92).
Redrawn from Kernell, Ducati, and Sjoholm (1975, figure 9).

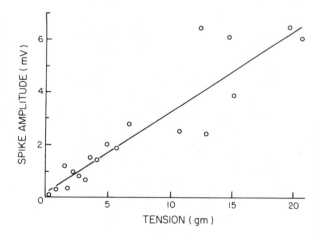

FIGURE 5.12. The relationship between the twitch tension surface recorded peak-to-peak (p-p) amplitudes in millivolts (mV) and the isometric force level in kilograms (kg) at which 25 motor units in the first dorsal interosseus muscle were recruited in one healthy human. Note the clear progressive increase in the surface amplitudes and twitch tensions of motor units recruited at progressively higher threshold levels. From unpublished observations of Brown and Yates.

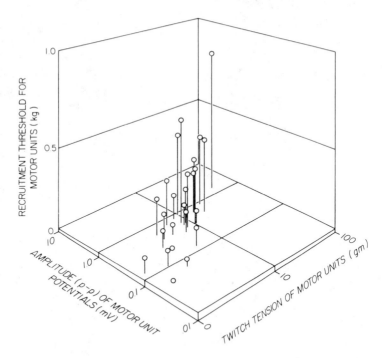

Clearly, the amplitude of MUPs recorded by either an intramuscular electrode or surface electrode does correlate with the tension of the MUs, although not necessarily with the innervation ratio of the MUs. This ratio cannot be measured in man, although it is possible to measure fiber density and assess the distributions of MFs in human MUs. Our ability to correlate MUP amplitudes and tensions is limited (Table 5.5).

ISOMETRIC CONTRACTION METHOD

In the early 1970s a new method was introduced that made it possible to measure the tensions and contraction times of single MUs recruited at various force levels in isometric contractions. In this method, the electrical and mechanical activities of single MUs were isolated from the activities of other MUs in the course of moderate to strong contractions by combining the use of highly discriminative intramuscular recording electrodes and electronic averaging (Figure 5.14). Discriminative electrodes are chosen because of their ability to record the spike discharges of only those MUs whose MFs are in the immediate vicinity of the recording electrode.

From among those few MUs with MFs generating spike potentials in the immediate vicinity of the recording surface of the electrode, one particular spike can be chosen on the basis of the force level at which it is recruited and its amplitude relative to that of other spikes recorded in the same site. Other MUP spikes with differing amplitudes can be excluded by using a window discriminator. Each time a spike occurs that exceeds the lower but not upper limits of the window, limits that are set for the operator, a pulse is generated by the window discriminator. The latter pulse is then used to trigger an electronic averaging device, which in turn pro-

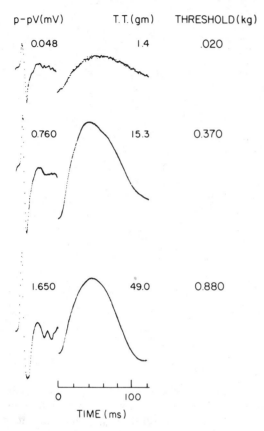

p–pV(mV)	T.T.(gm)	THRESHOLD(kg)
0.048	1.4	.020
0.760	15.3	0.370
1.650	49.0	0.880

TIME (ms)

FIGURE 5.13.   Representative motor unit action potentials (left) as recorded with surface electrodes and their recorded peak-to-peak (p-p) voltages in millivolts (mV), their corresponding twitches (middle) and twitch tension (TT) in grams (gm), as well as the threshold levels in kilograms (kg) at which these three motor units were recruited. The time scale applies to the twitch trace only.

As in Figure 5.11, there is progressive increase in the size expressed in twitch tension and spike amplitude of the motor units recruited at higher force levels. Both tension and spike traces are the electronic averages of the respective surface potential and tension records time locked to the activity of a single motor unit (see text and Figure 5.11).

gressively averages out the potentials and forces associated with the activities of all other MUs recruited to this point whose actions are not time locked to the chosen spike. The force

and amplitude records must be delayed to ensure that onsets of the MUP and twitch records are included in the average. Suitable discriminative intramuscular electrodes have included tungsten semimicro electrodes or bipolar, concentric, or Janus types. The leading off surfaces of the last three are between 25 to 75 μ in diameter. Possible errors in this technique include:

1. Synchronous discharges of two or more MUs. Such synchronization has been estimated to occur in as many as 15 and 20 percent of MUs (Buchthal and Madsen, 1950). This estimate is in our view, too high, but in any case such couplings between the discharges of MUs can be identified by special techniques and the records excluded (Milner-Brown, Stein, and Lee, 1975).

2. The tension contributions of two MUs are averaged together. This can happen when the amplitudes of two separate MUP spikes are so close to one another that both are included in the window. It is important, therefore, for the operator to ensure that the MUPs selected as trigger sources are indeed identical in shape as well as amplitude. Where two or more MUPs have similar amplitudes, the position of the intramuscular recording electrode must be adjusted to increase the relative amplitude differences between them.

3. Errors in measurements of MU force
   a. Fusion of twitches at rates of discharges over 7 to 8 Hz. Because the total contraction times of the MUs range from 70 to 100 ms or more, where the intertwitch interval is shorter than the total contraction time, successive twitches may superimpose or fuse. The result is that the amplitude of the averaged single twitch may be somewhat less than the true single twitch. This error could result in substantial error in the mea-

TABLE 5.5. Factors that Can Influence Correlations between Amplitudes of MUPs and Tensions Generated by their MUs

Factors that Primarily Affect Amplitude	Factors that Primarily Affect Tension
In surface recording, the depth of MUs below the surface	Firing frequency and fatigue characteristics of MUs
In intramuscular recordings, the number of MFs within the pickup territory of the electrode	Technical and physiological factors may make it difficult accurately to measure tensions generated by single MUs or the overall tension produced by the muscle such as
Diameters of MFs	Other synergistic muscles may contribute to overall tension recorded
	MUs recorded from may not usually act in the plane of the force transducer
In both surface and intramuscular recordings, distance between recording electrodes and MU	Muscle or MU may not be at optimal lengths for generation of their maximum territory
	Viscoelastic properties of tissues absorb some of the change in tension

Both Amplitude and Tension
Synchronous or near synchronous firing of two or more MUs (Milner-Brown, Stein, and Yemm, 1973a)

surement of twitch tensions, especially in abnormal states where the onset of firing frequencies may be appreciably higher (more than 10 Hz) and the total contraction times of the twitches longer. In such circumstances it may be impossible to record isolated twitches in single MUs by this technique. The incorporation of devices that automatically reject successive MU discharges when the interdischarge period is less than 90 to 100 ms does not entirely solve the problem, because some MUs just do not have onset frequencies as low as 10 Hz or less and the total contraction times of some may well exceed 100 ms.

b. The inclusion of in-series viscoelastic properties of the muscle and tendon. Part of the tension an MU generates is taken up by the viscoelastic properties of the muscle and tendon, skin, and subcutaneous tisses, and by the device used to record the force. The contributions of the viscoelastic properties of the tissues could well be changed in disease states, such that muscle tendon, skin, or other tissue could become more or less elastic compared to normal tissues.

c. Fatigue. Especially at high rates of firing, MUs can fatigue and their tensions decline. This would be expected most of all in the highest-threshold MUs, but appreciable declines could

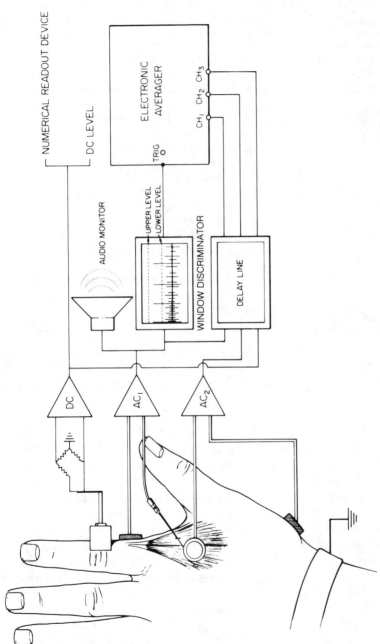

FIGURE 5.14.   General experimental arrangement for measuring the spike amplitudes and twitch tensions of single motor units recruited in the course of a steady isometric contraction. The tension is recorded by a force transducer, the strain gauge acting as one arm of a bridge circuit. The DC level of the output of the DC amplifier is proportional to the isometric tension exerted by the index finger against the transducer arm. The electrical potentials in the underlying first dorsal interosseus muscle are recorded by surface electrodes, the stigmatic electrode being located as close to the innervation zone of the muscle as possible.

The electrical activities of single motor units are also recorded by a discriminative intramuscular electrode (bipolar configuration, leading-off surfaces 25 to 50 μ in diameter or a tungsten microelectrode). The potentials associated with the activities of particular motor units are selected with the aid of a window discriminator on the basis of the force level at which they are recruited and their amplitude. Only potentials whose amplitudes fall between the operator-selected lower and upper amplitude levels may act as trigger sources for the electronic averager, which then averages out all other potentials and forces except those time locked to the trigger source potential. To avoid distortions of the onset of the mechanical and electrical events associated with the activity of the motor unit, both the potential and tension records should be delayed by a short interval prior to their entry into the electronic averager.

occur in lower-threshold MUs as well. It is the highest-threshold MUs, however, that make the largest demands on the recording system because their activities must be isolated from the activities of much larger numbers of other MUs, and more extended averaging is required. Such extended averaging would enhance apparent fatigue because of the need to maintain the contractions longer in order to average more potentials. Also, any tendencies toward impulse blocking or failures in neuromuscular transmission could degrade the averaged tensions and amplitudes of MUs when recorded by this technique.

d. Limitations in the capacity of the transducer to discriminate MU forces of the order of 1 gm or less when the overall force levels are of the order of 1 to 2 kg. At intermediate and high force levels, higher spring rates must be used in the transducers, rates that may make it harder to discriminate the lower tensions generated by some MUs. This could be particularly troublesome in abnormal states.

Whatever the errors and limitations, this method has been used to examine the recruit-ment orders of MUs in slow ramp and ballistic contractions, and the relative contributions of MU recruitment and rate coding of MUs to the overall tension development in muscles. This method has now been extended to look at a number of muscles, including the masseter, extensor digitorum communis, first dorsal interosseus, tibialis anterior, extensor digitorum brevis, and soleus muscles in man.

The most important observations derived from the use of this technique include:

1. Motor unit tension. There is a broad range in the tensions of MUs in muscles (Table 5.6). It is not known in man whether there is a true continuum in the tensions of the MUs, or whether MUs can be separated into distinct groups based on their tensions. If the latter were true, perhaps the divisions between the groups have been blurred by errors in technique.

2. Rates of MU discharge. In normal individuals, MUs begin to discharge at about 7 to 10 impulses per second. In isometric contractions, these rates can increase to 20 or more impulses per second as the strength of the contraction increases, there being an approximately linear relationship between the discharge rates and the level of isometric tension achieved (Mil-

TABLE 5.6.   Range in MU Tensions in Muscles

Muscle	Range in MU Tensions	Source
First dorsal interosseus	× 100 (0.1–10 gm)	Milner-Brown, Stein, and Yemm (1973a, 1973b, 1973c)
First dorsal interosseus	× 160 (0.18–30 gm)	Stephens and Usherwood (1977)
Extensor digitorum communis	× 5–10	Monster and Chan (1977)
Masseter	× 20 (11–205 gm)	Goldberg, Louis, and Derfler (1977)
Masseter	× 13–107 (0.1–33.6)	Yemm (1977)
Temporalis	15–30 × (0.3–30.3)	Yemm (1977)

ner-Brown, Stein, and Yemm, 1973c). In brisker (ballistic) contractions (Desmedt and Godaux, 1977a, 1977b, 1978, 1981) or alternating movements (Marsden, Meadows, and Merton, 1971; Grimby and Hannerz, 1968, 1976, 1977; Borg, Grimby, and Hannerz, 1978) these rates can become much higher—50 to 150 Hz—especially in the larger-tension MUs that have characteristically shorter contraction times and shorter periods of afterhyperpolarization in their parent motoneurons.

In general, however, the firing rates of MUs is somewhat lower, and in the course of prolonged maximal contractions they decline, perhaps to optimize the force output in fatiguing MUs (Bigland-Ritchie, Johansson, Lippold, and Woods, 1982).

In MUs with slower contraction times, individual twitches fuse at much lower frequencies and there would therefore be little apparent advantage to very high rates of discharge (Desmedt and Godaux, 1978; Burke, 1981).

3. Order of recruitment of MUs. The MUs are recruited in order of their tensions by increments in the force of contraction. Thus those that generate the least tensions and tend to have slower contraction times are recruited at the lowest force levels. Recruitment of larger-tension MUs is brought about by increments in the force of the muscle contraction (Milner-Brown, Stein, and Yemm, 1973a) (see Figures 5.12 and 5.13).

There is agreement that the conduction velocities of the lowest-threshold MUs are slower than those of higher-threshold MUs in both the first dorsal interosseus (Freund, Budingin, and Dietz, 1975) and the extensor digitorum brevis muscles (Borg, Grimby, and Hannerz, 1978). Moreover, the highest-threshold MUs are the most susceptible to fatigue; whereas the smaller-tension MUs recruited at lower threshold levels are fatigue resistant (Stephens and Usherwood, 1977). In the extensor digitorum communis muscle of the baboon (all fast-twitch MUs), however, there was no correlation between the conduction velocities and the tensions generated in single MUs (Eccles, Phillips, and Wu-Chien Ping, 1968).

Some investigators, however, have not been able to demonstrate good correlations in humans between the twitch tensions and the contraction times of MUs (Sica and McComas, 1971). This could depend to some extent on the muscle tested. For example, a reasonable correlation was demonstrable in the first dorsal interosseus muscle by Stein, Milner-Brown, and Yemm (1973a).

The force levels at which MUs are recruited are not fixed, but are a function of the type of movement and specifically the velocity of movement. Thus at the extreme as in a ballistic contraction in the first dorsal interosseus muscle where time from onset of contraction to the peak force is less than 0.15 second, MUs can discharge at a very high instantaneous rate (50 to 150 impulses per second). They begin to discharge just prior to onset of the contraction (Desmedt and Godaux, 1977a, 1977b). In such ballistic contractions, the thresholds at which MUs are recruited are much lower than in slower-amplitude contractions although the rank order of their recruitment is not altered. Sometimes apparent reversals were observed, possibly because the onset of twitches of the lower-threshold MUs in the distal muscles may have been delayed relative to the faster-conducting axons of the higher-tension MUs, even though at the level of the motoneuron, the lower-threshold and smaller-tension MUs were the first to be activated (Desmedt and Godaux, 1978).

In between the slow ramp increases in the force of a muscle contraction and the brisk ballistic contractions, the thresholds for recruitment or derecruitment of MUs vary with the speed of the contraction (rate of tension development), the absolute thresholds being lower the more rapid the contractions. The thresholds of MUs may also be appreciably higher when the muscle serves in a synergistic rather than primary role in a contraction (Desmedt and Godaux, 1981). There is also a tendency for the discharges of two or more MUs to become synchronized in manual laborers, weight lifters, and in other situations where muscles undergo strength training (Milner-Brown, Stein, and Lee, 1975).

Is the Recruitment Order Fixed?

Despite the now substantial evidence in humans and lower animals that a size principle governs the rank order of recruitment of MUs in muscle contraction, there is some evidence that to a very limited extent, modifications of this order are possible (see Phillips and Porter, 1977; Burke, 1981; Henneman and Mendell, 1981). Basmajian (1963) had claimed that humans could exercise considerable selection in their choice of MUs when aided by visual and auditory feedback. Others have not been able to confirm such a wide freedom of choice (Henneman, Shahani, and Young, 1976).

Grimby and Hannerz (1968) have, however, reported that subjects could change the recruitment order to a limited extent by certain strategies such as prior muscle stretch, unloading the muscle during contraction, vibration, or coactivating other muscles. Later, the same investigators also showed that in some instances, MUs that had high thresholds for recruitment in slow ramp contractions and whose axonal conduction velocities were high could be recruited at the outset of a contraction and sometimes to the exclusion of other MUs in rapid alternating or ballistic contractions in the extensor digitorum brevis (Grimby and Hannerz, 1968; 1977; Borg, Grimby, and

Hannerz, 1978). In addition, Kato and Tanji (1972) claimed that while the recruitment order among MUs with widely dissimilar recruitment thresholds could not be altered, the order could be altered among MUs with nearly identical thresholds, an observation noted also by Milner-Brown, Stein, and Yemm (1973b).

Such apparent alterations probably reflect the fact that muscles are called on to act in various ways depending on the task (Desmedt, 1980; Denier Van Der Gon, Gielen, Ter Haar Romeny, 1982). Moreover, not all parts of the same muscle serve the same purposes. Thus changes in the direction in which a muscle is called to act could change the selection of MUs to those best placed to achieve the required action. The selection of MUs therefore depends on the nature of the intended task and the relative recruitment thresholds of the MUs in the muscle (Person, 1974; Milner-Brown, Stein, and Yemm, 1973b; Desmedt, 1980; Burke, 1980, 1981). There is some evidence as well that when the inputs to a muscle are changed, the apparent recruitment order can be altered. Stephens, Garnett, and Buller (1978) and Datta and Stephens (1981) were able to show that changes in the recruitment patterns of MUs could be induced by cutaneous stimulation or altering the sensory feedback from the muscle. Similar alterations in response to changes in the sensory input have been demonstrated by Grimby and Hannerz (1968, 1976) in the human tibialis anterior muscle.

In summary, the apparent recruitment order depends not only on the inherent size of the motoneuron (or MU tension) but can be modified somewhat by sensory feedback from the periphery. Despite the latter qualifications, however, it remains true that in the simple case where muscles act as prime movers, MUs are recruited in order of their tensions; exceptions to the order for the most part are limited to MUs whose thresholds and sizes are reasonably close.

Mechanisms Underlying Recruitment Order

Two basic mechanisms are possible in the order of recruitment. It may depend on the properties of the motoneurons or on the densities and spatial distributions of the various inputs to the motoneurons, or on some combination of the two. It has been proposed (Henneman, 1957; Henneman, Somjen, and Carpenter, 1965a, 1965b) that the relative excitabilities of motoneurons depended on the sizes and hence, input resistances of the motoneurons (see review by Henneman and Mendell, 1981). In this model, equivalent spatially distributed and dense inputs could be expected to evoke larger postsynaptic transmembrane potentials at the initial segments of smaller compared to larger motoneurons. There is indeed a good correlation between the diameters of motoneurons and their input resistances. In most situations a variety of input sources, peripheral or central, produces equivalent recruitment orders of motoneurons.

There is, however, evidence that the order of recruitment can be modified and even reversed by altering the input signals originating in muscle stretch or cutaneous receptors. The latter evidence suggests that the inputs, both peripheral and central, may be important determinants of the order of recruitment. In most situations, however, the spatial and temporal patterns of these input signals are such that the order of recruitment remains consistent with the relative sizes of the motoneurons (Burke, 1980, 1981). In this model, the temporal coding, distribution, and densities of the various inputs to the motoneurons into the motoneuron pool may be as critical as the actual sizes of motoneurons in determining the rank order of recruitment. For example, the larger the number of synaptic connections a particular input makes on the motoneuron and the nearer this input is to the spike-generating zone of the motoneuron, the more likely the

motoneuron is to fire. This would contrast to situations in which there were fewer synaptic connections and these were projected to areas on the somal dendritic membrane that were more remote from the spike-generation zone. In the latter instance, the lower amplitudes and slower rise times of the EPSP(s) as seen at the initial segment tend to reduce the effectiveness of the input, as a drive to the motoneuron and the MU would appear to have a higher threshold. Beyond this, where the inputs to the motoneuron were equivalent in numbers of synapses and projection sites on the motoneuronal membranes, the magnitude of depolarization, for example in excitatory inputs, would be higher in smaller motoneurons because of their higher input resistances.

Until more is known about the termination sites, numbers of peripheral synaptic terminals, and the effectiveness of these synapses, the question about the relative importance of the properties of motoneurons and the nature of the inputs as the most primary determinants of recruitment order cannot be resolved. That not all investigators have been able to demonstrate strong correlations between MU tension and conduction velocity and hence, probably motoneuronal and axonal diameter, suggests that the mechanisms that govern recruitment order may be more complex than simply a matter of the sizes of the motoneurons (Goslow, Cameron, and Stuart, 1977). This whole question has been extensively and clearly reviewed by Henneman and Mendell (1981).

FORCE OF MUSCLE CONTRACTION

Four main factors govern the force of muscle contraction:

1. The numbers and sizes of MUs recruited
2. Muscle length
3. Patterns and firing frequencies of the MUs

4. Especially in primary diseases of muscle, the presence of any abnormalities in the contractile process

The relative importance of these factors varies among different muscles and the character of the movement. On the basis of his studies on the human first dorsal interosseus muscle, Stein (1974) has claimed that recruitment of MUs is the single most important mechanism by which the force of a muscle contraction is increased in weak contractions. As the strength of the contraction increases, however, the firing frequencies of MUs become more and more important, and once all or most of the MUs are recruited, it is the sole mechanism available for increasing the force. Thus in the first dorsal interosseus muscle, more than 90 percent of MUs have probably been recruited at isometric force levels below 1 kg and 80 percent at levels below 0.6 kg, whereas the maximum tension of which this muscle is capable in an isometric contraction is somewhere between 4 and 6 kg (Milner-Brown, Stein, and Yemm, 1973a). These observations were supported by the independent investigations of Tanji and Kato (1973).

Burke (1981) has also pointed out that the pattern of MU discharge can be a critical factor in the level of force generated. Thus in situations where there is no change in the overall rate at which motoneurons fire, "catchlike" step-ups in force can be achieved by double discharges at such short intervals that the two twitches overlap and fuse (Burke, 1981).

In ballistic contractions, the firing frequencies of MUs commonly reach high enough levels that successive twitches fuse, substantially increasing the overall force output of the muscle (Desmedt and Godaux, 1978). In the soleus muscle, the maximum force generated depends more on the MU recruitment than on rate coding.

In those MUs that fatigue, the force output may fall off in a sustained discharge. These are the same MUs that generate high tensions and can produce large quantal step-ups in tension, especially when their short-term firing frequencies result in fusion of twitches. Training these MUs can reduce their tendency to fatigue.

The magnitude of the tension that muscles or muscle groups can generate depends also on the length of the muscles. The connective tissues of muscle and tendon are in series with the contractile elements in the muscle and contribute to the viscoelastic properties of the muscle. The resistance to stretch of these elements increases as muscles are progressively lengthened. More critical is the degree to which the contractile elements, actin and myosin, overlap in the muscle, because this determines the number of cross bridges that can form between these elements (Gordon, Huxley, and Julian, 1966; Huxley, 1967, 1971, 1974). The critical dependence of maximum tension on muscle length is well illustrated by the effect changes in joint angle, and hence muscle length, have on the maximum tetanic tensions achieved by the soleus and tibialis anterior muscles in the human (McComas, Kereshi, and Quinlan, 1983).

Fatigue

Fatigue is a common complaint in neuromuscular and central motor disorders. The sense of being unable to generate or maintain a certain level of contraction is common too in healthy subjects in situations of excessive physiological or psychological stress. Muscle contraction is accompanied by a subjective "sense of the effort" necessary to achieve the intended contraction. In healthy subjects asked to make a maximum contraction, tension falls off gradually over time. This decline is accompanied by an increase in the sense of effort necessary to maintain the contraction and a growing sense of tiredness or fatigue.

The greatest tension that subjects can generate by a maximum voluntary effort and the falling off in this tension with a prolonged contraction are matched by the very similar maximum tensions and declines when these tensions are evoked by tetanic motor nerve or direct muscle stimulation. In most peripheral and muscle diseases, the declines in maximum tensions accompanying maximum voluntary contraction and supramaximal direct nerve or muscle stimulations also closely parallel one another. This contrasts with the situation in upper motoneuron weakness where the tensions generated in response to peripheral stimulation may be normal or near normal, but the patient experiences considerable difficulty reaching or maintaining similar tensions by voluntary effort alone. Similarly, in malingering and some psychiatric disorders the sense of effort may seem to be enhanced and be accompanied by grimacing and tightening of other muscles, whereas the contraction of the muscles to which the attention is directed is much more variable, and the tensions achieved are well below those achieved by peripheral stimulation. Proof that not all of the motoneuron pool has been recruited in such subjects may be brought out by stimulating the motor nerve supramaximally during the period of the maximum contraction. Such stimuli evoke twitches whose size is proportional to the sum of the tensions generated by the unrecruited MUs (see Merton, 1954 for principle of the method; and McComas, Kereshi, and Quinlan, 1983 for its application to functional weakness) (Figure 5.15).

What accounts for fatigue, or the subjective sense of increased effort required to sustain a maximum contraction in the face of weakening contraction despite the best efforts of normal subjects? Is fatigue central or peripheral in origin? Both are important questions. The question of whether fatigue is central or peripheral in origin has been examined by Merton (1954) in the adductor pollicis muscle. He demonstrated that the maximum tension achieved by voluntary contractions is very close to that which can be evoked by tetanic stimulation of the motor nerve. The subjective sense of effort was not a good guide to the force of the contraction, nor was the subject's sense that an extraordinary effort was being made necessarily accompanied by any measurable increase in force; indeed, at times the tension fell off.

In maximum voluntary contractions, the maximum tension could be maintained only for several seconds, after which the tension fell off, reaching about one-half of its original value by one minute. This fall in tension was accompanied by a parallel reduction in the tension evoked by tetanic nerve stimulation. Because Merton was unable to show any accompanying declines in electrical potentials in the muscle, he suggested that the progressive fall-off in tension was produced by change in the contractile apparatus itself, not changes in the capacities of nerve or muscle to transmit impulses or because of defects in neuromuscular transmission.

Others have claimed, however, that in the same muscle, there are declines in the amplitude of the M-potential at frequencies of stimulation over 50 Hz. Such decrements in M-amplitude could be produced by failures in neuromuscular transmission at some junctions, intermittent block of impulses in the presynaptic motor axons, especially in neurogenic disorders, or even conduction failures in the MFs themselves (see review by Burke, 1981). Reductions in electrical activity were less pronounced in maximum voluntary contractions than in tetanic nerve stimulation, although why this should happen is not clear (Bigland-Ritchie, Jones, and Woods, 1979; Jones, Bigland-Ritchie, and Edwards, 1979).

The whole question of central and peripheral mechanisms in fatigue needs to be looked at in human disease. Even though many of the issues cannot be resolved at this time, cer-

FIGURE 5.15.   Method for demonstrating incomplete recruitment of motor units despite a supposed maximum voluntary contraction in subjects with functional weakness.

(a) illustrates the principle of the method. In this normal subject, voluntary contractions (in this case, the plantar flexor muscles) of variable intensity up to maximum (top trace) are made. In the midst of the contraction, the motor nerve to these muscles is supramaximally stimulated and its twitch is recorded. Note that when the subject makes a maximum voluntary contraction an interpolated twitch is not detectible, indicating that the subject has presumably recruited all the available motor units in these muscles, none apparently remaining to be activated by the indirect stimulus.

(b), (c), and (d) Tracings from patients with functional weakness instructed to make a maximum voluntary contraction (top two plantar flexors of the foot and bottom one dorsiflexors of the foot). Not only are the submaximal tensions recorded, but the interpolated twitches are well retained. This indicates that for whatever reason, not all the motoneurons have been recruited by the subject despite his or her best effort. The horizontal calibration throughout is 2 s, but the vertical calibrations are 30 nm (a), 10 nm (b), 5 nm (c), and 4 nm (d).

From McComas, Kereshi, and Quinlan (1983).

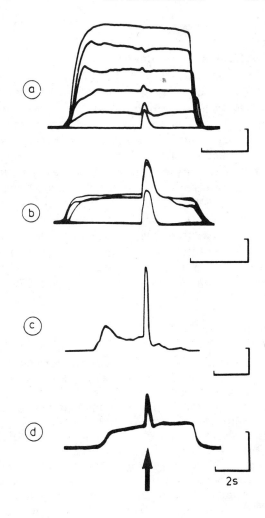

tain points are clear (see recent reviews by Bigland-Ritchie, 1983, and Edwards, 1983). Maximum voluntary contractions can generate tensions that closely approximate those achievable by high-frequency tetanic nerve or muscle stimulation. This means that humans are capable by their own voluntary efforts of forces that closely match those of which the peripheral apparatus is capable, and at these levels, there is no reserve available that can be brought out by any other stimulus. Once fatigue begins, maximum contraction may be better facilitated by reductions in the firing frequencies of MUs. Muscle fatigue in the healthy subject at least, is peripheral in origin and is probably accounted for by failures in neuromuscular transmission or conduction in the MFs themselves, as well as declines in the effectiveness of the contractile apparatus. Repetitive stimulation does increase the duration of the active state in muscle (Partridge and Benton, 1981), and this helps to compensate for the above in maintaining maximum voluntary contractions.

Effect of Training

Exercise increases the oxidative enzyme content of MFs, the degree of capillarization, and resistance to fatigue of muscle, and also may convert some FF-MUs to FR-MUs. No conversions to S-MUs have yet been demonstrated (Burke, 1981). Besides increasing the force of contractions, Burke (1981) has shown that there may be an actual increase in the conduction velocities of motor axons, at least in the cat (Walsh, Burke, Rymer, and Tsairis, 1978). Whether this is true in man is unknown. The frequency of synchronization between the discharges of single MUs has also been shown to be increased with strength training (Milner-Brown, Stein, and Lee, 1975).

References

Appelberg B, Emonet-Dénand F. Motor units of the first superficial lumbrical muscle of the cat. J Neurophysiol 1967;30:154–60.

Basmajian JV. Control and training of individual motor units. Science 1963;141:440–41.

Bergmans J. The physiology of single nerve fibers. Louvain, Belgium: Vander, 1970.

Bigland-Ritchie B. Changes in EMG and neural control during human muscle fatigue. Thirtieth Annual Meeting, American Association of Electromyography and Electrodiagnosis, Toronto, September 30–October 1, 1983.

Bigland-Ritchie B, Johansson R, Lippold CJ, Woods JJ. Changes of single motor unit firing rates during sustained maximal voluntary contractions. J Physiol 1982;328:27P.

Bigland-Ritchie B, Jones DA, Woods JJ. Excitation frequency and muscle fatigue: electrical responses during human voluntary contractions. Exp Neurol 1979;64:414–27.

Borg J, Grimby L, Hannerz J. Axonal conduction velocity and voluntary discharge properties of individual short toe extensor motor units in man. J Physiol 1978;277:143–52.

Boyd IA, Davey MR. Composition of peripheral nerves. Edinburgh: Livingstone, 1968.

Brandstater ME, Lambert EH. Motor unit anatomy. Type and spatial arrangement of muscle fibers. In: Desmedt JE, ed. New developments in electromyography and clinical neurophysiology. Basel: Karger, 1973:14–22.

Brodal A. Neurological anatomy. Oxford: Oxford University Press, 1981.

Brooke MH, Kaiser KK. Muscle fiber types: how many and what kind? Arch Neurol 1970;23:369–79.

Brooke MH, Kaiser KK. The use and abuse of muscle histochemistry. Ann NY Acad Sci 1974;228:121–44.

Buchthal F, Erminio F, Rosenfalck P. Motor unit territory in different human muscles. Acta Physiol Scand 1959;45:72–87.

Buchthal F, Guld C, Rosenfalck P. Multielectrode study of the territory of a motor unit. Acta Physiol Scand 1957a;39:83–104.

Buchthal F, Guld C, Rosenfalck P. Volume conduction of the spike of the motor unit potential investigated with a new type of multielectrode. Acta Physiol Scand 1957b;38:331–54.

Buchthal F, Madsen A. Synchronous activity in normal and atrophic muscle. Electroencephalogr Clin Neurophysiol 1950;2:425–44.

Buchthal F, Schmalbruch H. Spectrum of contraction times of different fibre bundles in the brachial biceps and triceps muscles of man. Nature 1969;222:89.

Buchthal F, Schmalbruch H. Contraction times and fiber types in intact human muscle. Acta Physiol Scand 1970;79:435–52.

Buchthal F, Schmalbruch H. Motor unit of mammalian muscle. Physiol Rev 1980;60:90–142.

Burke D, Skuse NF, Lethlean AK. Isometric contraction of the abductor digiti minimi muscle in man. J Neurol Neurosurg Psychiatry 1974;37:825–34.

Burke RE. Firing patterns of gastrocnemius motor units in the decerebrate cat. J Physiol 1968;196:631–54.

Burke RE. Motor units in mammalian muscle. In: Sumner AJ, ed. The physiology of peripheral nerve disease. Philadelphia: WB Saunders, 1980:133–94.

Burke RE. Motor units: anatomy, physiology, and functional organization. In: Brooks VB, ed. Handbook of physiology. The nervous system.

Vol. 2. Motor control. Bethesda, Md.: American Physiological Society, 1981:2345–422.

Burke RE, Levine DN, Zajac FE, Tsairis P, Engel WK. Mammalian motor units; physiological histochemical correlation in three types in cat gastrocnemius. Science 1971;174:709–12.

Burke RE, Strick PL, Kanda K, Kim CC, Walmsley B. Anatomy of medial gastrocnemius and soleus motor nuclei in cat spinal cord. J Neurophysiol 1977;40:667–80.

Burke RE, Tsairis P. Anatomy and innervation ratios in motor units of cat gastrocnemius. J Physiol 1973;234:749–65.

Carpenter MB, Sutin J. Human neuroanatomy. 8th ed. Baltimore: Williams & Wilkins, 1983.

Christensen E. Topography of terminal motor innervation in striated muscles from stillborn infants. Am J Phys Med 1959;38:17–30.

Close RI. Dynamic properties of mammalian skeletal muscles. Physiol Rev 1972;52:129–97.

Coërs C, Woolf AL. The innervation of muscle. Oxford: Blackwell, 1959.

Coërs C, Woolf AL. Pathological anatomy of the intramuscular motor innervation. In: Walton J, ed. Disorders of voluntary muscle. 4th ed. Edinburgh: Churchill-Livingstone, 1981:238–60.

Datta AK, Stephens JA. The effects of digital nerve stimulation on the firing of motor units in human first dorsal interosseus muscle. J Physiol 1981;318:501–10.

Denier Van Der Gon JJ, Gielen CCAM, Ter Haar Romeny, BM. Changes in recruitment threshold of motor units in the human biceps muscle. J Physiol 1982;328:28P.

Desmedt JE. Methodes d'études de la fonction neuromusculaire, chez l'homme: Myogramme isométrique, électromyogramme d'excitation et topographie de l'innervation terminale. Acta Neurol Psychiatr (Belg) 1958;58:977–1017.

Desmedt, JE. Patterns of motor commands during various types of voluntary movement in man. Trends Neurosci 1980;3:265–68.

Desmedt JE, Godaux E. Ballistic contractions in man: characteristic recruitment pattern of single motor units of the tibialis anterior muscle. J Physiol (Lond) 1977a;264:673–94.

Desmedt JE, Godaux E. Fast motor units are not preferentially activated in rapid voluntary contractions in man. Nature 1977b;267:717–19.

Desmedt JE, Godaux E. Ballistic skilled movements: load compensation and patterning of the motor commands. In: Desmedt JE, ed. Cerebral motor control in man: long loop mechanisms. Basel: Karger, 1978:21–55.

Desmedt JE, Godaux E. Spinal motoneuron recruitment in man: rank deordering with direction but not speed of voluntary movement. Science 1981;214:933–36.

Dubowitz V, Brook MH. Major problems in neurology, muscle biopsy. A modern approach. Vol. 2. Philadelphia: WB Saunders, 1973.

Eccles JC, Sherrington CS. Numbers and contraction values of individual motor units examined in some muscles of the limb. Proc R Soc Biol 1930;106:326–57.

Eccles RM, Phillips CG, Wu-Chien Ping W. Motor innervation, motor unit organization and afferent innervation of M. extensor digitorum communis of the baboon's forearm. J Physiol (Lond) 1968;198:179–92.

Edwards RHT. New techniques for studying human muscle function, metabolism and fatigue. Thirtieth Annual Meeting, American Association of Electromyography and Electrodiagnosis, Toronto, September 30–October 1, 1983.

Elliott HC. Studies on the motor cells of the spinal cord. I. Distribution in the normal human cord. Am J Anat 1942;70:95–117.

Elliott HC. Studies on the motor cells of the spinal cord. II. Distribution in the normal human foetal cord. Am J Anat 1943;72:29–38.

Feindel, W. Anatomical overlap of motor units. J Comp Neurol 1954;101:1–17.

Feinstein B, Lindegård B, Nyman E, Wohlfart G. Morphologic studies of motor units in normal human muscles. Acta Anatomica 1955;23:127–42.

Freund H. Motor unit and muscle activity in voluntary motor control. Physiol Rev 1983;63:387–436.

Freund HJ, Budingen HJ, Dietz VJ. Activity of single motor units from human forearm muscles during voluntary isometric contractions. J Neurophysiol 1975;38:933–46.

Goldberg LJ, Derfler B. Relationship among recruitment order, spike amplitude and twitch tension of single motor units in human masseter muscle. J Neurophysiol 1977;40:879–90.

Gordon AM, Huxley AF, Julian FJ. The variation in isometric tension with sarcomere length in vertebrate muscle fibers. J Physiol 1966;184:170–92.

Goslow GE, Cameron WE, Stuart DG. The fast-twitch motor units of cat ankle flexors. II. Speed-force relations and recruitment order. Brain Res 1977;134:47–57.

Grimby L, Hannerz J. Recruitment order of motor units on voluntary contraction: changes induced by proprioceptive afferent activity. J Neurol Neurosurg Psychiatry 1968;31:565–73.

Grimby L, Hannerz J. Disturbances in the voluntary recruitment order of low- and high-frequency motor units on blockades of proprioceptive afferent activity. Acta Physiol Scand 1976;96:207–16.

Grimby L, Hannerz J. Firing rate and recruitment order of toe extensor motor units in different modes of voluntary contraction. J Physiol (Lond) 1977;264:865–79.

Guth L. "Trophic" influences of nerve on muscle. Physiol Rev 1968;48:645–87.

Henneman E. Relation between size of neurons and their susceptibility to discharge. Science 1957;126:1345–46.

Henneman E, Mendell LM. Functional organization of motoneuron pool and its inputs. In: Brooks VB, ed. Handbook of physiology. The nervous system. Vol 2. Motor control. Bethesda, Md.: American Physiological Society, 1981:2423–507.

Henneman E, Olson CB. Relations between structure and function in the design of skeletal muscles. J Neurophysiol 1965;28:581–98.

Henneman EB, Shahani BT, Young RR. Voluntary control of human motor units. In: Shahani M. ed. The motor system: neurophysiology and muscle mechanisms. Amsterdam: Elsevier 1976:73–78.

Henneman E, Somjen G, Carpenter DO. Functional significance of cell size in spinal motoneurons. J Neurophysiol 1965a;28:560–80.

Henneman E, Somjen G, Carpenter DO. Excitability and inhibitability of motoneurons of different sizes. J Neurophysiol 1965b;28:599–620.

Huxley AF. The activation of striated muscle and its mechanical response. Proc R Soc Lond Biol 1967;178:1–27.

Huxley AF. The structural basis of muscular contraction. Proc R Soc Lond Biol 1971;178:131–49.

Huxley AF. Muscular contraction. J Physiol 1974;243:1–43.

Jones DA, Bigland-Ritchie B, Edwards RHT. Excitation frequency and muscle fatigue: mechanical responses during voluntary and stimulated contractions. Exp Neurol 1979;64:401–13.

Kato M, Tanji J. Volitionally controlled single motor units in human finger muscles. Brain Res 1972;40:345–57.

Kernell D, Ducati A, Sjoholm H. Properties of motor units in the first deep lumbrical muscle of the cat's foot. Brain Res 1975;98:37–55.

Kernell D, Sjoholm H. Recruitment and firing rate modulation of motor unit tension in a small muscle of the cat's foot. Brain Res 1975;98:57–72.

Krnjević K, Miledi R. Motor units in the rat diaphragm. J Physiol 1958;140:427–39.

Kugelberg E. Properties of rat hindlimb motor units. In: Desmedt JE, ed. New developments in electromyography and clinical neurophysiology. Basel: Karger, 1973:2–13.

Kuno M, Turkanis SA, Weakly JN. Correlation between nerve terminal size and transmitter release at the neuromuscular junction of the frog. J Physiol (Lond) 1971;213:545–66.

Marsden CD, Meadows JC, Merton PA. Isolated single motor units in human muscle and their rate of discharge during maximal voluntary effort. J Physiol 1971;217:12P–13P.

McComas AJ, Kereshi S, Quinlan J. A method for detecting functional weakness. J Neurol Neurosurg Psychiatry 1983;46:280–86.

Merton PA. Voluntary strength and fatigue. J Physiol (Lond) 1954;123:553–64.

Milner-Brown HS, Stein RB. The relation between the surface electromyogram and muscular force. J Physiol (Lond) 1975;246:549–69.

Milner-Brown HS, Stein RB, Lee RG. Synchronization of human motor units: possible roles of exercise and supraspinal reflexes. Electroencephalogr Clin Neurophysiol 1975;38:245–54.

Milner-Brown HS, Stein RB, Yemm R. The contractile properties of human motor units during voluntary contractions. J Physiol (Lond) 1973a;228:285–306.

Milner-Brown HS, Stein RB, Yemm R. The orderly recruitment of human motor units during voluntary isometric contractions. J Physiol 1973b;230:359–70.

Milner-Brown HS, Stein RB, Yemm R. Changes in firing rate of human motor units during linearly changing voluntary contractions. J Physiol (Lond) 1973c;230:371–90.

Monster AW, Chan H. Isometric force production by motor units of extensor digitorum communis muscle in man. J Neurophysiol 1977;40:1432–43.

Norris FH Jr, Gasteiger EL. Action potentials of single motor units in normal muscle. Electroencephalogr Clin Neurophysiol 1955;7:115–26.

Olson CB, Carpenter DO, Henneman E. Orderly recruitment of muscle action potentials. Motor unit threshold and EMG amplitude. Arch Neurol 1968;19:591–97.

Partridge LD, Benton LA. Muscle, the motor. In: Brooks VB, ed. Handbook of Physiology. The nervous system. Vol. 2. Motor control. Bethesda, Md.: American Physiological Society, 1981;2:43–106.

Person RS. Rhythmic activity of a group of human motoneurones during voluntary contraction of a muscle. Electroencephalogr Clin Neurophysiol 1974;36:585–95.

Peter JB. Histochemical, biochemical, and physiological studies of skeletal muscle and its adaptation to exercise. In: Podolsky RJ, ed. Contractility of muscle cells and related processes. Englewood Cliffs, N.J.: Prentice-Hall, 1971:151–73.

Phillips, CG, Porter R. Corticospinal neurones: their role in movement. London: Academic Press, 1977.

Reed AF. The nuclear masses in the cervical spinal cord of Macaca mulatta. J Comp Neurol 1940;72:187–206.

Romanes GJ. The motor cell columns of the lumbosacral spinal cord of the cat. J Comp Neurol 1951;94:313–63.

Romanes GJ. The motor pools of the spinal cord. In: Eccles JC, Schade JP, eds. Organization of the spinal cord. Amsterdam: Elsevier, North-Holland, 1964:93–119.

Rosenfalck P. Intra- and extracellular potential fields of active nerve and muscle fibers. Acta Physiol Scand 1969;75(suppl 321):1–168.

Sharrard WJW. The distribution of the permanent paralysis in the lower limb in poliomyelitis. J Bone Joint Surg 1955;37:540–58.

Sica REP, McComas AJ. Fast- and slow-twitch units in a human muscle. J Neurol Neurosurg Psychiatry 1971;34:113–20.

Sprague JM. A study of motor cell localization in the spinal cord of the rhesus monkey. Am J Anat 1948;82:1–26.

Stålberg E, Antoni L. Electrophysiological cross section of the motor unit. J Neurol Neurosurg Psychiatry 1980;43:469–74.

Stålberg E, Schwartz MS, Thiele B, Schiller HH. The normal motor unit in man. J Neurol Sci 1976;27:291–301.

Stålberg E, Trontelj JV. Single fiber electromyography. Old Woking: Mirvalle Press, 1979.

Stein RB. Peripheral control of movement. Physiol Rev 1974;54:215–43.

Stephens JA, Garnett R, Buller NP. Reversal of recruitment order of single motor units produced by cutaneous stimulation during voluntary muscle contraction in man. Nature (Lond) 1978;272:362–64.

Stephens JA, Usherwood TP. The mechanical properties of human motor units with special reference to their fatigability and recruitment threshold. Brain Res 1977;125:91–97.

Sterling P, Kuypers HGJM. Anatomical organization of the brachial spinal cord of the cat. II. The motoneuron plexus. Brain Res 1967;4:16–32.

Tanji J, Kato M. Recruitment of motor units in voluntary contractions of a finger muscle in man. Exp Neurol 1973;40:759–70.

Taylor A, Stevens JA. Study of human motor unit contractions by controlled intramuscular microstimulation. Brain Res 1976;117:331–35.

Thage O. The myotomes L_2-S_2 in man. Acta Neurol Scand 1965;(suppl 13):241–43.

Walsh JV, Burke RE, Rymer WZ, Tsairis P. Effect of compensatory hypertrophy studied in individual motor units in medial gastrocnemius muscle of the cat. J Neurophysiol 1978;41:496–508.

Wray SH. Innervation ratios for large and small limb muscles in the baboon. J Comp Neurol 1969;137:227–50.

Yemm R. The orderly recruitment of motor units of the masseter and temporal muscles during voluntary isometric contraction in man. J Physiol (Lond) 1977;265:163–74.

Young JL, Mayer RF. Physiological properties and classification of single motor units activated by intramuscular microstimulation in the first dorsal interosseus muscle in man. In: Desmedt JE, ed. Motor unit types, recruitment and plasticity in health and disease. Basel: Karger, 1981:17–25.

6 QUANTITATIVE ASSESSMENT OF THE OUTPUT OF MUSCLES AND MOTOR UNIT ESTIMATES

Two of the more valuable assessments that can be made in the assessment of neuromuscular diseases are measurements of the numbers of motor units (MUs) present in, and the maximum output of, a muscle or muscle group. Electrophysiological estimates of MU numbers are dealt with later in this chapter; the primary emphasis of the early part of the chapter is on quantification of muscle output.

Muscle output can be measured in a number of ways. The most important of these are shown in Table 6.1 and basically resolve into measuring and quantifying, in some way, the electrical activity or the force generated by muscle contraction.

In the clinic, muscle output is measured by grading the strength of maximum contractions of single muscles or groups of synergistic muscles acting across the same joint or in the same direction. While clinical gradings of muscle strength are approximate at best and depend critically on the ability or will of the patient to make a maximum effort, they are nonetheless invaluable. In the hands of experienced examiners the grades are reproducible. Moreover, clinical tests of strength are applicable

to many more muscles and muscle groups than are the more precise and quantitative methods, which are often not applicable to the very muscles most characteristically involved by some diseases. Clinical testing therefore establishes the general pattern of muscle weakness. Any more precise and quantitative assessments of muscle output should then be thought of as extensions of the more generally applicable but semiquantitative clinical assessments of strength, bulk, and the patient's efforts.

Assessment of voluntary contraction can be improved from the quantitative point of view by measuring the force generated by the muscle. These measurements are most easily carried out for the hand grip, biceps/brachialis, and jaw and ankle dorsiflexor and plantar flexor muscles. The forces generated in all these cases depend on muscle length, the subject's capacity to recruit all or most of the MUs, and the mechanical properties of the MUs themselves. The subject's effort can be bypassed by tetanic stimulation of the motor nerve. Comparison of a maximum voluntary and maximum tetanic stimuli evoked contrac-

TABLE 6.1.   Quantitative Methods for Measuring Output of Muscle(s)

Voluntary contraction
  Clinical grading of strength
  Quantitative measurement of force
  Measurement of electrical activity
    Surface recordings (integral of full wave rectified EMG activity)
    Intramuscular recordings
      Interference pattern—maximum contraction, 30% maximum contraction against
        fixed load
Indirect stimulation
  Single supramaximal stimulus
    Maximum twitch tension, maximum M-potential amplitude
  Tetanic stimulation
    Maximum tetanic tension
Direct stimulation
  Single stimulus
    Maximum twitch tension
  Tetanic stimulation
    Maximum tetanic contraction

tion is sometimes of diagnostic value (see Chapter 5).

Tetanic motor nerve stimulation is, however, an uncomfortable way to measure maximum force outputs of muscles, even when near-nerve or subcutaneous electrodes and sometimes local anesthetic block of the nerve proximal to the stimulus are used to reduce the stimulus currents and pain respectively. Such stimulation is most applicable to distal muscle(s) such as the adductor pollicis (Slomić, Rosenfalck, and Buchthal, 1968) or extensor hallucis brevis (Sica and McComas, 1971a) where the motor nerve and more important, the action of the respective muscles can be controlled and relatively well isolated from other muscles.

The maximum tetanic tension begins to fall off in the third and fourth decades of life (Burke, Tuttle, Thompson, Janney, and Weber, 1953).

The other principal way of quantitatively assessing muscle activity is by examining the associated electrical activity as recorded by surface or intramuscular electrodes in the course of a maximum voluntary contraction. The integral of the full wave rectified surface-recorded EMG is proportional to the force output of a muscle (see Chapter 7), but although this relationship holds true in normal muscles it may not apply to disease states. More commonly the electrical potentials generated by strong contractions are examined by studying the patterns produced by the interference of the various MU potentials with one another. The interference patterns so recorded by means of standard concentric needle electrode (leading-off surface about 0.07 mm^2) are governed by:

1.   Completeness of the recruitment. At maximum effort, all or most of the available MUs are recruited and discharge at or near their maximum frequencies (see Chapter 5). Subjects commonly experience difficulty maintaining the discharges of the highest threshold MUs, however, despite maximum efforts. Furthermore, as pointed out earlier, some subjects may not make a maximum effort or are incap-

able of such because of some central motor disorder or pain.

2. The number of MUs with muscle fibers (MFs) within the spike-detection zone (see Chapter 7) of the recording electrode. Changes in the distribution patterns of MFs within MUs such that large numbers of MFs sharing the same innervation become grouped together with an accompanying reduction in the overlap between the territories of neighboring MUs could also alter the recruitment patterns of MUPs. For example, any reduction in the degree of overlap between adjacent MU territories could reduce the number of MUs generating MF spikes within the pickup territory of the electrode. This could create the mistaken impression of a loss of MUs because of the reduction in the number of MUP seen in the interference patterns at that particular recording site. Moreover, the recruitment thresholds of MUPs could be altered by the restructuring of the innervation patterns of MUs. For example, where the MFs nearest to the recording electrode belong to normally higher-threshold MUs, subject may experience difficulty recruiting MUPs at that site although lower-threshold but more distantly originating MUPs may be seen in the recording. The preceding speculations receive some support from histochemical studies of muscle taken from the sites of actual recordings which have revealed close correlations between the firing patterns of the MUP, and the histochemical type of the MFs in the vicinity of the recording. Quantitative assessments of the relative recruitment thresholds of the MUPs were not, however, carried out in these studies (Warmolts and Engel, 1973). Interference patterns are additionally governed by the firing frequencies of the MUs that generate the MUPs and the amplitudes of the MUPs.

The latter depend on the numbers of MFs in each MU within the spike detection zone of the electrode, the degree of temporal dispersion between their potentials, and the diameters of these MFs.

In clinical practice, the interference patterns associated with maximum voluntary contractions are subjectively assessed for their fullness (number of spikes per unit time) and amplitudes. Such assessments are of value only when the abnormalities are striking and characteristic, as happens in well-developed neurogenic and primary muscle diseases. Much better and more reproducible is the method developed by Willison for quantifying the interference pattern both in terms of electrical activity produced and work required of the test subject (see Chapter 7).

Two other useful indices of the output of a muscle are the maximum twitch tension (Slomić, Rosenfalck, and Buchthal, 1968; Sica and McComas, 1971a) and, more commonly used in clinical practice, the maximum compound action potential as recorded by surface electrodes and generated by a muscle (M) or muscle group in response to a supramaximal stimulus delivered to the motor nerve (the maximum M-potential). Measurement of the maximum twitch tension is applicable mainly to the distal limb muscles while the maximum M-potential can be usefully and reproducibly recorded from a wide variety of muscles, including the facial, jaw, and proximal limb muscles.

THE COMPOUND M-POTENTIAL

The amplitude (or area) of the M-potential depends on three main variables, namely:

1. Position(s) and orientation of the electrodes in respect to the muscle

2. Numbers and diameters of MFs generating action potentials

3. Distances between these potential sources and the electrodes

The positions and orientations of the stigmatic and reference electrodes with respect to the MFs are critical. The initial postsynaptic currents in the innervation zone are inward across the postsynaptic membrane and extracellular electrodes in the immediate vicinity register initial negative deflections. Electrodes positioned outside this region record positive deflections because such regions act as current sources until such time as the conducted impulses reach the electrode. At that time the potential becomes negative, to return positive once the impulses have passed the recording site (the classical triphasic action potential) (see Figure 5.9).

For the measurement of maximum motor conduction velocities where recordings are made from a muscle (or muscle group), the latencies are measured between onset of the stimulus at various sites of stimulation proximal to the innervation zone and the onset of maximum M-potential. To this end, the stigmatic electrode should be positioned as close to the innervation zone as possible. This has the advantage also that all those MUs whose end-plate zones are similarly located are biphasic (negative-positive) and sum without phase cancellations between their negative phases (Figure 6.1). When the stigmatic electrode is not positioned over the end-plate zones of some of the MUs, however, phase cancellations between those MUPs may occur. This is because while the initial phases of those MUPs whose end-plate zones are in the immediate vicinity of the recording electrode are negative, other MUPs with more remotely placed end-plate zones may have initial positive phases. Such phase cancellations between MUPs reduce the amplitude of the M-potential, and the result is that the amplitude is not

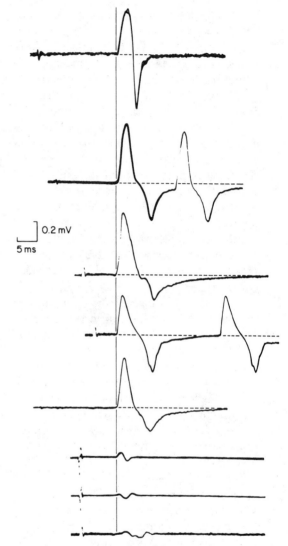

FIGURE 6.1.   Series of single thenar MUPs elicited at various distances from the motor point between the wrist and the proximal upper arm. All the motor unit action potentials were the first recruited in an all-or-nothing manner above motor threshold. F-responses were elicited in two of the MUPs. There is a 17-fold range in amplitudes of the above potentials (0.060 to 1.020 mV peak-to-peak). Note the biphasic (initial negative) character of the potentials here as recorded with the stigmatic electrode positioned over the end-plate zone.

proportional to the number of contributing MUPs.

Another good reason for positioning the stigmatic electrode over the end-plate zone is that the largest negative potential amplitudes are recorded here. The probable explanation for this rests with the initially high inward current densities in this region that are associated with onset of the postsynaptic action potential and subsequent enlargement of the zone of depolarization prior to separation of this wave of depolarization as the action potential conducts toward opposite ends of the MF.

For the stigmatic electrode to be as equidistant from as many of the MUPs in the muscle as possible, surface electrodes are preferable. McComas advocates the use of broad silver strip electrodes to cover as much of the end-plate zone as possible. This can be reasonably achieved for distal muscles or muscle groups such as the extensor digitorum brevis muscle (EDB) and thenar (T) or hypothenar (HT) groups (McComas, 1977) (Figure 6.2). Such surface electrodes cannot overcome the problem that more deeply placed MUs, even when of equivalent size, will register smaller-amplitude MUPs at the surface because of their greater distance from the electrodes.

The position of the reference electrode is critical also. In most subjects it is all but impossible to find a position in the hand or foot where the electrode will not see in volume, action potentials in the EDB, HT, or T muscles. Since the amplifier records the difference in potentials between those registered at the stigmatic and reference electrodes, the potential seen at the reference electrode can make an important contribution to the shape and size of the M-potential. For example, in recordings taken from the hand or foot where, in the case of belly tendon recording arrangements the reference electrode is positioned within 50 mm or so of the innervation zone, the reference electrode sees in volume the action potentials of the muscle as they conduct

at 2 to 4 m/s toward both ends of the muscle. The size of the potential seen by the reference electrode can be substantially reduced by moving the reference electrode further away as advocated by McComas and others (1974) (see Figure 6.2). Even in these relatively remote positions, for example, the fifth digit in the case of thenar recordings, the reference electrode still sees the thenar and lumbrical (first and second) potentials in volume.

Indeed, it is often difficult to find a position in the body where the potential as recorded at the reference electrode remains at zero potential, even when the reference electrode is positioned a considerable distance away from the active muscle(s). The effect of volume conduction on the potential seen at the reference electrode is of course, most apparent in higher gain recordings.

As alluded to above, other muscles than the group beneath the electrode, may also contribute to the M-potential. For example, the median nerve supplies the first and second lumbrical muscles whose potentials will be seen by both the stigmatic and reference electrodes, even when these are so placed as to record best from the T group (Figure 6.3). Such MUPs and their compound M-potential register as positive-negative or positive potentials at the thenar recording sites. Similarly, in the HT group recordings, other ulnar-innervated hand muscles, including the interossei, lumbricals, and adductor pollicis contribute to the HT M-potential; although the more distant the particular muscle, the lower the amplitudes of its potentials as recorded at the HT site (Figure 6.4).

In the human, the recordings are carried out in a volume conductor, and the muscle(s) from which the recordings are made cannot be isolated electrically from other muscle receiving innervation from the same motor nerve. Therefore potentials generated by these other muscles will be seen to some extent at both the stigmatic and reference electrodes,

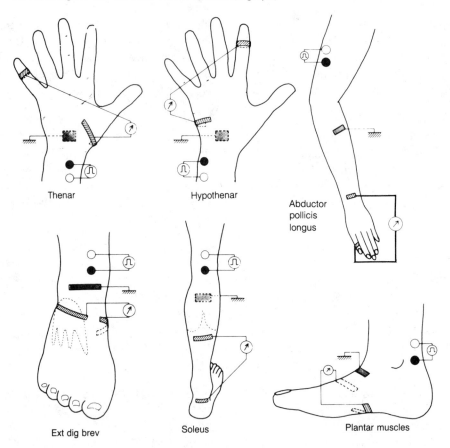

FIGURE 6.2.   Positions of surface electrodes, here thin silver strips, for recording the maximum M-potentials and component motor unit action potentials from the thenar, hypothenar, plantar, abductor pollicis longus, soleus, and extensor digitorum brevis muscles. The cathodal stimulating electrode distal in each case and the earth electrode is positioned between the stimulating and recording electrodes.
From McComas (1977, figure 6.2).

although of course the dominant contributors remain those muscles nearest to the electrodes.

The amplitude and area of the M-potential is also governed by the number of active MFs and their diameters that are nearest to the electrode(s). Theoretically, if one motoneuron innervated all the MFs in a muscle, its MU would generate the same M-potential as the normal number of MUs (about 100; see later discussion) for each intrinsic hand muscle. The M-potential is a product then of the number of MFs generating action potentials, not the number of MUs per se. Also, the larger the diameters of the MFs, the larger the recorded potentials for equivalent distances between the MFs and the recording electrodes.

Reductions in the number of active MFs could occur through loss of groups of MFs, as when transmission blocks in the parent motor

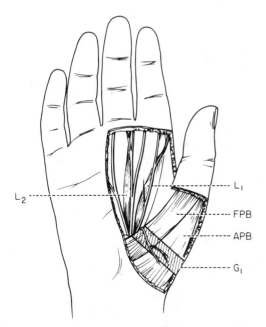

FIGURE 6.3. Median innervation of the hand to show the muscles most commonly supplied by the median nerve. These include the abductor pollicis brevis, all or part of the flexor pollicis brevis, the opponens pollicis (not seen), and the first and usually second lumbrical muscles. Note that an electrode positioned over the thenar innervation zone is remote from the median innervated lumbrical muscles. These lumbrically originating potentials are usually seen as positive by a stigmatic electrode positioned over the thenar muscles, becoming negative once this electrode is repositioned over the first and second lumbricals.

axon or the axon degenerates. The contributions of some MFs may also be lost through neuromuscular blocks, conduction failures in the sacrolemmal membrane itself as in periodic paralysis, or degeneration and loss of individual MFs as in many myopathies, leading to reductions in the amplitude of the M-response.

Reductions in the M-potential could also occur through phase cancellations among contributing MUPs where the relative latencies of the MUPs are sufficiently different that op-

posite phases in the MUPs overlap and cancel out to some degree when they sum in the M-potential. Similarly, less than optimal positioning of the stigmatic electrode, for reasons stated earlier, could result in unwanted phase cancellations among MUPs.

The intensity of the stimulus delivered to the motor nerve is also important. The stimulus must excite all the motor axons to evoke the maximum M-potential, but not be so large as to excite other nearby motor nerves and evoke M-potentials in other muscles whose potentials would also be seen by the recording electrodes.

The maximum M-potential could also be altered by movement of the underlying muscle with respect to the recording electrodes. The limb must therefore be carefully positioned and movement restricted if reproducible records are to be obtained for comparison to other subjects, and comparison of successive M-potentials evoked by a train of stimuli as in neuromuscular transmission testing (see Chapter 10).

The maximum M-potential evoked by supramaximal stimuli to the motor nerve, can also be used to quantitate muscle activity in proximal muscles as well, although the technical problems here are more troublesome. For example, unless the stimulus can be restricted to the motor innervation of a single muscle such as the axillary nerve for deltoid, the musculocutaneous nerve for biceps brachii, accessory nerve for trapezius, or long thoracic nerve for serratus anterior, the unavoidable spread of stimulus to the motor innervation of other muscles as occurs invariably with brachial plexus stimulation evokes electrical potentials in other muscles that are seen in volume by the recording electrodes. Furthermore, for the proximal muscles in the lower limb, such as iliac, psoas, and gluteus medius or maximus, the motor nerves are not accessible for stimulation.

In addition, proximal muscles are strong,

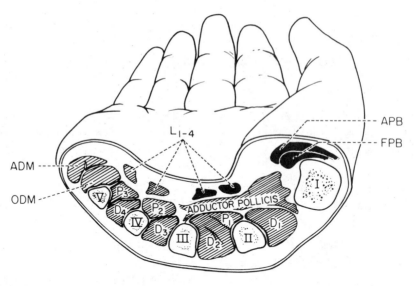

FIGURE 6.4.   Cross section of the hand through the midpalm to show the spatial extent of ulnar innervated muscles in the hand. Note that a surface electrode placed over the hypothenar group while spanning the abductor opponens and flexor digiti minimi cannot obviously cover the progressively more remote ulnar innervated muscles, of which the first dorsal interosseus, adductor pollici, and usually part of the flexor pollicis are the most laterally displaced.
P = palmar interossei (1–3).
D = dorsal interossei (1–4).
Ulnar innervated muscles are shown in hatched and median innervated muscles as solid black.

which makes it difficult to avoid movement artifacts associated with not only the actions of the muscle being recorded from, but with other muscles excited by, for example, stimulation of the brachial plexus.

ESTIMATIONS OF THE NUMBERS OF MUs IN MUSCLE(S)

One of the most desirable indices investigators would like to measure in peripheral nerve and to some extent muscle diseases is the number of MUs present. For example, estimates of the number of MUs could provide indications of the quantitative extent of mo-

toneuron or motor axon losses in serial studies, and the rates at which they are being lost, and would help to distinguish between wasting and weakness of fundamentally neurogenic as opposed to myogenic origin. Despite the clear desirability of determining the number of MUs in muscles, presently available techniques provide no more than rough indications. For example, the number of spikes in the maximum interference pattern provides only a very indirect indication because the recruitment pattern depends not only on the number of MUs recruited but on the firing frequencies of those MUs. Nonetheless, as pointed out in Chapters 7 and 8, automatic quantitative assessment of the interference pattern does provide a reliable way to distinguish between normal myopathic and neurogenic muscles.

The amplitude of the maximum M-potential indicated earlier is probably a better indication of the total membrane currents generated within a muscle than the number of MUs present and provides no direct indication of the contributions of individual MUPs to the whole M-potential. Because of collateral sprouting and reinnervation and possibly hypertrophy of MFs, the total membrane currents in muscle that have been denervated and that may have lost a substantial proportion of their normal complement of motoneurons may remain at normal or near normal levels. The M-potential amplitude in these cases therefore may not provide any indication of the underlying losses of motoneurons or motor axons except, for example, in the very early stages of a nerve crush before compensation within the muscle has taken place.

One approach to the problem of estimating the numbers of MUs in a muscle begins with the realization that the maximum M-potential is, after all, the sum of all the MUPs generated by those motor axons excited by the electrical stimulus. This being so, if a reliable measure could be obtained somehow of the mean amplitude of the component MUPs that together sum to produce the maximum M-potential, an estimate of the number of MUs (axons) present in the muscle could be made by simple division:

$$\text{Motor unit estimate} = \frac{\text{Maximum M-potential amplitude}}{\text{Mean MUP amplitude}}.$$

The next question, how to measure the mean MUP amplitude, could be dealt with by obtaining an average of the first several MUPs whose motor axons were excited above motor threshold (McComas, Fawcett, Campbell, Sica, 1971). Then, by simple division again:

$$\text{Mean MUP amplitude} = \frac{\substack{\text{Amplitude of the sum of} \\ \text{the first several MUPs} \\ \text{whose axons were} \\ \text{excited above threshold}}}{\substack{\text{Number of motor} \\ \text{axons so excited}}}.$$

In practice, the simplest way to examine the first several MU potentials with the lowest threshold to electrical stimulation is to stimulate at 1 Hz or a little less and to steadily increase the stimulus intensity. Once motor threshold is reached, the characteristic all-or-nothing potential corresponding to the activation of one MU can be readily detected (Figure 6.5). Further increases in the stimulus intensity excite other motor axons in the order of their thresholds, and the amplitude of the M-potential correspondingly increases with the addition of successively recruited MUPs. Once 5 to 10 successive amplitude increments can be reproducibly identified through several repetitions of the stimulus sequence, the mean MUP amplitude may be calculated by dividing the compound M-potential by the number of reproducible amplitude increments, which summing together, account for the compound M-potential. The motor unit estimate (MUE) is then calculated by dividing the amplitude of the maximum M-potential as elicited in response to a supramaximal stimulus delivered to the motor nerve by the mean amplitude increment of those MUPs whose axons were excited just above threshold.

McComas introduced and originally described this method for EDB, but later extended the method to other muscle groups (McComas, Fawcett, Campbell, and Sica, 1971; Sica, McComas, Upton, and Longmire, 1974; McComas, 1977). The EDB was originally chosen because this muscle is flat, relatively isolated from other muscles innervated by the same nerve, not too thick, and not covered by too much subcutaneous tissue. Also, the innervation zone occupies a relatively sim-

FIGURE 6.5.   Motor unit estimates in a healthy control (top) and diabetic subject (bottom). The maximum compound action potentials of the muscles as recorded with the stigmatic electrode positioned over the thenar innervation zone are shown on the left and are of similar size in both subjects. The quantum increases in the compound muscle potential as the stimulus was increased were substantially larger in the diabetic, indicating an increase in the mean motor unit action potential size and reduction in the number of motor units in the diabetic (about one-fifth the number in the control subject).

In both subjects, the intensity of successively delivered stimuli (I/s) was progressively increased until the first all-or-nothing thenar motor potential was recorded. Further increases in the intensity increased the proportion of "all" responses in this first motor axon to be excited until the threshold of the second motor axon was reached and its motor unit action potential became added to the first, resulting in a further incremental increase in the compound muscle potential.

In the above manner, further successive increases in the stimulus intensity increased the size of the compound muscle potential, each quantum increase in the latter signaling the activation of successively higher threshold motor axons whose individual thresholds in these two studies remained distinct and did not apparently overlap. Beyond the highest quantum increase in the compound M-potential shown, further increases in the stimulus intensity produced indications of alternation (see text).

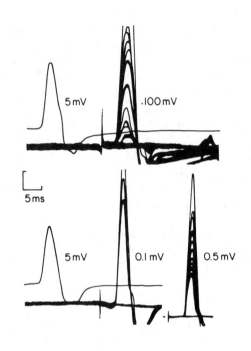

ple transverse band that can be readily identified physiologically and can be spanned by a strip electrode (see Figures 5.9 and 6.2).

In EDB, it can be shown by a combination of intramuscular and surface recordings that in healthy subjects at least, all MUs make a detectable contribution to the surface-recorded potential. There are problems, however, with the choice of this muscle. For example, terminal branches of the deep peroneal nerve go on to supply the dorsal interosseus muscles of the foot, and so it is important to keep the reference electrode away from this region. Also, part of the motor innervation to

EDB can come from a branch of the superficial peroneal nerve. This is said to occur in about 20 percent of subjects, an overestimate in our experience. When present, however, this anomalous innervation can contribute up to 30 percent to the EDB M-response (Lambert, 1969).

Fiber grouping has been seen in this muscle in healthy subjects early in life (Jennekins, Tomlinson, and Walton, 1972). This raises the question about whether EDB is a suitable muscle because the fiber grouping may be a consequence of repeated trauma to its motor nerve(s) at the level of the ankle. Be that as it may, the abnormalities described in certain disease states by the various motor unit estimation techniques, to be described in detail later, have been seen also in other muscles as well. Even if there were partial denervation and reinnervation in EDB, the abnormal estimates in certain diseases were much below the estimates in control subjects of equivalent age (McComas, Sica, and Upton, 1974).

The actual type of surface electrode chosen is probably not so important as it is that the electrodes be positioned properly with respect to the end-plate zone to avoid other muscle potentials as much as possible. There are, however, some important factors in the choice of suitable surface electrodes. For example, abrading and cleaning the skin in preparation for the use of electrode gel is time consuming and once on, the position of this type of electrode canot be easily adjusted to more optimal sites in order to obtain the highest amplitude and an initial negative response for the M-potential. We therefore have in our laboratory elected to use surface clip electrodes (Copeland Davies).

The electrode tips on clip electrodes can be sprung 15 to 30 mm apart and gently pinched onto the skin surface to reduce resistance of the electrode–skin junction and provide a stable low-noise recording. This does not cause bleeding. The main advantage is that the positions of these electrodes can be adjusted easily to optimize the recording site with respect to the innervation zone.

Theoretically more effective are the silver strip electrodes advocated by McComas, which are designed to cover the innervation zone better. Because the potentials generated by the underlying MUs are averaged out over the much larger surface areas of these electrodes (the electrode intersects a much larger number of different isopotential lines) and the amplitudes of MUPs and the maximum M-potentials are 10 to 30 percent below those with clip electrodes.

Although quite commonly used, the least desirable surface electrodes are small-diameter disk electrodes. These behave like point recording electrodes and cannot be oriented in the axis of the innervation zone. They also have all the disadvantages of the stick-on paste electrodes and none of the advantages of the strip electrodes.

Although physiological estimates of the number of MUs in EDB vary widely among subjects and even between tests by different observers on different days, they are in approximate agreement with anatomical estimates of MU numbers in this muscle. Physiological and anatomical estimates of MU numbers are shown in Tables 6.2 and 6.3.

These tables suggest that the physiological estimates of MU numbers with this incremental electrical stimulation technique are in reasonable agreement with anatomical estimates in the same muscles. The physiological estimates are approximate, however, and do depend on a number of factors (Table 6.4), all of which are important determinants of the reliability of the physiologic estimates. They are dealt with below.

Suitability of Muscles

The muscle(s) must not be so thick that the more deeply located MUs make only margin-

TABLE 6.2. Physiological Estimations of Numbers of MUs in Human Muscles

Muscle(s)	Estimate (± 1 SD)
Extensor digitorum brevis[1]	199 ± 60 (n = 41)
Soleus	846 ± 193 (n = 22)
Thenar[2]	340 ± 87 (n = 67)
Hypothenar[3]	380 ± 79 (n = 77)
Abductor pollicis longus[4]	421 ± 99 (n = 40)

[1]McComas, Fawcett, Campbell, and Sica, 1971; McComas (1977).
[2]Sica, McComas, Upton, and Longmire (1974).
[3]McComas, Sica, and Upton (1974).
[4]Defaria and Toyonaga (1978).

TABLE 6.3.   Anatomical Estimates of Numbers of Alpha Motor Axons

Muscle, Muscle Group	Estimated Numbers of Motor Axons	Investigators
Extensor digitorum brevis (human)	230,469	McComas (1977)
First lumbrical (human)	93, 98	Feinstein, Lindegård, Nyman, and Wohlfart (1955)
First dorsal interosseus (human)	119	
Abductor pollicis brevis (baboon)	43	Wray (1969)
Thenar muscle group (recurrent thenar motor branch)	203	Lee, Ashby, White, and Aguayo (1975)

The estimate for EDB is based on counts of the number of myelinated nerve fibers that exceeded 7 to 8 in the anterior tibial nerve, and the assumption that at least 100 of these nerve fibers pass on to the dorsal joints and interosseus muscles in the foot and 50 percent of the remainder are alpha motor axons.

ally detectable or no contributions to the surface-recorded potential. This problem would be magnified in any diseases where the sizes of the action currents associated with the discharge of their MUs were reduced through loss or atrophy of the MFs.

TABLE 6.4.   Important Factors Governing the Reliability of MU Estimates

Muscle(s) chosen are suitable for the study
Thresholds of the lowest-threshold motor axon do not overlap to any appreciable degree (important in the incremental stimulation technique)
MUPs are all uniform in size or failing this, the sample of MUPs selected are representative in their sizes and relative numbers of all the MUs in the muscle
Above assumptions hold true in disease(s) under study
No appreciable degree of conduction block between site of stimulation and the muscle
No appreciable degree of axonal branching proximal to the site of stimulation
Fluctuations in shapes and amplitudes of MUPs are not confused with the recruitment or derecruitment of motor axons by electrical stimulus
All MUs can make a detectible all-or-nothing contribution to the surface potential

Alternation among Motor Axons

For a motor nerve fiber, threshold can be defined as the stimulus intensity at which the motor axon generates an all-or-nothing action potential in response to the stimulus. This stimulus intensity is not a single level, but a range over which the probability of the all response increases from 0 to 100 percent (Figures 6.6 and 6.7).

The thresholds of individual motor nerve fibers at or just above motor threshold often appear to overlap to some extent, such that at any particular stimulus intensity the amplitude of the M-potential fluctuates in incremental or quantal steps (Brown and Milner-Brown, 1976a). This comes about because where the thresholds of two or more motor axons overlap, the number of these motor axons that develop an all response fluctuate from stimulus to stimulus, and depending on their number and the amplitudes of their MUPs, the M-potential amplitude will fluctuate (Figure 6.8).

In healthy human motor nerves, the number of sites where percutaneous stimuli are able to excite n (two or more) more axons in order of their respective excitabilities without indications of overlap between their thresh-

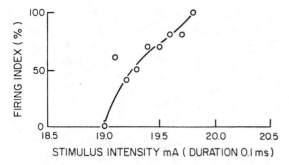

FIGURE 6.6. Changes in percentages of "all" responses in a single motor axon supplying the extensor digitorum brevis muscle. Trains of 100 constant-intensity stimuli were delivered percutaneously to the anterior tibial nerve just proximal to the ankle. The sequence repeated at successively higher stimulus intensities until the point was reached at which "all" responses occurred 100 percent of the time. Threshold here extended over a range of intensities between 19.0 to 19.8 in mA, over which the chance of an "all" response increased from 0 to 100 percent.

olds is illustrated in Table 6.5. At many sites no such overlap was apparent among thresholds of the first one to three motor nerve fibers excited above motor threshold. Beyond this stimulus intensity level, however, the thresholds of subsequently activated motor axons often do overlap and produce fluctuations in the amplitude of the M-potential even where the stimulus intensity is kept constant.

The relative excitabilities of motor nerve fibers may also differ depending on the frequency of stimulation because of variations among their recovery cycles, which can persist as long as 100 ms (Bergmans, 1970).

Differences in the Size (Amplitude and Area) of MUPs

Unfortunately, MUPs are not all similar in their amplitudes; indeed there is a 10- to 100-

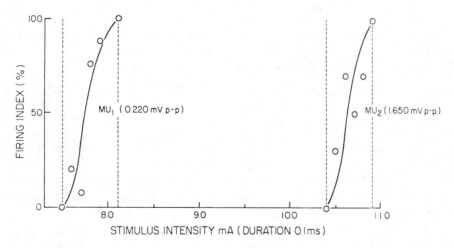

FIGURE 6.7. Range of stimulus intensities delivered to the median nerve over which the chance of an "all" response in the two remaining thenar motor axons (motor unit potentials) increased from 0 to 100 percent. Taken from a patient with amyotrophic lateral sclerosis. Note that the range of stimulus intensities here extended over 0.6 and 0.5 mA and that in this example at least, the thresholds of these two motor axons were widely separate. The peak-to-peak amplitudes in millivolts of these two corresponding motor unit action potentials are shown in brackets. Surface recording electrodes were used.

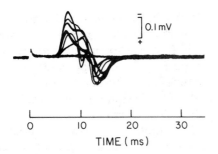

$$]\,0.1\,mV$$

TIME (ms)

FIGURE 6.8.   Fluctuations in amplitude of the compound muscle action potential when the thresholds of two or more axons overlap.

Shown are results of 100 successive constant-intensity stimuli delivered to the median nerve at the wrist. Surface electrodes (stigmatic over the innervation zone) were used to record the thenar motor potentials.

In this study, the amplitude fluctuated, there being no muscle potential (baseline) and several other potentials, each of whose shape and size were reasonably constant and must have corresponded to the activation of one or more of the axons whose motor unit action potentials, either singly or in combination with others of the motor unit action potentials, produced the various M-potential fluctuations. The observation of seven potential steps in reponse to such a long series of constant-intensity stimuli made it highly likely that three motor axons with overlapping thresholds accounted for all the potential fluctuations seen, some of the fluctuations being caused by alternation (see text). On the assumption that the largest of the potentials represents the sum of all three MUPs, the mean MUP is equal to the peak-to-peak amplitude of the largest of the compound muscle potentials divided by 3 (here equal to 0.127 mV) and not 0.054 mV as it would be if all the amplitude fluctuations were assumed to have been generated by the successive addition of progressively higher-threshold MUPs.

fold range in the thenar, hypothenar, and extensor digitorum brevis muscles (Figure 6.9). This being so, it is clearly important to know whether there is bias toward MUPs of any particular amplitude when threshold stimulation or another method is used to select the MUPs from which the mean MUP is calculated.

In the case where weak electrical stimulation with intensities just exceeding motor threshold is used to select the MUPs, the important factors governing selection of MUPs probably include the shape and durations of the stimulus pulse, the relative excitabilities of the various motor axons, and their relative proximities within the nerve trunk with respect to the cathodal electrode. For axons of equivalent excitability, those lying closest to the cathode would be expected to be the preferentially excited because of the stronger cathodal current nearest the overlying electrode.

The shape and duration of the stimulus pulse may be an important factor determining relative excitability among nerve fibers (Swett and Bourassa, 1981). For example, in unmyelinated nerve fibers of the crab, the rank order of excitation has been shown to depend somewhat on the duration of the stimulus. Thus brief stimuli (1 to 5 ms) preferentially activate the larger nerve fibers and longer stimuli (5 to 50 ms), the smaller fibers (Easton, 1952; Wright and Coleman, 1954). The apparently greater excitability of smaller fibers in respect to longer-lasting stimuli is probably explained by the greater degree of accommodation found in larger- compared to smaller-diameter nerve fibers. In this respect, Kugelberg and Sko-

TABLE 6.5.   Percentage of Stimulation Sites at which Successively Activated MUPs Could Be Obtained without Evidence of Overlap Between their Thresholds

	$n = 1$	$n = 2$	$n = 3$	$n = 4$	$n = 5$	$n = 6$
Total numbers of stimulation sites (169)	32	27	26	10	4	1

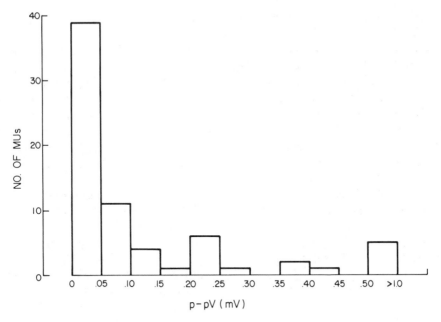

FIGURE 6.9. Range in peak-to-peak voltage (p-pV) in millivolts (mV) of hypothenar MUPs in 10 control subjects.
Note:

1. The preponderance of the smaller amplitude MUPs
2. The occasional presence of much higher-amplitude MUPs

The recordings were all done with surface electrodes and the histogram is based on only those MUPs whose motor axons could be excited without any evidence of alternation at various sites between the axilla and wrist.

glund (1946) noted that when the intensity of long-lasting stimulus pulse was gradually increased, single MUPs were activated in order, beginning with the lowest-amplitude and proceeding to progressively higher-amplitude MUPs. In this study the amplitudes of the MUPs of human motor axons were presumed to correlate closely with the diameter of the parent motor nerve fiber.

The question of relative excitabilities of nerve fibers of differing diameters and conduction velocities has not, however, been satisfactorily resolved so far in man. The question is important because there is a growing body of evidence in man, that the amplitude of MUPs as recorded with surface electrodes from distal muscle of the limbs do correlate positively with MU tension and the conduction velocities of the underlying motor axons (see Chapter 5). From animal experiments, larger-diameter nerve fibers should have lower thresholds (Erlanger and Gasser, 1937). If this principle can be applied to alpha motor axons, the lowest-threshold axons should be those with the largest diameters, smaller-diameter and presumably slower-conducting motor axons generating relatively lower MUP amplitudes possessing relatively higher thresholds to electrical stimulation.

It turns out, however, that this is not what

is seen at least in some human studies. For example, when percutaneous stimulation of motor nerves is carried out in man, it is the longer-latency MUPs that are recruited first, subsequent increases in the stimulus intensity recruiting progressively shorter-latency MU potentials (Hodes, Gribetz, Moskowitz, and Wagman, 1965; Podivinsky, 1965; Bergmans, 1970) in rank order of excitation from longer- to shorter-latency MUPs (Kadrie, Yates, Milner-Brown, and Brown, 1976) (Figure 6.10). This is paralleled by a corresponding ranking order of excitation in respect to MUP amplitude as well as from lower to higher amplitude MUPs as the intensity of the stimulus is increased (Figure 6.11). This phenom-

enon cannot be explained by stimulus advance because little or no subsequent change in the latencies of these single MUPs occurs despite large increases in stimulus intensity (Bergmans, 1970). One explanation put forward is that since in experimental nerve compression the more superficial nerve fibers are the earliest to be damaged by compression (Aguayo, Nair, and Midgley, 1971), these same motor axons may be among those excited first because they are nearest to the stimulating electrode, and because their conduction velocities would be slowed through the compression site, the latencies of their MUPs would be prolonged. This argument is hard to dismiss entirely, but would seem improbable in young subjects or in motor nerves such as the posterior tibial or radial nerves where the same phenomenon is just as readily seen but where the nerves are much less susceptible to compression injuries than are the median or ulnar nerves.

That the lower-amplitude MUPs were generated by smaller and not just more deeply placed MUs is suggested by the relatively longer latencies of the lower-amplitude MUPs compared to higher-amplitude MUPs when studied by weak electrical stimulation of motor nerves (Kadrie, Yates, Milner-Brown, and Brown, 1976; Brown and Milner-Brown, 1976a).

The above ranking order by amplitude and latency has been shown to apply to the first one to four motor axons excited, but whether this rule holds true for higher-threshold motor axons is not known. The important point here, however, is that weak electrode stimuli just exceeding motor threshold do appear preferentially to activate lower-amplitude MUPs, certainly much lower than are sometimes seen in strong isometric contractions or in the F-potentials in response to higher-intensity electrical stimuli.

Complicating the matter of the relative excitabilities of motor axons is the fact that lower-

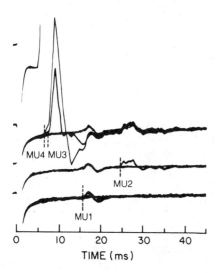

FIGURE 6.10.   Progressive recruitment of shorter-latency motor unit action potentials. Percutaneous stimulation of the anterior tibial nerve just proximal to the ankle and surface recordings of successively recruited MUPs MU1 to MU4 as the stimulus intensity was progressively increased from below upward.

Note that the first two motor unit action potentials (MU1 and MU2) here have substantially longer latencies than the next two (MU3 and MU4) recruited, and that as the stimulus intensity was increased there is little apparent shortening of the latencies of MU1 or MU2 through stimulus lead (see Chapter 3).

FIGURE 6.11. Peak-to-peak voltages (p-pV) in millivolts of the first, second, and third hypothenar MUPs whose axon thresholds were exceeded in turn by progressive increments in the stimulus intensity delivered to the ulnar nerve at various sites between the proximal upper arm and wrist. The vertical interrupted line denotes a change in scale factor for the p-pV of the motor unit action potentials.

Note the trend, which is significant at a *P* value <0.05 toward higher-amplitude motor unit action potentials as the stimulus intensity was increased.

From Kadrie, Yates, Milner-Brown, and Brown (1976).

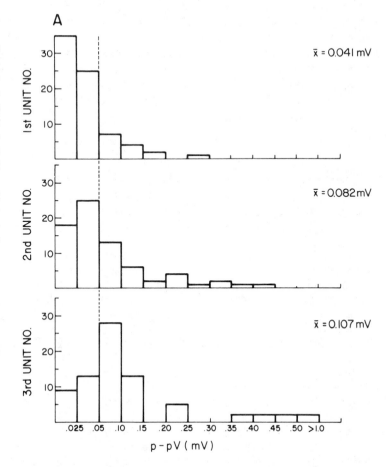

amplitude MUPs probably greatly outnumber the very large-amplitude MUPs. If motor axons were selected, therefore, irrespective of their diameters or the amplitudes of their MUPs, a preponderance of lower-amplitude MUPs would be expected in any small sample of MUPs used to calculate a mean MUP size. In this respect there is other evidence that percutaneous electrical stimuli just exceeding motor threshold when applied to the motor nerve excite some slower- as well as faster-conducting motor axons (Hodes, Gribetz, Moskowitz, and Wagman, 1965; Juul-Jensen and Mayer, 1966; Gilliatt, Hopf, Rudge, and Baraitser, 1976). Similarly, in human sensory nerves, even though some of the faster-conducting nerve fibers are excited by weak stimuli, so also are some of the slower conducting nerve fibers. Conversely, not all the faster-conducting nerve fibers may be excited until much higher-stimulus intensities are reached (Buchthal and Rosenfalck, 1966).

The question then of the relative excitabilities of motor axons of differing conduction velocity and MUP size, especially with respect to percutaneous stimulation, remains unsettled in man. The apparent bias toward the lower-amplitude and longer-latency MUPs of electrical stimuli just exceeding threshold runs contrary to our expectations based on studies of comparative nerve fiber excitabilities in vitro or in experimental animals where the nerve trunk was usually mounted directly on the stimulating electrodes (Figure 6.12).

Whatever the reasons for the bias of weak percutaneous electrical stimulation toward lower-amplitude and longer-latency MUPs in man, the fact remains that much higher-amplitude MUPs do in fact exist (Feasby and Brown, 1974; see Chapter 5), although their numbers relative to the smaller-amplitude MUPs is not known with any certainty in any human muscle, exclusion of these larger-amplitude MUPs from the calculation of mean MUP size means that the latter will be too low and the MUE correspondingly too high.

FIGURE 6.12.   In the case of direct nerve stimulation, while single nerve fibers are in general excited in order of their latencies from shorter to longer as the stimulus intensity is increased, there are occasional exceptions.

The single nerve fiber action potentials were recorded from a multifiber dorsal root filament in the cat in response to stimulation of the sciatic nerve in the thigh. The nerve was mounted directly on the stimulating electrode, here a tripolar arrangement (cathode central). The stimulus intensity increased from below upward, its intensity in volts is shown on the right.

Note that while the overall trend was for the nerve fibers to be excited in order of their latencies beginning with fiber 1 (F1) and ending with the fifth (F5) and sixth (F6) whose latencies were much longer, there were apparent minor exceptions among fibers. Thus the longer-latency F3 and F5 fibers were excited before the shorter-latency F4 and F6 fibers. Such apparent minor exceptions to the order of excitability probably reflect the relative positions of these fibers with respect to the stimulating electrodes as well as their specific excitabilities. There were, however, no exceptions to the threshold latency rule among fibers of widely dissimilar latencies, for example, F1 and F3.

Note also the progressive reduction in latency of F4 and F2 as the intensity was increased, probably because of stimulus lead or excitation of the nerve fiber progressively ahead of the position of the cathode as the intensity was increased and the resultant cathodal currents extended further down the nerve trunk. With such an electrode arrangement, the proximal anode may block impulses originating at the cathode when the stimulus intensity is too high (anodal block).

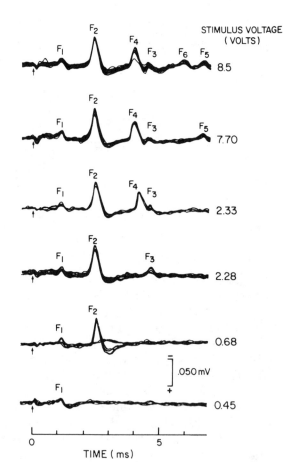

Validity of the Assumptions in Disease States

The factors that must hold for valid MUEs in healthy subjects must also hold true in diseases of nerve and muscle. In addition, special problems are presented by disease states. For example, the amplitudes of some MUPs as recorded on the surface may be so small in some diseases as to be undetectable with surface electrodes. Moreover, fluctuations in the shapes of MUPs may occur because of axonal or neuromuscular blocking, or because of greatly increased latency fluctuations at neuromuscular junctions within the MU. These fluctuations make it difficult to know whether alterations in the shape of the M-potentials represent fluctuations in the shapes of individual MUPs or changes in the number of component MUPs.

Conduction Block Distal to the Point of Stimulation

Transmission block in some of the motor axons between the site of stimulation and the muscle reduces the amplitude of the M-potential and results in a corresponding reduction in the MUE. This would not reflect any actual loss of motor axons (MUs) (Figure 6.13).

Axon Branching Proximal to the Point of Stimulation

In healthy subjects, there is probably very little branching of motor axons more than 50 to 150 mm proximal to the end-plate zone. For example, in EDB the mean MUP amplitude when the L5 root was stimulated directly was the same as when the peroneal nerve was stimulated at the fibular head (Figure 6.14). In some peripheral neuropathies, however, branching of motor axons at more proximal levels could develop, as for example, at the

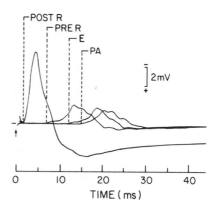

FIGURE 6.13.   Conduction block across carpal tunnel segment in patient with Guillain-Barrè polyneuropathy. Shown are maximum thenar compound action potentials elicited by supramaximal stimulation just distal (PostR) and proximal (PreR) to the retinaculum as well as in response to stimulation at the elbow (E) and proximal arm (PA). Note the substantial reduction in the size of the thenar M-potential as elicited proximal to the retinaculum compared to stimulation just dital to the carpal tunnel. The difference probably indicates conduction block in many of the median motor axons in the segment beneath the retinaculum.

site of a previous nerve crush or section. Stimulation of the motor nerve distal to the sites of branching could readily excite individual axon branches and not the whole MUP (see discussion of axon reflexes in Chapter 8). Axon reflexes, the electrophysiological sign of such branching, may not be recognized when any one of the following conditions prevails:

1. The longer-latency component is not seen or if seen, is thought to be a late linked component of the main MUP
2. The other axon branches have sufficiently higher thresholds such that the reflex nature of the late potential was not established by antidromic collision and block of the late potential at high stimulus intensities

FIGURE 6.14.   All-or-nothing step increments in the extensor digitorum brevis M-potential elicited by increases in the intensity of successive electrical stimuli delivered to the L5 ventral root (VR) and peroneal nerve at the fibular head (FH). Also shown are the corresponding maximum M-potentials evoked by supramaximal stimulation at the above two sites. The negative peak (−p) amplitudes or the mean MUPs elicited at the levels of the VR and FH were 0.029 and 0.028 mV respectively.

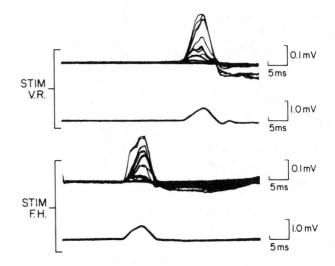

3. Impulse block occurs at the branch point because of an impedance mismatch at this site, in which case no late component would appear

It is interesting to note even in healthy subjects, that the mean amplitude of hypothenar MUPs excited by stimulation of the ulnar nerve proximal to the elbow was significantly larger than that of MUPs excited by stimulation distal to the elbow (Kadrie, Yates, Milner-Brown, and Brown, 1976). This suggests that even in health, some branching of motor axons may exist well proximal to the motor point, perhaps as a result of subclinical compression injuries of the ulnar nerve within the cubital tunnel or behind the medial epicondyle. Such injuries may lead to degeneration of some of the motor axons distal to the site of injury. The proximal ends of some of these motor axons could sprout to form two or more branches, and subsequently regenerate to reinnervate part of the denervated muscle. The thresholds of such branches may well differ sufficiently for graded electrical stimuli to excite the lowest-threshold branch only. The resulting muscle potential is gen-

erated by only that part of the complement of muscle fibers belonging to the MU that receive their innervation from the one branch stimulated.

Antidromic conduction of the impulse begun in the lowest-threshold branch, however, may on reaching the proximal point of branching, be orthodromically conducted throughout other axon branches belonging to the same MU, with the result that muscle fibers in the MU supplied by these other branches are activated as well. The latency of the latter potentials will depend on the conduction velocities of the respective axon branches and how proximally the site of branching is situated. These late components constitute the motor axon reflex. Proof that these late components do indeed constitute an axon reflex may be found in their disappearance when the stimulus intensity is increased to the point at which the thresholds of all the axon branches in the MU are exceeded. In the latter case, collisions between the reflexly conducted impulses in some branch(s) with antidromic impulses in the same branches, abolish the late axon reflex component(s) to the muscle potential.

Fluctuations in Shape and Size of MUPs

In healthy subjects, motor nerve stimulation at frequencies of 3 Hz or more produces an increase in the amplitude and shortening in the duration of MUPs (Kadrie and Brown, 1978a) possibly through enhanced synchronization between the action potentials of contributing single MFs and increases in the conduction velocities of these action potentials (Stålberg, 1976). In peripheral neuropathies synchronization could be enhanced through fiber grouping and consequent enhanced interactions between action currents of the MFs, akin to that described between nerve fibers (Katz and Schmitt, 1940). Conversely, such groupings could reduce the amplitude of MUPs through current shunting between adjacent MFs. Such theoretical possibilities have never been established.

At higher-stimulus frequencies, conduction block at branch points in intramuscular branches of the motor axons could result in decrements of the amplitudes of single MUPs (Stålberg and Trontelj, 1970; Desmedt, 1973; Ekstedt and Stålberg, 1973). In a like manner, transmission block at some of the neuromuscular junctions in the MU could reduce the number of MFs able to contribute their potentials to the overall MUP, in so doing reducing the amplitudes of MUPs especially at 3 to 5 Hz in myasthenia gravis (Kadrie and Brown, 1978b). Decrements in the amplitude of MUs are also characteristically seen in amyotrophic lateral sclerosis, but often at frequencies below 3 Hz (0.2 to 1 Hz) (Carleton and Brown, 1979) (Figure 6.15).

These fluctuations in the shapes and amplitudes of MUPs produced through repetitive stimulation of their motor axons result in increments or decrements in the M-potential that do not reflect changes in the number of MUPs, but rather changes in sizes of individual MUPs and hence their contribution to the M-poten-

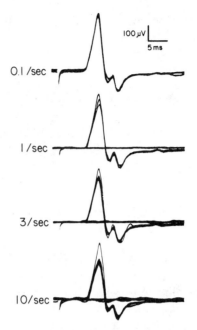

FIGURE 6.15. Changes in amplitude of a single thenar motor unit action potential (recorded by surface electrodes) from a patient with amyotrophic lateral sclerosis in response to stimulation at frequencies of 0.1 to 10 per second. Note the decrement in the amplitude even at one per second. Such decrements are never seen in normal human single motor unit action potentials.

tial. This can introduce errors in the estimates (Brown and Jaatoul, 1974; Carleton and Brown, 1979). One solution to this problem is to elicit the incremental responses in the M-potential not by increasing the stimulus intensity gradually over successive stimuli, but by beginning with an intensity that is already supramaximal for the first several motor axons, maintaining this intensity constant until such time as no more fluctuations occur, and then gradually reducing it to identify the successive decremental steps down in amplitude. This technique and the use of lower frequencies of stimulation help to avoid misleading fluctuations in the M-potential caused by neurogenic and synaptic block.

Where regeneration of motor axons has been complete or nearly complete, the MUE could well be in the normal range despite betrayal of the true situation by histochemical stains that reveal evidence of fiber grouping, or needle EMG studies that show clear electrophysiological vindication of reinnervation and fiber grouping.

Quantity of MUs that Contribute to the Surface Record

Theoretically, any shift of the territories of MUs toward more superficial or deep positions within the muscle could conceivably alter the amplitudes of MUPs even were there no change in the innervation ratios of MUs. Shifts toward deeper locations of MUs or the loss of significant numbers of MFs could have the affect of reducing the amplitudes of MUPs to below the levels at which their all-or-nothing potentials could be readily recognized on the surface, especially in the bulkier muscles.

Even in the normal extensor digitorum communis muscle Stålberg (1976) observed some MUs whose positions were so deep within the muscle that their MUPs were undetectable as recorded on the surface of the skin overlying the muscle. In primary muscle diseases, such as the dystrophies where the losses of muscle fibers from individual MUs may be substantial and the diameters of the MFs somewhat reduced, the MUPs may be difficult if not impossible to detect even in thin atrophic or small muscles. Figure 6.16 illustrates one such example from a patient with Duchenne muscular dystrophy. The problem posed by small or deeply positioned MUs in health and especially in muscle diseases has been recognized for a long time (Brown, Milner-Brown, and Drake, 1974), but the quantitative importance of the error to MUEs in

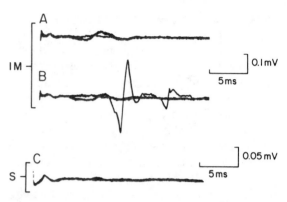

FIGURE 6.16. Intramuscular (IM) and surface (S) electrode recordings of extensor digitorum brevis motor unit action potentials elicited by electrical stimulation of the anterior tibial nerve just proximal to the ankle in a patient with Duchenne muscular dystrophy.

(A) and (B) clearly show the first two successive all-or-nothing motor unit action potentials elicited by increments in the stimulus intensity. In (C), only the first of the above two intramuscularly detected motor unit action potentials produced any detectable change in the surface recording, and even this was very small.

muscular dystrophies has never been properly investigated.

The MUEs probably become more accurate in the later stages of neurogenic disorders because the mean MUP amplitude is based on a much larger proportion of the total number of MUs. Indeed, in severe neurogenic disorders all the MUs that together sum to produce the maximum M-potential can be readily identified by incremental stimulation. Sometimes where the same axons can be stimulated at two or more sites, the conduction velocities in these motor axons can be measured (Figure 6.17). Such counts are very reproducible among testers and between examinations, and sometimes over extended periods between examinations, and sometimes over extended periods between examinations. Occasionally, it is even possible over several months to follow

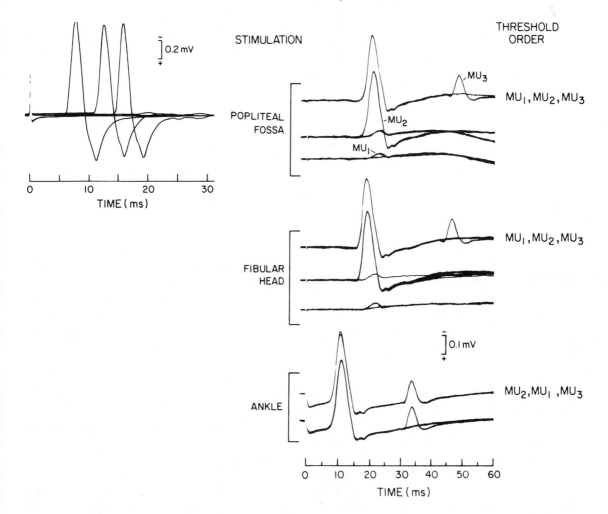

FIGURE 6.17.   (Left) Single remaining thenar motor unit action potential, recorded here with surface electrodes, in a patient with amyotrophic lateral sclerosis. The maximum motor conduction velocities between stimulation sites in the proximal upper arm and elbow and elbow and wrist were 46.0 and 45.6 m/s respectively, and were just below the 2-SD lower limits for maximum motor conduction velocities for these segments in healthy median nerves. The motor terminal latency was correspondingly prolonged to 5.6 ms. Peak-to-peak amplitude of this one remaining unit (1.52 mV) is just over 5 percent of the mean amplitude of the maximum thenar compound potential in controls.

(Right) Patient with Guillain-Barrè polyneuropathy 36 days following onset of paralysis. Shown are the three remaining extensor digitorum brevis motor unit (action) potentials whose axons remained excitable at the ankle, fibular head, and popliteal fossa levels. Shown here are their corresponding action potentials as recorded with a surface electrode. No more potentials could be detected with an intramuscular exploring electrode. The conduction velocities of all three potentials could be measured independently of one another. The velocities between the fibular head and ankle of MU1, MU2, and MU3 were 40.8, 36.3, and 25.3 m/s respectively, and between the popliteal fossa and fibular head 36.0, 40.0, and 32.7 m/s. The order in which these three potentials were excited as the stimulus intensity was increased is shown on the right.

the same MUP because of its distinctive shape, when care is taken to locate the recording electrodes in the same position.

Especially in healthy subjects, the technical, physiological, and statistical problems inherent in the incremental stimulation technique combine to make the MUEs very approximate. Such estimates can vary as much as 10 to 50 percent when repeated by the same examiner with the same technique, and by up to 100 percent between different trained electromyographers.

The inherent errors and limitations in the motor unit estimation technique no doubt account for some of the more obvious disagreements among practitioners regarding disease states, prime examples being myasthenia gravis and the muscular dystrophies. In these latter diseases McComas and co-workers reported abnormally low MUEs using the original incremental stimulation technique in EDB (McComas, Sica, and Currie, 1971; McComas, Campbell, and Sica, 1971; Sica and McComas, 1971; McComas, Sica, and Campbell, 1971; McComas, Sica, and Campbell, 1971; McComas, Sica and Brown, 1971; McComas, Brandstater, Upton, Delbeke, de Faria, and Toyonaga, 1977) and similar losses of MUs in other muscle, including the intrinsic muscles of the hand and soleus (McComas, Sica, and Upton, 1974). Ballantyne and Hansen (1974a, 1974b), however, reported normal estimates in myasthenia gravis and Duchenne, limb girdle, facioscapulohumeral, and myotonic muscular dystrophies.

OTHER METHODS FOR SELECTING MUPs FOR THE CALCULATION OF MEAN MU AMPLITUDE

The sample of MUPs on which the mean MUP amplitude is based is very small in relationship to the total number of MUs present in healthy subjects (5 percent or less) and there is normally a wide range in the amplitudes of MUPs in muscles. Thus it is vital to look at other possible ways of selecting MUs and MUPs on which to base the calculation of mean MUP amplitude besides the incremental stimulation technique already described (Table 6.6).

For example, spike-triggered averaging techniques may be used to isolate and measure the amplitudes of MUPs recruited throughout the course of weak, moderate and strong contractions. This helps to broaden the amplitude range of MUPs in the sample used to calculate the mean MUP amplitude (Figure 6.10). The true relative numbers of low-, mid-, and higher-threshold MUs are not known, however, and therefore how many MUPs of various sizes should be included in the sample is unknown.

There are other problems with using the isometric contraction method as a source of MUPs for the calculation of mean MUP size. For example, the maximum muscle compound action potential as elicited by electrical stimulation of the motor nerve is not equal to, but rather is somewhat less than, the sum of the peak-to-peak amplitudes of all the component MUPs. This results from the fact that because the conduction velocities and possibly residual latencies as well of motor axons are not the same, the latencies to the onset of their respective MUPs from onset of the stimulus will necessarily differ. Moreover, because the MUs themselves are not all positioned similarly within the muscle with respect to the recording electrodes, the times from onset of MUPs to their respective negative and positive peaks will differ. The overall result is that the peaks of the MUPs contribut-

TABLE 6.6.   Methods for Selecting MUs for Calculation of Mean MU Amplitude

Isolation of single MUPs recruited at various force levels in an isometric contraction
Isolation of single MUPs from the F-discharge
Multiple point stimulation to avoid alternation

ing to the maximum compound muscle action potential do not precisely correspond and the amplitude of the compound muscle potential is correspondingly somewhat less than if the peak amplitudes of the MUPs coincided in time. Unfortunately, there is no way properly to assign relative latencies to MUPs collected using the isometric contraction technique in such a way that their sum will correspond exactly to what it would be if their respective motor axons were stimulated at the same site as that used to elicit the maximum muscle compound action potential.

Another way of overcoming the problem posed by overlapping of motor axon thresholds is to stimulate the motor nerve at several sites along its length, accepting only those MUPs at each site whose axons have clear and distinct thresholds (Brown and Milner-Brown, 1976a; Milner-Brown and Brown 1976; Kadrie, Yates, Milner-Brown, and Brown, 1976). Often this limits the number of MUPs at any one site to three or fewer, but by combining MUPs at several sites it is possible to increase the sample size to 5 to 30 and avoid alternation in the bargain. That this method provides a representative sample of the MU population depends on whether such threshold stimulation biases the sample toward MUPs of any particular amplitude (see earlier discussion). Moreover, like the isometric contraction technique, it is impossible to reproduce the same latency differences among the MUPs as are incorporated in the maximum M-response.

The MUP sample may also be drawn from the F-response (Figure 6.18). This method is tricky and impractical as a way of securing MUPs, however, because it requires great care to select only those potentials in the F-response that meet the criteria for single MUPs, excluding others generated by combinations of MUPs (Feasby and Brown, 1974; Yates and Brown, 1979).

Ballantyne and Hansen (1974a, 1974b) modified the original technique by introduc-

ing the computer as a way to measure the areas of successively recruited MUPs. The MUE was then calculated by:

$$MUE = \frac{\text{maximum M-potential area}}{\text{mean MUP area}}.$$

The precision of the computer-assisted method is, however, more apparent than real. Our own experience with the use of a computer for the same purpose taught us that because an electronic average must be obtained for each successive MU increment, it is even harder to avoid the errors produced by alternation.

Modifications to the original method proposed by Panayiotopoulos, Scarpalezos, Papapetropoulos, and Michas (1973) appear to offer no advantages and have several important theoretical and practical limitations (Brown and Milner-Brown, 1976b).

EXPERIMENTAL COMPARISON OF PHYSIOLOGICAL AND ANATOMICAL ESTIMATES OF MU NUMBERS

There have been some attempts to correlate the physiological estimates of MU numbers based on the incremental stimulation technique and anatomical estimates of the numbers of motor axons innervating the same muscle (or muscle group). For example, in the rat soleus muscle, excellent correspondence was demonstrated between the physiological estimates based on incremental stimulation where the recordings were taken directly from the surface of the muscle and the anatomical estimates of the numbers of motor axons present (Eisen, Karpati, Carpenter, and Danon, 1974). Similar agreement between anatomical and physiological estimates have been shown in both normal and dystrophic mice for the soleus muscle (Law and Caccia, 1975).

Similarly, in the monkey extensor digitorum brevis muscle, basic agreement was shown between anatomical and physiological esti-

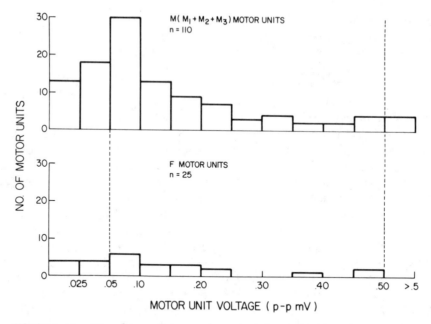

FIGURE 6.18.   Histograms of the peak-to-peak (p-p) amplitudes of individual hypothenar motor unit action potentials as recorded by surface electrodes.

(Top) The p-p amplitudes of the first (M1), second (M2), or third (M3) MUPs elicited by incremental increases in the stimulus intensity delivered to the motor nerve.

(Bottom) The p-p amplitudes of single motor unit action potentials in the F-response.

Note the wide range in the amplitudes of motor unit action potentials and the change in scale of the motor unit voltages indicated by vertical interrupted lines.

mates in normal muscles. The estimates failed to agree in one animal where the ventral root was damaged in the course of dorsal root section and ganglionectomy procedure (Peyronnard and Lamarre, 1977).

It is well to remember that substantial errors are also possible in anatomical estimates. For example, ganglionectomy and dorsal root section may damage some of the ventral root nerve fibers as was noted above. Moreover, in experiments where deafferentation procedures were not done, the proportions of sensory fibers in the motor nerve are only estimates, and could range from 40 to 60 percent

(Boyd and Davey, 1968). Axon branching proximal to the level at which the counts of motor axons were obtained cannot be excluded. Also, motor axons destined for other muscles innervated beyond the muscle could easily be included in the counts. For example, the motor nerve to the extensor digitorum brevis also innervates the dorsal interosseus muscles in the foot. In addition, uncertainties exist about just where the break occurs between large and smaller myelinated nerve fibers in the fiber size histogram (Lee, Ashby, White, and Aguayo, 1975). Anatomical estimates are themselves therefore very approximate and the apparent close correspondence between them and physiological estimation cannot be taken as conclusive evidence for the accuracy of the electrophysiological estimates.

In the human extensor digitorum brevis muscle, anatomical estimates of the numbers of motor axons were a little higher than physiological estimates in healthy subjects. Here, as pointed out above, the lateral terminal branch to the EDB does include some motor axons to the interosseus muscles of the foot. In other investigations good correlations were shown between physiological estimates of the number of EDB MUs and fiber densities (diameters > 4.6 μ) in the lateral fascicle of the deep peroneal nerve in various peripheral neuropathies. Actual counts of the numbers of larger myelinated nerve fibers were not obtained, however, and there was no assurance as to whether the connected nerve fibers were motor or sensory (Bolton, Gilbert, Girvin, and Hahn, 1979).

In the author's view, despite apparent agreements in both experimental animals and man between anatomical and physiological estimates, more comparative investigations are needed to sort out the discrepancies and to compare the MU counts technique with other quantitative electromyographic techniques for assessing muscle.

sequent modifications have a useful place in the evaluation of motoneuronal or axonal disorders. In these disorders, except in the earliest stages of reinnervation following nerve section or crush, all MUs make detectable contributions to the surface M-potential at least in distal limb muscles. This is not apparently always true in the primary disorders of muscle.

The methods are also sensitive ways to demonstrate MU losses at stages when muscle strength and maximum M-response amplitudes may be normal and there is no evidence of abnormal spontaneous activity in the muscle. Indeed, up to 80 to 90 percent of MUs may be lost with no change in the maximum twitch tension or M-potential generated by the muscle (McComas, Sica, Campbell, and Upton, 1971; Brown, 1973).

Practice with the method also provides the experience necessary to study the properties of single motor axons and neuromuscular transmission in single MUs (Desmedt and Borenstein, 1970; Kadrie and Brown, 1978a, 1978b; Carleton and Brown, 1979). These techniques, however, especially in healthy subjects, provide no more than a very approximate indication of the numbers of MUs present, and for technical reasons mentioned earlier, are applicable only to distal limb muscles.

Present Place of Motor Unit
Estimates in Electromyography

The original incremental stimulation technique is still the simplest to carry out in practice, and shares with its various subsequent modifications the fact that the procedure is readily tolerated by patients. These techniques, however, do not replace other quantitative methods in electromyography. In the author's view, the original method and sub-

Comparison to Other
Quantitative EMG Methods

The incremental stimulation technique for estimation of MU numbers has been compared to other quantitative assessments of MUP and the interference patterns as recorded with intramuscular needle electrodes (McComas and Sica, 1978). These measurements were made in distal muscles such as the extensor digitorum brevis and thenar muscles.

In disorders characterized by denervation, it was learned that the incremental stimulation technique was the more sensitive detector of denervation, demonstrating MU losses where the quantitative assessment of the intramuscularly recorded interference pattern was less sensitive. There were, however, examples where the MUEs were normal and the intramuscular EMG was abnormal. The latter happens where, despite degeneration in a proportion of the motor axons at some previous time, most or all of the motor axons subsequently are able to regenerate. The MUEs are most likely normal even though the needle electrode-recorded MUPs indicate changes in the innervation patterns of MFs.

The incremental stimulation technique is not yet applicable to the more proximal muscles in the limbs or trunk, although these same muscles are clearly accessible for intramuscular needle recordings. The two methods therefore provide complementary but different information about MU numbers and the changes in MU architecture.

SUMMARY

All the methods for estimating MU numbers have inherent theoretical and practical limitations. At this time, however, the easiest method remains the original one described by McComas in 1971. In our laboratory, the experience gained working with single motor axons and the undoubted pragmatic value of these tests as a sensitive detector of denervation has justified continued application of the technique. The methods are best combined with needle electromyography. It is hoped that in the future others will critically evaluate the strengths and weaknesses of the method pioneered by McComas and develop better methods than those presently available for estimating the numbers of MUs.

References

Aguayo A, Nair CPV, Midgley R. Experimental progressive compression neuropathy in the rabbit. Arch Neurol 1971;24:358–64.

Ballantyne JP, Hansen S. A new method for the estimation of the number of motor units in a muscle. I. Control subjects and patients with myasthenia gravis. J Neurol Neurosurg Psychiatry 1974a;37:907–15.

Ballantyne JP, Hansen S. Computer method for the analysis of evoked motor unit potentials. J Neurol Neurosurg Psychiatry 1974b;37:1187–94.

Bergmans J. The physiology of single human nerve fibers. Louvain, Belgium: Vander, 1970.

Bolton CF, Gilbert JJ, Girvin JP, Hahn A. Nerve and muscle biopsy: electrophysiology and morphology in polyneuropathy. Neurology 1979;29:354–62.

Boyd IA, Davey MR. Composition of peripheral nerves. Edinburgh: Livingstone, 1968.

Brown WF. Functional compensation of human motor units in health and disease. J Neurol Sci 1973;20:199–209.

Brown WF, Jaatoul N. Amyotrophic lateral sclerosis: electrophysiological study (number of motor units and rate of decay of motor units). Arch Neurol 1974;30:242–48.

Brown WF, Milner-Brown HS. Some electrical properties of motor units and their effects on the method of estimating motor unit numbers. J Neurol Neurosurg Psychiatry 1976a;39:249–57.

Brown WF, Milner-Brown HS. Letter to the editor. J Neurol Neurosurg Psychiatry 1976b; 39:929–30.

Brown WF, Milner-Brown HS, Drake J. Excerpta Medica International Congress Series No. 360 Recent advances in myology. Proceedings of the Third International Congress on Muscle Diseases. Newcastle-on-Tyne, September 1974.

Buchthal F, Rosenfalck A. Evoked potentials and conduction velocity in human sensory nerves. Brain Res 1966;3:1–122.

Burke WE, Tuttle WW, Thompson CW, Janney CD, Weber RJ. The relation of grip strength and grip-strength endurance to age. J Appl Physiol 1953;5:628–30.

Carleton SA, Brown WF. Changes in motor unit

populations in motor neurone disease. J Neurol Neurosurg Psychiatry 1979;42:42–51.

Defaria CR, Toyonaga K. Motor unit estimation in a muscle supplied by the radial nerve. J Neurol Neurosurg Psychiatry 1978;41:794–97.

Desmedt JE. The neuromuscular disorder in myasthenia gravis. In: Desmedt JE, ed. New developments in electromyography and clinical neurophysiology. Basel: Karger, 1973:241–304.

Desmedt JE, Borenstein S. The testing of neuromuscular transmission. In: Vinken PJ, Bruyn GW, eds. Handbook of clinical neurology. Amsterdam: Elsevier North-Holland, 1970;7:104–15.

Easton DM. Excitability related to spike size in crab nerve fibres. J Cell Comp Physiol 1952;40:303–15.

Eisen A, Karpati G, Carpenter S, Danon J. The motor unit profile of the rat soleus in experimental myopathy and reinnervation. Neurology 1974;24:878–84.

Ekstedt J, Stålberg E. Single-fiber electromyography for the study of the microphysiology of the human muscle. In: Desmedt JE, ed. New developments in electromyography and clinical neurophysiology. Basel: Karger, 1973:89–112.

Erlanger J, Gasser HS. Electrical signs of nervous activity. Philadelphia: University of Pennsylvania Press, 1937.

Feasby TE, Brown WF. Variation of motor unit size in the human extensor digitorum brevis and thenar muscles. J Neurol Neurosurg Psychiatry 1974;37:916–26.

Feinstein B, Lindegård B, Nyman E, Wohlfart G. Morphologic studies of motor units in normal human muscles. Acta Anatomica 1955;23:127–42.

Gilliatt RW, Hopf HC, Rudge P, Baraitser M. Axonal velocities of motor units in the hand and foot muscles of the baboon. J Neurol Sci 1976;29:249–58.

Hodes R, Gribetz I, Moskowitz JA, Wagman IH. Low threshold associated with slow conduction velocity. Arch Neurol 1965;12:510–26.

Jennekins FGI, Tomlinson BE, Walton JN. The extensor digitorum brevis: histological and histochemical aspects. J Neurol Neurosurg Psychiatry 1972;35:124–32.

Juul-Jensen P, Mayer RF. Threshold stimulation for nerve conduction studies in man. Arch Neurol 1966;15:410–19.

Kadrie HA, Brown WF. Neuromuscular transmission in human single motor units. J Neurol Neurosurg Psychiatry 1978a;41:193–204.

Kadrie HA, Brown WF. Neuromuscular transmission in myasthenic single motor units. J Neurol Neurosurg Psychiatry 1978b;41:205–14.

Kadrie HA, Yates SK, Milner-Brown HS, Brown WF. Multiple-point electrical stimulation of ulnar and median nerves. J Neurol Neurosurg Psychiatry 1976;39:973–85.

Katz B, Schmitt OH. Electric interaction between two adjacent nerve fibres. J Physiol 1940;97:471–88.

Kugelberg E, Skoglund CR. Natural and artificial activation of motor units—a comparison. J Neurophysiol 1946;9:399–412.

Lambert EH. The accessory deep peroneal nerve. A common variation in innervation of extensor digitorum brevis. Neurology 1969;19:1169–76.

Law PK, Caccia MR. Physiological estimates of the sizes and the numbers of motor units in soleus muscles of dystrophic mice. J Neurol Sci 1975;24:251–56.

Lee RG, Ashby P, White DG, Aguayo A. Analysis of motor conduction velocity in the human median nerve by computer stimulation of compound muscle action potentials. Electroencephalogr Clin Neurophysiol 1975;39:225–37.

McComas AJ. Neuromuscular function and disorders. Woburn, Mass.: Butterworths, 1977.

McComas AJ, Brandstater ME, Upton ARM, Delbeke J, deFaria C, Toyonaga K. Sick motoneurones and dystrophy: a reappraisal. In: Rowland LP, ed. Pathogenesis of human muscular dystrophies. Proceedings of the Fifth International Scientific Conference of the Muscular Dystrophy Association, Durango, Colorado. Amsterdam, Oxford: Excerpta Medica, 1977:180–86.

McComas AJ, Campbell MJ, Sica REP. Electrophysiological study of dystrophia myotonica. J Neurol Neurosurg Psychiatry 1971;34:132–39.

McComas AJ, Fawcett PRW, Campbell MJ, Sica REP. Electrophysiological estimations of the number of motor units within a human muscle. J Neurol Neurosurg Psychiatry 1971;34:121–31.

McComas AJ, Sica REP. Automatic quantitative analysis of the electromyogram in partially denervated distal muscles: comparison with motor unit counting. Can J Neurol Sci 1978;5:377–83.

McComas AJ, Sica REP, Brown JC. Myasthenia gravis: evidence for a "central" defect. J Neurol Sci 1971;13:107–13.

McComas AJ, Sica REP, Campbell HJ. "Sick" motoneurones. A unifying concept of muscle disease. Lancet 1971;1:321–25.

McComas AJ, Sica REP, Campbell MJ, Upton ARM. Functional compensation in partially denervated muscles. J Neurol Neurosurg Psychiatry 1971;34:453–60.

McComas AJ, Sica REP, Currie S. An electrophysiological study of Duchenne dystrophy. J Neurol Neurosurg Psychiatry 1971;34:461–68.

McComas AJ, Sica REP, Upton ARM. Multiple muscle analysis of motor units in muscular dystrophy. Arch Neurol 1974;30:249–51.

Milner-Brown HS, Brown WF. New methods of estimating the number of motor units in a muscle. J Neurol Neurosurg Psychiatry 1976;39:258–65.

Panayiotopoulos CP, Scarpalezos S, Papapetropoulos T, Michas C. Quantitative estimation of motor units using a new neurophysiological method. Minerva Med Greca 1973;1:195–99.

Peyronnard JM, Lamarre Y. Electrophysiological and anatomical estimation of the number of motor units in the monkey extensor digitorum brevis muscle. J Neurol Neurosurg Psychiatry 1977;40:756–64.

Podivinsky F. Effect of stimulus intensity on the rising phase of the nerve action potential in healthy subjects and in patients with peripheral nerve lesions. J Neurol Neurosurg Psychiatry 1965;30:227–32.

Sica REP, McComas AJ. An electrophysiological investigation of limb-girdle and facioscapulohumeral dystrophy. J Neurol Neurosurg Psychiatry 1971;34:469–74.

Sica REP, McComas AJ, Upton ARM, Longmire D. Estimations of motor units in small muscles of the hand. J Neurol Neurosurg Psychiatry 1974;37:55–67.

Slomić A, Rosenfalck A, Buchthal F. Electrical and mechanical responses of normal and myasthenic muscle. Brain Res 1968;10:1–78.

Stålberg E. Electrogenesis in dystrophic human muscle. In: Rowland LP, ed. Pathogenesis of human muscular dystrophies. Proceedings of the Fifth International Scientific Conference of the Muscular Dystrophy Association, Durango, Colorado. Amsterdam, Oxford: Exerpta Medica, 1976:570–89.

Stålberg E, Trontelj JV. Demonstration of axon reflexes in human motor nerve fibres. J Neurol Neurosurg Psychiatry 1970;33:571–79.

Swett JE, Bourassa CM. Electrical stimulation of peripheral nerve. In: Patterson MM, Kesner RP, eds. Electrical stimulation research techniques. New York: Academic Press, 1981:244–98.

Warmolts JR, Engel WK. Correlations of motor unit behavior with histochemical myofiber types in humans by open biopsy electromyography. In: Desmedt JE, ed. New developments in electromyography and clinical neurophysiology. Basel: Karger, 1973:35–40.

Wray SH. Innervation ratios for large and small limb muscles in the baboon. J Comp Neurol 1969;137:227–50.

Wright EB, Coleman PD. Excitation and conduction in crustacean single motor axons. J Cell Comp Physiol 1954;43:133–64.

Yates SK, Brown WF. Characteristics of the F-response. A single motor unit study. J Neurol Neurosurg Psychiatry 1979;42:161–70.

7 ELECTROMYOGRAPHY— NORMAL

Recording the electrical activity of muscles generated by voluntary contractions or in response to electrical stimulation of the motor nerves is a very important tool for the investigation of peripheral nerve and muscle disease. The potentials are produced by the action potentials of muscle fibers (MFs) and are necessarily recorded in volume in the extracellular space (see Chapter 3). The potentials may be recorded by introducing an electrode into the muscle subcutaneously or situating it on the skin over the muscle(s) being studied.

Because surface or subcutaneous electrodes are outside the muscle, motor unit potentials are attenuated in size compared to potentials recorded by intramuscular electrodes. Surface electrodes, however, are better placed to see the total electrical activity generated by the muscle, unlike smaller intramuscular electrodes that have more restricted pickup territories. Because the potentials recorded are more representative of the whole electrical activity in the muscle, surface electrodes are preferable when the objectives include measuring the electrical potentials generated by the whole muscle or motor conduction velocity and assessing conduction block (see Chapter 4).

The integral of the full-wave rectified surface electromyographic (EMG) record is proportional to the force generated by a muscle (Lippold, 1952; Bigland and Lippold, 1954a, 1954b; Libkind, 1968, 1969, 1972a, 1972b; Milner-Brown and Stein, 1975). Such measurements are, however, of little practical value in the EMG assessment of peripheral neuropathies or muscle diseases.

Needle electrodes bring the recording surfaces of the electrode into much closer proximity to individual motor units (MUs) and MFs. Thus it is much easier to appreciate changes in the distribution patterns of MFs accompanying myopathies and alterations in neuromuscular or intramuscular axonal transmission present in these diseases. Furthermore, although subcutaneous electrodes are able to detect the action potentials of single MFs, for example, fibrillation potentials, these are far better recorded by intramuscular electrodes. For these and other reasons, intramuscular electrodes have become the preferred tool for analysis of muscle activity in disease states. Chapters 8 and 9 deal with the types of abnormal potentials that may be recorded by means of these electrodes in various diseases. This chapter examines the priorities and objectives of needle electromyography, as outlined in Table 7.1, the derivation of the motor unit potential (MUP), the types of needle electrodes in common use and the kind of information that they can provide, and the associated techniques used to assess nerve and muscle function.

Most of these objectives can be achieved by the use of the conventional concentric needle electrode used in the majority of laboratories. Before looking at this electrode, however, it is necessary to review what is known about the normal MU territory and the distribution of MFs within that territory. Following this is a discussion of the relationship between changes in the transmembrane potential and extracellular potentials recorded in volume, with passage of the impulse along a single MF. With this as background, the discussion examines the derivation of the MUP, its normal values, and the changes it undergoes with maturation and aging. Following this is a review of the types of intramuscular electrodes and the extent to which they can meet the objectives outlined in Table 7.1.

TERRITORIES OF MUs AND DISTRIBUTIONS OF MFs

There is no direct anatomic evidence in the human to tell us about the numbers and locations of MFs within the territories of MUs. What we know about MU territories is based on the indirect evidence provided through earlier multielectrode recordings (Buchthal, Guld, and Rosenfalck, 1957a, 1957b; Buchthal, Erminio, and Rosenfalck, 1959; Buchthal, 1961; Rosenfalck and Buchthal, 1970; Buchthal and Rosenfalck, 1973). Recordings obtained through the use of a linear array of electrodes positioned at intervals along the side of the cannula were able to tell us about the transverse potential profiles of single MUs. By making certain assumptions about the proximity of the nearest MFs based on the rise times and amplitudes of the spikes at the two outermost electrodes registering a spike, estimates of the anatomical limits of the MU were made. Table 7.2 illustrates the values for MU territories obtained in a variety of muscles (see Figure 5.5). It is not known which

---

TABLE 7.1.   Objectives of Needle Electrode Examination in Muscle

Learning about the territories of MUs in the muscle including
    Transverse territory in the muscle occupied by single MUs
    Numbers and positions of single MFs within the MU territory
    Extent of overlap between adjacent MU territories
Determining concentrations (or densities) of MF belonging to the same MU within a particular region (spatial dimensions of which are governed by the shape and area of the recording electrode)
Learning about recruitment patterns of MUs within the muscle, including
    Thresholds for recruitment (mechanical properties of MUs including contraction times and tensions)
    Rates of discharge of MUs at threshold and rate changes as the tension is increased
    Completeness of recruitment pattern, i.e., numbers of MUs and their rates of discharge at maximum or present percentage of maximum contraction
Assessing transmission at neuromuscular junctions, including individual neuromuscular junctions
Detecting abnormal spontaneous or stimulus evoked potentials in individual MFs and MUs

TABLE 7.2.   Estimations of Diameters of Territories of MUs in Muscles Obtained through Use of Multielectrode

Muscle	Transverse territory of MU (mm + 1 SD)
Biceps	5.1 + 2.4
Extensor digitorum communis	5.5 + 2.1
Opponens pollicis	7.4 + 2.6
Tibialis anterior	7.0 + 3.0
Extensor digitorum brevis	11.3 + 4.1

From Buchthal (1961).

types of MUs these territories represent, but on the assumption that they were based on an analysis of only the first two or three recruited, they must represent only the lowest-threshold (type I) MUs.

The territories of some MUs are quite small, some being less than 2 mm in diameter. These may contain as few as 10 MFs (Buchthal and Rosenfalck, 1973). Between birth and adulthood, the transverse territories of MUs approximately double. Individual electrodes in this type of multielectrode can detect up to six separate and distinct MUPs. This suggests that the territories of at least six MUs overlap, although the true extent of overlap would probably be greater were it possible to include the highest-threshold MUs. Figure 7.1 illustrates the overlap of motor unit territories within the brachialis muscle.

Locations and Numbers of MFs in the MU

Further development led to the introduction of a multielectrode in which, through the use of much smaller diameter electrodes (25 μ) spaced at intervals in the side of the cannula, it was possible to resolve the action potentials of single MFs. Thus it was possible to locate and count the numbers of individual single MFs along an electrode tract through the territory of an MU (Stålberg, Schwartz, Thiele,

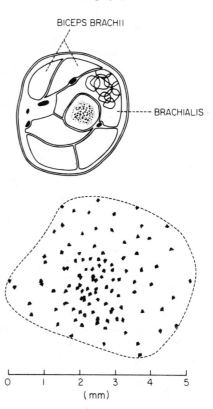

FIGURE 7.1.   Diagrammatic representation of the approximate cross-sectional territories of single motor units in the brachialis muscle in man.
(Top) Cross section of the mid-upper arm to show overlapping perimeters (or territories) of several motor units within the brachialis muscle. This muscle may contain upward of several hundred motor units.
(Bottom) Distribution of muscle fibers innervated by a single motoneuron in cross section. This particular motor unit has a transverse territory of about 5 mm. Muscle fibers belonging to this motor unit are scattered throughout the territory of the motor unit and intermingle with muscle fibers (not shown) that belong to as many as 10 to 30 other motor units. Most fibers in the motor unit have no neighboring muscle fibers belonging to the same motor unit, but occasional adjacent pairs or even three or more fibers showing the same motoneuronal innervation are found grouped together.
Note the tendency for the density of muscle fibers belonging to the same motor unit to increase toward the center of the motor unit territory.

and Schiller, 1976) (see Figure 5.7). Because of the short interelectrode distances and the high impedance of such electrodes, cross talk between adjacent electrodes can be a problem in this type of recording.

One solution to the technical problems associated with multielectrodes is to use two electrodes. First, one single-fiber EMG (SF-EMG) electrode is positioned near an MF belonging to the MU to be studied. This potential acts as a stable trigger source. A second SF-EMG electrode may then be inserted into the muscle in the vicinity of the first electrode. Single-fiber potentials recorded by this second electrode, which are time locked to the trigger source potential, can then be recorded as this second electrode is passed through the muscle territory of the motor unit in transverse calibrated steps. This tedious technique provides a view of the spatial distribution of single fibers belonging to one motor unit along a transverse corridor through the muscle.

Alternatively, the trigger source SF-EMG electrode may be coupled with the concentric needle electrode to record the spatially distributed electrical potentials associated with the activity of single motor units (Stålberg and Antoni, 1980). The larger leading-off surfaces of such electrodes, however, are less discriminative and probably record the compound potentials from as many as two or more muscle fibers belonging to the motor unit lying within this electrode's somewhat larger pickup territory. The pickup field of the electrode could well at times correspond to the group of muscle fibers innervated by major branches of the parent motor axon (Stålberg, 1982).

It is clear on the basis of the above studies as well as on histochemical maps of MFs belonging to single MUs in the rat (Edström and Kugelburg, 1968; Kugelberg, 1973; Brandstater and Lambert, 1969, 1973) and the cat (Doyle and Mayer, 1969) that in normal muscles at least, the territories of several MUs overlap in such a way that MFs that belong to

individual MUs intermingle with those of other MUs. There are seldom more than two, or at the most three, MFs immediately adjacent to one another that share the same innervation. This type of distribution precludes much interaction between the action currents of MFs in the same MU because of the insulation provided by other intervening MF belonging to other MUs. This may help prevent auto-reexcitation of MFs in the same MU (see Chapter 9).

Multielectrode studies do not provide any direct knowledge about innervation ratios of MUs or histochemical properties of the MFs in the MU.

Relationship Between Transmembrane and Extracellular Potentials that Accompany the Impulse

The MUP is the compound of the extracellular potentials of the MFs in the MU, but is weighted toward those MFs in the MU nearest to the electrode. This bias is critical to an understanding of the normal MUP and changes in the MUP in disease states. To begin, therefore, it is important to look at the relationship between the extracellular potential recorded by a point source electrode outside the MF and the corresponding transmembrane potential with passage of the impulse (Figure 7.2).

The most important points about the relationship between the transmembrane and extracellular potentials include:

1. The potential recorded just outside the muscle fiber is 1/10th to 1/100th the amplitude of the corresponding transmembrane potential.

2. There is a steep decline in the peak-to-peak voltage (p-pV) of the extracellular potential as the transverse (radial) distance between the muscle fiber and the

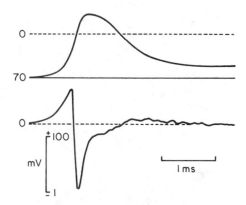

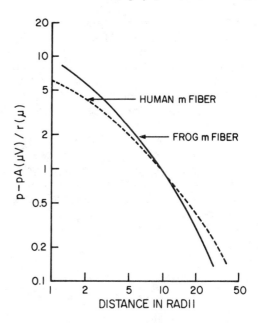

FIGURE 7.2. Parallel recordings of the changes in the transmembrane potential recorded with an intracellular electrode (top) and the extracellular potential as recorded just outside the membrane in the course of the action potential in a single muscle fiber.
Note:

1. The much larger size of the transmembrane potential in respect to the extracellular potential
2. The triphasic nature of the extracellularly recorded potential
3. The peak of the initial positive deflection corresponding to the onset of the inward sodium current directly opposite the extracellular electrode

In the middle of the muscle fiber the transmembrane current and therefore the size of the related locally recorded extracellular potential is equal to the first derivative of the internal longitudinal (or axial) current along the inside of the muscle fiber, and is therefore proportional to the second derivative of the membrane potential at that point.
From Katz and Miledi (1964, figure 10A).

FIGURE 7.3. Calculated radial decline in the peak-to-peak amplitude (p-pA) expressed as the p-pA divided by the radius of the fiber (V/μ) with increasing radial distance from the fiber measured in multiples of the radius of the muscle fiber. Calculations are shown for human and frog muscle fiber.

Note the steep radial decline in the amplitude of these potentials to about one-tenth to one-twentieth of the amplitude as measured just outside the fiber within 10 radii.
Adapted from Rosenfalck (1969, figure 16).

electrode increases (Figure 7.3). This decline is so steep that the amplitude of the potential declines to values less than 1/10th of that registered just outside the muscle fiber membrane at transverse distances of less than 0.5 mm.

3. Because of the progressive loss of the higher-frequency components of the potentials as the transverse distance be-

tween the electrode and the MF(s) increases, the rise time of the negative spike increases and the interpeak latencies increase (Figure 7.4).

4. The extracellular potential is triphasic. The initial positive peak recorded just outside the muscle fiber membrane corresponds to the onset of the change in sodium conductance and the abrupt increase in the inward sodium current.

5. The times when the transmembrane potential is at zero potential correspond to when the extracellular potential also crosses the zero potential baseline; these

FIGURE 7.4. Diagrammatic representation of changes in peak latencies of the extracellularly recorded triphasic action potential of a muscle fiber as the transverse distance between the fiber (bottom) and the recording site is increased. In this representation, the amplitudes of the potentials have been kept constant. As the transverse distance increases, there is a progressive displacement of the peak latencies of the potential, although the total duration of the potential remains constant, as do the zero-potential crossing times (one of which is indicated by a vertical interrupted line). λ = wavelength of the action potential.

Adapted from Rosenfalck (1969).

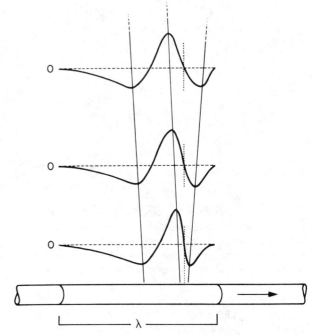

relationships do not change no matter what the distance is between the MF and the recording electrode.

6. Both potentials have identical durations.
7. The larger the diameters of MFs, the larger the amplitudes of the corresponding extracellular potentials. The diameters of MFs in large limb muscles range between 30 and 90 μ (average about 50 μ in man). In the newborn the diameters are much less (about 10 μ).

THE MOTOR UNIT POTENTIAL

The steep transverse decline in the p-p amplitude of the potential means that only those MFs in the MU within 0.5 mm of the electrode make much contribution to the MUP. Because the width of most MU territories can be as wide as 5 to 10 mm or more, it is clear that the majority of MFs belonging to an MU may make little or no contribution to the p-p amplitude of the MUP because they are too distant to register much of a potential at the electrode, even when the electrode is within the territory of the MU (Rosenfalck, 1969; Gath and Stålberg, 1976, 1978a, 1978b). Probably no more than 1 to 10 MFs in the normal MU generate the main spike of the MUP recorded by conventional concentric needle electrode. This represents less than 10 percent of the total number of MFs in the MU (Rosenfalck, 1969; Stålberg and Trontelj, 1979; Stålberg and Antoni, 1980).

The greater the number of MFs in the same MU that are within the immediate spike pickup territory of the electrode and the better these potentials coincide together in time, the larger the p-p amplitude of the spike. Hence changes in the normal intermingling pattern of MFs belonging to various MUs (see Chapter 5) to the grouping together of MFs belonging to the same MU would tend to increase the compound spike amplitude. The diameter of MFs is also important; the larger the diameter, the higher the p-p amplitude of the potential registered at a point an equivalent distance away.

In most muscles, the durations of MUPs are several times longer than the duration of single MF potentials (Figure 7.5). Just how long an MUP lasts from beginning to end (total duration) depends on those MFs whose potentials are most widely dispersed in time with respect to one another and that make a detectable contribution to the MUP. Temporal dispersion in the discharge times of MFs in the MU recorded near the end-plate zone then, depends on the longitudinal and transverse spatial scatter of end-plates in the MU. The more widely separate the end-plates, the more temporal dispersion there is in the discharge times of MFs in the MU because of the variations in the distances and conduction velocities between the presynaptic axons in the MU.

In the normal biceps muscle, the innervation zone is 10 to 30 mm wide. This degree of longitudinal scatter among the end-plates of single MUs could account for a range of several milliseconds in the times of arrival of the MU impulse at all the axon terminals throughout the MU territory and an equivalent dispersion in discharge times of their respective postsynaptic MFs (Buchthal, Guld, and Rosenfalck, 1957a; Buchthal, 1977, 1982).

The progressive increase in the duration of MUPs between birth and childhood is no doubt based on the expansion in the innervation zone, because of increases in diameters of MFs. Throughout adult life there is a progressive increase in the duration of MUPs (Figure 7.6) (measurements exclude polyphasic MUPs and potentials having linked components) and in the numbers of polyphasic MUPs. These two changes could reflect the progressive loss of motoneurons, endplate turnover, and processes of collaterali-

FIGURE 7.5. Comparative durations of single muscle fiber potentials (top) and MUPs (bottom) recorded in the region of the innervation zone with a standard concentric needle electrode. The recording bandwidth for all three recordings was 0.5 to 2,000 Hz.

Note the prepotential (PreP), which probably corresponds to the end-plate potential in this region, which precedes the main spike. The total duration of the single fiber potential was 4.0 ms or less than one-half of the two MUPs recorded in the same region. Durations are indicated by horizontal brackets.

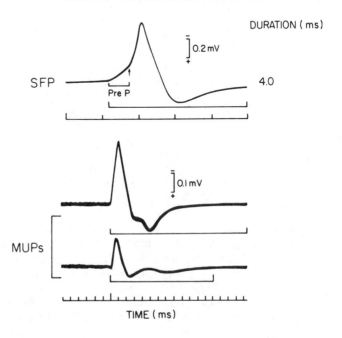

END-PLATE ZONE RECORDINGS

zation and reinnervation, particularly in the later decades.

Disease processes that increase the spatial distribution of the end-plate zone in the MU or change the relative conduction velocities in the terminal and preterminal branches of the presynaptic motor axon network would increase the temporal dispersion of the MF potentials and increase the duration of the MUP. Beyond the end-plate zone, the wider the variations among the conduction velocities of MFs in the MU and the more longitudinally distant the electrode is from the end-plate zone, the longer the durations of the MUP. In myopathies in particular, there is a tendency for wider variations among the diameters of single MFs, although whether this is quite as true among MFs in the same MU is unknown. Wider ranges among the diameters of MFs in the same MU, if expressed in equivalent variations among their conduction velocities, would tend to increase the temporal dispersion among MF potentials belonging to the same MU (see Chapter 8).

Duration also depends on the bandwidth of the recording system. By eliminating lower

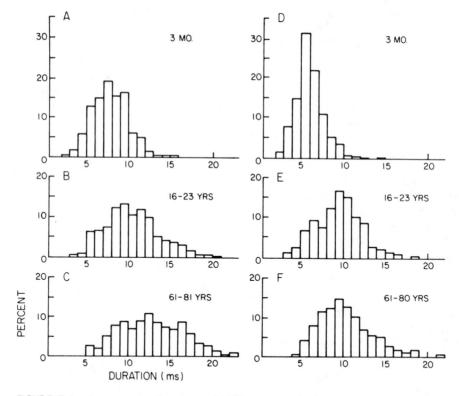

FIGURE 7.6.   Increases in durations of MUPs as recorded with standard concentric needle electrodes at three months and early and late adult life in a proximal muscle such as the biceps brachii (A–C) and a distal muscle such as the abductor digiti quinti (D–F). Note the progressive increase in MUP duration, especially between three months and early adult life, and also the wide range of MUP durations.
From Sacco, Buchthal, and Rosenfalck (1962, figure 2), reprinted with permission of the publisher. © 1962–75–75, The American Medical Association.

frequencies, high-pass filtering attenuates the contributions of more distant MF potentials in relation to MFs in the immediate vicinity of the electrode (Figure 7.7). This reduces the effective pickup territory of the electrode and reduces the chances of including some of the more distant and possibly more dispersed MF potentials with respect to those MF nearest to the electrode. This and the loss of the slower components of even those MFs near the electrode would tend to shorten the durations of MUPs.

The durations of successively recruited MUPs do not significantly differ even though there is an increase in the p-p amplitudes of the second and later MUPs compared to the first MUP recorded with intramuscular concentric needle electrodes. This observation fits with the recruitment patterns of MUPs discussed in detail in Chapter 5 (see also Buchthal, Pinelli, and Rosenfalck, 1954).

The number of phases in the MUP (number of baseline crossings) depends on the de-

gree of synchronization between the potentials of MFs and the numbers of these MFs in the immediate vicinity of the electrode. The greater the desynchronization, the more complex the compound potential. The degree of synchronization in turn depends on the longitudinal scatter of the end-plates and variations in conduction velocities of presynaptic axons and MFs in that part of the MU seen by the electrode.

Most MUPs in normal muscle are biphasic or triphasic (Table 7.3). Up to 10 percent of

TABLE 7.3. Numbers of Phases of MUPs in the Biceps

	Phases				
Age (years)	1	2	3	4	> 4
0–4	2	32	57	6	5
20–22	3	46	41	7	3

From Buchthal, Pinelli, and Rosenfalck (1954).

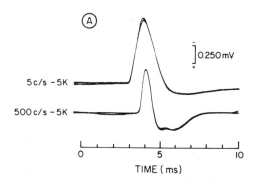

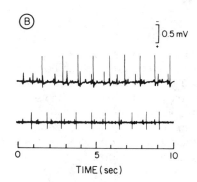

FIGURE 7.7. Recording of several voluntarily recruited MUPs by means of a conventional concentric needle electrode positioned in the vicinity of the innervation zone (note initial negative deflection of the potentials) to illustrate the effects of excluding the lower-frequency components of the signals by changing the high-pass filter from 5 c/s to 500 c/s (3 db down). (A) shows the impact on the largest of the MUPs seen in (B) of filtering out the lower-frequency components. This reduced the peak-to-peak amplitude by 21 percent and the total duration of this potential by 17 percent. The percentage of amplitude reductions was even greater for the smaller-amplitude MUPs (B) top; the overall effect tending to enhance some MUPs relative to others, presumably, for distance from the leading-off surface of the recording electrode.

those in control muscles are polyphasic (more than four baseline crossings).

Factors other than those mentioned above also alter the variables of MUPs. For example, the lower the temperature in the muscle, the slower the conduction velocities of impulses in the MFs and their presynaptic axons. Lower temperatures also prolong membrane currents and thus the action potential in single MFs. The result is a significantly longer duration of MUPs at lower temperatures (Figure 7.8).

Orientation of the electrode with respect to the MF nearest it is also important. Where the axis of the leading-off surface of the electrode is parallel to the MFs, the durations of MF potentials are shorter. The durations of recorded potentials are longer, however, where the axis of the electrode is perpendicular to the MFs.

Accurate assessment of MUP duration depends on the ability to recognize the true onset and termination times of the potential. The slower the onset or termination of the potentials and the higher the baseline noise, the more difficult it is to measure the true durations of the potentials. Accurate measurements of duration are made much easier when MUP triggered sweeps are combined with measures to delay the MUP by enough time

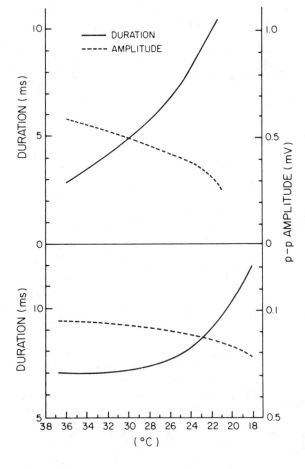

FIGURE 7.8.   Changes in duration and amplitude of two representative MUPs (top and bottom plots) as recorded with a concentric needle electrode as the temperature is reduced. Note the very substantial increase in duration, especially at the lower temperatures, and the general tendency to a parallel reduction in amplitude. Cooling also increases the safety factor for neuromuscular transmission. Redrawn from Buchthal, Pinelli, and Rosenfalck (1954, figure 2).

to recognize clearly its onset, electronic averaging of the potential, and recording the potential at a high enough gain to see its limits. Table 7.4 summarizes the main factors that change the values of the MUP. In short:

1. The nearer the MFs are to the electrode, the more MFs there are; the larger the diameters of those MFs and the better the degree of synchronization between their potentials, the higher the amplitude of the MUP will be.

TABLE 7.4. Factors Determining Amplitudes (p-p), Total Duration, and Number of Phases of MUPs

---

Amplitudes
Distance between the recording surfaces of the electrode and the MFs that generate the MUP
Number of MFs in the MU nearest to the electrode
Diameters of those MFs
Temporal coincidence between the action potentials of those MFs nearest to the electrode
Orientation of the electrode with respect to MFs generating the MUP
Type of electrode used
    Monopolar vs bipolar
    Area of the recording surface
    Shape of the recording surface
    Temperature of the muscle
    Bandwidth of the recording system

Duration
Longitudinal and transverse scatter of the end-plate zone in the MU
Conduction velocities of presynaptic motor axon branches
Neuromuscular delays
Conduction velocities of the MFs
Longitudinal distance between recording site and innervation zone
Temperature of the muscle
Bandwidth of the recording system
Type of electrode employed
    Bipolar or monopolar

Number of phases
Temporal coincidence between the action potentials of those MF nearest to the electrode
Number of MFs in the MU near the electrode

---

2. The less longitudinal scatter among the end-plates in an MU, the more similar the conduction velocities of their presynaptic axons and the MF; the higher the intramuscular temperature, the younger the subject; and the narrower the bandwidth of the recording system (especially at the low end), the shorter will be the duration of the MUP.

3. The greater the degree of synchronization between action potentials of these MFs nearest to the electrode, the less likely the potential is to be polyphasic.

TYPES OF EMG ELECTRODES

Because the qualities of the MUP and single MF potentials are dependent to some extent on the type of electrode used, it is important to look at the three intramuscular electrodes in common use and discuss their particular advantages and limitations.

Monopolar Needle Electrodes

Monopolar needle electrodes are made from stainless steel wire (0.3 to 0.5 mm in diameter) sharpened at the tip. The electrode is insulated except at the tip, the bare tip extending back 25 to 50 µ or more. A surface or subcutaneous electrode serves as the remote reference electrode. These needle electrodes work well; however, breakdowns in the insulation are common. This and the problem of maintaining a sharp tip makes them less durable than concentric needle electrodes.

For monopolar intramuscular electrodes of equivalent resistances to concentric needle electrodes, the amplitudes of MUPs are higher (durations the same) when recorded by the former compared to the latter. This advantage is achieved at the expense of enhanced pickup from other MUPs (Buchthal, Guld, and Rosenfalck, 1954).

Monopolar tungsten microelectrodes have been used by some investigators to stimulate single intramuscular motor axons, carry out microneuronographical recordings from human nerves, and isolate single MF spikes against a background of other EMG activity in isometric muscle contractions (see Chapter 5). For the last purpose, in our view, the SF-EMG electrode is easier to use. The tips of tungsten microelectrodes and their insulation are easily broken by insertion of the electrode through the skin unless a small nick is made at the outset with a sharp blade.

Concentric Needle Electrodes

Concentric needle electrodes were introduced by Adrian and Bronk in 1929 and are probably the most commonly used in routine electromyography in man. They consist of an outer needle cannula that serves as the reference electrode and a central core electrode that normally has a diameter of about 100 μ and is insulated from the outer cannula by epoxy

or equivalent insulating material (Figure 7.9). The tip is beveled, the area of the recording electrode surface depending on the angle of the bevel. The potentials so recorded depend on:

1. Surface area of the recording electrode (core).
2. Bandwidth of the recording system. To record MUP durations with the least distortion, the frequency limits should, as a minimum, extend between 2 and 2,000 Hz. At 2,000 Hz, however, the amplitude of the MUP is attenuated somewhat. It would be better to use a 10,000-Hz (3 db down) as the better upper limit, noting however, that the noise increases as the square root of the frequency.
3. Impedance of the electrode. This should be kept as low as possible to reduce the noise and avoid a possible impedance mismatch between the electrode and the first stage of the amplifier with consequent distortion of the frequency composition of the potential.

FIGURE 7.9. Diagrammatic representation of a transverse section through the territory of a motor unit illustrating the positions of the muscle fibers innervated by a single motoneuron. Superimposed on this are the sizes of a standard concentric needle electrode with its relatively large elliptical leading-off surface exposed in the bevel of the tip, and a single-fiber electrode with its single leading-off surface mounted in the side wall of the electrode. In both electrodes the recording electrode is separated from the cannula by epoxy resin insulating material. The diameters of the electrode cannulas are usually between 0.3 and 0.5 mm. The spike pickup territory of both electrodes covers only a fraction of the whole motor unit territory (see text).

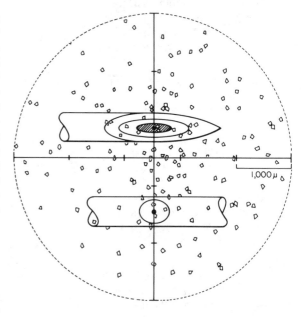

4. Volume conductor and filter characteristics of the muscle.

5. Depth of the needle. The cannula itself records a potential that can be up to 30 percent of the amplitude of the potential recorded by the core. This can be demonstrated when the cannula is made the active electrode and a remote subcutaneous electrode acts as the reference electrode. As more of the cannula enters the muscle, the area that is exposed to the muscle increases, and it tends to act more and more as a truly indifferent electrode the deeper into the muscle it is inserted. This is because more of the isopotential lines originating in the various voltage sources within the muscle cross and tend to average out over the cannula.

The importance of the orientation of a concentric electrode within the muscle on the amplitude and duration of the motor unit action potential has recently been stressed by Butler, Ball, and Albers (1982). These authors showed that when it was oriented perpendicular to the muscle fibers, the concentric electrode behaved like a monopolar electrode, although the amplitude and duration of the motor unit potentials were dependent on the depth of the electrode within the muscle. Unlike the bipolar arrangement, however, the amplitude and duration of the motor unit action potentials were increased when the cannula was oriented obliquely to the muscle fibers.

The primary advantage of concentric needle electrodes is that they are remarkably durable and hold up well to sterilization and repeated insertions. Observations made with them are very reproducible among laboratories, especially where the electrodes have been carefully prepared and maintained, special attention being paid to the bevel and the electrode surface. The design and the dimensions of the common concentric needle electrode are such that the spike component reflects the contribution of from one to at the most ten muscle fibers located nearest the recording electrode in normal muscle (Krnjevic and Miledi, 1958; Ekstedt, 1964; Rosenfalck, 1969). The duration of the MUP from onset to termination, however, reflects the volume-conducted electrical activity from a much larger number of muscle fibers in the MU. Indeed, possibly all the MFs in the smaller MUs could make some contribution to the MUP depending on the position of the electrode with respect to the MU.

More Selective Electrodes

The primary objective here is to so design the electrode as to best select the potentials generated by only those MFs in the immediate vicinity of the electrode, the purposes being to:

1. Study neuromuscular transmission at individual neuromuscular junctions.

2. Measure the conduction velocities of single MFs.

3. Lock onto the action potential generated by a SF, which then by acting as the trigger source, allows one to study other properties of the same MU, such as its contractile properties (see Chapter 5) and the size and shape of its potential as recorded with a second much larger recording electrode. Where there is much activity in other MUs, the forces or potentials time locked to the trigger source potential can be isolated from the background force or electrical activity by electronically averaging successive time-locked sweeps. This *spike-triggered averaging* is a valuable technique that makes it possible to examine the MUP and mechanical properties of the higher-threshold MUPs that in the normal course would be lost in the random background EMG activity (the interference pattern).

4. Estimate the number of MFs belonging to the MU, which are within the small pickup territory of this type of electrode.

There are three main strategies for making an electrode more selective. First, the electrode recording surface can be made much smaller. The primary advantage of smaller size is that the leading-off surface is immediately only to those MFs next to it. Larger electrodes can span several MFs, and so not only may a number of them be equally close to the electrode, but the potentials of single MFs will tend to average out over the extended leading-off surface because more of their isopotential lines will intersect the electrode. The tradeoff is that the smaller the diameter of the leading-off surface, the higher the impedance of the electrode. This in turn not only creates more electronic noise, but increases the capacitive leakages to ground and to other electrodes, such as the cannula or other small electrodes within the cannula. Such capacitive leakages between electrodes or their leads in the cannula or connecting cable degrade the potential amplitude and high-frequency (HF) components and leads to cross talk between electrodes. The last is mostly a problem when there are multiple high-impedance electrodes in an array close together. The effect of cross talk is that the potential may be seen at other electrodes, not through seeing the potential directly, but through interelectrode capacitive current leakages.

The practical lower limit to the diameter of a selective electrode in muscle is about 25 μ, or a little less than the diameter of some of the MFs. With this size electrode it is not unusual to record single MF action potentials with amplitudes of 10 to 20 mV, whereas the corresponding MUPs recorded by conventional concentric needle electrodes (dimensions 100 × 300 to 400) are usually of the order of 0.1 to 0.5 mV.

A second strategy is to use a bipolar arrangement (Buchthal, Guld, and Rosenfalck,

1954; Pollak, 1971; Hannerz, 1974a, 1974b; Andreassen and Rosenfalck, 1978) (Table 7.5). The closer the electrodes are together, the more cancellation there is of distant unwanted voltage sources. This is because the potentials generated by these sources tend to be very similar at the two electrodes, and the amplifier records the difference between the potentials registered at the electrodes. This same effect also applies, to some extent, to those potentials generated immediately opposite the electrodes in the pair, especially the slower components of these MF action potentials, which tend therefore to cancel out. The result is that SF potentials recorded by bipolar electrodes are generally somewhat shorter in duration and their amplitudes are reduced compared to monopolar recordings with electrodes of equivalent size. The optimal interelectrode distance for electrodes of 25 to 30 μ in diameter appears to be between 50 and 100 μ (see Table 7.5).

TABLE 7.5. Changes in p-p Voltage of Single MF Potentials and the Numbers of MFs within the Pickup Territory of the Electrode in Bipolar Electrode Recordings with Various Interelectrode Distances and in Unipolar Recordings

Distance between electrodes (μ)	p-pV (mV) MF action potential	Numbers of MFs within pickup territory of the electrode
Bipolar (Perpendicular to Long Axis of MFs)		
25	0.460	2–7
50	0.690	2–9
100	0.900	4–11
200	1.100	>15
Bipolar (Parallel to Long Axis of MFs)		
25	0.140	
50	0.250	5–9
100	0.490	
200	0.900	
Unipolar Recording		
	1.26	9–17

From Andreassen and Rosenfalck (1978).

Orientation of the electrode pair is also important. For example, when it is arranged perpendicular to the MFs, the amplitudes of the potentials are somewhat higher than when the electrode is orientated in the long axis of the MFs. Because of its long wavelength in relation to the interelectrode distance in the latter case, the potential tends to cancel out between the two electrodes.

The third strategy is to enhance the nearby MF potentials relative to more distant MFs by cutting out the lower-frequency components of the recording (Figures 7.7 and 7.10). This can be done by setting the high-pass filter at 200 to 500 Hz. This technique works because the more distant the MF source, the lower the frequency spectrum of its potentials as seen by the electrode (i.e, volume conduction acts as a low-pass filter). By filtering out the lower frequencies, the more remote MF potentials are diminished relative to the nearby MF potentials that have high-frequency components (the spike) and are not nearly so attenuated in amplitude as the more distant MF potentials. The strategy is not without its penalties, however, because there is some amplitude attenuation even for the nearby potentials and the effect can be to lose some amplitude-discriminating ability among different SF sources (Andreassen and Rosenfalck, 1978).

All the preceding strategies help the electromyographer to record as selectively as possible the activities of single MFs and MUs. The SF-EMG electrode itself is discussed later in this chapter. Other types of selective electrodes include implantable wire electrodes.

Basmajian (1973) has advocated the use of two wires, insulated except at their tip, inserted into the muscle with a needle carrier. The cannula is then withdrawn leaving the two fine-wire, low-mass electrodes within the muscle. The recording surface area is a function of the cross-sectional area of the wire and the extent to which the insulation has been stripped back from the tip. This type of elec-

FIGURE 7.10.   Effect of changing the bandwidth on the shape and duration of a single MUP as recorded from the extensor digitorum communis muscle with a conventional concentric needle electrode in a patient with polymyositis. Bandwidths:

Top	0.5 to 5,000 Hz	
Middle	500 to 5,000 Hz	all 2 db down
Bottom	2 to 200 Hz	

Note that because of the fast-frequency components, the spike component is hardly altered at all by changing the high-pass filter to 500 Hz, although the same maneuver severely attenuated the lower-frequency components of the MUP, especially the slow initial positive, thereby appreciably shortening the overall duration of the MUP.

Just the opposite happened, however, when the filter was set so as to exclude the higher-frequency components but pass the lower frequencies (bottom). The potentials were electronically averaged (n = 64).

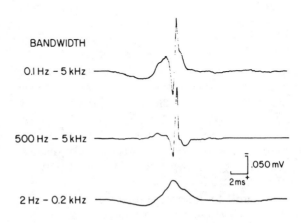

BANDWIDTH

0.1 Hz – 5 kHz

500 Hz – 5 kHz

.050 mV

2 ms

2 Hz – 0.2 kHz

trode has the advantages that it provides a relatively high degree of discrimination in the selection of individual MUPs and good positional stability in the muscle, especially if the little hook is left on the end of the electrode. These electrodes are suitable for long-term stable recordings, such as kinesi-esthesiological studies, from selected sites in a muscle. These electrodes are tricky to insert, however, and the operator must be careful to avoid abrasions of the insulation. The electrodes may break and it is very hard to adjust their position once they are in place. It is possible, however, to modify their design in order to permit some adjustment and optimize the recording from different MUPs (Andreassen and Rosenfalck, 1978). Improved versions include electrodes described by Hannerz (1974a) and Andreassen and Rosenfalck (1978).

SINGLE-FIBER NEEDLE ELECTROMYOGRAPHY

The cannula of the SF electrode is 0.5 mm or less in diameter (see Figure 7.9). Its cross-sectional area is about 100 times that of a single MF (Ekstedt, 1964). Therefore to help limit damage to MFs in the course of the electrode tract, the electrode bevel must be as sharp as possible.

The leading-off surface of the recording electrode is mounted on the side of the cannula opposite the bevel so that the electrode records from MFs pushed aside by the bevel but left intact. The diameter of the recording electrodes is small (25 to 30 μ) and their number and arrangement vary depending on the requirements of the investigator. By the use of various combinations and orientations of these electrodes on the side of the cannula it is possible to determine the orientation of the MFs with respect to the long axis of the cannula, measure the conduction velocities of single MF action potentials, and work out the potential fields about single MFs in the muscle (Ekstedt, 1964; Stålberg, 1966).

Earlier in this chapter, it was pointed out that electrodes 25 to 50 μ in diameter represent the reasonable lower limits for recording MF action potentials as selectively as possible. Electrodes much smaller in diameter increase the impedance too much with little improvement in selectivity for recording single MF action potentials. The optimal diameters seem to be close to those of the MFs.

Bipolar electrodes with interelectrode distances between 60 and 200 μ are even more selective in isolating the action potentials of single MFs, an advantage further enhanced by filtering out the lower-frequency components (500 Hz and lower). The amplitudes of such action potentials, however, are less than with monopolar techniques (Andreassen and Rosenfalck, 1978) (Table 7.5). In SF-EMG, it sometimes improves the recording qualities of the electrode to pass a brief current (about 10 to 20 MA) through the electrode in order to reduce its impedance, as recommended for concentric needle and single-fiber electrodes by Ekstedt (1964) and for concentric needle electrodes by Buchthal, Guld, and Rosenfalck (1954).

The SF electrode is inserted into the muscle perpendicular to the direction of the MFs to ensure maximum selectivity for the recording of single MF action potentials. This is even more important when bipolar electrodes are used. The subject is then asked to make a contraction, at which time the electrode is moved to a point in the muscle at which one or more potentials meeting the criteria for single MF action potentials are clearly identifiable. The position of the electrode can then be fine tuned to enhance the amplitude of the potential(s) as much as possible.

The oscilloscope sweep is triggered by the MF potential, and the delayed potentials are displayed on one of the channels of the oscilloscope. At each site in the muscle where potentials meeting the criteria for single MF potentials are detected, the numbers of these potentials are counted (the fiber density).

When one or more potentials are found that are linked to the triggering potential, measurements of their variations in discharge times with respect to one another can be made (the jitter). Use of this technique requires knowledge of the characteristics of single-fiber action potentials as recorded with this type of electrode.

Characteristics of Single-Fiber Action Potentials as Recorded by SF-EMG Electrodes

Principal characteristics of SF action potentials as recorded by SF-EMG are as follows (see Ekstedt, 1964; Stålberg and Trontelj, 1979):

1. SF potentials are smooth biphasic spikes. There are no discontinuities in the main part of the potential to suggest the presence of other MF potentials (Figure 7.12). The initial positive phase is sometimes absent near the end-plate zone. The potentials may terminate in a longer-lasting, low-amplitude positive phase.

2. The p-p amplitude of SF potentials recorded by the SF electrode are much higher than the amplitudes of MUPs SF potentials recorded by concentric needle electrodes (because of the larger areas of the central core electrode in the latter, 0.015 to 0.070 mm, versus about 0.002 mm in the SF-EMG electrode) (Figure 7.11). For example, the mean amplitude SF potential is 5.6 mV (range, 0.7 to 25.2 mV) when the position of the electrode is adjusted. These values are much higher than the amplitudes of MUPs recorded (random insertion) by concentric needle electrodes (Buchthal, Guld, and Rosenfalck, 1954). There, only 2 percent of the potential amplitudes exceeded 0.7 mV and none exceeded 1.0 mV in an SF recording. There is also steep transverse decrement in the amplitude of SF potentials as

the distance between the MF source and the electrode increases (see Figure 7.3).

3. The duration of the main spike is brief (mean, 0.470 ms; range, 0.265 to 0.8 ms). This is much shorter than the longer durations of MUPs or even single MF potentials as recorded by the larger concentric needle electrode because of the deliberate attenuation of the lower-frequency components of the potential, the closer proximity of the MF, and the smaller area of the recording electrode in the SF-EMG technique.

4. The rise times of single MF spikes are short (less than 0.150 ms; range, 0.067 to 0.200 ms).

5. Where there are two or more SF electrodes present in the cannula and they are close enough together to record the same spikes, the action potentials they record have simultaneous baseline intersections. Moreover, when the long axis of the MF is perpendicular to the electrode pair, similar declines in the amplitudes of the potential are seen at both electrodes as the distance between the MF and the electrodes increases. This criterion is not necessary in service laboratories.

It is possible to record SF action potentials with conventional concentric needle electrodes. Their amplitudes, however, even when the electrode position is adjusted to obtain the maximum amplitude, are much lower than those recorded by the SF-EMG electrode. It is also harder to isolate individual spike components from the composite MUP. Sometimes the contributions of individual SF spikes can be seen as discontinuities superimposed on the otherwise smooth main MUP and can be recognized by their variations in latencies with respect to the main potential or when their latencies separate them clearly from the main MUP (linked potentials). Single-fiber contributions to the main MUP can be enhanced also by borrowing a trick from SF-

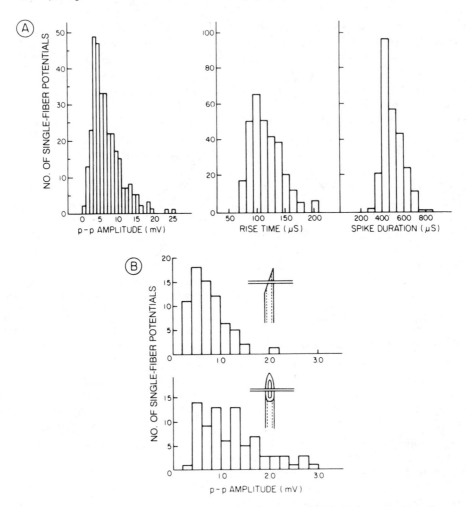

FIGURE 7.11. Spike peak-to-peak amplitude, rise time (initial positive peak to negative spike peak), and spike durations of single-fiber potentials as recorded with a single-fiber electrode (A) whose position was adjusted for optimal spike amplitude.

Note the very high amplitude of some of the potentials, the brief rise times, and very short spike durations as compared with motor unit spike potentials. The comparable single-fiber potentials as recorded with a conventional concentric needle electrode are generally much lower in amplitude (B) because of the much larger leading-off surface of these electrodes. Even so, the amplitudes were significantly altered by changing the orientation of the leading-off surface with respect to the muscle fiber (see insets).

From Ekstedt (1964, figures 32 and 39).

EMG techniques, namely, filtering out lower-frequency components of the signal (1,000 Hz or less). In our experience it is relatively easy to record SF action potentials from the orbicularis oculi and other facial muscles with standard concentric needle electrodes by filtering out the lower frequencies and thereby enhancing the MF potentials nearest the electrode.

Technical Factors in the Recording System that Alter Characteristics of SF Potentials

The characteristics of SF potentials recorded by SF-EMG electrodes are altered by changes in the distance between the MF and the electrode, the type of recording (bipolar or unipolar), capacitive cross talk between electrode leads, and the impedance of the electrodes. For example, the shorter the interelectrode distance in a bipolar electrode, the shorter the durations of the SF potentials recorded. Also, where leads run together for an appreciable distance within the cannula there may be appreciable interelectrode capacitances (of the order of 8 to 10 micro-microfarads between the leads). This capacitance may be further increased (by about 5 to 10 micro-microfarads) in the input cable of the amplifier. The effect of all this capacitance is that sometimes the cross-talk signal at one or more electrodes in an array can exceed the volume-conducted spike recorded at that point. When the impedance of the electrodes is too high, the higher-frequency components of the signal may be shunted by stray capacitances to ground. For this reason it is important to keep electrode resistances as low as possible (Ekstedt, 1964). It is also important because of the high impedances of SF-EMG electrodes to use amplifiers that have high enough input impedances and low input capacitances; suitable values being about 250 megohms and 10 to 15 micro-microfarads respectively, measured at the input connector of the electrode cable with the amplifier.

The Double Spike and Multiple Spike

At about one-third of the locations in normal muscles where potentials meeting the criteria for SF potentials are recorded, a second potential meeting the same criteria and clearly separate from the triggering potential can be recorded (see Figure 7.12). This second spike has a number of characteristics, namely:

1. Its characteristics are not identical to those of the triggering potential. This means that the second potential in the pair is not simply a repetitive discharge in a single muscle fiber.
2. Because the second potential is time locked to trigger the source potential, the two potentials must be generated by MFs

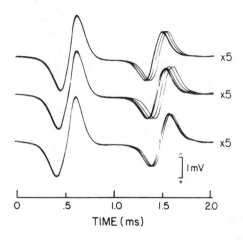

FIGURE 7.12.   The double spike and jitter phenomena. Shown are pairs of single muscle fiber potentials as recorded with a single-fiber EMG electrode from the orbicularis oculi muscle. The initial potential in the pair served here as the trigger source. Hence all the fluctuations in latency at the two neuromuscular junctions are seen as the fluctuations in latency of the second fiber with respect to the earlier constant trigger source potential. The bandwidth of the recording was 500 to 10,000 Hz (2 db down), and in each of the recordings, five successive discharges are superimposed. The calculated jitter values of the recordings from below upward are 13, 32, and 22, μsec respectively.

Note the smooth biphasic shape of the above potentials with no discontinuities to suggest the presence of other fiber potentials.

innervated by the same motoneuron. This view receives further support from the constant coupling of these potentials observed at various firing frequencies.

3. The firing times of the two potentials vary somewhat with respect to one another, a phenomenon for which the word *jitter* has been coined.

Normally, there is a very small variation in latency at the neuromuscular junction between the arrival of the presynaptic spike and the onset of the MF action potential. The *jitter* is produced by the combined effect of the variations in latency at the two neuromuscular junctions. Because one of the potentials acts as the constant trigger source, however, the combined variations in latency at the two junctions are expressed solely by the variation in latency of the second (jittering) potential with respect to the constant trigger source potential.

This jitter value or interspike interval variation is a measure of the safety factor of neuromuscular transmission at the two neuromuscular junctions. When this safety factor is reduced, the variation in the interpotential interval increases and at the limit, one of the impulses may block when its EPP no longer reaches the threshold level necessary to generate a muscle fiber action potential.

interpreted to mean that the two potentials originate in the split portions of a muscle fiber. This phenomenon is especially common in the muscular dystrophies, where jitter is not increased by neuromuscular blocking agents. Changes in jitter in neuromuscular diseases are described in Chapter 10.

Jitter can be quantified by measuring the range of the difference in latencies between the trigger source potential and the second potential. Such a method, however, provides only a measure of the worst case represented by the maximum difference in latency between the two potentials. It is better therefore to measure the mean consecutive difference in latencies of 50 to 100 potential pairs. This measurement is facilitated by on-line devices that automatically calculate the jitter as the sum of the latency differences of consecutive numbers of spike pairs minus 1. In this type of automatic calculation, the number of pairs is usually limited to 50 and 100 to eliminate longer-term changes in the interspike interval (Ekstedt, Nilsson, and Stålberg, 1974; Stålberg and Trontelj, 1979; Jablecki, 1978).

A simple manual method is to store 5 to 10 consecutive potential pairs, measure the range in the latency difference, and multiply this value by 0.37. The jitter values obtained by this calculation are very close to those obtained by automatic devices (see Figure 7.12).

Measurement of Jitter

Jitter is best expressed as the mean consecutive difference (MCD) in the latency between two time-locked spikes and is of the order of 5 to 50 μsec in normal muscle (see Figure 7.12) (Stålberg and Ekstedt, 1973). Between 27 and 30°C, jitter is linearly related to temperature, diminishing as the temperature increases. As might be expected, jitter is increased by neuromuscular blocking agents. Occasionally the jitter between two MF action potentials is very small (< 5 μsec), an observation that has been

Measurement of Fiber Density

In the extensor digitorum communis (EDC) muscle, the mean number of MF spikes per electrode recording site is less than two (1.4 to 1.5). This value increases beyond the sixth decade of life, and is increased especially in neurogenic disorders where sometimes many spikes are observed (Stålberg and Ekstedt, 1973; Stålberg, Schwartz, and Trontelj, 1975; Thiele and Stålberg, 1975; Schwartz, Stålberg, Schiller, and Thiele, 1976) The mean fiber density (FD) is also increased in many primary muscle diseases. Such increases result for the most part from the twin processes of denervation and reinnervation and the consequent grouping together of MFs innervated by the same MU. Such fiber grouping leads to an increase in the number of MFs innervated by the same motoneuron within the restricted pickup territory of the SF electrode.

Axonal Conduction

The presence of intramuscular axonal branching and sometimes conduction block in motor axons can be detected with the SF-EMG electrode (Stålberg and Ekstedt, 1973). Conduction block in axons is common in amyotrophic lateral sclerosis and other neurogenic disorders.

Single-fiber EMG has provided important new evidence about changes in the distribution of MFs in single MUs, neuromuscular transmission at single junctions, changes in axonal and MF conduction and axonal branching, and insights into changes in MUPs in peripheral nerve and muscle diseases.

The technique demands attention to recording technique, proper maintenance of the electrode, and experience in the use of the method in muscles and disease states. Electrodes and the appropriate instrumentation are now commercially available and should make this valuable technique much more generally practicable in EMG laboratories.

MACRO NEEDLE ELECTROMYOGRAPHY

The single-fiber EMG electrode is highly selective and reflects the activities of only those muscle fibers within the immediate vicinity of the recording electrode. Even the standard concentric needle electrode sees but a small proportion of the muscle fibers in the motor unit, at least with respect to the spike components of the MUP. What was needed in electromyography was a recording electrode that would more truly reflect the electrical activities of all the muscle fibers in the motor unit. To this end two types of recording electrodes have been employed. The first, the surface electrode was discussed in detail in Chapter 6. The second, the macro needle electrode, has only recently been introduced into electromyography (Stålberg and Trontelj, 1979; Lang and Falck, 1980; Stålberg, 1980, 1982, 1983; Stålberg and Fawcett, 1982) but already promises to make a very important contribution to the electromyographical analysis of peripheral nerve and muscle disease, particularly when combined with single fiber electromyography as well.

The macroelectrode consists of a modified single fiber EMG electrode in which the 25-μ recording surface is exposed in a side part of the cannula 7.5 mm back from the tip of the electrode (Stålberg, 1980, 1983). The cannula itself serves as the macro electrode. To ensure a standardized recording surface, the cannula is insulated to within 15 mm of the tip of the needle. Thus the single-fiber electrode is placed centrally in the macro electrode recording surface presented by the exposed distal 15 mm of the cannula. The single-fiber recording surface is thereby so placed that if the triggering muscle fiber is in the center of the motor unit, 7.5 mm of the macro recording surface being exposed on both sides of the recording site. In this position the macroelectrode surface is so placed as to span the transverse territories of most motor units in health and disease.

By adjusting the position of the electrode within the muscle, single-fiber potentials from different motor units may be selected and the associated macro MUPs obtained by electronically averaging the potentials recorded by the macroelectrode that are time locked to the single-fiber spike acting as the trigger source. Macro EMG potentials so obtained are more representative of all the muscle fibers in the motor unit than are conventional concentric needle electrode recordings because not only does the recording surface span a much larger part of the transverse territory of the motor unit, but there is relatively greater attenuation of the higher-frequency components generated by muscle fibers nearest to the electrode as compared to more distant generators compared to the case of the concentric and even more so, single-fiber electrode.

There is some indication that the fractionated appearance of some macro-recorded MUPs reflects the activities of subpopulations of muscle fibers innervated by branches of the motor axon within the muscle. Computer simulation studies (Nandedkar and Stålberg, 1983) suggest that the amplitude and area of the macro-recorded MUP is related to the number of muscle fibers in the motor unit. As might be expected, the amplitude of the macro MUP is highest near the end-plate zone where any temporal scatter in the firing times of the component muscle fibers would be mostly dependent on the spatial scatter of the end-plates. Moving further away from the end-plate zone, differences in the conduction velocities of the various muscle fibers in the motor unit could be expected to add to the temporal dispersion of single-fiber potentials in the motor unit. This probably explains the lower-amplitude of macro MUPs recorded at a distance away from the end-plate zone. Reinnervation could be expected to increase macro MUP amplitudes through increasing the number of muscle fibers in the motor unit, although the large size of the recording surface would make these potentials less dependent on whether the muscle fibers were grouped or distributed throughout the motor unit territory. Even so, the computer simulation studies suggest that for a given number of muscle fibers in the motor unit, the amplitude of the macro-recorded MUP is higher the more compact the territory of the motor unit is.

Macro EMG is a new technique whose values and limitations are presently being explored. The technique provides a much better measure of the electrical activity of the whole MU than any of the electromyographic techniques available today. It is most powerfully exploited when combined with single-fiber EMG that provides critical additional information about fiber density, terminal and preterminal axonal conduction and neuromuscular transmission within the motor unit.

AUTOMATIC AND SEMIAUTOMATIC ANALYSIS OF EMG ACTIVITY

Measurements of the values of individual MUPs and the complex patterns of EMG activity brought out by maximum contractions are valuable electrophysiological diagnostic tools in the assessment of peripheral nerve and muscle disease. The isolation and manual measurement of 10 to 20 independent MUPs in several muscles is tedious. Without such measurements and quantification, however, it is sometimes very hard to be certain whether or not abnormalities exist or whether the primary disorder is neurogenic or myogenic. The reasons for this are as follows:

1. There is a broad range of MUP durations and amplitudes even in normal muscles (Figures 7.13 and 7.14). This makes it impossible to base judgments on a few MUPs as to whether there have been changes in amplitude or duration. To establish clearly that there has been a change, there must be some statistical analysis of a large enough number of MUPs generated by separate and distinct MUs to make a significant statement about possible important departures from normal age-corrected values for the muscle being examined.

2. The number of polyphasic MUPs is sub-

FIGURE 7.13.   Range in durations and amplitudes of MUPs as recorded with a concentric needle electrode from the biceps. Note the truly wide range in amplitudes and durations of single MUPs in healthy muscle. (Recording bandwidth 2 to 10,000 Hz)
From Buchthal, Guld, and Rosenfalck (1954, figure 6).

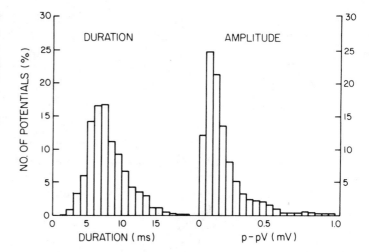

stantial even in healthy muscles (up to 10 percent).

3. There are no truly satisfactory ways manually to measure interference patterns; i.e., it is impossible to measure a mean amplitude or number of spikes properly by hand.

Therefore to address the problems and limitations in manual EMG analysis, several automatic methods have been introduced in the last 20 years as aids to the quantification and analysis of the electromyogram. The purposes of these methods include:

1. For single MUPs, the automatic measurement of MUP variables such as duration, amplitudes, number of phases, and rates of discharge (Bergmans, 1971; Lee and White, 1973)

2. For the interference patterns, measurement of the mean amplitudes, number of spikes, interspike intervals, etc. (Fitch and Willison, 1965; Hayward and Willison, 1973, 1977; Hayward, 1977; Fuglsang-Frederiksen, Scheel, and Buchthal, 1976, 1977)

Automatic Measurement of MUP Variables

Numerous methods and devices are available for the automatic measurement of several MUP variables. In all, selection of the MUs or MUPs is under the control of the operator, in that the operator selects the sites where recordings are made and in some methods, can choose which MUPs to include in the sample. The last point is important, because while there is no significant trend in the durations of MUPs in relation to recruitment order, the amplitudes of the higher-threshold MUs do tend to be higher even in needle electrode recordings, where in addition, the position of the leading-off surface of the electrode with respect to the spike sources in the MU is so critical.

Essential to any automatic analysis of MUPs are provision for MUP-triggered sweeps and an adequate delay in the signal to visualize the true onset of the potential. It also helps to have available a window discriminator so that the operator can select an MUP with a particular amplitude out of the background activities of others with amplitudes that may exceed or be below that of the target MUP. Mea-

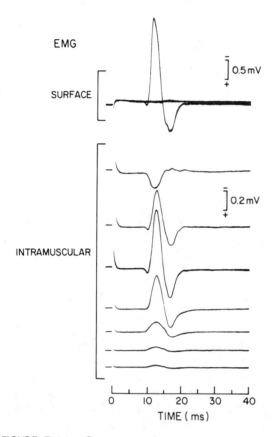

EMG

SURFACE

⌐
⌐ 0.5 mV
+

INTRAMUSCULAR

⌐
⌐ 0.2 mV
+

0   10   20   30   40

TIME (ms)

FIGURE 7.14.   Changes in the intramuscularly re-corded MUP as the electrode (in this case a standard concentric needle) is moved at 2-mm intervals trans-versely through the extensor digitorum brevis muscle while stimulating its parent motor axon just proximal to the ankle. Stimuli are so adjusted as to excite this one motor axon only (see all-or-nothing response as recorded with a surface electrode positioned near the innervation zone). Note that the shape and size of the intramuscularly recorded potential are heavily dependent on their position within the territory of the motor unit. The intramuscularly recorded MUP was detectable in this example over a transverse territory of 16 mm (not all recording sites shown here).

surements can be made of the first, second, or perhaps even third MUP recruited at each site before moving to another site in the mus-cle at least 10 mm or more distant (trans-versely) to avoid looking at potentials gener-ated by the same MUs, but as seen by the electrode still within the pickup territory of the electrode. In each muscle, at least 10 or, probably better, 20 MUPs can be isolated and measurements made of their main values prior to statistical analysis of these and comparison to control values for the same muscle, in the same decade of life, at more or less the same temperature, and as recorded by electrodes with the same electrical and physical charac-teristics.

Electronic averaging of operator-selected MUPs helps to reduce the background elec-tronic noise and the asynchronous activities of other MUPs. In so doing, it becomes much easier to measure the durations of the MUPs precisely and prepare the way for automatic measurement and statistical analysis of the potentials.

One of the major stumbling blocks to au-tomatic computer-assisted MUP measure-ments is the method by which onset and ter-mination times are identified in single MUPs. It was pointed out earlier that these parts of the potentials can be very indistinct and merge almost imperceptibly, with the baseline po-tential, sometimes over several milliseconds. Electronic averaging helps to resolve the MUPs better but does not solve the problem. To date, each method establishes arbitrary criteria as to what represents a significant de-parture from the baseline potential and hence onset or termination of potential (Bergmans, 1971, 1973, 1979; Lee and White, 1973; Ko-pec, Hausmanowa-Petrusewicz, Rawski, and Wolynski, 1973; Kopec and Hausmanowa-Pe-trusewicz, 1976). The threshold levels at which significant baseline departures are judged to have occurred has an important influence on the durations of the MUPs; the higher the threshold levels, the shorter the measured du-rations of the potentials. For this reason it is very helpful if provision is made for the print-out of all MUPs included in the calculation, together with indications on the potentials of precisely where the measurements were made.

Overall, the computer-assisted systems must be as easy to operate as possible because this is only one part of the whole EMG and should not take disproportionate amount of available time. The system must recognize that the operator's eyes are engaged by the visual monitor and that there is one hand on the needle electrode.

Several commercial devices are available that provide automatic analysis of MUP values (Kopec and Hausmanowa-Petrusewicz, 1976; Sica, McComas, and Ferreira, 1978). Results with these methods compare very well in precision with established manual measurements (Fuglsang-Frederiksen, Scheel, and Buchthal, 1976, 1977). The duration of MUPs obtained by the automatic techniques may not correspond to those established (Buchthal, 1957) with more traditional methods, however (Sica, McComas, and Ferreira, 1978).

Automatic Analysis of Interference Pattern (Method of Willison)

The method to be described provides an automatic analysis of the EMG interference patterns brought out by contractions against a standard load (Fitch and Willison, 1965; Hayward and Willison, 1973; Hayward, 1977), or which are 30 percent of the maximum tension the subject is able to generate (Fuglsang-Frederiksen, Scheel, and Buchthal, 1976). The EMG activity is recorded through intramuscular needle electrodes whose position in the muscle has been adjusted to where the amplitudes of the potentials are maximum. The interference patterns so recorded are functions of the number of MUs recruited, firing frequencies of the MUs, amplitudes as well as numbers of phases and durations of the MUPs recruited, and the positions of MFs belonging

to the various recruited MUs with respect to the needle electrode.

Analysis of the EMG involves the generation of two derived pulses, a frequency (or time) pulse and an amplitude pulse (Figure 7.15). The frequency or turns pulse is generated every time the EMG signal changes polarity by more than 100 μV, and the voltage pulse every time the potential level changes by 100 μV, whatever the direction. The numbers of respective turns and voltage pulses per unit time (usually 5 seconds) are counted, and values obtained for the numbers of turns per second and the mean voltage per turn.

In the healthy subject, there is little significant change in the turns count or voltage pulses with age, but there is an obvious increase in the numbers of turns and voltage with increasing load. Hence it is clearly important to standardize the force at which the calculations are carried out. This procedure has been used by others and compared with the traditional method of manual measurement of MUP amplitudes, durations, and numbers of phases in neurogenic and primary muscle diseases.

In primary muscle diseases, Fuglsang-Frederiksen, Scheel, and Buchthal (1976) reported that the most frequent abnormality was an increase in the ratio of the number of turns per unit amplitude at forces that were 30 percent of the maximum obtainable. False positive results were observed when the load was fixed at the same preset standard levels as used in controls. Other abnormalities included an increase in the number of turns per unit time at 30 percent force levels, an increase in the incidence of short time intervals between turns, and in most, an overall decline in the mean voltage (see Chapter 8). In myopathies, this basic pattern is explained by the need to recruit more MUs that must fire at higher frequencies to achieve a force equivalent to a normal muscle or a predetermined percentage of maximum force possible for the muscle(s).

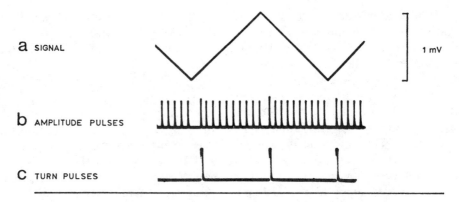

FIGURE 7.15.   Method of Fitch and Willison (1965) for quantifying the EMG activity
as recorded with a needle electrode in the muscle. Two pulse trains are derived
from the EMG. First, amplitude pulses are generated (b) whenever the signal, a
calibration signal here (a) changes by 0.1 mV, and turns pulses (c) are generated
every time the potential changes direction, changes in direction of less than 0.12
mV being ignored. The total counts of the two sets of impulses are then used to
derive the frequency of turn pulses or numbers of potentials per second, as well as
the mean amplitude of each potential in mV. The turns frequency and their mean
amplitude are increased by increasingly forceful contractions.
From Hayward and Willison (1973, figure 1).

The fact that many MUPs have multiple spike components adds to the number of turns counted. Overall, the incidence of abnormalities was about the same as the diagnostic yield from the conventional methods, although the results for some patients were normal with one test and abnormal with the other. It should be noted that in some patients who had primary muscle diseases, higher-amplitude MUPs were sometimes seen (Rose and Willison, 1967).

In neurogenic diseases (Hayward and Willison, 1977) the most characteristic abnormality was an increase in the mean amplitude without any change in the turns count. In these diseases the higher mean amplitude value probably results from the recruitment of MUPs of higher than normal amplitude. The increase in amplitude was greater, the weaker the muscle, although the increases were no greater in amyotrophic lateral sclerosis than in other neurogenic disorders. Fuglsang-Frederiksen, Scheel, and Buchthal (1976), again using forces that were 30 percent of the maximum, observed the same increase in the mean amplitude but also noted an increase in the incidence of long intervals between turns and a reduction in the number of turns at 30 percent force levels compared to normal. The prolonged MUP durations at lower intramuscular temperatures were associated with reductions in the number of turns. By analogy, the lower turn counts in neurogenic disease could be a product of the prolonged MUP durations so characteristic of the diseases.

Willison's method has important advantages and some disadvantages. It does provide for reproducible measurements derived from the EMG that are at least as sensitive as the equivalent cumbersome manual measurements of single MUP values and interference patterns that demand a lot more time to make the same distinction, namely, to distinguish between neurogenic and myogenic diseases. The method provides reproducible figures that are of diagnostic value, but it is sometimes not clear how these figures relate to actual changes in the MU numbers, the MUPs, or the firing frequencies of the MUs. Also, it is not applicable to more than a few readily tested muscles such as the biceps, triceps, or foot dorsiflexors, and represents a detailed analysis of the electromyographic patterns recorded from the very limited pickup territories recordable by intramuscular electrodes. Differences in these patterns in different parts of the muscle could exist, and the observed recruitment patterns may not be directly related to the measured forces of contraction. For the latter, the electromyographer would have to exclude the contributions of synergistic muscles. Overall, the method seems to be worthwhile, practical, quantitative for distinguishing the three main categories of MUPs, namely, normal, neurogenic, and primary muscle diseases. More experience is needed in various diseases, however, and at different stages of these diseases before the value of the technique can be properly assessed.

Semiautomatic methods have the potential of greatly increasing the accuracy of EMG analysis in service laboratories. There, many have found the conventional manual methods too time consuming and tedious for day-to-day work and have therefore opted for the easier but much less accurate and potentially very biased method of simply "eyeballing" the free-running EMG activity or MUP-triggered traces. There has as yet been no agreement about selection criteria for MUPs or the best methods to measure their values. Moreover, there is no broad experience with these methods in certain disease states, and few comparative studies have been conducted regarding the relative accuracies of the methods, each originator tending to market his own.

For the present therefore, it is probably ad-visable to wait until the issue is better resolved before investing in the expenses these methods entail. The methods also create an important communication problem, because the values of MUPs and interference patterns obtained by the different techniques cannot be directly compared to well-established values for these same muscles obtained by the original manual measurements. This makes it harder for laboratories to compare observations and communicate their results. In contradistinction to the automatic or semiautomatic analytical methods applied to concentric needle electromyography, the automatic devices designed to measure jitter and fiber density are of undoubted help and do not suffer from the same problems.

References

Adrian ED, Bronk DV. Discharge of impulses in motor nerve fibers. J Physiol 1929;67:119–51.

Andreassen S, Rosenfalck A. Recording from a single motor unit during strong effort. IEEE Trans Biomed Eng 1978;25:501–8.

Basmajian JV. Electrodes and electrode connectors. In: Desmedt JE, ed. New developments in electromyography and clinical neurophysiology. Basel: Karger, 1973:502–10.

Bergmans J. Computer-assisted measurement of the parameters of single motor unit potentials in human electromyography. In: Desmedt JE, ed. New developments in electromyography and clinical neurophysiology. Basel: Karger, 1973:482–88.

Bergmans J. On the practical feasibility of automatic analysis of single motor unit potential parameters with computer assistance. Acta Neurol Scand 1979;73(suppl):307.

Bergmans J. Computer-assisted on-line measurement of motor unit potential parameters in human electromyography. Electromyography 1971;11:161–81.

Bigland B, Lippold OCJ. Motor unit activity in the voluntary contraction of human muscle. J Physiol 1954a;125:322–35.

Bigland B, Lippold OCJ. The relation between force, velocity and integrated electrical activity in human muscles. J Physiol 1954b;123:214–24.

Brandstater ME, Lambert EH. A histochemical study of the spatial arrangement of muscle fibers in single motor units within rat tibialis anterior muscle. Bull Am Assoc Electromyogr Electrodiagn 1969;82:15–16.

Brandstater ME, Lambert EH. Motor unit anatomy. In: Desmedt JE, ed. New developments in electromyography and clinical neurophysiology. Basel: Karger, 1973:14–22.

Buchthal F. An introduction to electromyography. Oslo: JW Cappelen, 1957.

Buchthal, F. The general concept of the motor unit. Publ Assoc Nerv Ment Dis 1961;38:28–30.

Buchthal F. Diagnostic significance of the myopathic EMG. In: Rowland LP, ed. Pathogenesis of human muscular dystrophies. Proceedings of the Fifth International Scientific Conference of the Muscular Dystrophy Association, Durango, Colorado. Amsterdam, Oxford: Excerpta Medica, 1977:205–18.

Buchthal F. Fibrillations: clinical electrophysiology. In: Culp WJ, Ochoa J, eds. Abnormal nerves and muscles as impulse generators. New York: Oxford University Press, 1982:632–62.

Buchthal F, Erminio F, Rosenfalck P. Motor unit territory in different human muscles. Acta Physiol Scand 1959;45:72–87.

Buchthal F, Guld C, Rosenfalck P. Action potential parameter in normal human muscle and their dependence on physical variables. Acta Physiol Scand 1954;32:200–18.

Buchthal F, Guld C, Rosenfalck P. Multielectrode study of the territory of a motor unit. Acta Physiol Scand 1957a;39:83–104.

Buchthal F, Guld C, Rosenfalck P. Volume conduction of the spike of the motor unit potential investigated with a new type of multielectrode. Acta Physiol Scand 1957b;38:331–54.

Buchthal F, Pinelli P, Rosenfalck P. Action potential parameters in normal human muscle and their physiological determinants. Acta Physiol Scand 1954;32:219–29.

Buchthal F, Rosenfalck P. On the structure of motor units. In: Desmedt JE, ed. New developments in electromyography and clinical neurophysiology. Basel: Karger, 1973:71–85.

Butler BP, Ball RD, Albers JW. Effect of electrode type and position on motor unit action potential configuration. Muscle Nerve 1982;5:S95–S97.

Doyle AM, Mayer R. Studies of motor units in the cat. Bull Sch Med Univ Maryland 1969;54:11–17.

Edström L, Kugelberg E. Histochemical composition, distribution of fibers and fatigability of single motor units. J Neurol Neurosurg Psychiatry 1968;31:424–33.

Ekstedt J. Human single muscle fiber action potentials. Acta Physiol Scand 1964;61(suppl 226):1–96.

Ekstedt J, Nilsson G, Stålberg E. Calculation of the electromyographic jitter. J Neurol Neurosurg Psychiatry 1974;37:526–39.

Fitch P, Willison RG. Automatic measurement of the human electromyogram. J Physiol 1965;178:28–29P.

Fuglsang-Frederiksen A, Scheel U, Buchthal F. Diagnostic yield of analysis of the pattern of electrical activity and of individual motor unit potentials in myopathy. J Neurol Neurosurg Psychiatry 1976;39:742–50.

Fuglsang-Frederiksen A, Scheel U, Buchthal F. Diagnostic yield of the analysis of the pattern of electrical activity of muscle and of individual motor unit potentials in neurogenic involvement. J Neurol Neurosurg Psychiatry 1977;40:544–54.

Gath I, Stålberg E. Techniques for improving selectivity of electromyographic recordings. IEEE Trans Biomed Eng 1976;23:467–72.

Gath I, Stålberg E. The calculated radial decline of the extracellular action potential compared with in situ measurements in the human brachial biceps. Electroencephalogr Clin Neurophysiol 1978a;44:547–52.

Gath I, Stålberg E. On the volume conduction in human skeletal muscle: in situ measurements. Electroencephalogr Clin Neurophysiol 1978b;43:106–10.

Hannerz J. Discharge properties of motor units in relation to recruitment order in voluntary contraction. Acta Physiol Scand 1974a;81:374–84.

Hannerz J. An electrode for recording single motor unit activity during strong muscle contractions. Electroencephalogr Clin Neurophysiol 1974b;37:179–81.

Hayward M. Automatic analysis of the electromyogram in healthy subjects of different ages. J Neurol Sci 1977;33:397–414.

Hayward M, Willison RG. The recognition of myogenic and neurogenic lesions by quantitative EMG. In: Desmedt JE, ed. New developments in electromyography and clinical neurophysiology. Basel: Karger, 1973:448–53.

Hayward M, Willison RG. Automatic analysis of the electromyogram in patients with chronic partial denervation. J Neurol Sci 1977;33:415–23.

Jablecki CK. Single-fiber electromyography. Minimonograph 6. Rochester, Minn.: American Association of Electromyography and Electrodiagnosis, 1978.

Katz B, Miledi R. Propagation of electric activity in motor nerve terminals. Proc R Soc Biol 1964;161:453–82.

Kopec J, Hausmanowa-Petrusewicz I. On-line computer application in clinical quantitative electromyography. Electromyogr Clin Neurophysiol 1976;16:49–64.

Kopec J, Hausmanowa-Petrusewicz I, Rawski M, Wolynski M. Automatic analysis in electromyography. In: Desmedt JE, ed. New developments in electromyography and clinical neurophysiology. Basel: Karger, 1973:477–81.

Krnjevic K, Miledi R. Motor units in the rat diaphragm. J Physiol (Lond) 1958;140:427–39.

Kugelberg E. Properties of the rat hind-limb motor units. In: Desmedt JE, ed. New developments in electromyography and clinical neurophysiology. Basel: Karger, 1973:2–13.

Lang AH, Falck B. A two-channel method for sampling averaging and quantifying motor unit potentials. J Neurol 1980;223:199–206.

Lee RG, White DG. Computer analysis of motor unit action potentials in routine clinical electromyography. In: Desmedt JE, ed. New developments in electromyography and clinical neurophysiology. Basel: Karger, 1973:454–61.

Libkind MS. II Modelling of interference bioelectrical activity. Biophysics 1968;13:811–21.

Libkind MS. III Modelling of interference bioelectrical activity. Biophysics 1969;14:395–98.

Libkind MS. IV Modelling of interference bioelectrical activity. Biophysics 1972a;17:124–30.

Libkind MS. V Modelling of interference bioelectrical activity Biophysics 1972b;17:130–37.

Lippold OCJ. The relationship between integrated

action potentials in a human muscle and its isometric tension. J Physiol (Lond) 1952;117:492–99.

Milner-Brown HS, Stein RB. The relation between the surface electromyogram and muscular force. J Physiol 1975;246:549–69.

Nandedkar S, Stålberg E. Simulation of macro EMG motor unit potentials. Electroencephalogr Clin Neurophysiol 1983;56:52–62.

Nandedkar S, Stålberg E. Simulation of single muscle fibre action potentials. Med Biol Eng Comput 1983;21:158–165.

Pollak V. The waveshape of action potentials recorded with different types of electromyographic needles. Med Biol Eng 1971;9:657–64.

Rose AL, Willison RG. Quantitative electromyography using automatic analysis. Studies in healthy subjects and patients with primary muscle disease. J Neurol Neurosurg Psychiatry 1967;30:403–10.

Rosenfalck P. Intra- and extracellular potential fields of active nerve and muscle fibres. Acta Physiol Scand 1969;75(suppl 321):1–168.

Rosenfalck P, Buchthal F. On the concept of the motor subunit. Int J Neurosci 1970;1:27–37.

Sacco G, Buchthal F, Rosenfalck P. Motor unit potentials at different ages. Arch Neurol 1962;6:44–51.

Schwartz MS, Stålberg E, Schiller HH, Thiele B. The reinnervated motor unit in man. A single-fibre EMG multielectrode investigation. J Neurol Sci 1976;27:303–12.

Sica REP, McComas AJ, Ferreira JCD. Evaluation of an automatic method for analysing the electromyogram. Can J Neurol Sci 1978;5:275–81.

Stålberg E. Propagation velocity in human muscle fibres in situ. Acta Physiol Scand 1966;70(suppl 287):1–112.

Stålberg E. Macro EMG, a new recording technique. J Neurol Neurosurg Psychiatry 1980;43:475–82.

Stålberg E. Macro-electromyography in reinnervation. Muscle Nerve 1982;5:S135–38.

Stålberg E. Recent techniques and current practical electromyography. In: Serratruce G, Gastraut JL, Pouget J, eds. Electromyography seminar, Marseilles, France, 1982.

Stålberg EV. Macro EMG. Minimonograph 20.

Rochester, Minn.: American Association of Electromyography and Electrodiagnosis, 1983.

Stålberg E, Antoni L. Electrophysiological cross section of the motor unit. J Neurol Neurosurg Psychiatry 1980;43:469–74.

Stålberg E, Antoni L. Computer-aided electromyography. In: Desmedt JE, ed. Progress in Clinical Neurophysiology. Basel: Karger, 1983;10:186–240.

Stålberg E, Ekstedt J. Single-fibre EMG and microphysiology of the motor unit in normal and diseased muscle. In: Desmedt JE, ed. New developments in electromyography and clinical neurophysiology. Basel: Karger, 1973:113–29.

Stålberg E, Fawcett PRW. Macro EMG in healthy subjects of different ages. J Neurol Neurosurg Psychiatry 1982;45:870–78.

Stålberg E, Schwartz MS, Thiele B, Schiller HH. The normal motor unit in man. A single-fibre EMG multielectrode investigation. J Neurol Sci 1976;27:291–301.

Stålberg E, Schwartz MS, Trontelj JV. Single-fibre electromyography in various processes affecting the anterior horn cell. J Neurol Sci 1975;24:403–15.

Stålberg E, Trontelj JV. Single-fibre electromyography. Surrey, England: Mirvalle Press, 1979.

Thiele B, Stålberg E. Single-fibre EMG findings in polyneuropathies of different aetiology. J Neurol Neurosurg Psychiatry 1975;38:881–87.

8 NEEDLE ELECTROMYOGRAPHIC ABNORMALITIES IN NEUROGENIC AND MUSCLE DISEASES

Several variables of motor unit potentials (MUPs) including their amplitudes, durations and numbers of phases as well as the interference patterns brought out in maximum muscle contractions have been used to distinguish between primary neurogenic and muscle diseases (Kugelberg, 1947, 1949; Buchthal, 1957, 1970) (Figures 8.1 and 8.2). In making such distinctions, it is well to remember that there is a wide range in the amplitudes and durations of MUPs even in normal subjects (see Chapter 7). Both values are influenced by alterations in muscle and temperature and by increasing age.

Therefore, to establish whether or not MUPs are normal, muscles should be warm (>34°C), measurements made of at least 20 MUPs recorded at at least 10 or more separate sites per muscle, and the values compared to age-matched control values. This is easier said than done, because two or more MUPs recorded at separate sites in the muscle could have the same motor unit (MU) source unless the recording sites are at least 10 to 20 mm apart. Even here the MU source could be the same unless simultaneous macro or surface electromyographic (EMG) recordings are done to exclude this possibility.

Manual measurement of the characteristics of as many as 10 to 20 separate MUPs per muscle is a tedious task and because of this, is not done by most electromyographers. Short of such quantification, however, it is impossible sometimes to know whether or not the amplitudes and durations of MUPs are normal. The observation of occasional complex MUPs is of little value because as many as 3 to 10 percent (up to 25 percent in deltoid; Buchthal, 1977) of intramuscular MUPs in control limb muscles have more than four phases. Moreover, without coherent EMG techniques it is hard to visualize in a constant manner the whole MUP and in particular to recognize linked potentials (Figure 8.3). For these reasons there is a real need to adopt coherent techniques in combination with am-

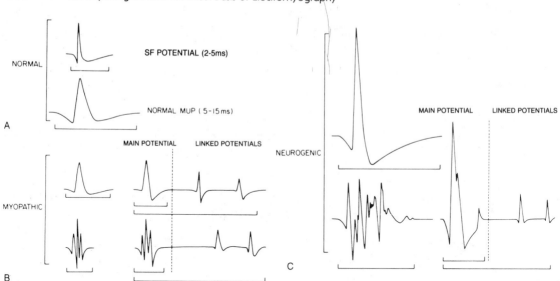

FIGURE 8.1.   General pattern of changes in MUPs as recorded with a standard concentric needle electrode in primary muscle and neurogenic diseases (B and C) in comparison to normal single muscle fiber and MUPs (A). Single muscle fiber action (SF) potentials are smooth biphasic and triphasic potentials with durations between 2 to 5 ms. In normal muscles, the range in durations of single motor unit action potentials (MUP) is wide (5 to 15 ms) and depends on the muscle, the age of the subject, and the temperature of the muscle (see Figure 7.8). Most motor unit action potentials are biphasic and triphasic, fewer than 10 percent possessing more than four phases. Other potentials separated by an interval from the main potential but obviously time locked to the latter are called linked potentials.

In most instances of primary diseases of muscle (B) there is an increase in the proportion of shorter duration motor unit action potentials, many of which are composed of multiple spike components and more than four phases. In other instances, the duration and shape of the motor unit action potentials suggest that the potential may be generated by a single muscle fiber only within the pickup territory of the recording electrode. Other muscle fibers belonging to the same motor unit are possibly distant or too weak a voltage source (possibly their diameters are too small) to be detected.

Despite the shorter mean duration of the main motor unit action potential complex, many such potentials are linked to other action potentials that precede or follow the main potential by an appreciable interval. In some such instances the overall duration (main and linked components combined) or the motor action potential may be very prolonged (30 to 60 ms), as has been reported in Duchenne dystrophy.

In neurogenic disease (C) there is usually an increase in the proportion of longer-duration motor unit action potentials, many of whose amplitudes are increased as well. Also, as in myopathic disorders, linked potentials are common.

In both neurogenic and primary muscle diseases, changes in the shape of the main potentials as well as fluctuations in latency and blocking of spike components in the main action potential or its linked components are probable indications of reduced safety factors for neuromuscular transmission, blocking of neuromuscular transmission, or blocking of impulses in presynaptic axons. The longer latencies of the linked components are indications of slowed conduction in immature axon collaterals or small-diameter muscle fibers or both, as well as possibly increased spatial scatter of the end-plates.

The relatively low amplitudes of many of the longer-latency linked action potentials possibly indicate that these potentials are generated by muscle fibers whose diameters are reduced through immaturity or some degenerative process.

The durations of the whole motor unit potential, or, in the case of those motor unit potentials with linked potentials, the main potential, are indicated by the horizontal brackets.

FIGURE 8.2. Histogram of motor unit action potential durations as recorded with a concentric needle electrode in a normal subject (right) and a patient with polymyositis (left). Note the preponderance of shorter-duration MUPs in polymyositis but also the wide range of durations even in the normal (2 to 17 ms).
Redrawn from Buchthal and Pinelli (1953, figure 1).

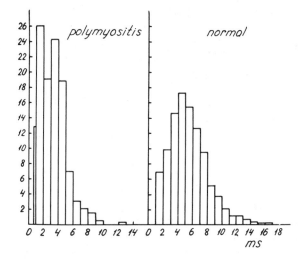

plitude discrimination to help the operator to visualize and select MUPs, automatic or semi-automatic devices to measure the numbers of phases (baseline crossings), durations, and amplitudes of these MUPs, as well as the means to analyze the significance of any apparent departures from normal values established for the particular type of electrode and

recording technique employed, muscle selected, and age of the subject.

Even when care is taken to measure and quantify the MUP values, sometimes it is just not possible on the basis of needle electromyographic examination alone to distinguish primary muscle disease from neurogenic diseases. This problem is especially true in the

FIGURE 8.3. Motor unit action potential from the deltoid muscle of a patient with Duchenne muscular dystrophy. The recording was made by means of a standard concentric needle electrode. (A) A free-running oscilloscope sweep was used and the links between the three potentials are not readily appreciated. (B) and (C) The first spike in the potential complex served to trigger the oscilloscope and the complex was delayed, enabling the examiner to see all three spike components, which are now clearly seen as components of one whole potential, the intercomponent intervals being quite constant. Before (C) and (D), the electrode was slightly rotated, this action attenuating the second component, while altering very little the size or shape of the first and third components. From Desmedt and Borenstein (1976, figure 2).

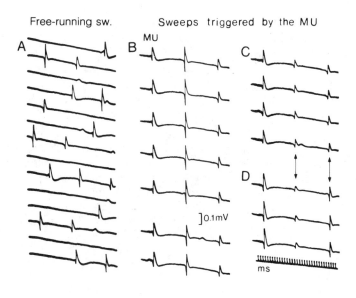

late stages of primary muscle diseases and in those muscle diseases where recurrent cycles of denervation and reinnervation are prominent epiphenomena. Despite the latter reservation, in most situations it is possible to make distinctions between neurogenic and primary muscle diseases. To this end, certain abnormalities in the needle electromyographic patterns have become established as pointing to a primary muscle disease (Figures 8.1, 8.2, 8.3 and 8.4). These are shown in Table 8.1. (For review see Buchthal, 1977; Stålberg and

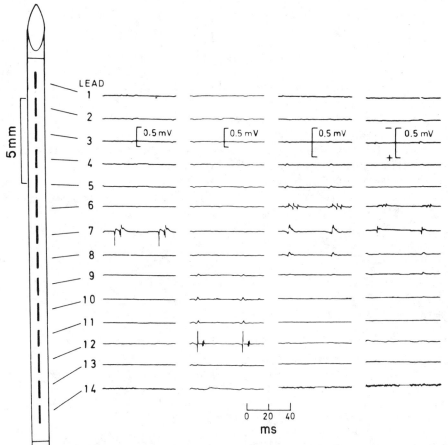

FIGURE 8.4. Territories of four motor unit action potentials from a patient with Duchenne muscular dystrophy as recorded with a multielectrode similar to that in Figure 5.6. Note that the transverse territories of these potentials are much smaller compared to those of motor unit action potentials in amyotrophic lateral sclerosis. The amplitudes of the Duchenne motor unit action potentials were also comparatively smaller. In most instances the Duchenne potentials consist of multiple distinct spikes, and in all four instances, two successive discharges of the motor unit potentials are seen.
From Buchthal (1977, figure 6).

TABLE 8.1.   Needle Electromyographic
Changes in Muscle Disease

Individual MUPs
*Shorter mean MUP duration (Figures 8.1 and 8.2)
   (excludes MUPs with linked potentials)
Reductions in MUP amplitude (Figures 8.1, 8.3, 8.4,
   8.5)
  Criterion unreliable
  Sometimes amplitudes increased
*Increased incidence of early or late linked
   potentials (Figures 8.1, 8.3, 8.4)
  (Seen in both neurogenic and muscle diseases)
SF-EMG changes
  Increased jitter
  Increased incidence of neuromuscular blocking
  Decreased jitter (?fiber splitting)
  Increased fiber density
MU territory
  Reductions in MU territory (multielectrode
   recordings) (Figures 8.4, 8.5)
Macro EMG
  Reduced amplitudes (and areas) of MUPs
  Increased proportion of fractionated-appearing
   MUPs
Abnormal spontaneous activity
  Fibrillation potentials
   Sometimes in dystrophies
   Most common in polymyositis
  Positive sharp waves
   Sometimes in dystrophies
   Most common in polymyositis
  Bizarre high-frequency discharges
   Nonspecific
   True myotonia (see Chapter 9)
Recruitment changes
  *Complete (+/− lower amplitudes) recruitment
   pattern in weak or wasted muscle (Figure
   8.6)
  May be reduced recruitment in very late stages
  Automatic analysis—recruitment (30 percent
   maximum force)
   Increase in number of turns
   Increase in ratio of turns to mean amplitude
   Increase in incidence of short time intervals
    between turns

---

*Most important.

Trontelj, 1979; Warmolts and Wiechers, 1980; Hayward, 1980; Ludin, 1980; Swash and Schwartz, 1981; Buchthal and Kamieniecka, 1982).

The amplitude of the main spike component(s) of the MUP depends on the numbers and diameters of muscle fibers that are within the immediate spike pickup territory of the electrode (diameter <1 mm). On the other hand, the duration of an MUP is controlled by the larger number of muscle fibers belonging to the MU whose potentials just exceed the detection limits of the recording electrode and system (Rosenfalck, 1969). Of all the variables of individual MUPs, shorter durations are the best criteria of a myopathy (Kugelberg, 1949; Buchthal and Pinelli, 1953; Buchthal, 1977; Hayward, 1980; Buchthal and Kamieniecka, 1982), amplitude being of much less value because it is so dependent on the distance between the electrode and the muscle fibers (Rosenfalck, 1969).

In normal muscle the longitudinal and transverse scatter of end-plates in each MU is probably the main reason behind the observation that MUPs exceed by 3 to 10 times the duration of single muscle fiber potentials (see Chapter 7).

Differences among the conduction velocities of muscle fibers belonging to the same MU and within the pickup territory of the electrode would also contribute to the longer duration of the MUP compared to a single fiber potential. The wider the range of their conduction velocities, the more temporal dispersion would be expected in the compound sum of their single fiber potentials to make the MUP. This last factor is probably more important in myopathies where there is a wider scatter in the diameter of muscle fibers. Differences among the conduction velocities of muscle fibers in the MU would also tend to increase progressively the MUP duration as the longitudinal distance was increased between the innervation zone and the recording site.

The characteristically shorter durations of MUPs in myopathies is best explained by a random loss of muscle fibers from MUs (Buchthal, 1977) (see Figures 8.1, 8.2, and 8.9). Because the duration of MUPs depends on those muscle fibers whose action potentials are the most widely separated in time and that exceed detection limits of the recording system, random losses of muscle fibers must at some point include some of those muscle fibers, which through wide separation of their end-plates in the MU or possibly differences between their conduction velocity, govern MU duration. This simple model readily explains the reductions in MU territories, reduced amplitudes of MUPs within those territories (Buchthal, Rosenfalck, and Erminio, 1960), and reduction in mean MUP duration.

The matter is not, however, as simple as the model implies, because the increased variations among the diameters of muscle fibers as is characteristic of myopathies (Swash and Schwartz, 1981) might be expected to increase the degree of temporal dispersion among single fiber potentials in the MU. Furthermore, such a simple model of random fiber loss alone would predict a reduction in fiber density (FD), not the increases in FD so characteristic in single-fiber (SF) EMG recordings in many of the muscular dystrophies (Stålberg, Trontelj, and Janko, 1974; Stålberg and Trontelj, 1979). One other hypothesis sometimes mentioned to explain the shorter MUP duration is that the spatial extent of MU territories is reduced through the muscle atrophy in myopathic diseases, muscle fibers sharing the same innervation coming to lie closer to one another. While this could indeed bring the muscle fibers belonging to individual MUs nearer together, it would not alter any temporal dispersion through differences among the conduction velocities of the muscle fibers or through the longitudinal scatter of their end-plates.

Recent macro EMG studies have shown that in myopathies increased numbers of lower amplitude MUPs are found. In addition, some of the MUPs have a more fractionated appearance. The increased fiber density so commonly seen in single-fiber EMG recordings in the face of normal or reduced macro EMG-recorded MUPs is quite in keeping with the twin concepts of a general fall out of muscle fibers from the motor unit accounting for the reduced macro EMG MUP and splitting of muscle fibers and reinnervation of regenerated muscle fibers in some regions of the motor unit accounting for the increased fiber densities seen with single-fiber EMG recordings.

Polyphasic potentials (more than four phases) make up to 2 to 10 percent (sometimes even higher in muscles such as the deltoid) of MUPs in control muscles. These percentages are much higher in the muscular dystrophies, congenital myopathies, and polymyositis (Buchthal, 1977) (Figures 8.1, 8.4, and 8.5). Some of these polyphasic potentials are examples of so-called linked potentials where there are often appreciable intervals (>5 ms) between the main and the linked potentials or among linked potentials.

The shorter-duration polyphasic potentials (those without linked components) probably result from random losses of muscle fibers or an increase in temporal dispersion among their respective potentials or both. The simple shape of the main spike of most MUPs depends on the near synchronous sum of 2 to 20 individual muscle fiber potentials. Loss of muscle fibers, especially if there is any degree of temporal dispersion introduced through increased differences among the conduction velocities of the muscle fibers or end-plate scatter, would tend to desynchronize the sum of the contributing potentials and increase the number of phases.

The very long-duration polyphasic potentials (usually with linked components) are common in muscle diseases (Desmedt and

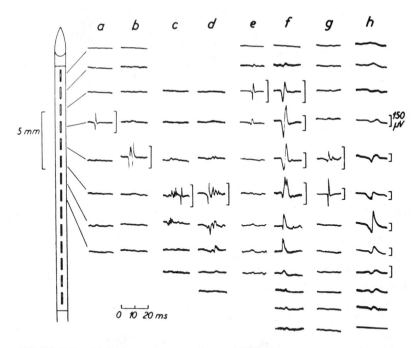

FIGURE 8.5. Multielectrode recordings of MUPs in various types of primary muscle diseases to illustrate the often polyspike—(a), (e), and (g)—character and sometimes short durations of such motor unit action potentials as well as the reduced transverse territories of many of these myopathic motor unit action potentials. The recording in (h) is from a normal subject, while those in (a) and (b) are from Duchenne muscles, (c) and (d) from limb girdle dystrophic muscles, (e) and (f) from patients with facioscapulohumeral type of dystrophy, and (g) from a patient with myotonic dystrophy. The multielectrode used was similar to that used in Figures 5.6 and 8.4. From Buchthal, Rosenfalck, and Erminio (1960, figure 2).

Borenstein, 1974; Buchthal, 1977). Such linked components could come about in some instances by fiber splitting and the perhaps very unequal conduction velocities of the split components or, probably more often, through collateral axon sprouts of unequal length, diameter, or degree of myelination. Where the conduction velocity of the axon sprouts or their muscle fibers is different from others in the MU or where their end-plates are widely separate, time intervals between the main potential and linked potentials may be appreciable.

As in neurogenic disease where collateralization takes place, jitter is most abnormal and the incidence of neuromuscular blocking is most common in those components separated from the main potential by the longest time intervals. This suggests that these collaterals and their end-plates and muscle fibers are the most immature. This concept is supported perhaps by their usually lower amplitudes, suggesting that they were generated by smaller-diameter muscle fibers. Sometimes the linked potential precedes the main potential.

In muscle diseases, the tensions that individual MUs can generate could be reduced through possible uncouplings between electrical and mechanical events in the muscle, changes in or losses of contractile elements, or actual losses of some muscle fibers in the

MUs. To generate the requisite level of tension, subjects would have to recruit more MUs and increase the rates of discharge of these MUs. These two mechanisms taken together with the high incidence of complex MUPs in muscle disease combine to explain the complex interference patterns seen in weak contractions (Figure 8.6).

FIGURE 8.6.   Interference patterns as recorded by a standard concentric needle electrode in the course of a maximum voluntary contraction. Recordings were made from the biceps brachii muscle of a patient with polymyositis (top), a normal subject (bottom), and from the tibialis anterior in a patient with an L5 root entrapment (middle).

In the normal subject, the number of spikes per unit time is a function of the numbers of motor units recruited that generate potential spikes within the pickup territory of the electrode and the firing frequency of these motor unit action potentials.

In the patient with polymyositis, the peak amplitude of the action potential was reduced, but the number of spike components was similar and in other similarly affected muscles even increased despite obvious weakness because of the recruitment of polyphasic (polyspike) motor unit action potentials.

In the case of L5 root entrapment, despite a maximum effort, a reduced number of motor unit action potentials was recruited, producing the less spiky appearance of the interference pattern compared to normal. Such incomplete recruitment patterns may be the result of conduction block in some of the motor axons, degeneration of some motoneurons or their axons, an apparent loss of motor unit action potentials through fiber grouping with a reduced overlap between adjacent motor unit territories, a possible relative increase in the proportion of higher-threshold motor units within the pickup territory of the electrode, a central motor disorder impairing recruitment, or simply lack of effort on the part of the subject.

Increases in mean or peak amplitude of the interference pattern may indicate increased amplitude of the component MUPs and hence increased fiber densities and possibly fiber hypertrophy (see text).

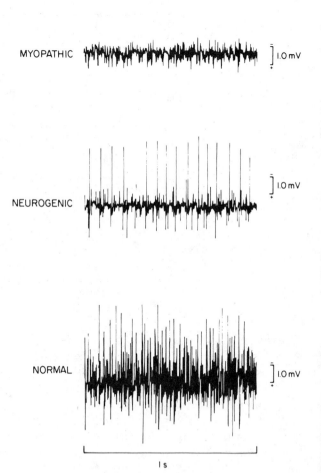

Fibrillation potentials that are sometimes seen in these diseases are explicable in some situations at least, by necrosis or degeneration of segments of muscle fibers in such a way as to separate viable segments of muscle fibers from their original innervation.

Ectopic impulse generation and ephaptic transmission between muscle fibers or split portions of muscle fibers could account for the other examples of abnormal spontaneous activity such as the bizarre repetitive discharges (BRD) sometimes seen in these diseases. The BRD that are especially common in polymyositis and Duchenne dystrophy are seen in neurogenic disorders as well. Fiber splitting is not confined to muscle diseases, but is seen in neurogenic disease and in normal subjects near tendinous insertions and especially in bipennate muscles (Swash and Schwartz, 1981). The myotonic phenomenon is discussed in Chapter 9.

The preceding classic alterations in the values of single MUPs and MU recruitment, although characteristic of most muscle diseases, are not seen in all muscle diseases or at all stages in the evolution of these diseases. For example, in advanced stages, the number of detectable independent MUPs is sometimes much fewer than normal, and the interference patterns are consequently incomplete despite a maximum contraction. Indeed, at the near terminal stages of involvement of a muscle, there may be electrical silence in the muscle.

In the later stages of polymyositis or sometimes in the muscular dystrophies, amplitudes of some of the remaining MUPs can be increased and their durations longer than normal. These "neurogenic-looking" MUPs could develop through the tendencies toward clustering together of muscle fibers innervated by the same motoneuron, in turn a product of reinnervation and the subsequent progressive maturation of these MUPs as the active disease progresses (Pinelli and Buchthal, 1953; Heathfield and Williams, 1960; Campbell,

1961; Mechler, 1974; Swash and Schwartz, 1981).

Even in the intermediate stages of some muscle diseases, electromyographic patterns may not be typical of the so-called myopathic pattern. For example, in limb girdle and facioscapulohumeral dystrophies, MU territories may be in the normal range, the amplitudes of their MUPs normal or even increased, and their MUP durations in the normal range (Buchthal, Rosenfalck, and Erminio, 1960). In this respect it is of interest that at least in some cases of limb girdle dystrophy there is evidence of motoneuron loss (Tomlinson, Walton, and Irving, 1974).

Short-duration MUPs are not exclusive to the preceding primary muscle diseases but may be seen in other disorders as well. Examples include:

1. Disorders of neuromuscular transmission. In the Lambert-Eaton syndrome and myasthenia gravis, neuromuscular block at some proportion of the neuromuscular junctions in each MU could explain the lower amplitudes and shorter durations sometimes seen in MUPs.
2. Periodic paralysis. In these disorders some of the muscle fibers may be inexcitable and hence incapable of contributing their action potentials to the whole MUP.
3. Earliest stages of reinnervation of a muscle following transection of the motor nerve. In the early period of reinnervation, the MUPs are characteristically low in amplitude and short in duration. This is explained by the as yet very low innervation ratios of MUs and the presence of immature neuromuscular junctions at which transmission may block intermittently. Shortly thereafter, as the innervation ratios increase, MUP durations increase, sometimes to values many times normal because of the wide temporal dispersion in the discharges of the compo-

nent muscle fibers, which in turn is primarily a result of the very slow conduction velocities in the as yet immature and poorly myelinated presynaptic axons.

Overall, EMG techniques do provide accurate means by which to distinguish between primary neurogenic and muscle diseases. The most reliable EMG predictors of muscle disease are shortening of the mean MUP duration and complete but lower-amplitude recruitment patterns, especially in weak or wasted muscles. When taken together with the observation of increases in the number of turns, ratio of turns to mean amplitude, in the incidence of short time intervals between turns in contractions (30 percent of maximum force), these classic abnormalities correlate very well with histologic evidence of a primary muscle disease (Fuglsang-Frederiksen, Scheel, and Buchthal, 1976; Hayward, 1980; Buchthal and Kamieniecka, 1982; see also Chapter 7).

NEEDLE EMG CHANGES IN NEUROGENIC DISEASE

The main needle electromyographic characteristics of neurogenic disorders are shown in Table 8.2.

Degeneration of motoneurons or their motor axons and the subsequent processes of collateralization and reinnervation change the innervation patterns of single MUs in muscle. From a random pattern in which the territories of as many as 10 or more MUs overlap (Kugelberg, 1973; Brandstater and Lambert, 1973; Buchthal and Rosenfalck, 1973) there develop strong tendencies toward the grouping together of muscle fibers that belong to the same MU (Karpati and Engel, 1968; Morris and Woolf, 1970; Kugelberg, Edstrom, and Abbruzzese, 1970) and less overlap between adjacent territories. In some instances there could be changes in the overall number of muscle fibers per MU (innervation ratio). The

TABLE 8.2.   Needle Electromyographic Changes in Neurogenic Disease

Individual MUPs
  Increased mean MUP duration
  Increased in MUP amplitudes
  Increased incidence of linked (pre- or post-)
      potentials (Figure 8.1)
    Nonspecific
  Increased variability of MUP shape

SF-EMG
  Increased jitter
  Increased incidence of neuromuscular blocking
  Increased fiber density
  Increased incidence of axonal blocking

Macro EMG
  Increased amplitude (and area) of MUPs

MU territory
  Increases in MU territory (multielectrode
      recordings) (Figures 8.7, 8.8)

Abnormal spontaneous activity (see Chapter 9)
  Fasciculation
  Fibrillation
  Positive sharp waves
  Bizarre high-frequency discharges

Recruitment changes
  Discrete pattern in maximum contraction (Figure
      8.6)
  Increase in mean amplitude
Automatic analysis—recruitment (30% maximum
      force)
  Decrease in number of turns
  Increase in mean amplitude

main consequences of changes in innervation patterns are increases in the concentration or numbers of muscle fibers that belong to individual MUs within certain regions of the muscle. In these regions the FD measured by the SF-EMG electrode and the amplitudes of MUPs would be expected to be highest, but these changes are not measurements of the overall innervation ratios in the MUs (Kugelberg, Edstrom, and Abbruzzese, 1970; Kugelberg, 1973).

In some neurogenic disorders the MU territories are increased (Erminio, Buchthal, and

Rosenfalck, 1959) (Figures 8.7 and 8.8), and perhaps in some of these instances the innervation ratios are increased. In amyotrophic lateral sclerosis, however, some MUs whose MUP amplitudes are as high as those recorded by standard concentric needle electrodes do not

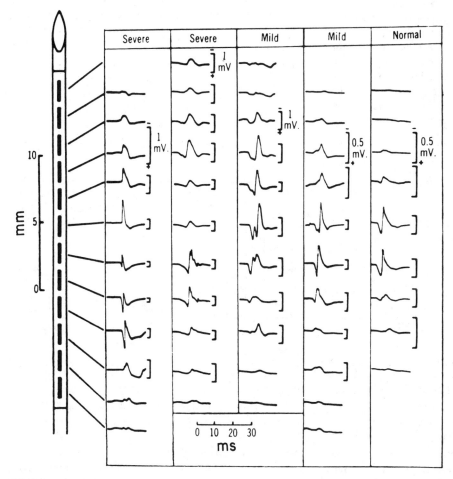

FIGURE 8.7.   Increases in the transverse territories of tibialis anterior motor units in amyotrophic lateral sclerosis as recorded by a multielectrode compared to a normal MUP recorded from the same muscle (far right). Note the generally greater transverse extent of the muscle over which the spike components of the MUP can be recorded in amyotrophic lateral sclerosis.

The spatial decline in spike amplitude with distance and possible cross talk between adjacent recording leads in the cannula would all tend to increase the apparent spatial extent of the MUP in situations where the strength of local current sources was increased through any tendency to grouping of muscle fibers innervated by the same motor unit or hypertrophy of the muscle fibers.

Also, as with normal motor units, the apparent transverse territory depends on where the electrode passes through the actual territory of the motor unit as well as the actual arrangement of the muscle fibers within the muscle, whether parallel, unipennate, bipennate, or multipennate.

FIGURE 8.8. Histogram of the transverse territories and maximum amplitudes of MUPs in the biceps brachii of normal subjects (top) and patients with amyotrophic lateral sclerosis (bottom). Note the clear increase in amplitude and transverse territories of many MUPs in amyotrophic lateral sclerosis while at the same time there is still substantial overlap in the sizes and spatial extents of many of the MUPs in the controls and patients.

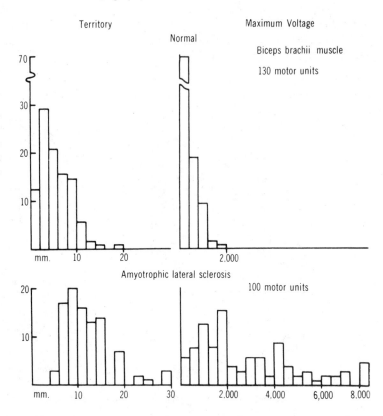

generate high tensions (Milner-Brown, Stein, and Lee, 1974). This observation is in keeping with the accepted view that the MUP amplitudes recorded with standard needle electrodes correlate best with the packing densities of muscle fibers in MUs (Swash and Schwartz, 1981), not the overall innervation ratios of these MUs. Indeed, there is even some debate about whether the MU territories are increased in amyotrophic lateral sclerosis and various polyneuropathies despite increases in FD (Schwartz, Stålberg, Schiller, and Thiele, 1976).

Characteristically, in most neurogenic disorders, the durations and amplitudes of macro EMG-recorded MUPs are increased, reflecting probably, in most instances, increases in the innervation ratios of motor units in these diseases (Stålberg, 1983).

One of the other morphological characteristics of neurogenic disease, the presence of groups of angular atrophic muscle fibers with dark pyknotic nuclei, probably has no electrophysiological correlate since these fibers most likely are irreversibly denervated (Swash and Schwartz, 1981) and no longer excitable.

The processes of collateralization and reinnervation are no doubt primary sources of prolonged MUP durations through extension of the MU innervation zone longitudinally, and perhaps transversely, and the presence of motor axon collaterals. The variable lengths, diameters, and degree of myelination (Coërs and Woolf, 1959; Wohlfart, 1958) of these motor axon collaterals all contribute to increase the degree of temporal dispersion among the individual muscle potentials contributing to the MUP.

The same mechanisms operate to explain the presence of linked potentials in neurogenic disease, and where the collaterals and their end-plates are immature, the neuromuscular transmission abnormalities are expressed as increased variability in the shapes, concentric needle-recorded MUPs, increased jitter, neuromuscular blocking, and axonal block in SF-EMG recordings. The latter abnormalities are most prominent in rapidly progressive or recent neurogenic disorders, greater stability being shown in the more slowly progressive or mature neurogenic disorders.

Changes in the recruitment patterns of MUs in neurogenic disease are readily explicable on the basis of the MU losses and changes in variables of individual MUPs. Thus in a well-established neurogenic disorder the pattern of recruitment characteristically is more discrete, and the mean amplitude of the potential is usually increased (Figure 8.8). To compensate for the losses of MUs, the firing frequencies including onset frequencies of MUs are often increased. This is a compensatory mechanism also seen in muscle diseases, where to achieve the requisite force, MUs must fire at higher frequencies compared to normal.

In muscle diseases the problem is primarily one of reduced force outputs per MU because of the loss of muscle fibers and possible electromechanical uncoupling or destruction of contractile elements. In neurogenic diseases there are simply fewer MUs available to generate the necessary force. Added to both classes of disease, especially the latter, are losses of contributing muscle fibers through neurogenic and neuromuscular block. It must be stated also that even in neurogenic disease, electromechanical uncoupling or other abnormalities in the contractile apparatus could contribute to the weakness (Milner-Brown, Stein, and Lee, 1974).

Reductions in the number of available MUs and the degree of overlap between adjacent MU territories could change recruitment patterns and amplitudes of MUPs in other ways. For example, it is known that higher-threshold MUPs have higher amplitudes than lower-threshold MUPs. In diseases in which there are appreciable losses of MUs, some of the higher-threshold MUPs could be among those recruited at apparently lower thresholds. In this case the higher amplitudes are not abnormal. This phenomenon is sometimes seen in acute Guillain-Barré polyneuropathy where through conduction block in large numbers of motor axons, higher-threshold MUPs are more apparent in the interference pattern. This is seen at too early a stage to explain these high-amplitude potentials on the basis of changes in MU innervation patterns.

The fiber grouping so characteristic of reinnervation in muscle biopsy material could also affect the recruitment patterns of MUPs. For example, reductions in the degree of overlap between adjacent MU territories could reduce the number of MUs within the pickup territory of the recording electrode and hence the number of MUPs recruitable in those regions, even though there may have been no overall loss of MUs (Figure 8.9). Moreover, if the needle electrode was situated among a group of type II muscle fibers, the MUPs recorded at this site could all have higher thresholds and the patient could well experience some difficulty activating and maintaining the discharges of these MUs. Alternatively, MUPs recorded in a type I zone could be expected to be recruited and their discharges maintained with less effort (Warmolts and Mendell, 1979).

Other possible causes of more discrete recruitment patterns besides actual loss of MUs or reduced overlap of MU territories are conduction block, central motor disorders such as the pyramidal syndrome (see Chapter 12), or simply lack of a full effort. The last two possibilities are betrayed by greater irregularities in discharges of MUs.

FIGURE 8.9. Models of alterations in muscle fiber distribution patterns and motor unit territories in primary muscle and motoneuronal or axonal diseases. (Left) Highly simplified normal motor unit illustrating the scattered distributions of muscle fibers within its transverse territory. Occasional muscle fibers (about one-third) are close enough to one another to be recorded as distant pairs of single muscle fiber potentials with a single-fiber EMG recording electrode. (Middle) In primary muscle disease the transverse territories of single motor units may be reduced. The innervation ratios of most motor units are probably reduced as well; however, the fiber density may be increased through the process of collateralization and reinnervation.

(Right) In neurogenic disorders, the classic changes include increases in the transverse territories within muscles occupied by single motor units, sometimes substantial increases in fiber density, and an increase in the innervation ratios of motor units, although the last is supposition because it cannot be directly measured in man. Not all neurogenic disorders are accompanied by an increase in the territory occupied by motor units in the muscle; indeed, in some instances the territory may actually be reduced, although there is usually an increase in fiber density or grouping.

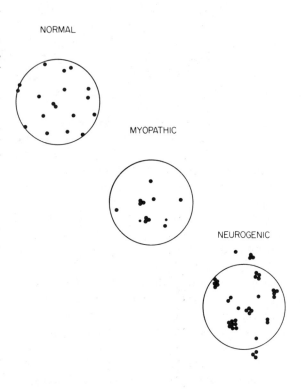

PATTERNS OF EMG ABNORMALITIES

The particular patterns of EMG abnormalities observed, some of which have already been discussed, are dependent on a number of factors (Table 8.3).

Completeness of Lesions

Obviously, where all the motor innervation has been interrupted, peripheral collateralization and reinnervation by intact motor axons is not possible, and recovery depends solely on how complete the subsequent regeneration is. The latent period is governed by the distance between the point of interruption and the muscle as well as the condition of the nerve at the site of the injury (see Chapter 2; also Seltzer, 1980).

Time Interval Between Injury and EMG

The initial period following injury is dominated by degenerative changes, progressive loss of excitability in the degenerating motor axons, failures in neuromuscular transmission, and denervation of muscle fibers (see also Chapter 11 for discussion of acute facial palsy). In man it takes between 7 and 10 days in the case of proximal muscles, and 3 to 4 weeks in the case of distal limb muscles, for fibrillation to develop following root lesions causing wallerian degeneration distal to the

TABLE 8.3. Factors that Govern Patterns of EMG Abnormalities in Neurogenic Disease

---

Completeness of the original injury, for example, a crush or transection injury

Time interval between
  Original injury and the EMG
  Onset of the illness and the EMG

Progressive or nonprogressive nature of the disorder

If progressive, rate of progression
  Rates of degeneration of motoneurons or their axons

Capacity of other motor axons to take on innervation of denervated muscle fibers

---

injury. Only once denervation develops does the process of collateral sprouting and reinnervation take place. Similarly, in neurogenic diseases of short duration (less than four weeks) such as acute axonal neuropathies, evidence of reinnervation may not develop for several weeks.

Whether or Not the Disorder Is Progressive

Progressive disorders may continue to show evidence of ongoing axonal or motoneuronal degeneration through the presence of denervation activity (fibrillation) and instabilities of neuromuscular transmission. In long-standing and nonprogressive disorders (examples being old polio or a previous neuralgic amyotrophy) fibrillation is usually infrequent and instabilities in the shapes of MUPs are less common.

In the course of a progressive neurogenic disease, the MU population could include:

1. Normal MUs and their MUPs. In most muscles there is a broad range of MUP amplitudes (although not durations), higher-amplitude MUPs having higher thresholds for recruitment (Milner-Brown and Stein, 1975).

2. Enlarged normal MUs. Here normal MUs, through collateral sprouting and reinnervation could increase their innervation ratios and possibly their territories as well. The MUPs associated with these MUs could exhibit:
    a. Increased territories
    b. Increased fiber densities (SF-EMG) (Figure 8.9)
    c. Increased amplitudes and durations
    d. Increased incidences of late linked potentials
    e. Increased jitter and impulse block in immature axon sprouts and neuromuscular junctions
    f. Axonal blocking in immature axon sprouts and neuromuscular junctions

3. MUs in the process of degeneration. These MUPs could be expected to show:
    a. Shorter durations and lower amplitudes (this may not be true if the MU undergoing degeneration is one whose innervation ratio had previously been increased through collateralization)
    b. Variations in shapes and amplitudes
    c. Increased incidences of axon blocking

The above simple model predicts that there would be a wide range in the amplitudes, durations, and shapes of MUPs in neurogenic disease. The situation could be even more complex if the processes of degeneration and collateral sprouting were to take place in different axonal branches of the same MU at the same time.

Evolution of the classic pattern in neurogenic disease takes time. For example, the reinnervation pattern that follows acute idiopathic facial palsy is characterized by an initial prolongation in MUP duration, and as maturation proceeds, by progressively shorter durations and higher amplitudes of the MUPs (see Chapter 11). This contrasts with the state in acute poliomyelitis where MUP amplitudes have been observed to increase as early as one to four weeks, but increases in the MUP durations appear to take longer to develop.

Rate of Progression

The more rapid the progression of the neurogenic disease, the greater the demands on the collateralization process to keep pace with the rate of denervation, and the greater the incidence of variabilities in MUPs, fibrillation, increased jitter, and neurogenic and neuromuscular blocking.

The preceding abnormalities are characteristic of rapidly progressive neurogenic disorders and could be indicative of motor axons and neuromuscular junction undergoing degeneration. Except for the fibrillation, however, they probably point more to very active collateralization and the subsequent establishment of many immature axon sprouts and neuromuscular junctions (Stålberg, Schwartz, and Trontelj, 1975; Thiele and Stålberg, 1975; Schwartz, Stålberg, Schiller, and Thiele, 1976). Impulse block is thought to be indicative of reinnervation within three to six months of the recording (Hakelius and Stålberg, 1974).

Acute axonal neuropathies are sometimes accompanied by the appearance of complex, often shorter-duration MUPs whose shape varies in successive discharges (Pinelli and Buchthal, 1951). Sometimes these potentials are so brief as to suggest they have been generated by a single muscle fiber. In single MUs, little is known about the time interval between the earliest abnormalities in neuromuscular transmission and axonal conduction and the end stage when all innervation is lost in the MU in motoneuronal or axonal diseases. The whole process could take a matter of only hours to, at the most, one to two days when motor axons are severed. The process of degeneration probably takes much longer in dis-

orders such as amyotrophic lateral sclerosis and even longer in the neuronal hereditary neuropathies.

Similar instabilities in MUPs, increased jitter, and blocking are seen in the first MUPs recordable in nearby reinnervated muscle following a previous nerve crush or section. The above abnormalities must here reflect the immature nature of the axons and end-plates.

Capacity of other Motor Axons to Reinnervate Denervated Muscle Fibers

One of the hallmarks of collateralization and reinnervation is the increase in FD as recorded by the SF-EMG electrode. In normal muscle, there are usually only one or two muscle fibers that generate spikes within the spike-detection zone of the SF-EMG electrode. In neurogenic disease this number (see Figure 8.9) can be much higher (4 to 10 muscle fibers). This is not seen, however, in all neurogenic diseases. For example, fiber densities have been reported to be normal in the uremic and diabetic neuropathies (Thiele and Stålberg, 1975).

The normal FD in these disorders could mean that the capacities of motor axons (motoneurons) to sprout and reinnervate nearby denervated muscle fibers is somehow reduced. This is a question that needs to be addressed in other axonal neuropathies as well.

NEEDLE ELECTROMYOGRAPHIC ABNORMALITIES IN DEMYELINATING NEUROPATHIES

The most characteristic abnormalities in the acute demyelinating neuropathies such as Guillain-Barré and diphtheritic polyneuropathies are listed in Table 8.4. Conduction block

TABLE 8.4.   Needle EMG Changes in
Demyelinating Neuropathies

Reductions in numbers of recruitable MUs
Sometimes increased numbers of polyphasic and
    long-duration MUPs
Sometimes neurogenic blocking
Repetitive discharge of MUPs
Changes indicative of denervation and reinnervation

---

in the acute paralytic stage is probably the main cause of weakness and incomplete recruitment patterns in these diseases. Whether or not this is apparent in weak contractions depends on the lower-threshold MUs being among those whose impulses are blocked. The lowest-threshold MUs generally have the slowest conduction velocities and may be among those whose motor axons are blocked earliest (Sumner, 1980; Sumner, Saida, Saida, Silberberg, and Asbury, 1982). Such a preferential block of the slower-conducting motor axons could well explain the earlier recruitment of higher-amplitude, normally higher-threshold MUPs and explain the apparent increased amplitude of macro EMG-recorded MUPs seen early in Guillain-Barré polyneuropathy. The conduction block could be rate dependent and only manifest at higher rates of discharge (see Chapter 2).

The MUPs could become abnormal in demyelinating neuropathies because of axonal degeneration and subsequent reinnervation or through demyelination and conduction delays in the intramuscular motor branches. The latter could prolong the durations and increase the numbers of phases of MUPs. Also, demyelination in intramuscular motor axon branches could produce neurogenic blocking.

In Guillain-Barré polyneuropathy, some degree of axonal degeneration is common. Hence the neurogenic abnormalities in MUPs outlined earlier can, as a result, be seen in this disease as well.

Linked Potentials

One of the most important advances in clinical electromyography has been the introduction of MUP-triggered sweeps, which makes it much easier to identify potentials that are time locked to the main potential even though the interval between the main and linked potentials is sometimes as long as 50 ms or more. These linkages are usually impossible to recognize in the auto or time-trigger modes because of the long intervals that sometimes separate the main and linked potentials (LPs).

Recognition of LPs is helped by superimposition of multiple traces or faster displays of successive potentials. In order to see the earliest components of the potential, the potential should be delayed. For most purposes, delays of 5 to 10 ms are all that are necessary, although occasionally they must be as long as 25 to 50 ms in order to see any LPs that precede the trigger source potential. Window discriminators that make it possible, within limits, to select MUPs of a given amplitude from the background activity of other MUPs are also very helpful in analysis of MUPs and recognition of LPs. These windows have upper and lower amplitude limits that can be set by the operator, with only those MUPs whose amplitudes are within the window being able to act as trigger sources.

Other names attached to LPs include satellite potentials, late components of MUPs, parasite potentials, and coupled discharges. The term *late linked potentials* (LLP), although descriptive of the most common situation, namely, where these potentials follow the main MUP, does not describe the less common situation where the linked potentials precede the main potential. The simple term linked potential is therefore preferable to the more exclusive term late linked potential.

The distinction between the so-called LPs and the main MUP is sometimes not clear.

This happens sometimes when the main potential is very prolonged and often complex, or where no clear interval exists between the main potential(s) and earlier or later potentials. Buchthal (1977) has suggested some arbitrary criteria by which such prolonged polyphasic potentials can be distinguished from those of shorter duration in myopathies.

Early measurements of MUP durations in healthy subjects and in neurogenic and muscle diseases did not appreciate the true incidence of LPs and because of this, underestimated the mean durations of MUPs. Indeed, in some instances, multiphasic MUPs were, by design, excluded from the populations of MUPs used to calculate the mean MUP durations.

In the muscular dystrophies the incidence of LPs has been reported to be as high as 47 percent (Lang and Partanen, 1976; Borenstein and Desmedt, 1973; Desmedt and Borenstein, 1976). Frequently, LPs possess amplitudes and durations that suggest they could be generated by single muscle fibers. They often also exhibit excessive jitter and even impulse block. The latter suggests that some of these LPs originate at immature neuromuscular junctions, the longer intervals between the main and linked potentials being explained by wide separation of their respective end-plate zones, slow conduction in motor axon collaterals, and possibly, differences in the conduction velocities of muscle fibers generating the various components. The increased jitter and possibly block in turn reflect the immaturity of the neuromuscular junctions.

Linked potentials are also very common in neurogenic disorders, as might be expected (Borenstein and Desmedt, 1973). In these, as in primary muscle fiber disorders, the time intervals between the main MUP and linked potentials may be very long (of the order of 50 to 60 ms).

Other Coupled Discharges

Linked potentials are examples of couplings between components belonging to the same MU. Other examples of coupled discharges include:

1. The synchronous discharge of two or more motoneurons. Synchronization between the discharges of two or more MUs has been observed in some healthy subjects (Milner-Brown, Stein, and Lee, 1975).
2. Doublet, triplet, and multiplet discharges (see Chapter 9).
3. Ephaptic transmission between two or more motor axons or muscle fibers (see Chapter 9).
4. Axon reflexes. Because the thresholds of axon branches are sometimes quite distinct from one another, stimuli intense enough to excite one branch only may, by antidromic conduction to the branch point, reach other branch(es) and by orthodromic conduction in these reach the muscle to evoke a response in those muscle fibers innervated by these branches. These phenomena are called axon reflexes.

Most branching in motor axons is distal in location, the majority taking place in the muscle itself (Eccles and Sherrington, 1930; Wray, 1969). In healthy humans, however, it is not uncommon to observe axon reflexes whose branch points are as much as 100 to 150 mm proximal to the motor point (Stålberg and Trontelj, 1970).

Following transection and surgical reunion of a nerve trunk, axon reflexes commonly occur in the nerve trunk distal to the transection site. The branch points, estimated by looking for the level proximal to which the stimulus evokes only the compound direct M-response and not both the direct and reflex components, are most often at or near the level of the transection. In some cases the branches even pass to different muscles (Esslen, 1960). Axon reflexes are sometimes also demonstrable in entrapment neuropathies, particularly where the neuropathy is of long duration and there is evidence of prior wallerian degeneration, denervation, and reinnervation.

Split Muscle Fibers

Split muscle fibers are sometimes seen in normal muscle fibers, especially when these are hypertrophic and at the musculotendinous junctions. They are even more common in hypertrophic muscle fibers of primary muscle and neurogenic diseases (Swash and Schwartz, 1981). Possibly in such split fibers, action potentials propagating along the muscle fiber could, on reaching the split, continue into the split components, provided these are viable and have intact sarcolemmal membranes. Because there is one common end-plate, impulses in the splits would be tightly time locked and could be expected to exhibit very little jitter between them (Stålberg and Ekstedt, 1973). Moreover, because the diameters of the split segments would probably be smaller than those of the parent muscle fibers, their conduction velocities should be less and their latencies longer than in adjacent normal-diameter muscle fibers.

CORRELATIONS BETWEEN EMG AND MUSCLE BIOPSIES

Precise neuromuscular diagnosis demands the correlation of evidence obtained from history and physical examination, pattern of inheritance, muscle enzyme measurements, EMG and nerve conduction studies, and often muscle and nerve biopsies. When evidence from EMG and biopsy is comprehensive and quantitative, these techniques can have a high predictive value in making the primary distinction of whether there is a disorder in the peripheral nerves or muscles; in the case of muscle or sometimes nerve biopsies, it is frequently possible even to make a precise diagnosis (Swash and Schwartz, 1981). Neither EMG nor muscle biopsy provides direct evidence about the innervation ratios of MUs, although EMG, unlike muscle biopsy, is able to provide some indirect electrophysiological indications of the probable transverse territories within a muscle occupied by single MUs, the extent of overlap between adjacent MU territories, and the loctions and concentrations of muscle fibers belonging to single MUs (Figure 8.9). These values may all be altered in muscle or peripheral nerve disorders where for any reason, muscle fibers have become denervated and have subsequently acquired new innervation.

Muscle biopsies can indicate changes in the patterns and relative numbers of the various types of muscle fibers based on their histochemical properties, the diameters of muscle fibers, the presence of necrotic and regenerating muscle fibers, and the nature of any cellular infiltrate. In addition, they sometimes indicate the presence of characteristic structural alterations within muscle fibers, some of which may be very helpful in reaching a specific clinical diagnosis. Table 8.5 lists the more important histological criteria of neurogenic and primary myopathic diseases.

These histological criteria have proved to be the most reliable indicators of neurogenic or myogenic disease. Clearly, the type grouping in the neurogenic biopsy correlates with increased fiber densities and perhaps the higher amplitudes of MUPs noted in some of these diseases, but the atrophic or angular fibers may well be inexcitable and contribute

TABLE 8.5.   Histological Evidence Pointing to Primary Myogenic or Neurogenic Diseases

Myogenic	Neurogenic
Presence of necrotic muscle fibers (in the absence of selective type I or II fiber atrophy)	Type grouping (in absence of any fiber type preponderance)
Presence of regenerating muscle fibers	Presence of atrophic dark/angular fibers, singly or in groups
Increase in variability of muscle fiber diameters	
+/− Increase in fibrosis	+/− Target fibers
+/− Inflammatory cell infiltrates (polymyositis)	

Adapted from Dubowitz and Brooke (1973), Swash and Schwartz (1981), and Buchthal and Kamieniecka (1982).

nothing to the EMG recording. There is no known physiological correlate of target fibers. In both primary and neurogenic diseases, as has been pointed out earlier in the consideration of each, the most important sources of increased jitter and neurogenic and neuromuscular blocking are immature axonal sprouts and their newly formed end-plates.

Disagreements between the results of biopsy and EMG examinations are largely explained by sampling errors, the so-called neurogenic epiphenomena in some muscle diseases, and sometimes the very early or late stages of these diseases.

References

Borenstein S, Desmedt JE. Electromyographical signs of collateral reinnervation. In: Desmedt JE, ed. New developments in electromyography and clinical neurophysiology. Basel: Karger, 1973:130–40.

Brandstater ME, Lambert EH. Motor unit anatomy. In: Desmedt JE, ed. New developments in electromyography and clinical neurophysiology. Basel: Karger, 1973:14–22.

Buchthal F. An introduction to electromyography. Copenhagen: Gyldendalske Boghandel, Nordisk Forlag, 1957.

Buchthal F. Electrophysiological abnormalities in metabolic myopathies and neuropathies. Acta Neurol Scand 1970;46(suppl 43):129–76.

Buchthal F. Diagnostic significance of the myopathic EMG. In: Rowland LP, ed. Pathogenesis of human muscular dystrophies. Proceedings of the Fifth International Scientific Conference of the Muscular Dystrophy Association, Durango, Colorado. Amsterdam, Oxford: Excerpta Medica, 1977:205–18.

Buchthal F, Kamieniecka Z. The diagnostic yield of quantified electromyography and quantified muscle biopsy in neuromuscular disorders. Muscle Nerve 1982;5:265–80.

Buchthal F, Pinelli P. Muscle action potentials in polymyositis. Neurology 1953;3:424–36.

Buchthal F, Rosenfalck P. On the structure of motor units. In: Desmedt, JE ed. New developments in electromyography and clinical neurophysiology. Basel: Karger, 1973:71–85.

Buchthal F, Rosenfalck P, Erminio F. Motor unit territory and fiber density in myopathies. Neurology 1960;10:398–408.

Campbell EDR. Single large motor unit action potentials in myopathies. Proc R Soc Med 1961; 54:421–23.

Coërs C, Woolf AL. The innervation of muscle—a biopsy study. Oxford: Blackwell, 1959.

Desmedt JE, Borenstein S. Regenerative phenomena in muscular dystrophy and polymyositis: an electromyographic study. In: Milhorat AT, ed. Exploratory concepts in muscular dystrophy. No. 333, International Congress Series. Amsterdam: Excerpta Medica, 1974:555–59.

Desmedt JE, Borenstein S. Regeneration in Duchenne muscular dystrophy: electromyographic evidence. Arch Neurol (Chicago) 1976;33:642–50.

Dubowitz V, Brooke MH. Muscle biopsy—a modern approach. London: WB Saunders, 1973.

Eccles JC, Sherrington CS. Numbers and contraction values of individual motor units examined in some muscles of the limb. Proc R Soc Biol (Lond) 1930;106:326–55.

Erminio F, Buchthal F, Rosenfalck P. Motor unit territory and muscle fiber concentration in paresis due to peripheral nerve injury and anterior horn cell involvement. Neurology 1959;9:657–71.

Esslen E. Electromyographic findings on two types of misdirection of regenerating axons. Electroencephalogr Clin Neurophysiol 1960;12:738–41.

Fuglsang-Frederiksen, Scheel U, Buchthal F. Diagnostic yield of analysis of the pattern of electrical activity and of individual motor unit potentials in myopathy. J Neurol Neurosurg Psychiatry 1976;39:742–50.

Hakelius L, Stålberg E. Electromyographical studies of free autogenous muscle transplants in man. Scand J Plast Reconstr Surg 1974;8:211–19.

Hayward M. Electrodiagnosis of the muscular dystrophies. Br Med Bull 1980;36:127–32.

Heathfield KWG, Williams JRB. Diagnosis of polymyositis. Lancet 1960;1:1157–61.

Karpati G, Engel WK. Type grouping in skeletal muscle after experimental reinnervation. Neurology (Minneap) 1968;18:447–55.

Kugelberg E. Electromyography in muscular disorders. J Neurol Neurosurg Psychiatry 1947;10:122–33.

Kugelberg E. Electromyography in muscular dystrophy. J Neurol Neurosurg Psychiatry 1949;12:129–36.

Kugelberg E. Properties of the rat hind-limb motor units. In: Desmedt JE, ed. New developments in electromyography and clinical neurophysiology. Basel: Karger, 1973:2–13.

Kugelberg E, Edstrom L, Abbruzzese M. Mapping of motor units in experimentally reinnervated rat muscle. J Neurol Neurosurg Psychiatry 1970;33:319–29.

Lang AH, Partanen VSJ. "Satellite potentials" and the duration of motor unit potentials in normal neuropathic and myopathic muscles. J Neurol Sci 1976;27:513–24.

Ludin HP. Electromyography in practice. New York: Stratton-Thieme, 1980.

Mechler F. Changing electromyographic findings during the chronic course of polymyositis. J Neurol Sci 1974;23:237–42.

Milner-Brown HS, Stein RB. The relation between the surface electromyogram and muscle force. J Physiol 1975;246:549–69.

Milner-Brown HS, Stein RB, Lee RG. Contractile and electrical properties of human motor units in neuropathies and motor neurone disease. J Neurol Neurosurg Psychiatry 1974;37:670–76.

Milner-Brown HS, Stein RB, Lee RG. Synchronization of human motor units: possible roles of exercise and supraspinal reflexes. Electroencephalogr Clin Neurophysiol 1975;38:245–54.

Morris CJ, Woolf AL. Mechanism of type I muscle fiber grouping. Nature (Lond) 1970;226:1061–62.

Pinelli P, Buchthal F. Duration, amplitude and shape of muscle action potentials in poliomyelitis. Electroencephalogr Clin Neurophysiol 1951;3:497–504.

Pinelli P, Buchthal F. Muscle action potentials in myopathies with special regard to progressive muscular dystrophy. Neurology 1953;3:347–59.

Rosenfalck P. Intra- and extracellular potential fields of active nerve and muscle fibres. Act Physiol Scand 1969;75(suppl 321):1–168.

Schwartz MS, Stålberg E, Schiller HH, Thiele B. The reinnervated motor unit in man. A single-fibre EMG multielectrode investigation. J Neurol Sci 1976;27:303–12.

Seltzer ME. Regeneration of peripheral nerve. In: Sumner AJ, ed. The physiology of peripheral nerve disease. Philadelphia: WB Saunders, 1980:358–431.

Stålberg EV. Macro EMG. American Association of Electromyography and Electrodiagnosis. Minimonograph 20. Rochester, Minn.: American Association of Electromyography and Electrodiagnosis, 1983.

Stålberg E, Ekstedt J. Single-fibre EMG and microphysiology of the motor unit in normal and diseased muscle. In: Desmedt JE, ed. New developments in electromyography and clinical neurophysiology. Basel: Karger, 1973:113–29.

Stålberg E, Schwartz MS, Trontelj JV. Single-fibre electromyography in various processes affecting the anterior horn cell. J Neurol Sci 1975;24:403–15.

Stålberg E, Trontelj JV. Demonstration of axon reflexes in human motor nerve fibres. J Neurol Neurosurg Psychiatry 1970;33:571–79.

Stålberg E, Trontelj JV. Single-fibre electromyography. Surrey, England: Mirvalle Press, 1979.

Stålberg E, Trontelj JV, Janko M. Single-fibre EMG findings in muscular dystrophy. In: Hausmanowa-Petrusewicz I, Jedrzejowska H, eds. Structure and function of normal and diseased muscle and peripheral nerve. Warsaw: Polish Medical Publishers, 1974:185–90.

Sumner AJ. The physiological basis for symptoms in Guillain-Barré syndrome. Ann Neurol 1980;9(suppl):28–30.

Sumner AJ, Saida K, Saida T, Silberberg DH, Asbury AK. Acute conduction block associated with experimental antiserum-mediated demyelination of peripheral nerve. Ann Neurol 1982;11:469–77.

Swash M, Schwartz MS. Neuromuscular diseases. Berlin: Springer-Verlag, 1981.

Thiele B, Stålberg E. Single-fibre EMG findings in polyneuropathies of different aetiology. J Neurol Neurosurg Psychiatry 1975;38:881–87.

Tomlinson BE, Walton JN, Irving D. Spinal cord limb motor neurones in muscular dystrophy. J Neurol Sci 1974;22:305–27.

Warmolts JR, Mendell JR. Open-biopsy electromyography. Arch Neurol 1979;36:406–9.

Warmolts JR, Wiechers DO. Myopathies. In: Johnson EW, ed. Practical electromyography. Baltimore: Williams & Wilkins, 1980:110–34.

Wohlfart G. Collateral regeneration in partially denervated muscle. Neurology (Minneap) 1958;8:175–80.

Wray SH. Innervation ratios for large and small limb muscles in the baboon. J Comp Neurol 1969;137:227–50.

9 NORMAL AND ABNORMAL SPONTANEOUS ACTIVITY IN MUSCLE

Normally impulses originate only at the cell body or initial segment in motoneurons or the receptor end-organs in sensory fibers. Similarly, in muscle, all impulses in the muscle fibers begin at the end-plate zone. In resting muscle the only spontaneous potentials usually detectable are the miniature end-plate potentials in the immediate vicinity of the endplates. Ongoing impulse activity originating in stretch receptors as well as possibly other mechanoreceptors in the muscles might theoretically be detectable in intramuscular recordings, but the low density of such afferents in most regions of the muscle as well as the relatively small diameters of such fiber ($<20~\mu$) makes ongoing activity in the various muscle afferents an unlikely source of spontaneous activity recordable by the conventional concentric needle electrode.

In contracting muscle where impulses in alpha motor axons might be expected to add to the chorus of recorded activity within the muscle, the progressive tapering of the diameters of the axons as they branch and rebranch prior to reaching their end-plates would tend to weaken their strength as electrogenic sources still further. There is a wide variety of nerve fibers present within muscle, including the motor efferents (alpha and gamma motor axons) and the remaining 50 to 60 percent of the nerve fibers made up of various afferents, some discharging at rest and others in relation to muscle contraction. Regardless of this, the asynchronous nature of their discharges, their relative weakness as electrogenic sources and low concentrations except in the immediate vicinity of the motor point, and course of the nerve to the innervation zone, make nerve fibers most unlikely sources of recordable potentials, especially with the relatively large leading-off surfaces of most intramuscular electrodes used in service electromyography.

Electrical stimulation of motor nerves that is intense enough to evoke a relatively well-synchronized volley in the nerve may result in detectable nerve action potentials preceding the muscle (M) potential by 1.5 to 2 ms (see Figure 3.16). The amplitudes of such nerve action potentials are usually small (less than 0.1 mV) when recorded by the standard concentric needle EMG electrode even in the immediate vicinity of the motor point.

The synchronous discharges of large numbers of MFs, such as results when motor nerves are stimulated supramaximally, may reexcite the intramuscular motor axons and evoke small antidromic volleys in the nerve trunk because of the strong electrical currents set up in the muscle by the intense MF activity (Buller and Proske, 1978). Such antidromic volleys would naturally follow after the antidromic impulses in the motor axons produced directly by the nerve stimulus itself.

Except for such well-synchronized volleys in motor nerves as those that follow strong electrical stimulation of the motor nerve, we have not been able to detect a presynaptic potential preceding the MF action potentials in the end-plate zone. This holds true even when MF spike-triggered sweeps and electronic averaging techniques were used (Brown and Varkey, 1981).

Muscle fibers themselves are therefore the source of all the potentials recorded in muscles. The one exception is the small prepotential mentioned above, preceding the synchronous M-response to an electrical motor nerve stimulus.

Normally spontaneous potentials in MFs are detectable only in the end-plate zone (Wiederholt, 1970; Brown and Varkey, 1981). Outside the end-plate zone, subcutaneous electrodes record no spontaneous potentials; however, introduction of a needle into the muscle triggers discharges in MFs. Such insertional activity is usually brief but may become excessive in amount and duration in the presence of denervation, the myotonias, polymyositis, and some of the muscle dystrophies (Figure 9.1).

It is important to examine the role of the needle electrode in producing or increasing the frequency of abnormal or normal spontaneous activity. Needle insertion certainly increases the frequency of miniature end-plate potentials (MEPPs) in the end-plate zone. Indeed, Blight and Precht (1980) have claimed that earlier estimates of MEPP frequency were too high, the higher frequencies being produced by the mechanical irritation of the nearby recording electrode. Certainly the bi-

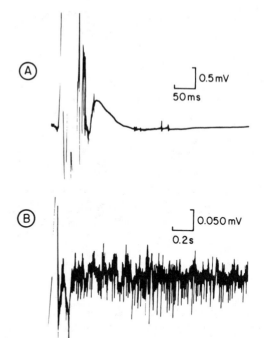

FIGURE 9.1.   Insertional activity recorded outside the innervation zone in a normal muscle (A). The burst of electrical discharges usually lasts between 50 and 250 ms depending on the vigor of the insertion and the size and sharpness of the needle. In contrast, insertion in a denervated muscle (B) produces a prolonged shower, in this case, of predominantly positive sharp waves lasting longer than the usual insertion-evoked electrical discharges.

phasic end-plate spikes in the end-plate zone seem to be produced solely by insertion of the needle electrode into the region; their discharge frequencies and numbers fall off to zero levels over several minutes.

The amount of insertional activity in and outside the end-plate zone depends on the size and sharpness of the electrode; large, dull, or burred needles producing a good deal more injury potentials and other insertional activity than smaller, sharp electrodes.

In this chapter attention is first directed toward the normal spontaneous and evoked electrical activity in the end-plate zone. Subsequent sections deal with abnormal spontaneous and provoked activity originating in motoneurons or their axons, or in the MFs themselves.

ELECTRICAL ACTIVITY IN THE END-PLATE ZONE

In contrast to intramuscular recordings outside the innervation zone where no spontaneous electrical activity is present at rest, spontaneous activity is present in the innervation zone. This activity takes two forms (Table 9.1 and Figure 9.2). Both of these potentials have irregular discharge frequencies that can be increased by needle movement and blocked by neuromuscular blocking agents. The low-amplitude negative potentials are MEPPs. The other biphasic all-or-nothing potentials are MF action potentials. This conclusion is based on the observations that these biphasic potentials can be blocked by neuromuscular blocking agents, outside the innervation zone these potentials have initial positive phases, and the durations and amplitudes of these potentials are identical to single MF action potentials and fibrillation potentials. The negative prepotentials seen at the outset of the biphasic potentials could be the extracellular equivalent of the end-plate potential (EPP). This last view is suggested by variations in the time of onset of the main negative spike with respect to the prepotential and sometimes periodic blocking of the negative spike in disorders of neuromuscular transmission. In support of the above hypothesis, the prepotentials are never seen outside the innervation zone.

What triggers the biphasic potentials in the innervation zone is not known. Perhaps the intramuscular electrode triggers potentials in the motor axon terminals or preterminals, or disrupts nearby MFs. The latter could release potassium into the extracellular space and depolarize the nerve terminals. Both mechanisms could increase MEPP frequencies and through suprathreshold EPPs trigger postsynaptic muscle fiber action potentials (Brown and Varkey, 1981).

Recently, Partanen and Nousiainen (1983) have put forward the idea that the end-plate spikes are really generated by the action potentials of intrafusal muscle fibers as driven by gamma motoneurons. Intrafusal muscle fibers are clearly another potential source for spontaneous activity outside the end-plate zone. Muscle spindles, however, are usually

TABLE 9.1.   Spontaneous Activity at the End-Plate Zone

	Biphasic Potentials	Monophasic Potentials
Amplitude	0.1 to 0.5 mV (p-p)	0.01 to 0.1 mV
Duration	1–5 ms	Up to 5 ms
Phases	Biphasic; initial negative phase	Monophasic, negative
Prepotentials	Yes	No
Discharge pattern	Irregular; triggered by needle electrode	Irregular; frequency increased by electrode movement
Origin	Postsynaptic action potential in single muscle fibers +/− preceding EPP	MEPP
Effect of denervation	Disappear	Disappear

FIGURE 9.2.   (A) Miniature end-plate potentials as recorded by a glass microelectrode in the region of the end-plate in the rat hemidiaphragm. These potentials when recorded intracellularly are monophasic-positive and vary in size, most being somewhere between 0.2 and 1.0 mV in amplitude. Occasionally, so-called giant potentials 2 to 3 mV in amplitude may be seen (one such potential is shown here in the top trace). The potentials in this case triggered the oscilloscope sweep and were themselves delayed in order to see their entire time course. The above potentials were recorded at − 70 mV.

(B) Similar recording to the above but from a fiber where the miniature end-plate potential amplitudes were a little smaller (bottom trace of the two). In the upper trace of the pair, the electrode was withdrawn slightly until it was just extracellular (EC). Note the reversal in the polarity of the potentials (now monophasic-negative) and the halving of the amplitude.

(C) The MEPPs as recorded in the immediate vicinity of the end-plate zone in a human muscle with a standard concentric needle electrode. In such recordings the potentials are monophasic and negative. Note that the amplitudes of such potentials are about one-tenth of what they are recorded with intracellular electrodes.

(D) Two examples of biphasic (negative-positive) spikes as recorded in the immediate vicinity of the end-plate zone in a human muscle. The negative spikes are usually preceded by a prepotential (PreP), which probably corresponds to the end-plate potential (EPP).

The MEPPs (top) and biphasic potentials (bottom) served to trigger the oscilloscope sweeps and were themselves delayed in order to see the entire time courses of the potentials.

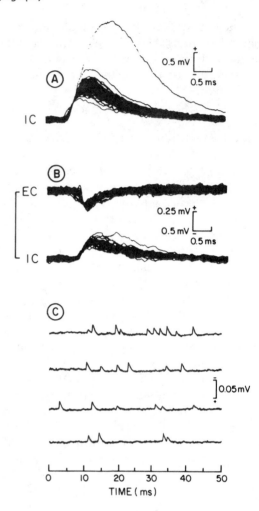

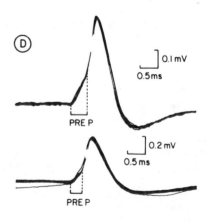

distributed widely throughout muscles and not preferentially in the region of the end-plate zone for the extrafusal muscle fibers. The biphasic spikes so characteristically recorded in close proximity to miniature end-plate potentials must arise, therefore, in extrafusal not intramuscle fibers, as was earlier proposed by Brown and Varkey (1981). Also, we have not noticed any alteration in the discharge frequency of the biphasic potentials induced by moderate passive stretch or voluntary contraction of the muscle, such as to suggest these potentials were generated by the intrafusal muscle fibers or their associated nerve fiber afferents.

ABNORMAL SPONTANEOUS AND PROVOKED ELECTRICAL ACTIVITY IN MUSCLE

Many types of abnormal electrical activity have now been described in muscle. Some of these originate in the motoneuron, peripheral axon, or axon terminals, while others originate in the muscle itself (see Culp and Ochoa, 1982). In common, these abnormal electrical discharges originate in most instances at ectopic sites and may involve ephaptic transmission.

Ectopic Impulse Generation and Ephaptic Transmission

Normally in peripheral nerves and muscle fibers, as stated earlier, impulses originate only at the receptor end-organs, motoneurons, or end-plates. Transmission between motoneurons and their MFs is through chemical transmission at the neuromuscular junction, there being no ephaptic or direct electrical connections among nerve fibers in the nerve trunk or among MFs. The intermingling of MFs belonging to separate MUs would discourage much interaction between the action currents belonging to the same MU.

The following conditions are necessary for direct electrical transmission to take place between excitable axons or muscle fibers:

1. There should be close proximity between the axons or MFs to minimize current leakages between adjacent excitable membranes into the extracellular space.
2. The postephaptic axon or MF should have a higher-input impedance in relation to the current source (i.e., a large fiber can better act as a current source to excite a small fiber than can a small fiber ephaptically drive a larger fiber).
3. In the case of spontaneous discharges, there should be a pacemaker source to trigger the impulses.
4. Favoring ephaptic transmission would be any conditions that increase the excitability of the postephaptic fiber.

The preceding conditions are met in peripheral nerve where the axons are amyelinated as in the dystrophic mouse (Huzier, Kuno, and Miyata, 1975; Rasminsky, 1978, 1982) or in experimental demyelination of the fifth cranial nerve (Burchiel, 1980). In muscle, the reorganization of MUs and the consequent closer opposition of MFs belonging to the same MU would increase the chance of significant interactions taking place between the action currents of MFs in the same MU. In a similar manner, the split portions of split MFs would be in tight opposition to one another.

Favoring both ectopic impulse generation and ephaptic transmission would be any conditions that altered the properties of the sodium channels, or hyperpolarized the membrane in such a way as to reduce sodium channel inactivation and therefore membrane accommodation (Bergmans, 1982). Other factors known to increase the excitability of axon and MFs membranes are:

1. Reductions in concentrations of serum ionized calcium.
2. Ischemia, especially in the immediate postischemic period (Kugelberg, 1946; Ochoa and Torebjork, 1980; Gilliatt, 1982).
3. Compression. For example, acute compression of dorsal root ganglia and chronic injury of dorsal roots have been shown to produce ectopic spontaneous discharges in these structures (Howe, Calvin, and Loeser, 1976; Howe, Loeser, and Calvin, 1977).
4. Depolarizations. Partial depolarizations of the membranes as long as these did not enhance accommodation could temporarily increase the excitability of the membrane. Such partial depolarizations could be produced by trains of impulses and the subsequent accumulation of potassium in the extracellular space just outside the membrane.

Examples of probable ectopic impulse generation are shown in Table 9.2.

TABLE 9.2.   Abnormal Spontaneous Activity in Nerve and Muscle

In motor axons
Fasciculation
The neuromyotonias
Doublets, triplets, and multiplets
Tetany
Myokymia
Hemifacial spasm
Postischemic fasciculation
Tetanus
Stiff-man syndrome
In muscle fibers
Fibrillation
Myogenic fasciculation
Bizarre repetitive discharges (BRD)
Cramp
Myotonia

FASCICULATION

Fasciculation is the spontaneous twitch caused by the discharge (in neurogenic disease) of the whole motor unit (MU), or groups of neighboring MFs not necessarily sharing the same innervation (benign fasciculation). Where the MUs are not too deep and the subcutaneous tissue is not too thick, the twitches can be seen. In deeper locations, they can be felt and sometimes even heard with a stethoscope. By contrast, the contractions of single MFs such as are present in fibrillating MFs cannot be seen except when these occur in the most superficial MFs, and here only where the surface of the muscle itself can be visualized directly.

Fasciculation potentials (FPs) as recorded by skin, subcutaneous, or intramuscular electrodes have durations, amplitudes, and territories similar to MUPs and are commonly followed by a slow potential, probably produced by the twitch-evoked mechanical displacement of the electrode. Fasciculation is common in the orbicularis oculi muscle in tense or tired but otherwise healthy persons, in heavily exercised muscles, and sometimes in other muscles sporadically for no obvious reason. In all these cases, the fasciculation is benign.

Fasciculation can also be seen in peripheral nerve, and root entrapment syndromes, motoneuronal diseases (Figure 9.3) including amyotrophic lateral sclerosis and Jacob-Creutzfeldt disease, axonal neuropathies, thyrotoxicosis, and cholinesterase poisoning. Benign fasciculation is thought to be of primary myogenic origin (Stålberg and Trontelj, 1982). The current suggestion is that pacemaker MFs ephaptically activate adjacent MFs (not necessarily in the same MU) to produce well-synchronized discharges of multiple MFs and a visible twitch. Ephapsis between adjacent MFs is suggested by the low jitter values between coactivated MFs. These fasciculations are not

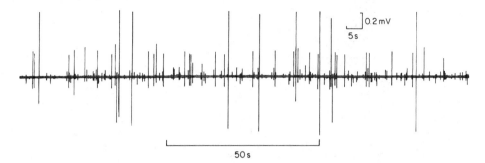

]0.2 mV
5 s

50 s

FIGURE 9.3. Fasciculations as recorded from the deltoid muscle of a patient with amyotrophic lateral sclerosis. On the assumption that potentials of identical spike amplitude are very likely to have been generated by the source, there are at least 10 separate and distinct potentials in the recording within the pickup territory of the standard concentric recording electrode, used here to record the potentials. The discharge frequency of individual potentials varied from as low as 0.005 per second to as high as 1 per 10 seconds, higher frequencies tending to be seen in the lower-amplitude spikes in this disease. Bandwidth of recording was 100 to 5,000 Hz (2 db down).

the discharges of single MUs but of MFs more related by their close proximity to one another than by their innervation. What triggers the pacemaker fibers is unknown.

There is considerable debate about the site of origin and the electrogenesis of the FP in neurogenic disease (Figure 9.4). Postulated sites include the motoneuron and various sites in the peripheral motor axon, including the axon terminals or the preterminals themselves. Our present knowledge and hypotheses about the site(s) of origin are based on the results of spinal anesthesia, section of or local anesthetic block of peripheral nerves, and studies of the actions of various compounds (see reviews by Ludin, 1976; Roth, 1982; and Wettstein, 1979).

For example, it is known that section of motor axons can lead to the development of dendritic spikes in the so-called chromatolytic neuron (Eccles, Libet, and Young, 1958; Kuno and Llinás, 1970; Kuno, Miyata, and Muñoz-Martinez, 1974a, 1974b; Kuno, 1975). These dendritic spikes can trigger action potentials in the motoneurons. (Some chromatolytic

neurons can be made to generate action potentials by weak excitatory postsynaptic potentials (EPSPs) or even stimulation of single 1a afferents, which suggests that their thresholds are much lower than those of normal motoneurons.) Whether a similar but less complete chromatolytic reaction in the motoneurons occurs in degenerative diseases of the motoneurons and leads to spontaneous discharges there is unknown. In keeping with a possible origin in the motoneurons themselves are the observations that spinal anesthesia can abolish about one-half of FPs (Swank and Price, 1943) and that FPs may be synchronous in separate muscles in the same segmental distribution. Of course the latter observation does not exclude the possibility of ephaptic transmission between motor axons of the same spinal segmental origin, in the roots, or even proximal peripheral nerves, or even the possibility of fasciculation in a single motor axon that branches proximal to the motor points of both muscles.

The interesting suggestion has even been made that FPs can develop in spinal moto-

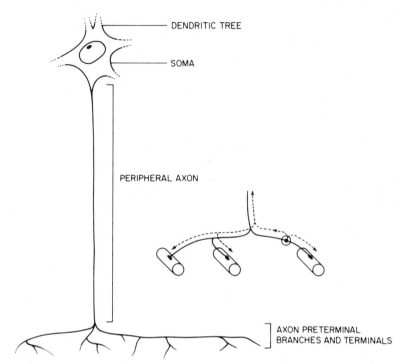

DENDRITIC TREE

SOMA

PERIPHERAL AXON

AXON PRETERMINAL
BRANCHES AND TERMINALS

FIGURE 9.4.   Postulated sites of origin of fasciculation potentials include the motoneuron dendritic tree or soma, any number of sites along the peripheral axon, and perhaps most commonly in the preterminal and terminal branches. In the latter sites spontaneous spikes antidromically invade the motor axon to reach other branches of the terminal motor axon tree (see arrows in insert).

neurons that have been "centrally denervated" by a suprasegmental lesion (King and Stoop, 1973).

At the other extreme is the view that the majority of FPs originate at sites in the intramuscular motor axon terminals or preterminals (Stålberg and Trontelj, 1970; Roth, 1978a, 1978b, 1982). Impulses generated at these sites could, by antidromic invasion, activate the remainder of the peripheral branches of the MU, and so the whole MU (Figure 9.4). Such a mechanism seems to be the best explanation for the FPs induced by anticholinesterase and cholinergic compounds (Eccles, Katz, and Kuffler, 1941; Meadows, 1971). Such compounds could depolarize the motor axon terminals and generate action potentials at these

sites. Ectopic impulse generation at the same sites in various degenerative diseases of the motoneurons and axons could underlie many of the FPs in these diseases, although the precise electrogenic mechanisms responsible for the ectopic and spontaneous generation of impulses are unknown as yet. They may share some mechanisms in common with penicillin afterdischarges (Noebels and Prince, 1977).

If the ectopic site of origin of the FP is constant, there may be little change in shape in the FP between potentials. Where the site of origin changes or there are multiple sites of origin, however, the shape could change from FP to FP in the same MU (Stålberg and Trontelj, 1982). Changes in the shape of the same FP could also reflect intermittent axonal and neuromuscular blocks in the terminal and preterminal axonal network and at the various neuromuscular junctions respectively (Stålberg and Trontelj, 1982).

Possible origins of FPs at other sites in motor axons between the motoneuron cell bodies and the intramuscular axon terminals have been suggested by techniques in which the motor nerves have been sectioned (Forster, Borkowski, and Albers, 1946) or blocked by local anesthetic drugs (Forster and Albers, 1944). Unfortunately, in the latter experiments, the completeness of the block was not tested electrophysiologically.

Using a collision technique in which the FPs themselves were used to trigger a stimulator whose pulses could be delivered at various sites along the course of the motor axon, Roth (1978a, 1978b) claimed that the majority of FPs originated within the distal arborization of the motor axon within or close to the muscle. On the other hand, Wettstein (1979), employing a similar technique, reported that many FPs originated much more proximally along the motor axon.

Conradi, Grimby, and Lundemo (1982) showed that widespread fasiculation in patients with amyotrophic lateral sclerosis may be abolished by nonparalytic doses of the synthetic curare derivative (Pavulon) and sometimes increased by neostigmine. Because of the similarity to fasciculations produced through cholinesterase inhibitors, the authors suggest that the fasciculations in amyotrophic lateral sclerosis may have a similar peripheral origin. Acetylcholine receptors are known to be present in the membranes of motor axon terminals. Spontaneous spike generation at these sites augmented through the effects of circulating acetylcholine could, by variable antidromic invasion of the rest of the terminal branches of the motor axon, possibly account for the fasciculation seen in amyotrophic lateral sclerosis and other neurogenic diseases.

It seems clear at this time that FPs may begin in ectopic sites at multiple levels, although probably the majority originate in the motor axon terminals or preterminals as suggested by Roth (1982) (Conradi, Grimby, and Lundemo, 1982). Whatever the level of origin, in some cases it has been shown that activity in sensory fibers can provoke fasciculation in some cases (Sinderman, Conrad, Jacobi, and Prochazka, 1973). Such interactions could be transsynaptic at the level of the motoneuron or ephaptic in the peripheral axons.

In the human, there are no characteristics of benign FPs that reliably distinguish them from MUPs in the same muscle. Even in amyotrophic lateral sclerosis, FPs are often indistinguishable in their amplitudes, shapes, and durations from other MUPs in the same muscle, although many FPs cannot be recruited by the patient. In one study of those fasciculating MUPs that could be recruited voluntarily, the firing patterns of the potentials were said to be similar to those of lower-threshold MUPs (Conradi, Grimby, and Lundemo, 1982). Trojaborg and Buchthal (1965) pointed out that the interpotential intervals between FPs in amyotrophic lateral sclerosis are on the whole longer than in benign fasciculation, although this is of little practical value to the electromyographer.

There are then no reliable ways of distinguishing benign FPs from the so-called malignant FPs seen in a variety of neurogenic diseases. Only the other features (see Chapter 8) in the EMG allow the electromyographer to establish whether or not a neurogenic disease is present and hence by extension whether or not the fasciculation is benign.

THE NEUROMYOTONIAS

The neuromyotonias are characterized by cramps, impaired muscle relaxation, and often fasciculation and myokymia (see Gamstrop and Wolfart, 1959; Isaacs, 1961, 1964, 1967; Hughes and Matthews, 1969; Gardner-Medwin and Walton, 1969; Wallis, VanPoznak, and Plum, 1970; Welch, Appenzeller, and Bicknell, 1972; Isaacs and Frere, 1974; Irani, Purohit, and Wadia, 1977; Negri, Caraceni, and Boiardi, 1977; Lutschg, Jerusalem, Ludin, Vassella, and Mumenthaler, 1978; Lublin, Tsairis, Streletz, Chambers, Riker, VanPoznak, and Duckett, 1979; Warmotts and Mendell, 1980; Lance, Burke, and Pollard, 1979; Stohr, 1981). The main pathophysiological characteristics include (see Bergman's 1982 review):

1. Fasciculation
2. Asynchronous continuous MU discharges sometimes at high frequencies (>100 Hz)
3. Doublets, triplets, and multiplets
4. Blocking by neuromuscular blocking agents diphenylhydantoin or carbamazepine, not blocked by spinal anesthesia or local anesthetic blocks of peripheral nerve trunks, especially when the latter are proximal in location
5. Provocation by mechanical tapping, especially near the motor point; and polarizing currents applied over the distal motor nerve
6. Prolonged myotonic-like voluntary contractions

These physiological observations point to the peripheral motor axons as the sites of origin of spontaneous and provoked impulses. The sites are in all likelihood distal in location. This belief is based on observations that percussion and polarizing currents delivered to the nerve are most effective in provoking the discharges when applied to the distal segments of the motor nerves, and while motor conduction velocities are often normal, the motor terminal latencies are prolonged. Bergmans (1982) has suggested that perhaps the distal motor axons are in a hyperpolarized state and therefore more susceptible to repetitive discharge because of their reduced accommodations.

The basic mechanisms responsible for the neuromyotonia in these disorders may vary somewhat depending on the nature of the primary diseases. Some cases apparently occur sporadically, others are hereditary, while still others are associated with an obvious peripheral neuropathy. Some cases exhibit little spontaneous activity but do show prominent electrical or natural stimulus-evoked activity. Some have followed heavy exposure to insecticides, and localized forms may be seen in local entrapment neuropathies (Stohr, 1981).

Doublets, Triplets, and Multiplets

Doublets, triplets, and multiplets are characterized by repetitive MUP discharges (or single muscle fiber potentials in the case of SF-EMG recordings) at short intervals (see Simpson, 1969; Partanen and Lang, 1978; Partanen, 1978, 1979; Stålberg and Trontelj, 1982) (Figure 9.7). The interval between the first and second discharges ranges between 4 and 10 ms and that between the second and third between 15 and 30 ms (Stålberg and Trontelj, 1982). They often occur in short spontaneous bursts, but are also commonly evoked by electrical stimulation of the nerve. These repetitive discharges or afterdischarges are common in the neuromyotonias, tetany, and amyotrophic lateral sclerosis. In the last they sometimes occur in association with fasciculation. They have been described also in Guillain-Barré polyneuropathy.

Tetany

Spontaneous and provoked contractions in muscles are common in the presence of low concentrations of ionized serum calcium (see Kugelberg, 1948; Layzer and Rowland, 1971). The contractions may be provoked by hyperventilation, tapping the peripheral nerves, or tourniquet occlusion of the blood supply to limbs. Discharges of MUPs at 5 to 30 Hz in long trains or shorter bursts, as well as afterdischarges in the form of doublets, triplets, and multiplets are common in the EMG. The tetanic contraction increases in intensity as more MUs join the asynchronous discharge.

Loss of accommodation and other evidence of hyperexcitability of motor axons in the presence of low serum levels of ionized calcium (Solandt, 1936; Kugelberg, 1944, 1948) readily explain the heightened responses to mechanical taps delivered to the nerves (Chvostek's sign) and ischemia (Trousseau's sign). In the case of the latter, the more proximal the location of the tourniquet on the limb, the easier it is to induce tetanic contraction. This observation and the results of local anesthetic blocks at multiple levels suggest that the ectopic impulses can originate at multiple sites in the motor axons. Some of the discharges possibly originate in the muscle fibers themselves (Stålberg and Trontelj, 1982).

Myokymia

Myokymia is a special kind of involuntary spontaneous contraction characterized by continuous rippling or quivering actions in a muscle or group of muscles. They may be seen in the calf muscles of healthy individuals following vigorous exercise. Myokymia may also occur in the face in association with pontine tumors or multiple sclerosis, following an acute idiopathic facial palsy, or in Guillain-Barré polyneuropathy (Daube, Kelly, and Martin, 1979). Less often, the condition may be seen in limb muscles, many of which have radiation-induced plexopathies or myelopathies. Less commonly associated conditions include other chronic disorders of the spinal cord, multiple sclerosis, inflammatory polyradiculoneuropathies, ischemic neuropathy, and diffuse vasculitis (Albers, Allen, Bastron, and Daube, 1981).

In EMG recordings from affected muscles,

the characteristics of myokymic discharges are bursts of potentials between which there are periods of silence, the grouped discharges recurring in a semirhythmic manner. The numbers and frequency of discharges of individual potentials in the burst, and burst duration and frequency are quite variable. The shapes and sizes of individual potentials in the burst suggest they are generated by part or all of the motor unit. Indeed, such discharges can deplete the active muscle fibers of their glycogen and reveal the innervation patterns of single motor units in muscle (Williamson and Brooke, 1972). Myokymic discharges, including the multiplets or grouped motor unit action potentials in tetany, cannot, as a rule, be voluntarily altered. Other spontaneous discharges such as bizarre repetitive discharges are not grouped but consist in most cases of repetitive discharges of complex potentials at very regular intervals, the train of discharges beginning and ending abruptly. Neuromyotonic discharges that are also spontaneous do not recur in the rhythmic or semirhythmic fashion of myokymic discharges; they tend to discharge at substantially higher rates (over 200 Hz) as compared with the 50 Hz or less characteristic of myokymic bursts.

The precise electrophysiological origins of myokymic activity are unknown. They are probably similar to those of hemifacial spasm and the neuromyotonic discharges discussed earlier, that is, ectopic, spontaneous impulses such as those seen in experimentally injured, compressed (Granit, Leksell, and Skoglund, 1944), or demyelinated nerves (Van Zandycke, Martin, Vande Gaer, and Van den Heyning, 1982; Burchiel, 1981). Such discharges in experimentally demyelinated regions may be exacerbated by reduced calcium ion concentrations (Brick, Gutmann, and McComas, 1982), although no studies of this have been made in human myokymia.

Unlike the neuromyotonias where the majority of the spontaneous discharges appear to have a distal origin in the motor axon or its terminal branches, local anesthetic blocking studies of patients with postirradiation plexopathies and myokymia affecting limb muscles reveal a more proximal origin for the discharges, probably at the site of the irradiation injury (Albers, Allen, Bastron, and Daube, 1981).

In facial myokymia, isolation of motoneurons of the seventh nerve by destruction of presynaptic interneurons, interruption of descending corticobulbar or other supranuclear connections, and direct irritation of the motoneurons or their extensive axon processes in the brainstem have all been suggested as possible explanations for the spontaneous discharges in those instances where there were lesions in the brainstem (see Van Zandycke, Martin, Vande Gaer, and Van den Heyning, 1982).

Hemifacial Spasm

Hemifacial spasm is characterized by twitches or tonic contractions and synchronous or near synchronous discharges in separate facial muscles (Auger, 1979) (Figure 9.5). There are three main types including an idiopathic group, some in which there is compression of the seventh nerve by aberrant vessels, vascular malformations near the brainstem, or cerebellopontine angle tumors, and others that develop following Bell's palsy or trauma (surgical or otherwise) to the seventh nerve.

In hemifacial spasm, MUPs may discharge at rates as high as 150 to 400 impulses per second, while at other times, trains of 2 to 10 impulses at 20 Hz per second are seen (Figure 9.6). Characteristically, there is a high degree of synchronization between the bursts in separate facial muscles. Sometimes the bursts can be triggered by antidromic volleys evoked by an electrical stimulus delivered to the seventh nerve. In the idiopathic group, for which no cause can be established after intensive investigation including vertebral arteriography, the

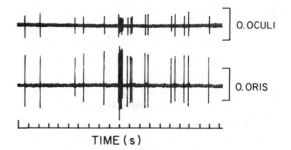

FIGURE 9.5. Spontaneous discharges in the orbicularis oculi and oris muscles in a patient nine months following a previous idiopathic facial palsy. Note the synchrony between the discharges in both these widely separate muscles. Such discharges probably originate in abnormal spontaneous discharges in one or more motor axons, other neighboring fibers being activated by ephaptic transmission (see text).

voluntary MUP recruitment patterns, MUPs, and motor terminal latencies in the seventh cranial nerve are usually all normal and there is no fibrillation in the facial muscles. In some of the other cases, however, there is evidence of axonal degeneration and the related denervation and reinnervation patterns in the EMG.

The precise pathogenesis of the abnormal spontaneous discharges in hemifacial spasm or the probably related facial myokymic discharges is not known. Reasonable speculations include ectopic impulses originating in trigger zone(s) in seventh nerve motor axons in their course through or beyond the brainstem. Naturally passing impulses in seventh nerve afferents might trigger abnormal trains of impulses in the motor axons by ephaptic transmission. This would result in a sort of artificial synapse as originally described by Granit, Leksell, and Skoglund (1944) in experimentally compressed and injured nerves, between the motor axons and afferents that are in the seventh nerve (see Chapter 11). Repetitive discharges in motor axons triggered by single passing impulses in the same axons and ephaptic transmission between nearby

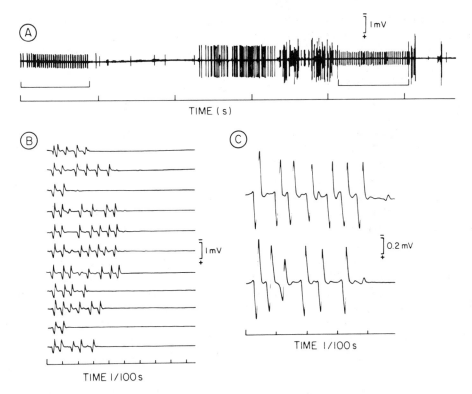

FIGURE 9.6.   Intramuscular concentric needle electrode recording from the frontalis muscle from a patient with hemifacial spasm (idiopathic variety).

(A) Overall character of the discharges as recorded over 5 to 6 seconds. The activity consists of bursts of potentials, individual bursts in this case lasting 1–2 seconds. The interburst period varies considerably. Each potential in the bracketed bursts actually consists of repetitive spikes (2 to 7), the first spike of which was used to trigger the oscilloscope sweep in (B) and (C). Successive potentials in the burst are shown in a roster display on an expanded time base in (B) and (C). The gain is increased in (C). Such discharges probably are caused by spontaneous activity at one or more sites in the motor axon, each spike in the motor axon being followed by a variable number of spikes following the initial one.

motor axons could also serve to multiply the extent and numbers of MU discharges in the facial muscles, as was suggested in the early 1950s (Woltman, Williams, and Lambert, 1951; Williams, Lambert, and Woltman, 1952). It is also possible that the impulses could be generated in the seventh nerve motoneurons (Hjorth and Willison, 1973), perhaps following axonal injury or central lesions partially deafferenting these motoneurons as suggested by Ferguson (1978), although there is no direct evidence to support the latter hypothesis. Hopf and Lowitzsch (1982) presented evidence supporting an origin in the seventh nerve as distal as the internal auditory meatus.

Janetta, Hackett, and Ruby (1970) claimed that compression of the seventh nerve by aberrant vessels is an important mechanism, and they advocated decompression. The benefit of such surgery, however, may not be related so much to decompression as the attendant mild trauma to the nerve (Auger, Piepgras, Laws, and Miller, 1981).

In some cases of hemifacial spasm with no prior history of facial palsy, needle electromyographic recordings from various facial muscles on the affected side have shown a higher proportion of hypercomplex MUPs and linked potentials. Also, single-fiber EMG recordings revealed increased fiber densities. No fibrillation potentials were seen in these muscles. These observations suggest that at one time there had been axonal degeneration in some of the facial motor axons and the subsequent reinnervation patterns account for the altered EMG potentials. Of course, such axonal degeneration could have been produced through lesions affecting the seventh motor axons in their intramedullary as well as their extramedullary course.

Tetanus

The spontaneous and excessive discharges of MUs that characterize tetanus could have several origins. One hypothesis for which there is no direct experimental support is that there is impaired Renshaw inhibition of alpha motoneurons (Brooks, Curtis, and Eccles, 1957; Curtis and DeGroat, 1968).

There is in addition, evidence of involvement of motor end-plates (Duchen, 1973) and peripheral nerves, including sensory fibers (Shahani, Astur, Dastoor, Mondkar, Bharucha, Nair, and Shah, 1979). The spontaneous motor discharges in tetanus may then originate in both the spinal cord and the peripheral motor axons.

Stiff-Man Syndrome

The disorder of stiff-man syndrome is characterized by increased muscle tone and spasms

often brought on by excitement or movement. Unlike the Isaac syndrome, the proximal muscles are more involved than distal muscles. Tendon reflexes in this disorder are normal (Spehlmann and Norcross, 1979; Olafson, Mulder, and Howard, 1964; Gordon, Jauszko, and Kaufman, 1967).

The continuous MU discharges persist at rest, although the level of spontaneous MU activity is somewhat reduced in sleep and even absent in rapid eye movement stages of sleep. The MUPs are normal. Fibrillations and fasciculations, afterdischarges, and other evidence of enhanced motoneuronal-axonal or muscle membrane excitability are absent. Conduction velocities are normal. The spontaneous discharges are reduced by spinal anesthesia, which suggests an origin in the motoneurons themselves. Diazepam in high doses does reduce the level of spontaneous activity, but carbamazepine and diphenylhydantoin do not.

Here as in tetanus the postulated basis is thought to be impaired recurrent inhibition of the motoneurons, possibly through loss of the Renshaw interneurons. As in tetanus, there is no pathological support for this hypothesis.

Intraspinal lesions may also produce rigidity in muscles innervated by the same spinal segments (Penry, Hoefnagel, Vanden Noort, and Denny-Brown, 1960; Rushworth, Lishman, Hughes, and Oppenheimer, 1961), possibly through destruction of the interneurons and "isolation" of the motoneurons. Experimental spinal cord ischemia produces a similar picture of rigidity and extensively destroys spinal interneurons (Gelfan and Tarlov, 1959, 1963).

Fibrillation Potentials

Fibrillation potentials are spontaneous, short-duration, biphasic or triphasic action potentials recorded outside the end-plate zone. They are most often seen in neurogenic diseases

(Figure 9.7), but sometimes occur in primary muscle diseases. Their electrical characteristics are described in Table 9.3. Their simple triphasic or biphasic shape, short durations, and steep radial decline in amplitude all stamp these as the action potentials of single MFs (Buchthal and Rosenfalck, 1966; Stålberg and Trontelj, 1982; Buchthal, 1982a, 1982b). Whether or not they are sometimes generated by two or more MFs in close proximity to one another is unknown, but such has been suggested to account for the occasional more "irregular" shapes (discontinuities on rising or falling phases) and slightly longer-duration fibrillation potentials (Buchthal, 1982a).

Fibrillation activity is reduced by cold, abolished by ischemia, and is resistant to tetrodotoxin (TTX) (see Chapter 1). In keeping with its origin in the muscle membrane itself, neuromuscular blocking agents do not alter fibrillation.

Electrogenic Origin of Fibrillation

Experimental investigations reveal two types of fibrillation (Li, Shy, and Wells, 1957; Thesleff, 1963, 1982; Belmar and Eyzaguirre,

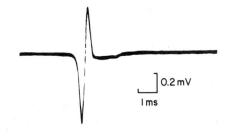

FIGURE 9.7. Fibrillation potential to show its triphasic character as recorded outside the end-plate zone with a single-fiber EMG electrode. Note the short duration and smooth shape, which strongly suggest generation by a single muscle fiber. Because of the relatively close proximity of the fiber to the small recording electrode leading-off surface, the amplitude of this fibrillation potential exceeded 1.0 mV, or 5 to 10 times the usual amplitude recorded with larger concentric needle electrodes.

1966; Purves and Sakmann, 1974a, 1974b; Smith and Thesleff, 1976). In one type the action potentials are triggered by regular oscillations of the membrane potential (Li, Shy, and Wells, 1957; Thesleff and Ward, 1975). These are most often centered about the old end-plate region. The depolarization phases

TABLE 9.3. Electrical Characteristics of Fibrillation Potentials

Shape	Smooth	
Number	Biphasic—positive-negative	Recorded
of phases	Triphasic—positive-negative-positive (Figure 9.7)	Outside end-plate zone
	Biphasic—negative-positive Irregular (5%)	Recorded in vicinity of end-plate zone
Amplitude	0.0–0.5 mV (p-p) (may be >1 mV recorded by SF-EMG electrode)	
Localization	Sharp radial decline in amplitude	
Discharge Pattern	Regular or Irregular	
Frequency	Increased by needle movement but present in subcutaneous recordings	

Adapted from Buchthal and Rosenfalck (1966) and Buchthal (1982a).

of these oscillations progressively increase until threshold is reached and action potentials are triggered at regular intervals. The cause of the regular oscillations is unknown, but changes in the properties of the sodium channels could underlie them.

The other type of fibrillation is characterized by action potentials that are triggered at irregular intervals by spikelike prepotentials (0.15 to 10 mV), most of which seem to originate in the region of the old end-plate (Figures 9.8 and 9.9). The prepotentials do not themselves propagate and they are not blocked by curare. The latter suggests they are not mediated through the action of acetylcholine, even though acetylcholine has been known to

be released by Schwann cells upon direct stimulation at denervated amphibian end-plates (Dennis and Miledi, 1974). The prepotentials are blocked by tetrodotoxin (TTX), indicating their dependence on sodium channels, and may originate in the transverse tubular systems (Purves and Sakmann, 1974b; Smith and Thesleff, 1976). Both types of fibrillation are enhanced in the presence of low concentrations of extracellular calcium ion.

Both types exhibit rhythmic cycles in their activity, periods of active discharge alternating with periods of quiescence (Thesleff, 1982). The latter could explain the absence of fibrillation in some denervated muscle fibers (Buchthal, 1982a, 1982b).

FIGURE 9.8. Varieties of intracellularly recorded potentials in the mouse diaphragm 9 to 10 days following denervation.
A = single discrete subthreshold depolarization.
B = complex subthreshold depolarization.
C = subthreshold depolarization that exceeded threshold and triggered postsynaptic action potentials.
D = fibrillation potentials lacking a prepotential, here recorded in the region of the tendon.
From Smith and Thesleff (1976, figure 2).

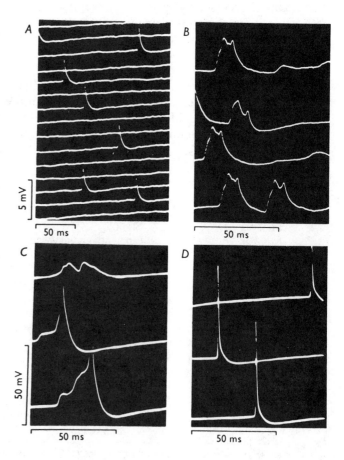

FIGURE 9.9. (A) Unitary potentials recorded in the innervation zone in a severely denervated human muscle. The complex nature of the potentials and their shape strongly suggest they are the equivalent of the spontaneous depolarizations noted in Figure 9.8B. Regenerative spikes may originate in some of these complex potentials.
(B) Potentials shown over a 2-second period to illustrate their high frequency (over 30/s).
(C) Just outside the above region, only triphasic potentials with the characteristics of single muscle fiber potentials were seen.
(D) The fibrillation potentials with a much lower firing frequency (just over 2/s).

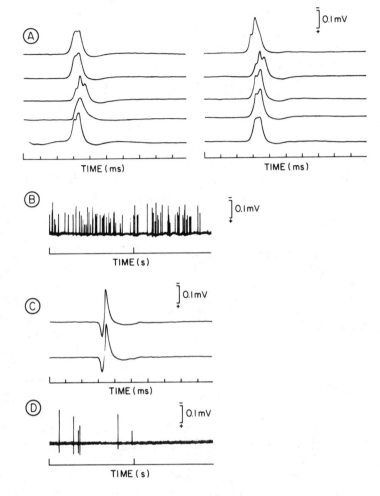

The Occurrence of Fibrillation in Various Diseases

Table 9.4 outlines the major categories of nerve and muscle diseases in which fibrillation occurs and some in which there is debate about its presence. Fibrillation most characteristically develops following section of a motor nerve, and is one of four major developments in the denervated muscle. The other changes are partial membrane depolarization, the development of TTX-resistant action potentials, changes in the time course of the action potential, and the appearance of extrajunctional acetylcholine receptors (see Chapter 2).

The latent period between transection of motor axons and the subsequent development of fibrillation in muscles innervated by these axons depends on the length of those motor axons distal to the transection. For example, fibrillation develops in the proximal arm muscles as early as one to two weeks, but not for three to four weeks in the intrinsic hand muscles in cases where the respective motor roots have been avulsed. Preceding the development of fibrillation, there may be an increase in the insertional activity (Lambert, 1960; Buchthal, 1962). On the other hand, fibrilla-

TABLE 9.4.   Causes of Fibrillation

Section or crush of motor nerves
Degeneration of motoneurons or axons
   See Chapter 2
      Motoneuron diseases
      Root lesions, plexopathies, peripheral
         neuropathies

Muscle disease	Including dystrophies (Duchenne and myotonic dystrophy)
	Polymyositis
	Myoglobinuria
	Congenital myopathies
	Muscle trauma

?Conduction block

?Neuromuscular transmission block
   Myasthenia gravis
   Botulinum toxin poisoning
Hyperkalemic periodic paralysis
Increase in fibrillation in denervated muscle
induced by
   Acetylcholine
   Norepinephrine
   Reductions in concentration of extracellular
     calcium ion

tion can persist for many years in a muscle where there has been a previous neurogenic lesion, although these potentials are seldom frequent at such late stages.

The development of fibrillation in the various motoneuronal and motor axonal diseases is to be expected. It is common in some primary muscle diseases (Humphrey and Shy, 1962; Buchthal, 1967, 1982a, 1982b), in which its origin is perhaps more puzzling. Possible explanations include denervation of viable segments of muscle fibers through segmental necrosis as could occur in Duchenne dystrophy and polymyositis (Desmedt and Borenstein, 1975), the failure of regenerated but isolated muscle fibers to acquire innervation because they are too far away from the innervation zone, changes in the properties of the muscle membrane such as to make them more excitable and capable of spontaneous impulse generation, and possibly direct neural damage as could occur to intramuscular axon branches in polymyositis or through a coexistent hereditary defect in the axons or motoneurons as suggested by McComas (1977). By disrupting the continuity of muscle fibers and separating portions of them from their innervation, trauma to muscle could induce fibrillation activity, as has been experimentally produced (Desmedt and Borenstein, 1975; Desmedt, 1978; Partanen and Danner, 1982).

Whether or not blocking transmission of impulses in motor axons can produce fibrillation in circumstances where the axons themselves remain intact remains uncertain. The problem here is that many of the experiments to test this question run the danger of damaging the motor axons by direct trauma at the site of experimental compression, local anesthetic, or tetrodotoxin block (see review by Harris, 1980). The weight of evidence at the present time is that fibrillation does not develop as a consequence of conduction block alone, provided there has been no wallerian degeneration (McComas, Jorgensen, and Upton, 1974; Gilliatt, Westgaard, and Williams, 1978), even though in the latter experimental model some degree of extrajunctional sensitivity to acetylcholine did develop.

The occurrence of fibrillation in poisoning with botulinum toxin and in myasthenia gravis is dealt with in Chapter 10; hyperkalemic periodic paralysis is discussed later in this chapter.

Acetylcholine, norepinephrine, and reduced concentrations of extracellular calcium ions are all known to increase the number of fibrillating muscle fibers.

Not all the short-duration simple biphasic and triphasic potentials in muscle diseases need be fibrillation potentials, although their characteristics stamp them as being generated by single muscle fibers. For example, the very short-duration MUPs sometimes seen in polymyositis, thyrotoxic myopathy, hyperkalemic periodic paralysis, Duchenne dystrophy, and myasthenia gravis no doubt reflect reductions in the numbers of muscle fibers that contribute to the MUP, and this could sometimes reach the point at which MUPs recorded by intramuscular electrodes at certain sites within the muscle appears to be generated by single muscle fibers alone.

Positive Sharp Waves

Positive sharp waves are closely related to fibrillation potentials and were described in 1949 by Jasper and Ballem. The electrical characteristics of these potentials are given in Table 9.5.

The significance of positive sharp waves is similar to that of fibrillation potentials. Often positive sharp waves precede the appearance of fibrillation potentials by one to two days following nerve transection.

TABLE 9.5.   Characteristics of Positive Sharp Waves

Characteristic	Description
Pattern	Most are biphasic waves and have initial sharp and brief positive phase, and a later longer-lasting and slower negative phase (Figure 9.10). (Sometimes one or two negative spikes are observed superimposed on the initial positive potential or on the later slow negative potential.)
Amplitude	Similar to fibrillation potentials but sometimes reaches several mV
Duration	10 to 30 ms and sometimes longer
Discharge pattern	Regular or irregular
Localization	Sharp decline in amplitude as transverse distance increases

Their precise electrogenic origin is unknown. Sometimes a typical fibrillation potential is seen to evolve into a positive sharp wave through a progressive decline and eventual disappearance of the sharp wave negative spike in the progressively deepening initial positive wave. At the same time, the slow negative afterpotential develops. It seems probable that in these instances the inward sodium current in the immediate vicinity of the electrode progressively declines to the point of block, leaving the outward passive current just preceding the blocked action potential and a later hyperpolarization. Why the late negativity should last so long in some instances is not clear (Figure 9.10). Sometimes when the concentric needle electrode passes through and shortly beyond the end-plate zone, the negative-positive spikes and even miniature end-plate potentials reverse polarity, becoming positive-negative or wholly positive and simulating positive sharp waves (Figure 9.11).

Bizarre Repetitive Discharges

Bizarre repetitive discharges (BRD) are complex potentials within muscle often consisting of multiple spike components, the whole complex firing at frequencies as low as 5 Hz to as

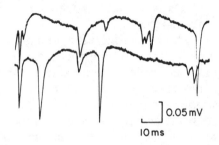

0.05 mV

10 ms

FIGURE 9.10.   Positive sharp waves, here recorded with a standard concentric needle electrode. Note the relatively long duration of the second negative phase.

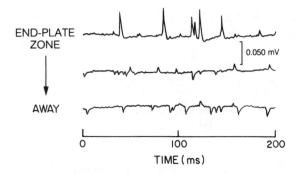

FIGURE 9.11.   Inversion of the polarity of miniature end-plate potentials as the recording electrode (here a standard concentric needle electrode) is passed a very short distance (less than 1 mm) beyond the immediate site of origin of the miniature end-plate potentials. The resultant positive potentials have durations and shapes similar to the miniature end-plate potentials but are of opposite polarity and as befits the increased distance from the source and the fact that the more active of the recording surfaces is most probably the cannula; their amplitudes are appreciably lower.

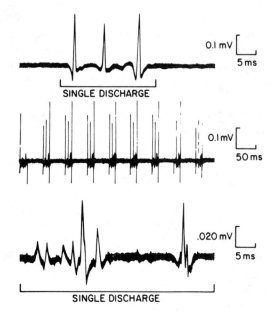

FIGURE 9.12.   Example of a bizarre repetitive discharge with a low firing frequency (18 repetitions per second). The individual three-spike components in this discharge are shown at the top, and a train of such discharges is in the middle. In most instances such discharges begin and stop abruptly. In the course of such repetitive discharges the interdischarge periods are often remarkably constant. Sometimes blocking of individual spike components in the discharge may be seen. Occasionally, however, greater variability in the interburst period occurs. Very commonly such bursts are composed of many spike components, as is shown for one such burst (Bottom).

high as 100 Hz or more. At the higher firing frequencies, especially, individual spike components may intermittently block. Characteristically, the discharges onset and terminate abruptly (Figure 9.12). In some cases discharges firing at similar frequencies may be found in needle electromyographic explorations of the same region in the muscle carried out several days apart. This suggests the presence of relatively stable pacemaker source within the muscle.

In SF-EMG recordings the potentials consist of up to 10 spike components that exhibit very low interspike jitter values, although slowly progressive changes in the intervals between spike components may be observed. The probable electrogenic source of these potentials is a pacemaker muscle fiber whose spontaneous impulses ephaptically excite adjoining muscle fibers (Stålberg and Trontelj,

1982; Trontelj and Stålberg, 1983). These BRD have been described in a variety of muscle and peripheral nerve diseases.

Cramp

Cramp is a painful, involuntary, sustained contraction of a muscle brought on especially when the muscle is contracted forcefully in a shortened state. The most common example in healthy humans is seen when the gastrocnemius and soleus muscles are forcefully contracted in the plantar flexed position (Layzer and Rowland, 1971). The cramp is relieved by firm massage and, even better, by forceful passive stretching of the firmly contracted muscle.

Cramp is sometimes preceded and terminated by scattered fasciculations. The EMG in cramp is characterized by high-frequency discharges of MUPs in irregular bursts that extend to different areas in the muscle. Although the discharges can be blocked by local anesthesia of the motor nerves, they can be reelicited by tetanic stimulation beyond the block. Cramp could be caused by the autoreexcitation of MFs produced by intense action currents of MFs in a strong contraction. The scattered fasciculations seen sometimes in association with the cramp may possibly be generated in a manner similar to that postulated for benign fasciculation.

Myotonia

The true myotonic phenomenon is characterized by prolongation of a voluntary contraction despite an attempt to relax the muscle(s). Similar prolonged contractions can be brought out by tapping the muscle or inserting an electrode into the muscle.

The myotonic discharge is characterized by a burst of potentials that progressively increases and then decreases in frequency and amplitude (Figure 9.13). These discharges are not blocked by neuromuscular transmission blocking agents, and hence must originate in the muscle membrane and not in the motor axons or motoneurons.

Recorded by concentric needle electrodes and triggered by movement of the electrode through the muscle, the myotonic potentials are often biphasic (positive-negative) spikes,

less than 5 ms in duration, or monophasic (positive) potentials that last longer (5 to 10 ms). Both potentials represent action potentials in single MFs, although the near synchronous discharge of groups of MFs nearest to the recording surface of the electrode cannot be excluded. Table 9.6 lists those clinical disorders in which myotonia may be seen.

Electrochemical Basis of the Myotonia Phenomenon

Normally a single impulse in the presynaptic motor axon is followed by only a single impulse in the postsynaptic muscle fiber. The fact that repetitive discharges do not occur in the muscle fiber is a tribute to the fact that the membrane leaks chloride ions as well as potassium ions into the extracellular space contained within the transverse tubular network as the impulse conducts along the transverse tubular membrane. Were chloride ions not to accompany potassium ions into the tubular space, the resulting accumulation of potassium ions within the confined space afforded by the tubular network could raise the potassium ion concentration sufficiently, even after a few impulses, to depolarize the tubular membrane to the point where repetitive discharges occur and prolonged contraction of the fiber follows in response to a single presynaptic impulse. The enhanced chloride conductance accompanying the impulse helps, therefore, to stabilize the membrane and prevent reactivation and repetitive firing of the tubular membrane following passage of the presynaptically induced impulse along the tubular membrane.

The central role of chloride conductance in preventing repetitive discharges in the tubular membrane and the resultant prolonged contractions of the muscle fiber suggests that reduced chloride conductance, whether from reduced numbers of chloride channels or malfunction of the chloride channels them-

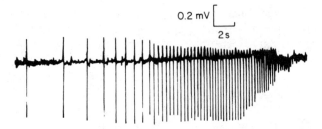

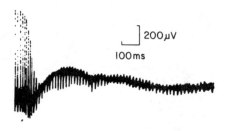

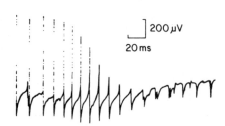

FIGURE 9.13. (Left) Myotonic discharge as recorded with a standard concentric needle electrode and elicited by lightly tapping the electrode, here inserted into the extensor digitorum communis muscle. In this case, slight movement of the electrode triggered a burst of positive-negative discharges whose frequency increased to a maximum of about seven impulses per second, the amplitude falling off eventually, probably corresponding to progressive depolarization of the muscle fiber. (Right) Myotonic discharge also triggered by tapping the electrode, but here consisting of repetitive negative-positive spikes shown on slower (above) and faster (below) time bases.

TABLE 9.6.   Myotonic Disorders in Humans

Myotonic Disorder	Presumed Underlying Defect
Hereditary	
Myotonic dystrophy	Possible defect in cation channels or lipid matrix of membrane
Myotonia congenita	Reduced chloride conductance possibly
Autosomal recessive	due to reduced numbers or functional
Autosomal dominant	abnormalities of the chloride channels
(Thomsen's disease)	
Paramyotonia congenita	Possible defect in cation channel function
without periodic paralysis	
Chondrodystrophic myotonia	Unknown
Acquired	
Drug induced	
Azacholesterols	Defective lipid matrix of the membrane and possible secondary abnormalities of cation channel function
Monocarboxylic acids	Reduced chloride conductance
Other	
Hypothyroidism	Unknown

Derived in part from Munsat and Scheife (1979), McComas (1977), and Bryant (1982).

selves, could explain the myotonia characteristic of human myotonic dystrophies or drug-induced myotonias. Indeed, mathematical modeling of muscle fiber membranes has shown that repetitive discharges of the membrane may be induced where its chloride conductance has been reduced by as little as 10 percent (Adrian and Marshall, 1976; Barchi, 1975, 1982). It turns out, at least in myotonia congenita and the myotonia produced through exposure to monocarboxylic acids, that a reduction in chloride conductance is probably the main mechanism responsible for the myotonia. The increased membrane resistance of myotonic membranes may partly be explained by the reduced chloride conductance of these membranes, although this would not of course explain the increased resistance of other myotonic membranes where the chloride conductance is not so reduced.

In other myotonic disorders the causes are less clear. For example, reduced chloride conductance has not been shown in myotonic dystrophy (Lipicky, 1977) or paramyotonia (Hayes and Thrush, 1972). In these latter myotonic disorders the abnormality may rest in a disorder of the voltage-dependent cation channels, sodium, potassium, or calcium, especially the last, although to date this has not been proved (Bryant, 1982).

The mechanism of the myotonia induced by the asa cholesterols is not known but may somehow be tied up with the replacement of cholesterol in the membrane by desmosterol, which accumulates because its conversion to cholesterol is prevented through the action of these drugs. The other cholesterol synthesis inhibitor, clofibrate, may act more directly through reducing chloride conductance in the membrane (Bryant, 1982). The presumed underlying mechanisms for some of the myotonias are listed in Table 9.6. Otherwise, in the human myotonias, the muscle membrane sensitivity to acetylcholine, as well as the end-plate potentials, are all normal (Hofmann and Smith, 1970).

The question of a possible neural contribution to myotonia has been discussed by McComas (1977).

The myotonic discharges are triggered by presynaptic nerve stimulation, insertion of a needle, and mechanical taps, but do not occur spontaneously. For example, microelectrode recordings just outside myotonic muscle fibers prior to puncturing the membrane do not reveal any fluctuations in the nearby muscle fiber membrane potentials. Puncture of the membrane, however, is accompanied by a burst of action potentials whose frequency and amplitude subsequently decline until, in some cases, the discharge abruptly ceases. Such recordings reveal the failure of the membrane to repolarize fully between action potentials. In some instances the membrane becomes progressively depolarized to the point at which the impulses finally stop, perhaps because of the cumulative inactivation of the sodium channels by the progressive depolarization of the membrane.

Other factors may alter myotonia. For example, drugs such as procainamide, quinine, and phenytoin, which block voltage-dependent sodium channels, will reduce the propensity to myotonia in both experimentally induced and naturally occurring myotonia. Also, increasing the extracellular sodium or potassium ion concentrations or reducing the extracellular calcium or magnesium concentrations may aggravate any tendency toward myotonia. The environmental temperature is yet another important factor affecting myotonia. Many patients with myotonia dystrophia or myotonia congenita report that cold aggravates the condition and increases the sense of stiffness in muscles, while warmer temperatures or repetitive activity (warming up) will reduce the myotonia (Walton and Gardner-Medwin, 1981). In vitro studies (Bryant, 1982), however reveal, contrary to what might be expected from the above clinical observations, that reducing the temperature of the muscle reduces the degree of repetitive activity in muscle fibers.

Overall, much remains to be learned about the biophysical basis of the myotonic phenomenon. Even in myotonia congenita, where reduced chloride conductance is held to be the major defect responsible for the myotonia, other abnormalities such as enhanced potassium conductance may play a part and of course the postulated underlying defects in cation channels in other myotonias remains to be confirmed.

DISORDERS OF HYPOEXCITABILITY

Periodic Paralyses

The periodic paralyses (PP) are characterized by attacks of weakness in which the muscle becomes inexcitable when directly stimulated electrically. The reason for such a loss of excitability is probably explained by alterations in the permeability properties of the membrane, of which more will be said later. In these disorders the main electrophysiological abnormalities (Buchthal, 1970; Engel, 1977; McComas, 1977; McComas and Johns, 1981) include in the EMG (Buchthal, 1970):

1. Normal motor (and sensory) conduction velocities
2. Reduced maximum muscle compound action potential amplitudes
3. Reduced amplitudes and durations of individual MUPs (sometimes to the point at which they may be generated by as few as one remaining excitable MF
4. True myotonic discharges and fibrillation potentials (some cases of hyperkalemic periodic paralysis and paramyotonia congenita)

At the level of muscle fibers they include:

1. Unresponsiveness of muscle fibers to direct and indirect stimulation
2. Normal end-plate potentials (EPPs) (Engel, 1981)
3. Reductions in membrane resistance (Engel and Lambert, 1969; McComas, Mrozek, and Bradley, 1968; Engel, 1977)
4. Depolarization of the membrane potential to -60 mV or less during the attack and to a lesser extent between attacks (Creutzfeldt, Abbott, Fowler, and Pearson, 1963)
5. Correction of transmembrane potential by procaine (Hofmann and Smith, 1970) and choline replacement of sodium
6. Restoration of action potentials by hyperpolarization
7. Normal contractions may be induced by direct application of calcium ions to MFs stripped of their sarcolemmal membranes (Engel and Lambert, 1969); this indicates the essential intactness of the contractile mechanisms of the muscle fibers

Morphological studies reveal, in all varieties of PP, dilatation of the sarcoplasmic reticulum as well as proliferation of the transverse tubular system producing central cavities within the MFs (Engel, 1977).

The basic mechanisms in these diseases, including both the primary and secondary varieties of the hypokalemic and hyperkalemic PP as well as the normokalemic type, are not as yet fully understood. The defect in the muscle must lie in the sarcolemmal or transverse tubular membranes or both, in view of the normal EPPs and responsiveness of the contractile apparatus to the direct application of calcium ions. Also, the lower membrane resistances and reduced transmembrane potential characteristic of PP are best explained by excessive leakiness of the membrane to sodium ions (increased sodium permeability).

The resulting progressive depolarization of the membrane to -60 mV or below could inactivate enough sodium channels to block generation and transmission of action potentials and would thus readily account for the lack of any response to direct as well as indirect stimulation.

In keeping with the above hypothesis is the observation that the impulse may be restored by artificially hyperpolarizing the membrane, partially blocking sodium channels by procaine or replacing extracellular sodium loss by choline.

Layzer (1982) suggested that, at least for hypokalemic PP, the membrane potential is stabilized between attacks through an accelerated action of sodium-potassium (Na-K) pump. In increasing the efflux of sodium ions, such an enhanced pumping action also pumps potassium inward against its concentration gradient, and in so doing reduces the extracellular potassium concentration. The latter, if reduced to too low a level, may shut off the Na-K pump, the resulting progressive depolarization of the membrane eventually blocking impulse generation. The shutdown of the pump in the face of a critically reduced extracellular concentration of potassium ions would in this model be enhanced by any stimulus that initially stimulates the pump, such as insulin, exercise, salt loading, and epinephrine. This model is not so clearly applicable directly to the hyperkalemic or normokalemic varieties of PP.

Despite apparent similarities in the membrane conductances and membrane potentials among the various PP, there are important differences among them in their urinary excretion of sodium, potassium, and chloride ions, and water in the attacks, in addition to other clinical differences in the nature of the attacks and the factors that precipitate the attacks (see Engel, 1977).

The progressive blocking of action potential generation in single MFs readily accounts for the reductions in the amplitude of the maximum compound action potentials and the reduced amplitudes and durations of the MUPs.

Contracture

Contracture may be defined as contraction of a muscle accompanied by electrical silence. The resultant muscle shortening is thus not preceded by any conductance changes in the outer or transverse tubular membranes. Contracture is characteristic of some of the glycogen storage diseases such as McArdle's disease and phosphofructokinase deficiency, and has also been seen in chronic alcoholic patients during heavy bouts of drinking. The contracture of the glycogen storage diseases may be brought on by exercise or experimentally induced ischemia.

Contracture may develop under the two latter conditions, but electrical discharges in the muscle do not accompany the contracture and venous blood lactate fails to rise. In these diseases, absence of a particular enzyme and overaccumulation of glycogen may be shown by muscle biopsy and histochemical techniques (Dubowitz and Brooke, 1973). The lack of adenosinetriphosphate in these disorders possibly interferes with the reuptake of calcium ions by the sarcoplasmic reticulum and in so doing provokes continued muscle contraction. Similar contractures can be produced by the metabolic inhibitors such as iodoacetate and dinitrofluorobenzene (Layzer and Rowland, 1971).

Repetitive supramaximal stimulation of motor nerves causes a rapid decrement in the amplitude of the maximum M-potential and cramp with no accompanying electrical activity in the glycogen storage diseases (Dyken, Smith, and Peake, 1967). The MUPs, recruitment patterns, and spontaneous activity in the end-plate zone are normal, however.

References

Adrian RH, Marshall MW. Action potentials reconstructed in normal and myotonic muscle fibers. J Physiol 1976;258:125–43.

Albers JW, Allen AA, Bastron JA, Daube JR. Limb myokymia. Muscle Nerve 1981;4:494–504.

Auger RG. Hemifacial spasm: clinical and electrophysiologic observations. Neurology 1979; 29:1261–72.

Auger RG, Piepgras DG, Laws ER Jr, Miller RH. Microvascular decompression of the facial nerve for hemifacial spasm: clinical and electrophysiological observations. Neurology 1981;31:346–50.

Barchi RL. An evaluation of the chloride hypothesis. Arch Neurol (Chicago) 1975;32:175–80.

Barchi RL. A mechanistic approach to the myotonic syndromes. In: Proceedings of a Symposium to Honor Dr. E. H. Lambert, Mayo Clinic, Rochester, Minnesota, April 1982. Muscle Nerve 1982;5:S60–S63.

Belmar J, Eyzaguirre C. Pacemaker site of fibrillation potentials in denervated mammalian muscle. J Neurophysiol 1966;29:425–41.

Bergmans J. Repetitive activity induced in single human motor axons: a model for pathological repetitive activity. In: Culp WJ, Ochoa J, eds. Abnormal nerves and muscles as impulse generators. Oxford: Oxford University Press, 1982: 393–418.

Blight AR, Precht W. "Spontaneous" quantal release of transmitter absent in vivo. Abst Soc Neurol Sci 1980;6:601.

Brick JF, Gutmann L, McComas CF. Calcium effect on generation and amplification of myokymic discharges. Neurology (NY) 1982;32:618–22.

Brooks VB, Curtis DR, Eccles JC. The action of tetanus toxin on the inhibition of motor neurones. J Physiol (Lond) 1957;35:655–72.

Brown WF, Varkey GP. The origin of spontaneous electrical activity at the end-plate zone. Ann Neurol 1981;10:557–60.

Bryant RH. Abnormal repetitive impulse production in myotonic muscle. In: Culp WJ, Ochoa J, eds. Abnormal nerves and muscles as impulse generators. Oxford: Oxford University Press, 1982:702–25.

Buchthal F. The electromyogram. World Neurol 1962;3:16–34.

Buchthal F. Electrophysiological differences between myopathy and neuropathy. In: Milhorat AT, ed. Proceedings of the International Conference Convened by the Muscular Dystrophy Association of America, New York. International Congress Series no. 147. New York: Excerpta Medica, 1967:207–16.

Buchthal F. Electrophysiological abnormalities in metabolic myopathies and neuropathies. Acta Neurol Scand 1970;46(suppl 43):129–75.

Buchthal F. Fibrillations: clinical electrophysiology. In: Culp WJ, Ochoa J, eds. Abnormal nerves and muscles as impulse generators. Oxford: Oxford University Press, 1982a:632–62.

Buchthal F. Spontaneous electrical activity: an overview. In: Proceedings of a Symposium to Honor Dr. E. H. Lambert, Mayo Clinic, Rochester, Minnesota, April 1982. Muscle Nerve 1982b;5:S52–S59.

Buchthal F, Rosenfalck P. Spontaneous electrical activity of human muscle. Electroencephalogr Clin Neurophysiol 1966;20:321–36.

Buller AJ, Proske U. Further observations on backfiring in the motor nerve fibers of a muscle during twitch contractions. J Physiol 1978; 285:59–69.

Burchiel KJ. Abnormal impulse generation in focally demyelinated trigeminal roots. J Neurosurg 1980;53:674–83.

Burchiel KJ. Ectopic impulse generation in demyelinated axons: effects of $PaCO_2$, pH and disodium edetate. Ann Neurol 1981;9:378–83.

Conradi S, Grimby L, Lundemo G. Pathophysiology of fasciculations in ALS: as studied by electromyography of single motor units. Muscle Nerve 1982;5:202–8.

Creutzfeldt OD, Abbott BC, Fowler WM, Pearson CM. Muscle membrane potentials in episodic adynamia. Electroencephalogr Clin Neurophysiol 1963;15:508–19.

Culp WJ, Ochoa J, eds. Abnormal nerves and muscles as impulse generators. Oxford: Oxford University Press, 1982.

Curtis DR, DeGroat WC. Tetanus toxin and spinal inhibition. Brain Res 1968;10:208–12.

Daube JR, Kelly JJ, Martin RA. Facial myokymia with polyradiculoneuropathy. Neurology (NY) 1979;29:662–69.

Dennis MJ, Miledi R. Electrically induced release of acetylcholine from denervated Schwann cells. J Physiol 1974;237:431–52.

Desmedt JE. Muscular dystrophy contrasted with denervation: different mechanisms underlying spontaneous fibrillations. Electroencephalogr Clin Neurophysiol 1978;34:531–46.

Desmedt JE, Borenstein S. Relationship of spontaneous fibrillation potentials to muscle fiber regeneration in human muscular dystrophy. Nature 1975;258:531–34.

Dubowitz V, Brooke MH. Muscle biopsy: a modern approach. London: WB Saunders, 1973.

Duchen LW. The effects of tetanus toxin on the motor end-plates of the mouse. J Neurol Sci 1973;19:160–68.

Dyken ML, Smith DM, Peake RL. An electromyographic diagnostic screening test in McArdle's disease and a case report. Neurology (Minneap) 1967;17:45–50.

Eccles JC, Katz B, Kuffler SW. Nature of the "endplate" potential in curarized muscle. J Neurophysiol 1941;4:362.

Eccles JC, Libet B, Young RR. The behaviour of chromatolysed motoneurones studied by intracellular recording. J Physiol 1958;143:11–40.

Engel AG. Hypokalemic and hyperkalemic periodic paralysis. In: Goldensohn ES, Appel SH, eds. Scientific approach to clinical neurology. Philadelphia: Lea & Febiger, 1977:1742–65.

Engel AG. Metabolic and endocrine myopathies. In: Walton J, ed. Disorders of voluntary muscle. 4th ed. Edinburgh: Churchill Livingstone, 1981:664–711.

Engel AG, Lambert EH. Calcium activation of electrically inexcitable muscle fibers in primary hypokalemic periodic paralysis. Neurology (Minneap) 1969;19:851–58.

Ferguson JH. Hemifacial spasm and the facial nucleus. Ann Neurol 1978;4:97–103.

Forster FM, Albers BJ. Site of origin of fasciculations in voluntary muscle. Arch Neurol Psychiatry 1944;51:264–67.

Forster FM, Borkowski WJ, Albers BJ. Effects of denervation on fasciculations in human muscle. Arch Neurol Psychiatry (Chicago) 1946;56:276–83.

Gamstrop I, Wolfart G. A syndrome characterized by myokymia, myotonia, muscular wasting and

increased perspiration. Acta Psychiatr Neurol Scand 1959;34:181–93.

Gardner-Medwin D, Walton JN. Myokymia with impaired muscular relaxation. Lancet 1969; 1:127–30.

Gelfan S, Tarlov IM. Interneurones and rigidity of spinal origin. J Physiol 1959;146:594–617.

Gelfan S, Tarlov IM. Altered neuron population in L7 segment of dogs with experimental hindlimb rigidity. Am J Physiol 1963;205:606–16.

Gilliatt RW. Paresthesiae. In: Culp WJ, Ochoa J, eds. Abnormal nerves and muscles as impulse generators. Oxford: Oxford University Press, 1982:477–89.

Gilliatt RW, Westgaard RH, Williams IR. Extrajunctional acetylcholine sensitivity of inactive muscle fibers in the baboon during prolonged nerve pressure block. J Physiol 1978;280:499–514.

Gordon EE, Jauszko DM, Kaufman L. A critical survey of stiff-man syndrome. Am J Med 1967;42:582–99.

Granit R, Leksell L, Skoglund CR. Fiber interaction in injured or compressed region of nerve. Brain 1944;67:125–40.

Harris AJ. Trophic effects of nerve on muscle. In: Sumner AJ, ed. The physiology of peripheral nerve disease. Philadelphia: WB Saunders, 1980:195–220.

Haynes J, Thrush DC. Paramyotonia congenita, an electrophysiological study. Brain 1972; 95:553–58.

Hjorth RJ, Willison RG. The electromyogram in facial myokymia and hemifacial spasm. J Neurol Sci 1973;20:117–26.

Hofmann WW, Smith RA. Hypokalemic periodic paralysis studied in vitro. Brain 1970;93:445–74.

Hopf HC, Lowitzsch K. Hemifacial spasm: location of the lesion by electrophysiological means. In: Proceedings of a Symposium in Honor of Dr. E. H. Lambert, Mayo Clinic, Rochester, Minnesota, April 1982. Muscle Nerve 1982; 5:S84–S88.

Howe JF, Calvin WH, Loeser JD. Impulses reflected from dorsal root ganglia and from focal nerve injuries. Brain Res 1976;116:139–44.

Howe JF, Loeser JD, Calvin WH. Mechanosensitivity of dorsal root ganglia and chronically injured axons: a physiological basis for the radicular pain of nerve root compression. Pain 1977;3:25–41.

Hughes RC, Matthews WB. Pseudo-myotonia and myokymia. J Neurol Neurosurg Psychiatry 1969;39:11–14.

Humphrey JG, Shy GM. Diagnostic electromyography. Arch Neurol 1962;6:17–30.

Huzier P, Kuno M, Miyata Y. Electrophysiological properties of spinal motoneurones of normal and dystrophic mice. J Physiol 1975;248:231–46.

Irani PF, Purohit AV, Wadia NH. The syndrome of continuous muscle fibre activity. Acta Neurol Scand 1977;55:273–88.

Isaacs H. A syndrome of continuous muscle fibre activity. J Neurol Neurosurg Psychiatry 1961;24:319–25.

Isaacs H. Quantal squander. S Afr J Lab Clin Med 1964;10:93–95.

Isaacs H. Continuous muscle fibre activity in an Indian male with additional evidence of terminal motor fibre abnormality. J Neurol Neurosurg Psychiatry 1967;30:126–33.

Isaacs H, Frere G. Syndrome of continuous muscle fibre activity. S Afr Med J 1974;48:1601–07.

Janetta PJ, Hackett E, Ruby JR. Electromyographic and electron microscopic correlates in hemifacial spasm treated by microsurgical relief of neurovascular compression. Surg Forum 1970;21:449–51.

Kugelberg E. Accommodation in human nerves. Acta Physiol Scand 1944;8(suppl 24):1–105.

Kugelberg E. "Injury activity" and "trigger zones" in human nerves. Brain 1946;69:310–24.

Kugelberg E. Activation of human nerves by ischemia. Arch Neurol Psychiatry 1948;60:140–52.

Kuno M. Responses of spinal motor neurones to section and restoration of peripheral motor connections. Cold Spring Harbor Symp Quant Biol 1975;40:457–63.

Kuno M, Llinás R. Enhancement of synaptic transmission by dendritic potentials in chromatolysed motoneurones of the cat. J Physiol 1970;210:807–21.

Kuno M, Miyata Y, Muñoz-Martinez EJ. Differential reaction of fast and slow alpha-motoneurones to axotomy. J Physiol 1974a;240:725–739.

Kuno M, Miyata Y, Muñoz-Martinez EJ. Properties of fast and slow alpha motoneurones following motor reinnervation. J Physiol 1974b;242:273–88.

Lambert EH. Electromyography. In: Glasser O, ed. Medical physics. Chicago: Year Book Publishers, 1960:251–56.

Lance JW, Burke D, Pollard J. Hyperexcitability of motor and sensory neurons in neuromyotonia. Ann Neurol 1979;5:523–32.

Layzer RB. Periodic paralysis and the sodium-potassium pump. Ann Neurol 1982;11:547–52.

Layzer RB, Rowland LP. Cramps. N Engl J Med 1971;285:31–40.

Li CL, Shy GM, Wells J. Some properties of mammalian skeletal muscle fibers with particular reference to fibrillation potentials. J Physiol 1957;135:522–35.

Lipicky RJ. Studies in human myotonic dystrophy. In: Rowland LP, ed. Pathogenesis of human muscular dystrophies. Amsterdam: Excerpta Medica 1977.

Lublin D, Tsairis P, Streletz LJ, Chambers RA, Riker F, VanPoznak A, Duckett SW. Myokymia and impaired muscular relaxation with continuous motor unit activity. J Neurol Neurosurg Psychiatry 1979;42:557–62.

Ludin HP. Electromyography in practice. New York: Stratton-Thieme, 1976:59–62.

Lutschg J, Jerusalem F, Ludin HP, Vassella F, Mumenthaler M. The syndrome of "continuous muscle fibre activity." Arch Neurol (Chicago) 1978;35:198.

McComas AJ. Neuromuscular function and disorders. Woburn, Mass.: Butterworths, 1977.

McComas AJ, Johns RF. Potential changes in normal and diseased muscle cell. In: Walton J, ed. Disorders of voluntary muscle. Edinburgh: Churchill Livingstone, 1981:1008–29.

McComas AJ, Jorgensen PB, Upton ARM. The neurapraxic lesion: a clinical contribution to the study of trophic mechanisms. Can J Neurol Sci 1974;1:170–79.

McComas AJ, Mrozek K, Bradley WG. The nature of the electrophysiological disorder in adynamia episodica. J Neurol Neurosurg Psychiatry 1968;31:448–52.

Meadows JC. Fasciculation caused by suxamethonium and other cholinergic agents. Acta Neurol Scand 1971;47:381–91.

Munsat TL, Scheife RT. Myotonia. In: Klawans

HL, ed. Clinical neuropharmacology. New York: Raven Press, 1979:83–107.

Negri S, Caraceni T, Boiardi A. Neuromyotonia. Report of a case. Eur Neurol 1977;16:35–41.

Nielsen VK, Friis ML, Johnsen T. Electromyographic distinction between paramyotonia congenita and myotonia congenita: effect of cold. Neurology 1982;32:827–32.

Noebels JL, Prince DA. Presynaptic origin of penicillin after-discharges at mammalian nerve terminals. Brain Res 1977;13:59–74.

Ochoa JL, Torebjörk HE. Paraesthesia from ectopic impulse generation in human sensory nerves. Brain 1980;103:835–53.

Olafson RA, Mulder DW, Howard FM. Stiff-man syndrome: a review of the literature, report of three additional cases and discussion of pathophysiology and therapy. Mayo Clin Proc 1964;39:121–44.

Partanen JV, Danner R. Fibrillation potentials after muscle injury in humans. In: Proceedings of a Symposium to Honor Dr. E. H. Lambert, Mayo Clinic, Rochester, Minnesota, April 1982. Muscle Nerve 1982;5:S70–S73.

Partanen JV, Nousiainen U. End-plate spikes in electromyography are fusimotor unit potentials. Neurology 1983;33:1039–43.

Partanen VSJ. Double discharges in neuromuscular diseases. J Neurol Sci 1978;36:377–82.

Partanen VSJ. Lack of correlation between spontaneous fasciculations and double discharges of voluntarily activated motor units. J Neurol Sci 1979;42:261–66.

Partanen VSJ, Lang AH. An analysis of double discharges in the human electromyogram. J Neurol Sci 1978;36:363–75.

Penry JK, Hoefnagel D, Vanden Noort S, Denny-Brown D. Muscle spasm and abnormal postures resulting from damage to interneurones in spinal cord. Arch Neurol 1960;5:500–12.

Purves D, Sakmann B. The effect of contractile activity on fibrillation and extra-junctional acetylcholine sensitivity in rat muscle maintained in organ culture. J Physiol 1974a;237:157–82.

Purves D, Sakmann B. Membrane properties underlying spontaneous activity of denervated muscle fibers. J Physiol 1974b;239:125–53.

Rasminsky M. Ectopic generation of impulses and cross-talk in spinal nerve roots of "dystrophic" mice. Ann Neurol 1978;3:351–59.

Rasminsky M. Ectopic excitation, ephaptic excitation and autoexcitation in peripheral nerve fibers of mutant mice. In: Culp WJ, Ochoa J, eds. Abnormal nerves and muscles as impulse generators. Oxford: Oxford University Press, 1982:344–62.

Roth G. Intranervous regeneration of lower motor neuron. I. Study of 1153 motor axon reflexes. Electromyogr Clin Neurophysiol 1978a;18:225–88.

Roth G. Intranervous regeneration of lower motor neuron. II. Study of 1153 motor axon reflexes. Electromyogr Clin Neurophysiol 1978b;18:311–51.

Roth G. The origin of fasciculations. Ann Neurol 1982;12:542–47.

Rushworth G, Lishman WA, Hughes JT, Oppenheimer DR. Intense rigidity of the arms due to isolation of motoneurones by a spinal tumour. J Neurol Neurosurg Psychiatry 1961;24:132–42.

Shahani M, Astur FD, Dastoor DH, Mondkar VP, Bharucha EP, Nair KG, Shah JC. Neuropathies in tetanus. J Neurol Sci 1979;43:173–82.

Simpson JA. Terminology of electromyography. Electroencephalogr Clin Neurophysiol 1969;26:224–26.

Sinderman F, Conrad B, Jacobi HM, Prochazka VJ. Unusual properties of repetitive fasciculations. Electroencephalogr Clin Neurophysiol 1973;35:173–79.

Smith JW, Thesleff S. Spontaneous activity in denervated mouse diaphragm muscle. J Physiol 1976;257:171–86.

Solandt DY. The measurement of "accommodation" in nerve. Proc R Soc Biol 1936;119:355–79.

Spehlmann R, Norcross K. Stiff-man syndrome. In: Klawans HL, ed. Clinical neuropharmacology. New York: Raven Press, 1979:109–21.

Stålberg E, Trontelj JV. Demonstration of axon reflexes in human motor nerve fibres. J Neurol Neurosurg Psychiatry 1970;33:571.

Stålberg E, Trontelj JV. Abnormal discharges generated within the motor unit as observed with single-fiber electromyography. In: Culp WJ, Ochoa J, eds. Abnormal nerves and muscles as impulse generators. Oxford: Oxford University Press, 1982:443–74.

Stohr M. Repetitive impulse-induced EMG discharges in neuromuscular diseases. Ann Neurol 1981;9:204.

Swank RL, Price JC. Fascicular muscle twitchings in amyotrophic lateral sclerosis. Their origin. Arch Neurol Psychiatry 1943;49:22–26.

Thesleff S. Spontaneous electrical activity in denervated rat skeletal muscle. In: Gutmann E, Hnik P, eds. The effect of use and disuse on neuromuscular functions. Prague: Publishing House of Czechoslovak Academy of Sciences, 1963.

Thesleff S. Fibrillation in denervated mammalian skeletal muscle. In: Culp WJ, Ochoa J, eds. Abnormal nerves and muscles as impulse generators. Oxford: Oxford University Press, 1982:678–94.

Thesleff S, Ward MR. Studies on the mechanism of fibrillation potentials in denervated muscle. J Physiol 1975;244:313–23.

Trojaborg W, Buchthal F. Malignant and benign fasciculations. Acta Neurol Scand 1965;41(suppl 13):251–54.

Trontelj J, Stålberg E. Bizarre repetitive discharges recorded with single-fiber EMG. J Neurol Neurosurg Psychiatry 1983;46:310–16.

Van Zandycke M, Martin JJ, Vande Gaer L, Van den Heyning P. Facial myokymia in the Guillain-Barré syndrome: a clinicopathologic study. Neurology (NY) 1982;32:744–48.

Wallis WE, VanPoznak A, Plum F. Generalized muscular stiffness fasciculations and myokymia of peripheral nerve origin. Arch Neurol 1970;22:430–39.

Walton JN, Gardner-Medwin D. Progressive muscular dystrophy and the myotonic disorders. In: Walton J, ed. Disorders of voluntary muscle. Edinburgh: Churchill-Livingstone, 1981:481–524.

Warmotts JR, Mendell JR. Neurotonia: impulse-induced repetitive discharges in motor nerves in peripheral neuropathy. Ann Neurol 1980;7:245–50.

Welch, LK, Appenzeller O, Bicknell JM. Peripheral neuropathy with myokymia-sustained muscular contraction and continuous motor unit activity. Neurology 1972;22:161–69.

Wettstein A. The origin of fasciculations in motoneuron disease. Ann Neurol 1979;5:295–300.

Wiederholt WC. "End-plate noise" in electromyography. Neurology (Minneap) 1970;20:214–24.

Williams HL, Lambert EH, Woltman HW. The problem of synkinesis and contracture in cases of hemifacial spasm and Bell's palsy. Ann Otol Rhinol Laryngol 1952;61:850–70.

Williamson E, Brooke MH. Myokymia and the motor unit. Arch Neurol 1972;26:11–16.

Woltman HW, Williams HL, Lambert EH. An attempt to release hemifacial spasm by neurolysis of the facial nerve. Proc Staff Meet Mayo Clin 1951;26:236–40.

10 NEUROMUSCULAR TRANSMISSION— NORMAL AND ABNORMAL

Primary neuromuscular transmission diseases such as myasthenia gravis are uncommon. Much more common are the abnormalities in neuromuscular transmission sometimes seen in neurogenic and primary muscle diseases. This chapter reviews the basis of normal neuromuscular transmission, points out where abnormalities in transmission could develop, and discusses the various diseases in this category. The basic abnormalities are explained and types of clinical tests of neuromuscular transmission are covered, with emphasis on their values and limitations.

STRUCTURE OF THE NEUROMUSCULAR JUNCTION

Before proceeding to a discussion of neuromuscular transmission disorders in man, it is necessary to review briefly the structure of the neuromuscular junction and presynaptic and postsynaptic mechanisms in neuromuscular transmission. There have been several recent reviews of the subjects and the reader is encouraged to examine them for more detail

(Lambert, Okihiro, and Rooke, 1965; Katz, 1966, 1969; Hubbard, 1973; Gage, 1976; Gauthier, 1976; Kuffler and Nicholls, 1976; Lester, 1977; Heuser and Reese, 1977; Martin, 1977; Takeuchi 1977; Miyamoto, 1978; Fambrough, 1979; Lindstrom and Dau, 1980; Ceccarelli and Hurlbut, 1980; Peter, Bradley, and Dreyer, 1982; Tauc, 1982; Llinás, 1982).

The basic elements of the neuromuscular junction are illustrated in Figures 10.1 and 10.2. End-plates are localized about half-way between the origin and insertion of individual muscle fibers (MF), although the overall pattern of the innervation zone in whole muscles may be quite complex depending on patterns of origin and insertion of all the MFs within the muscle (see Chapter 5). In normal muscle there is but one end-plate per MF, but in 2 to 3 percent of normal MFs and in states of reinnervation the incidence of multiple innervation of MFs may be higher.

Just proximal to the end-plate region the motor axon breaks up into a number of terminal branches, their terminal expansions; the presynaptic terminals contain vesicles, mitochondria, and cytoskeletal elements. This

FIGURE 10.1.   Drawing of the neuromuscular junction of the frog. The preterminal axon is invested by the myelinated processes of Schwann cells, while the terminal axon is invested by Schwann cell cytoplasm only. The axon terminal in the frog lies in a longitudinal depression on the surface of the muscle fiber. The immediate potsynaptic membrane is thrown into folds to form synaptic clefts. The number of acetylcholine receptors inserted in the membrane is highest in the crests of the folds immediately opposite the axon terminal.

The expanded view shows the transverse depression in the axon terminal opposite the postsynaptic clefts. On either side of these depressions are the active sites to which the acetylcholine-containing presynaptic vesicles attach. The active sites may also correspond to the sites of entry of Ca++ ions into the axon terminal, a prerequisite for acetylcholine release.

In the mammal, the contact zone is not linearly arranged as here, but is ellipsoid and the postsynaptic folds are not so regularly arranged.

Longitudinal section through a terminal axon branch lying in a corresponding longitudinal depression in the muscle fiber (top). The myelin sheath ends proximal to the terminal axon branch, which is invested by Schwann cell cytoplasmic processes only. The postsynaptic membrane opposite the axon terminal branch is thrown into transverse folds opposite which are parallel rows of intramembranous particles (bottom). The latter probably correspond to the active sites at which

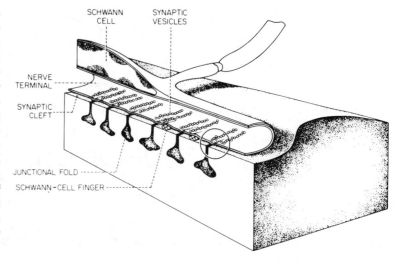

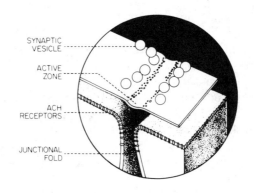

exocytosis of the acetylcholine-containing vesicles takes place. Such active sites may be where Ca++ ions enter the axon terminal, a necessary prerequisite for the release of acetylcholine.

The density of acetylcholine (ACh) receptors is highest at the crests of the junctional folds. In the gap (synaptic cleft) between the axon terminal and postsynaptic membrane is a matrix containing molecules of acetylcholinester-

ase. This substance not only intercepts and destroys a large proportion of the ACh before it reaches ACh receptors, but through the same action helps to destroy ACh released following its coupling with and activation of the ACh receptor. Thus the possibility of recombination of freed ACh molecules with other ACh receptors in the immediate vicinity is limited.

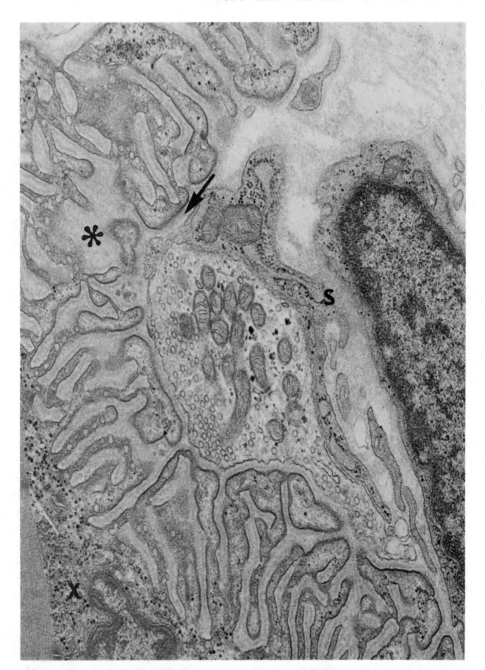

FIGURE 10.2.   Electron micrograph illustrates a normal human end-plate including the axon terminal containing mitochondria and synaptic vesicles, the synaptic cleft *(arrow)*, the postjunctional folds and clefts *(asterisk)*, and the underlying sarcoplasm *(x)*. Shown also is the investing Schwann cell including its cytoplasmic processes *(s)* and nucleus (top).

From Engel and Santa (1971, figure 1).

whole terminal arborization pattern impresses itself into a gutterlike depression on postsynaptic MF, the *primary synaptic cleft*. From this primary cleft, *secondary clefts* extend outward in a radial fashion throwing the postsynaptic membrane into a number of folds (Figure 10.1), the crests of which contain the highest concentrations of acetylcholine receptors (ACh-Rs) and lie directly opposite—across the primary cleft—the release sites of the ACh in the axon terminals.

The whole end-plate forms an ellipsoid structure that varies somewhat in size ($<$ 30 by 70 μ) and shape (Coërs and Woolf, 1959; Zacks, 1964; Padykula and Gauthier, 1970; Santa and Engel, 1973; Fardeau, 1973). Some evidence, at least in the rat and mouse, shows that the total postsynaptic membrane area is appreciably higher in the larger-diameter, faster-twitch MFs than in the smaller-diameter and slower-twitch red fibers (Duchen, 1971a). This may reflect the need for a larger end-plate current (EPC) in the larger MFs because of their lower input resistances (Kuno, Turkanis, and Weakly, 1971).

Freeze fracture studies reveal the presence of parallel double rows of intramembranous particles in the presynaptic membrane (Ellisman, Rash, Staehelin, and Porter, 1976; and review by Ceccarelli and Hurlbut, 1980) at which sites are clustered the synaptic vesicles. It is at these active sites that exocytosis of vesicles has been observed (Heuser, Reese, Dennis, Jan, Jan, and Evans, 1979; Heuser and Reese, 1981) and it has been suggested that the intramembranous particles may correspond to the actual calcium channels. In keeping with this hypothesis is the observation that the magnitude of the maximum calcium current in the presynaptic terminal of the squid giant axon is a function of the number of such intramembranous particles (Pumplin, Reese, and Llinás, 1981).

Similarly, on the crests of the postjunctional folds are other intramembranous particles that probably correspond to the ACh-R sites and are found in densities of 1,000 to 3,000 per square micron, the overall number of ACh-Rs being estimated to be about 1 to 5×10^7 based on estimates of the number of α-bungarotoxin sites on the human end-plate (Fambrough, Drachman, and Satyamurti, 1973). The ACh-Rs are also present in the extrajunctional membrane, although their densities are much lower than in the junctional folds and their properties may not be identical (Fambrough, 1979).

Covering the MF membrane and Schwann cells and investing the axon terminals are basement membranes (lamina), which fuse to form one membrane within the synaptic cleft. At normal end-plates, however, Schwann cell processes do not enter the synaptic cleft, which is about 500 Å wide.

SYNTHESIS AND BREAKDOWN OF ACh

Acetylcholine is synthesized primarily in the axon terminals themselves, although there is clear evidence that it can be synthesized elsewhere in the axon and motoneuron as well. It has been shown to be released from the regenerating tips of motor axons (Decino, 1981). The enzyme *choline-O-acetyltransferase*, produced in the motoneuron cell body and transported to the axon terminals, catalyses the combination of the two substrates *choline* and *acetyl coenzyme A* to form ACh. The stores of choline in the axon terminal are very limited and depend on reuptake of choline from the axon terminal following degradation of the ACh under the action of *acetylcholinesterase* (AChE) in the synaptic cleft or from choline in the plasma itself. Estimates suggest that about one-half of the choline produced as a consequence of this breakdown can be recaptured by the terminal. Choline must be actively transported across the terminal membrane, however, and this can be blocked, experimentally at least, by *Hemicholinium-3* and its analogs (Elmqvist and Quastel, 1965). Choline uptake is greatly accelerated by nerve stimulation and so is able to keep pace with release at stimulus rates as high as 20 Hz.

PRESYNAPTIC MECHANISMS IN NEUROMUSCULAR TRANSMISSION

In the amphibian, there is clear evidence that the impulse in the presynaptic axon directly invades the axon terminal (Katz and Miledi, 1965), but whether the impulse directly reaches the terminals or is electrotonically conducted to the terminals at all mammalian end-plates is not known. The site at which the myelin sheath terminates just proximal to the axon terminals may, because of the lower resistance and higher capacitance of the preterminal and terminals, represent a region where conduction of the impulse is less secure and hence more likely to block and prevent release of ACh. This does not happen at normal neuromuscular junctions. Presynaptic axonal conduction block may, however, reduce the safety factor for neuromuscular transmission (Hatt and Smith, 1976).

Microelectrodes inserted into the immediate end-plate region record spontaneous *miniature end-plate potentials* (MEPPs), which in the human intercostal muscle when corrected for a transmembrane potential of −80 mV have amplitudes of close to 1 mV (0.94 ± 0.026 mV). These potentials occur irregularly at about 0.2 to 0.03 per second (Engel, Lambert, and Gomez, 1977). Electrical stimulation of the nerve terminals or increases in concentrations of extracellular calcium or potassium ions increase the frequencies of these MEPPs (Liley, 1956a, 1956b; Hubbard, 1961, 1963; Hubbard and Schmidt, 1963; Hubbard, Jones, and Landau, 1968; Hubbard and Willis, 1968).

Recorded in the extracellular space in the immediate innervation zone by the much larger conventional EMG electrodes, these potentials are monophasic-negative and their amplitudes are one-tenth or less of the accompanying changes in transmembrane potential (Figure 10.3). The frequencies of the MEPPs in such recordings are often much higher, probably because of the irritative effect of the large EMG electrode that could depolarize the axon terminals directly or through disrupting cellular membranes and increasing the local concentrations of extracellular potassium ions (Figure 10.3). Such electrodes could also see MEPPs from several end-plates.

These MEPPs correspond to the release of one quantum of a package of ACh, which in turn undoubtedly corresponds to the release of one vesicle, in most cases, into the synaptic space. Estimates suggest that, at least at the frog and rat end-plates, there are 5,000 to 10,000 molecules of ACh per vesicle (Kuffler and Yoshikami, 1975; Fletcher and Forrester, 1975).

In response to a presynaptic impulse in the motor axon, there develops a near synchronous release of large numbers of quanta (about 100 to 200 in the amphibian and about 50 at

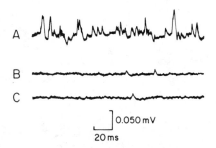

FIGURE 10.3. End-plate recording, human tibialis anterior just after insertion (A) of the needle and one (B) and two (C) minutes later. Note the high frequency of the miniature end-plate potentials (MEPPs) in (A), many being compounded of several unitary MEPPs just after insertion of the electrode (here a standard concentric needle), while a short time later—(B) and (C)—far fewer MEPPs are seen.

human neuromuscular junctions) (Figure 10.4). The multiquantal release produces an *end-plate potential* whose amplitude exceeds by two to three times the amplitude necessary to depolarize the postsynaptic membrane to threshold and produce an action potential in the MF.

Proof that nerve stimulus-evoked ACh transmitter release is multiquantal rests with the clear demonstration that when neuromuscular transmission is partially blocked by lowering the extracellular calcium ion concentration (or increasing the magnesium ion concentration) to the level at which all EPPs are subthreshold, sometimes no EPP at all occurs in response to a presynaptic stimulus. In these circumstances it can be shown that the amplitudes of EPPs vary in quantal steps, the amplitude in response to any one presynaptic impulse being some multiple 0, 1, 2 . . . n of the mean MEPP (Martin, 1955, 1966, 1977; Elmqvist and Lambert, 1968; Katz, 1966; Katz and Miledi, 1972). The distribution of EPP amplitudes in these circumstances follows a Poisson distribution. The relationship be-

tween the amplitude of the EPP and the number of quanta is not, however, linear because the nearer the EPP amplitude approaches the *equilibrium potential for the EPP* (-20 to -10 mV), the lower the resultant membrane currents. This happens because as pointed out in Chapter 1, the actual transmembrane membrane currents are a function not only of the membrane conductance for a particular ion species, but the driving force; namely, the difference between the equilibrium potential for the ion and the actual transmembrane potential. Hence as the amplitude of the EPP approaches the equilibrium potential of the EPP, the driving force for the ionic currents, here dominated by sodium ions, diminishes. Therefore the magnitude of the transmembrane current diminishes despite the same increase in membrane conductance.

Release of ACh has been shown to depend on prior inward movement of calcium ion into the axon terminal (see Katz and Miledi, 1968; and review by Katz, 1969; Miledi, 1973) and can be blocked by clamping the presynaptic terminal at the calcium equilibrium potential

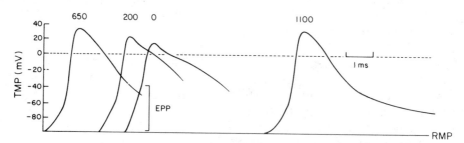

FIGURE 10.4.   Postsynaptic muscle fiber potentials recorded with an intracellular electrode both in the immediate vicinity of the end-plate (O) and at various distances on either side of the end-plate, 200 and 650 μ respectively in one direction and 1,100 μ in the opposite direction. Note the hump on the rising phase of the potential, which is of highest amplitude in the immediate vicinity of the end-plate (here close to 60 mV in amplitude) and which falls off rapidly in size on either side of the end-plate. The reduction in spike amplitude and subsequent hump in the falling-off phase of the action potential as recorded near the end-plate are caused by the short-circuiting of the membrane in this regon as a result of increases in ionic conductance produced through the actions of acetylcholine.

Redrawn and adapted from Fatt and Katz (1951).

or in the presence of very low concentrations of extracellular calcium ions. The quantal content of the EPP conversely can be increased by increasing these concentrations.

Hyperpolarization of the axon terminals produced by repetitive stimulation of the motor axon terminals increases the amplitude of the presynaptic spikes. It also serves to increase the amplitudes of EPPs, probably through increasing the influx of calcium into the axon terminals, thereby increasing the quantal content of the EPP (Hubbard and Schmidt, 1963). This latter mechanism may explain the *post-tetanic potentiation* (PTP) seen shortly after a strong muscle contraction or tetanus motor nerve stimulus (see later discussion).

Just how the calcium influx triggers the release of ACh is unknown at this time. This stage takes an appreciable time (about 0.5 ms of a total neuromuscular delay of 0.75 ms), however, and shows remarkable temperature dependence. Thus cooling the muscle to 7°C can increase this delay to as long as 6 ms.

Acetylcholine crosses the synaptic gap in as short a time as 50 μsec. One-third to one-half of the ACh is destroyed by AChE in the matrix of the space. Acetylcholinesterase is present on both the presynaptic and postsynaptic membranes, but is not bound to the ACh-Rs themselves. The remainder of the ACh then binds to the ACh-Rs briefly (about 100 to 200 μsec), in which time the protein somehow changes its physicochemical properties such that the ion channel linked to the receptor site increases its conductance; primarily to sodium and to a lesser extent potassium and possibly also calcium ions (the rate of sodium-to-potassium conductance is about 30 : 1). These channels are not blocked by tetrodotoxin, although the latter does block extrajunctional sodium channels.

There is also now, clear evidence that ACh may be released in a nonquantal form (Katz and Miledi, 1977; Tauc, 1982) and these leakages may be substantial.

POSTSYNAPTIC MECHANISMS IN NEUROMUSCULAR TRANSMISSION

The precise relationship between the ACh-Rs and the ion channel is unknown. Whatever the connection, the channel remains open only about 1 to 1.5 ms and then closes spontaneously (inactivation). One single quantum of ACh has been estimated to open about 1,000 channels. Dissociation of the ACh-R–ACh complexes releases some ACh, which, provided it is not broken down by AChE, is able to recombine with other ACh-R, thus prolonging the end-plate current (EPC) (Katz and Miledi, 1973).

Indeed, in the absence of AChE or when it has been blocked by anticholinesterases, repeated activation of ACh-R by the available ACh can substantially prolong the EPC. This causes reexcitation of MF action potentials until such time as the ACh eventually leaks out of the synaptic space (Katz and Miledi, 1973).

Prolonged exposure of the end-plate to ACh results in progressive reduction in the EPC through possible inactivation of the ACh-R on ionic channels, a process called *desensitization*. The time course of the accompanying EPP and MEPP are appreciably slower than the corresponding EPCs because of the cable properties, particularly the high capacitance of the MFs (Gage, 1976) (Figure 10.5).

STORAGE OF ACETYLCHOLINE

There is evidence that ACh is stored in at least two forms: an immediately available store and slower-release form (see review by Hubbard, 1973). For example, even at stimulus frequencies as low as 0.1 Hz, the successive EPPs in response to the stimulus train decline in amplitude to reach steady-state values whose amplitudes are dependent on the frequency of stimulation. Progressively higher frequencies of stimulation do not continue to

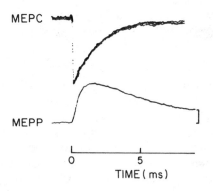

FIGURE 10.5. Relationship of the time course of the miniature end-plate current (MEPC) as recorded with an extracellular electrode and the corresponding miniature end-plate potential (MEPP) as shown for two MEPPs. Note that the MEPC reaches its peak rapidly and is over while the MEPP has not returned to its resting potential level. These delays reflect the resistive and capacitative properties of the membrane. Adapted from Gage (1976).

increase the amount of ACh released per unit time. Eventually, frequencies are reached at which the amount of ACh released per unit time achieves an upper limit, although changes in the quantal content of individual EPPs may be dependent on stimulus frequency. These observations have suggested that there is a relatively small store of ACh available for immediate release. Beyond this store, however, there is another store from which ACh can be mobilized to meet the needs of synaptic transmission, but there is an upper limit to the rate at which ACh can be released from this store.

These observations help to explain the changes in EPP amplitude at various frequencies of stimulation at normal neuromuscular junctions as well as some of the failures of neuromuscular transmission in disease states where the *safety factor for neuromuscular transmission* may be lower. In such circumstances, reduction in the quantal content of the EPP, even at low frequencies of stimulation (0.1 to 5 Hz), may reduce the amplitude

of the EPP to below the levels at which an action potential can be generated in the MF.

In the human, EPPs and EPCs are not measurable by current techniques, only the postsynaptic action potentials in the MFs that are recorded as single fiber potentials with single-fiber electromyography (SF-EMG) or as compound motor unit potentials (MUPs) or the maximum compound M-potential, the last from whole muscles or groups of muscles. Failures of neuromuscular transmission are then signaled by single-fiber blocking in the SF-EMG technique or reductions in the compound MU or maximum M-potentials. Techniques to assess these changes are discussed in detail later.

The preceding account of neuromuscular transmission is summarized by Figure 10.6, which also suggests a number of sites where neuromuscular transmission could become disturbed. Abnormalities at certain of these sites produced specific diseases of neuromuscular transmission to be discussed later in this chapter. Disorders of neuromuscular transmission are classified in Table 10.1 according to whether the abnormality, known or presumed is presynaptic, postsynaptic, or both.

Because of its central importance to any discussion of neuromuscular transmission disorders, myasthenia gravis is discussed first. This is followed by a review of the available clinical methods of testing neuromuscular transmission and finally by discussions of the other disorders, illustrating for each its unique features and the types of abnormalities to be seen in clinical testing.

MYASTHENIA GRAVIS

There have been several important advances in our understanding of myasthenia gravis (MG) over the last decade. Previous speculation that the neuromuscular transmission abnormalities were presynaptic in origin has

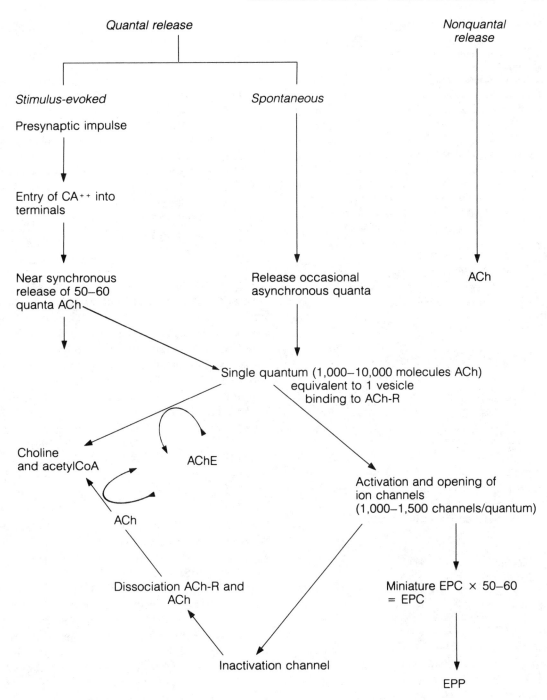

FIGURE 10.6.

TABLE 10.1.   Classification of Disorders of Neuromuscular Transmission

Presynaptic
    Eaton-Lambert syndrome
    Toxins
        Botulinum
        Clostridium tetani
        Tick
        Black widow spider
        Scorpion
    Congenital
        Possible abnormal synthesis of ACh
            Deficiency of AChE with small nerve
                terminals and reduced ACh release
    Secondary to
        Peripheral neuropathies
        Amyotrophic lateral sclerosis
        Multiple sclerosis
        Primary muscle diseases
Postsynaptic
    Myasthenia gravis (autoimmune)
    Congenital
        Prolonged ACh-R opening time
        ?Abnormal ACh-R
    Drug induced
        Antibiotics—tetracycline, oxytetracycline, D-
            penicillamine, anticholinesterases, curare
Combined Presynaptic and Postsynaptic Actions
    Anticonvulsants
    Antibiotics
        Polymyxin group
        Aminoglycosides—streptomycin, neomycin,
            kanamycin
        Monobasic amino acids—lincomycin,
            clindamycin
        Procainamide and quinidine
        Lithium
        β-Adrenergic blocking agents
Cation-induced neuromuscular disorders
    Magnesium
    Calcium

proved to be incorrect, the primary abnormality being destruction of the end-plate receptors by antibodies directed against the receptor proteins. Untrastructural studies clearly show that while there are wide variations among end-plates in the extent of the abnormalities seen in MG, the most characteristic abnormalities include:

1. Reductions in total postsynaptic membrane area (Figure 10.7) are apparent in the "simplification" of the postsynaptic membrane, namely, shallower secondary clefts and loss of folds.
2. There is, however, no change in the number of vesicles per unit area of the axon terminals.
3. Some immature or simple neuromuscular junctions with nearby regenerating axons may be seen.

These abnormalities clearly point to the possibility of denervation at some end-plates, and reinnervation and the establishment of miniature end-plates in other instances. The most important abnormalities, namely, loss of ACh-Rs (Fambrough, Drachman, and Satyamurti, 1973; Engel, Lindstrom, Lambert, and Lennon, 1977; Lindstrom and Lambert, 1978) and postsynaptic membrane through antibodies directed at the receptors have now received clear support. Not only are circulating antibodies to ACh-Rs demonstrable in most patients with MG, but immunoglobulin G (IgG) and complement have been localized to the end-plate region in the human disease and its close experimental analogs (Kelly, Lambert, and Lennon, 1978; Engel, Lambert, and Howard, 1977; Sahashi, Engel, Lindstrom, Lambert, and Lennon, 1978). Plasma exchange has not produced dramatic resolution of the clinical or electrophysiological abnormalities (Campbell, Leshner, and Swift, 1980) even though there were reductions in the antireceptor antibody levels. In this regard it is interesting that serum containing ACh-R taken from patients with MG has been shown to produce physiological abnormalities reminiscent of MG in experimental animals (Oda, Korenaga, and Ito, 1980; Pagala, Tada,

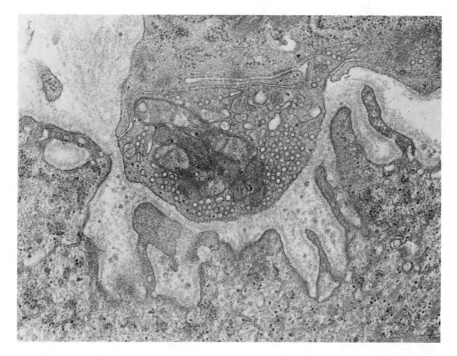

FIGURE 10.7.   Electron micrograph of an end-plate in myasthenia gravis. The postsynaptic membrane is highly simplified, there being far fewer folds than is normal. The nerve terminal, however, is filled with synaptic vesicles (top). (Magnification × 22,500)
From Engel and Santa (1971, figure 6), and reprinted with the permission of the publisher, The New York Academy of Sciences.

Namba, and Grob, 1982; Murali, Pagala, Tada, Namba, and Grob, 1982). Myasthenic immunoglobulins have also been shown to accelerate the breakdown of ACh-Rs in tissue culture (Kao and Drachman, 1977).

The ACh-R antibodies may not be detectable in mild or pure ocular forms of human MG. Levels of antibodies do, however, correlate to some extent with changes in severity of clinical involvement in individual patients (Vincent and Newsom-Davis, 1980; Lindstrom and Dau, 1980; Tindall, 1981); although other studies have not been able to show any apparent correlation between plasma ACh-R antibody levels and the clinical state

of the myasthenia (Roses, Olanow, McAdams, and Lane, 1981).

The absence of axon terminals at some end-plates and presence of some "new" immature end-plates and regenerating axons suggest that in some instances the destruction of the end-plate may be so severe as to denervate the MF; while in other instances recovery is indicated by regenerative phenomena. Similar changes have been seen in experimental autoimmune MG (Engel, Tsujihater, Lambert, Lindstrom, and Lennon, 1976), although the acute mononuclear infiltrates and intense degenerative changes seen early in that disorder are not seen in MG.

Physiological and Pharmacological Abnormalities in MG

Table 10.2 shows the main characteristics of MG. The very reduced amplitudes of some of the MEPPs, to within the noise levels of the recording system in some instances, probably accounts for some of the reports of reduced MEPP frequencies (Dahlbäck, Elmqvist, Johns, Radner, and Thesleff, 1961).

The primary basis of the physiological abnormalities in MG is progressive depletion of ACh-R. The identical abnormalities are also seen at end-plates where the ACh-Rs have been blocked by α-bungarotoxin (Satya-murti, Drachman, and Slone, 1975). The loss of receptors clearly explains the reduction in the amplitudes of the MEPPs and EPPs and reduced safety factor for neuromuscular transmission that results. Elementary interactions between ACh and ACh-R are normal, however (Ito, Miledi, Vincent, and Newsom-Davis, 1978). Despite the normal quantal content of the EPP and the normal elementary ACh–ACh-R interaction, amplitudes of EPPs are reduced because fewer receptors are available to bind with the ACh. In addition, larger losses of ACh could occur through increased leakages out of the wider synaptic clefts.

Because the amplitudes of EPPs normally

TABLE 10.2.   Physiological Characteristics of Neuromuscular Transmission in Myasthenia Gravis

Primary
  Presynaptic
    Normal MEPP frequency[1,2]
    Normal quantal content of EPP[1,2]
  Postsynaptic
    Normal
      Transmembrane potential[1,2]
      Input resistances of MFs[1,2]
      Membrane time constant[2]
    Normal interactions ACh–ACh-R[3]
    Elementary EPP (single channel), amplitude, and time course are normal
    Reduced amplitudes of
      EPP especially in response to a stimulus train (Figure 10.9)
      MEPP[1,3,4] amplitude proportional to ACH receptor surface[4]
Reductions in the safety factor for neuromuscular transmission with
  Increased variability in neuromuscular transmission delay[2]
  Subthreshold EPPs and failures of neuromuscular transmission[2]
Secondary changes
  Functional denervation   →   Fibrillation (uncommon)
    There have been no demonstrated increases in extrajunctional ACh sensitivity or
        tetrodotoxin-resistant action potentials[3]
  Formation of new immature end-   →   Reduced safety factor for neuromuscular
    plates and reinnervation   transmission

[1]Elmqvist, Hofmann, Kugelberg, and Quastel (1964).
[2]Elmqvist (1973).
[3]Ito, Miledi, Vincent, and Newsom-Davis (1978).
[4]Engel, Lindstrom, Lambert, and Lennon (1977).

exceed threshold in MF by two to three times, even substantial reductions in EPPs may not produce subthreshold EPPs and failures of neuromuscular transmission (Figure 10.8). Where the amplitudes of the EPPs just exceed threshold in response to single stimuli, however, the normal reduction in the quantal content of the EPP in response to a train of stimuli (see earlier section) may lead to some of the EPPs falling below threshold levels and producing transmission failure.

Curare, a drug that acts postsynaptically, produces post-tetanic changes very similar to those at myasthenic end-plates. In both, a brief tetanic stimulus (50 to 100 impulses per second for 10 seconds) often produces and increases the amplitudes of EPPs evoked by test stimuli delivered shortly after the tetanus. This *post-tetanic potentiation* (PTP) lasts but a short time, especially when the tetanus is brief, and is characteristically followed by a period of *depression* whose duration and degree can be

FIGURE 10.8. Diagrammatic representation of changes in the end-plate potential (EPP) (crosshatched) and the development of an action potential in a muscle fiber as they would appear if recorded in the end-plate zone by an intracellular electrode. (A) Normal neuromuscular junction. Repetitive stimulation (S1, S2 . . . Sn) results in a progressive decline in the EPP because of reduction in its quantal content. Because the amplitude of the EPP continues to exceed threshold for generation of an action potential in the muscle fiber, impulse blocking does not occur. No decrement in the overall size of the MUP or maximum M-potential would be expected. (B) The same progressive reduction in quantum content of the EPP in situations where postsynaptic responsiveness to the released acetylchline may be reduced, for example, through reduced numbers of ACh-R. The amplitude of the EPP may become so reduced as to result in failure of some EPPs to reach the critical threshold levels necessary to trigger a postsynaptic action potential in the muscle fiber (responses to the fourth and fifth stimuli here). Such impulse blocking is characteristically preceded by an increase in the variability in onset time of muscle fiber action potential with respect to the presynaptic stimulus. When they affect a significant proportion of the end-plates, such failures in neuromuscular transmission can account for the sometimes clinically apparent fatigue as well as for decrements in the maximum M-potential or sizes of individual MUPs seen in response to repetitive stimulation or activation. (C) Conversely, in disorders such as the myasthenic syndrome, the quantal content of the EPP is often so low at onset of a stimulus train as to fall below the threshold level of depolarization of the postsynaptic

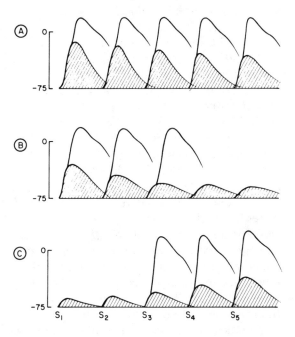

muscle fiber necessary to trigger an action potential. Successive stimuli lead to progressive increases in the quantum content of the EPP until, after several impulses, the EPP amplitude exceeds the threshold at which action potentials are triggered and transmission is restored. Such effects, when extended to a significant proportion of end-plates in a muscle, account for the incremental increases in the maximum M-potential at stimulus frequencies of over 20 Hz and the sometimes clinically appreciable increase in strength occasionally seen in the myasthenic syndrome.

increased by lengthening the duration of the tetanus. This depression is probably equivalent to *post-tetanic exhaustion* (PTE) and perhaps to depletion of the immediately available stores of ACh. The PTP may also be produced by brief intense voluntary contraction, with an increase in the amplitude(s) of the maximum M-potential evoked by a single or brief train of stimuli delivered just after this exercise in comparison to the preexercise amplitudes.

Even if EPPs do not fall below threshold, there may be increased fluctuations in the time interval between the stimulus (or presynaptic pulse) and the generation of action potentials in the MFs. These are the basis of increases in jitter and impulse block at single neuromuscular junctions seen in SF-EMG studies and the decrements in the maximum M-potential in response to a train of stimuli.

Loss of ACh-Rs is not the only cause of neuromuscular transmission failures in MG. For example, levels of anticholinesterase drug that are optimal at some myasthenic end-plates may produce cholinergic block at other end-plates through a process of desensitization, while at other end-plates the drug level may be inadequate to restore neuromuscular transmission. Furthermore, corticosteroids sometimes used in the treatment of MG may themselves produce failures in neuromuscular transmission and destruction of end-plates.

The degree to which end-plates are affected can vary widely within individual MUs. There may also be appreciable differences among MUs in the severity of the neuromuscular transmission disorder, perhaps reflecting differences in the safety factors for neuromuscular transmission among the types of MUs. On clinical evidence alone, it is also apparent that not all muscles are affected to the same degree. The fact that the levator palpebrae and extraocular muscles are among those most commonly affected may reflect their persistent tonic activity in the waking states unlike some of the limb muscles. Also, the safety factor for neuromuscular transmission at normal and abnormal neuromuscular junctions is increased when muscles are cooled somewhat, as in the intermediate and especially distal, acute motor, and bulbar muscle, temperature being maintained at core temperature. Clearly too, the occasional immature neuromuscular junctions seen in this disease may add to the complement of end-plates with reduced safety factors for transmission.

The preceding outline of the basic physiological neuromuscular transmission abnormalities in MG provides the necessary background for the material to come.

TESTS OF NEUROMUSCULAR TRANSMISSION

Table 10.3 shows the tests of neuromuscular transmission available, each one of which is discussed in turn.

The most conventional way to assess neuromuscular transmission is to measure changes in amplitude of the maximum compound M-potential (MCMP) in response to supramaximal stimulation of the motor nerve. For such evaluations surface electrodes are employed because they best reflect the activities of the whole muscle or group of muscles. The amplitude of the MCMP in such recordings depends most importantly on the number of MFs that generate action potentials in the underlying muscle(s), the temperature of the muscle, and the degree of temporal dispersion in the summation of the component action potentials.

Repetitive stimulation of the motor nerve in healthy humans produces characteristic changes in the amplitude and duration of the MCP (Figure 10.9) whose magnitude depends on frequency of stimulation. The general order of magnitude of these changes at various stimulus frequencies is outlined in Table 10.4.

Increases in peak-to-peak amplitude at 5-

TABLE 10.3. Clinical Tests of Neuromuscular Transmission

Evaluation of changes in the maximum M-potential evoked by supramaximal stimulation
of motor nerves
  Evaluation of M-potentials in response to single stimuli and trains of stimuli at 1, 3, 10,
  20 per second
  Examination of poststimulus changes in the M-potential looking for
    Post-tetanic potentiation (PTP)
    Post-tetanic exhaustion (PTE)
  Evaluation of changes in M-potential when stimulation is combined with strategies to
    reduce to safety factor for neuromuscular transmission such as
    Exercise or tetanic stimulation
    Ischemia
    Curare, systemic or regional
    Warming the muscle(s)
Evaluation of neuromuscular transmission at individual neuromuscular junctions by
  SF-EMG
  Measurement of variations of neuromuscular delays (jitter)
  Assessment of incidence of neuromuscular blocking
  Assessment of numbers of independent spike generators belonging to the same MU
    within the immediate vicinity of the electrode (fiber density)
Other electrophysiological tests
  Stapedius reflex
  Ocular movement
  Intraocular pressure

to 20-Hz stimulation are probably the result of increases in the degree of synchronization between the action potentials of all the contributing MFs. Such *pseudofacilitation* contrasts with increases in the p-p amplitude of M-potentials through real increases in the numbers of contributing MFs to the M-potential, *true facilitation*. Decrements in amplitude at higher frequencies of stimulation are probably the product of progressive axonal and neuromuscular block.

In the evaluation of changes in the M-potential in reponse to repetitive stimulation it is vital to be aware of and to control technical errors. For example, movements of the underlying muscle(s) with respect to the recording electrodes can produce spurious changes in the shape and amplitude of M-potentials, especially at higher frequencies of stimulation where successive twitches may fuse. It is also important to ensure that the electrical stimulus remains supramaximal throughout the stimulus program and does not extend to other nearby motor nerves whose muscle responses could contribute significantly to the recorded potential. To these ends, care should be taken to prevent movement of the affected part of the limb as much as possible. The stimuli to the nerve should all be at least 110 to 120 percent supramaximal and careful attention should be paid to the actions of other muscles and muscle groups to ensure that their actions do not interfere with the recording. The last is particularly a problem in testing proximal muscles where it is hard to prevent extension of the stimuli to other motor axons when, for example, the brachial plexus is stimulated at Erb's point. It is far better to stimulate the musculocutaneous or accessory nerves separately and record their

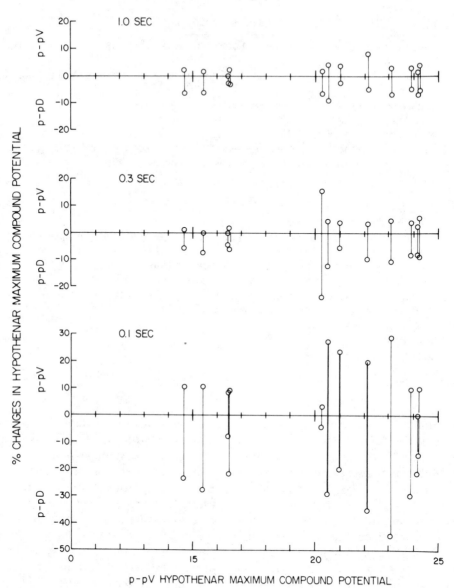

FIGURE 10.9.   Percentage changes of the fifth compared to the first maximum M-potential (here hypothenar) peak-to-peak voltage (p-pV), and peak-to-peak duration (p-pD) at stimulus intervals of 1.0, 0.3, and 0.1 second. Note the reciprocal relationship between the changes in p-pV and p-pD; as p-pV increases, p-pD decreases in keeping with the enhanced degree of synchronization between discharges of component single muscle fiber potentials contributing to the M-potential. The amplitude of the maximum M-potential in the 12 controls included in this study are shown also, but there is no obvious relationship between the magnitude of the M-potential and changes in the potential in response to repetitive stimulation.
From Kadrie and Brown (1978a, figure 5).

TABLE 10.4.   Changes in the Maximum
M-Potential in Response to Repetitive
Supramaximal Stimulation of the Motor Nerve

Frequency of Stimulation (stimuli/second)	Changes in M-Potential (p-p amplitude and duration)
1 or less	Little or none
2–3	There may be reductions in the p-p amplitude, maximum by the fourth or fifth potential in the train; these should not exceed 10%
5–50	Lower frequencies May be 10–20% increases in p-p amplitude Higher frequencies There may be reductions in the p-p amplitude by as much as 50% at 50-Hz stimulation

Based on studies of Desmedt (1961), Lambert, Rooke, Eaton, and Hodgson (1961), Lambert (1966), Slomić, Rosenfalck, and Buchthal (1968), Desmedt and Borenstein (1970), Ozdemir and Young (1971, 1976), and Kadrie and Brown (1978a, 1978b).

biceps, brachialis, and trapezius M-potential respectively.

The temperature of the muscle is also important to record and, especially in the more distal muscles, to try and keep above 35°C (Borenstein and Desmedt, 1973, 1974, 1975; Ricker, Hertel, and Stodieck, 1977). The reason for this is that the safety factor for neuromuscular transmission is reduced at higher temperatures because, although there is an increase in MEPP frequency, the amplitudes of the EPPs are reduced, possibly through an increase in the activity of ACh-E and an enhanced breakdown of ACh (Hubbard, Llinás, and Quastel, 1969). Higher temperatures also reduce the safety factor for neuromuscular

transmission through presynaptic blocks of impulse propagation in the presynaptic axon terminals. The probability of such blocks was greatly enhanced in the presence of high extracellular Ca^{++} ion concentrations (Eusebi and Miledi, 1983). Increases in muscle temperature also shorten the duration and increase the amplitude of the M-potential through shortening the duration of the membrane currents in the MFs.

In MG the maximum M-potential amplitude in response to single motor nerve stimuli is normal except in the more severely affected muscles and patients (Harvey and Masland, 1941a, 1941b; Desmedt, 1961; Lambert, Rooke, Eaton, and Hodgson, 1961; Slomić, Rosenfalck, and Buchthal, 1968; Desmedt and Borenstein, 1970, 1976a; Ozdemir and Young, 1971, 1976; Desmedt and Borenstein, 1976b; Stålberg, 1980; Stålberg and Sanders, 1981). Also, the maximum motor conduction velocities are normal although there may be a significant prolongation of motor terminal latencies (Slomić, Rosenfalck, and Buchthal, 1968; McComas, Sica, and Brown, 1971; Kadrie and Brown, 1978b).

Often there is a characteristic decrement in the amplitude of the maximum M-potential in excess of that seen in normal muscle (>10 percent), best seen at 2 to 3 stimuli per second and which reaches its maximum by the fourth to sixth potential in the train, following which there is often partial or full recovery (Figure 10.10). At this frequency of stimulation there is little or no pseudofacilitation and the basic defect in neuromuscular transmission is not masked by mobilization of transmitter, both of which occur at higher frequencies of stimulation.

The fact that the maximum M-potential evoked by single stimuli is usually in the normal range suggests that at most neuromuscular junctions the EPP exceeds threshold levels required for generation of action potentials in the postsynaptic MFs. Only when the quantal content of the EPP is reduced through repet-

FIGURE 10.10.   Changes in the thenar maximum M-potential in response to supramaximal stimulation at 3 per second (8 stimuli in the train) both before exercise and at intervals of 10 seconds and 2 and 6 minutes following a 30-second period of maximal voluntary contraction of the thenar muscles. In this patient there was a 68 percent reduction in peak-to-peak amplitude (p-pA) of the maximum M-potential. Shortly after the period of exercise, however, not only was the p-pA of the first M-potential in the train increased by 35 percent, but the decrement was reduced to 50 percent *(posttetanic potentiation)*. After a longer interval, here 2.5 minutes, the situation had reversed so that the p-pA of the first M-potential was reduced below that in the preexercise period and the magnitude of the decrement was now even greater, 76 percent *(posttetanic exhaustion)*. By 6 minutes following exercise, the percentage of decrement had not yet recovered to preexercise values, but the first M-potential had almost returned to its preexercise size. In this study in which the temperature of the thenar muscle group was 35°C, posttetanic potentiation was more pronounced than posttetanic exhaustion, although the reverse may be seen, the magnitude of each being critically dependent in many patients on muscle temperature and duration of exercise.

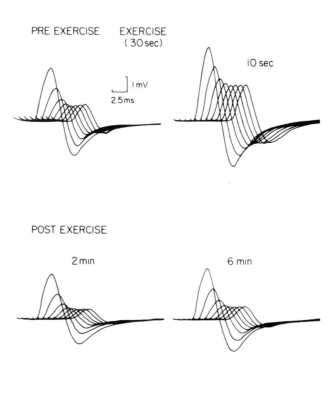

itive stimulation does the EPP, at any appreciable number of the end-plates, fall below threshold and transmission fail as a consequence (Figure 10.9). This usually happens within the first stimuli in MG, after which release often recovers sufficiently for EPP amplitudes once again to exceed threshold levels and be sufficient to generate MF action potentials.

Unfortunately, this relatively simple test often fails to reveal any abnormal decrements, especially when applied to the distal limb muscles (Ozdemir and Young, 1976; Stålberg and Sanders, 1981). The latter, although the easiest to test for technical reasons

(they are smaller, movement is easier to control, and stimulus can be isolated to the desired motor nerve), are less likely to show abnormal decrements than are the more proximal muscles. For this reason, others have advocated testing proximal muscles routinely where even the results in more distal muscles are normal or produce equivocal results (Ozdemir and Young, 1971, 1976; Desmedt and Borenstein, 1976a).

It is precisely because the EPPs' amplitudes exceed by such a wide margin the threshold levels required to generate action potentials in the MFs (by two to three times), that neuromuscular transmission can persist even in the presence of substantial loses of ACh-Rs. To unmask the abnormalities in neuromuscular transmission in such situations it is sometimes necessary to employ strategies to reduce the safety factor further to the point at which the abnormalities produced by the disease express themselves by clear failures in transmission. Such strategies should not, under the conditions of the test, so reduce the safety factor for neuromuscular transmission that transmission fails at normal end-plates. Common strategies for reducing the safety factor are shown in Table 10.3.

Increasing Muscle Temperature

It was pointed out earlier that warming the muscle reduces the safety factor for neuromuscular transmission (Figure 10.11). This phenomenon has been emphasized by several investigators (Desmedt, 1961; Slomić, Rosenfalck, and Buchthal, 1968; Borenstein and Desmedt, 1975; Desmedt and Borenstein, 1970, 1976a, 1977; Ricker, Hertel, and Stodieck, 1977; Krarup, 1977a, 1977b; Stålberg, 1980).

Exercise

Prior *exercise* may also reveal abnormalities in neuromuscular transmission. There are two ways to achieve this: through a brief (10 to 30 seconds) period of maximum voluntary contraction (Lambert, Rooke, Eaton, and Hodgson, 1961) or a brief tetanic stimulus delivered to the motor nerve (30 to 100 stimuli per second for 2 to 10 seconds as in Desmedt and Borenstein, 1970). Following this exercise program, test stimuli may be delivered at intervals beginning within 10 seconds of the end of the exercise and repeating at 1- to 2-minute intervals for 4 to 10 minutes. The test train

most suitable is probably a short train of 5 to 10, supramaximal stimuli delivered at 3 per second.

Following such a program there may be a short period of *facilitation* or *potentiation* demonstrable, evident as early as 10 seconds following exercise and ending within 10 to 30 seconds. This brief period of *post-tetanic potentiation* (PTP) may be evident as an increase in the p-p amplitude of the maximum M-potential or a lesser degree of decrement in the M-potential in response to the test 3 per second stimulation.

This earlier period is succeeded by a depression, the *post-tetanic exhaustion* (PTE), which reaches its peak between 2 and 4 minutes after the exercise period. This depression is characterized by a reduction in the p-p amplitude of the M-potential and a larger decrement in its amplitude in response to the test train of stimuli. Both PTF and PTE have been observed in partially curarized muscle and at end-plates blocked by α-bungarotoxin.

The basis of PTE is not known at this time, but it may be the equivalent of the weakness patients experience with exercise in MG. Both PTF and PTE are two distinct processes that overlap somewhat in time, although the period of exhaustion lasts much longer. Their relative contributions in the postexercise period can be altered by changing the intensity or duration of the exercise (Stålberg, 1980). For example, in MG of moderate degree, a 20-second period of exercise may suffice to produce PTF but not PTE, whereas when the MG is more severe, a similar period of exercise may produce no PTF, PTE being dominant even in the early postexercise period. The preceding may explain the earlier observations of Ozdemir and Young (1976) that PTF was not seen in some myasthenics when the muscle was exercised for as long as 30 seconds; rather a decrement developed that was in every way reminiscent of PTE, but instead of beginning a minute or so later, began as

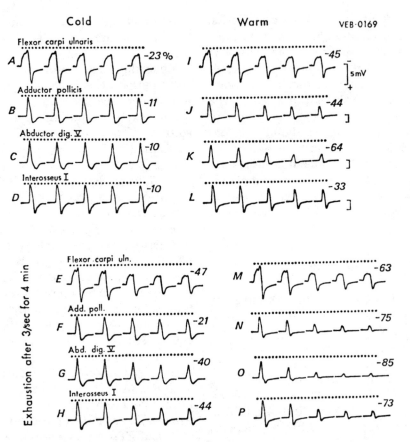

FIGURE 10.11.   Female patient, 26 years of age with generalized myasthenia gravis. Effect of temperature on neuromuscular transmission. Shown are the percentage decrements in the fifth compared to the first maximum M-potentials as elicited by stimulation at 3 per second of the ulnar nerve at the elbow in rested muscle—(A) through (D)—and following a period of stimulation at 3 per second for four minutes in which the intramuscular temperatures were 31 to 32°C—(A) through (H).

(I) through (L) illustrate the decrement, this time following warming of the muscle to 35 to 37°C, for rested muscles and following the period of repetitive stimulation at 3 per second for four minutes (M) through (P). Note that the decrement was greatly enhanced by warming the muscles as well as by prior exercise.

From Borenstein and Desmedt (1973, figure 8).

early as 10 to 15 seconds following the period of exercise.

Of the two methods of exercising the muscle, voluntary contraction is obviously the least distressing to the subject but has the disadvantage of depending on the subject's effort. Tetanic supramaximal nerve stimulation provides a more constant and reproducible exercise, but is more distressing, at least in some subjects. Desmedt claims that the use of near-nerve stimulating electrodes helps to diminish the discomfort experienced by some patients with tetanic supramaximial stimulation by allowing a more optimal position with respect to the motor axons, and the use of much less intense stimuli.

Ischemia

Ischemia was reported by Harvey and Masland (1941a) to increase the decrement in MG; such decrements exceeding any seen at equivalent times in control muscles exposed to ischemia for the same time. Desmedt and others subsequently developed a test protocol that combined ischemia and repetitive supramaximal stimulation in order to increase the sensitivity of the repetitive stimulation test and enhance the ability of the latter test to detect neuromuscular transmission problems in MG. Their protocol has been called the *two-step test* (Desmedt and Borenstein, 1976a, 1977).

In the initial step, the nerve is supramaximally stimulated at 3 per second for a period of 4 to 5 minutes (a total of 720 to 900 stimuli). In the second step, the preceding mild and controlled form of exercise is repeated, this time in combination with a 4- to 5-minute period of ischemia. Decrements are looked for during the initial period of stimulation to the subsequent period of ischemia and following the ischemia.

In normal rested hand muscles, significant decrements do not develop in the period of nonischemic stimulation, although decrements up to 50 percent may develop during the period of ischemia. This latter may be caused by ischemic axonal block rather than progressive failures of neuromuscular transmission, at least in healthy subjects. It should be noted here, however, that when stimulation at 3 per second is carried out for pro-longed periods (7 to 15 minutes or more) even in the absence of ischemia, decrements may develop even in healthy subjects.

Abnormal increases in jitter and perhaps impulse block may develop toward the end of the 4- to 5-minute period of ischemia in control subjects (Stålberg and Ekstedt, 1973). Provided the ischemia lasts no more than 4 to 5 minutes, however, abnormal decrements do not subsequently occur.

These observations in healthy subjects stand in contrast to those myasthenics in whom abnormal decrements in the p-p amplitude of the maximum M-response may develop both during and after the period of mild exercise alone (step 1). Even larger decrements in p-p amplitude may be seen following the period of combined ischemia and exercise. The second (ischemia) step may thus enhance any abnormalities present in the first step, or even bring out a decrement not apparent before the ischemic period.

The durations and frequencies of the stimulation as well as the duration of the ischemia were chosen by Desmedt to enhance the neuromuscular defects as much as possible, while at the same time avoiding as many technical problems as possible. Thus stimulation of 3 per second was chosen as their optimal frequency for MG. The period of ischemia was kept to 4 to 7 minutes because longer periods can produce decrements in the postischemic period even in normal muscles. Ischemia may also induce conduction block in the nerve. Hence the longer the period of ischemia, the shorter must be the distance between the site of stimulation and the end-plate zone to minimize this problem (see Chapter 2).

Regional Curare Test

The combination of neuromuscular blocking agents and repetitive stimulation has been advocated as yet another way to reduce the safety factor for neuromuscular transmission and increase the sensitivity of the repetitive stimulation test (Rowland, Aranow, and Hoefer, 1961; Horowitz, Jenkins, Kornfeld, and Papatestas, 1975, 1976; Hertel, Ricker, and Hirsch, 1977; Brown, Charlton, and White, 1975). This is especially important in patients who have ocular myasthenia only and no apparent involvement of other muscles as judged by their responses to repetitive stimulation of respective motor nerves. In some of these patients, latent disorders of neuromuscular transmission can be revealed in these apparently normal muscles by reducing the safety factor for neuromuscular transmission by the use of neuromuscular blocking agents combined with repetitive stimulation. Even one-tenth of the normal curarizing dose injected into the systemic circulation of patients with ocular myasthenia often produces clinically apparent weakness in limb muscles where none was obvious before or would be obvious in healthy subjects (Rowland, Aranow, and Hoefer, 1961). Such systemic injections of neuromuscular blocking agents carry the risk of respiratory failure, however. Therefore, to regionalize exposure, the agent may be injected into the circulation beyond an occlusive tourniquet.

In the regional test (Horowitz, Jenkins, Kornfeld, and Papatestas, 1976), 0.2 mg of *d*-tubocurarine (in 20 ml of 0.9 percent saline solution) is injected into a forearm vein after inflating a proximal pneumatic tourniquet sufficiently to occlude the circulation totally to and from the arm beyond the tourniquet. After a period of six and one-half minutes, the tourniquet is released and test trains of stimuli are delivered to the motor nerves at various intervals to look for abnormal decrements in end-plates exposed to the tubocurarine.

Of critical importance in selection of the appropriate muscles to be tested is distribution of the muscle involvement in MG (see review by Simpson, 1981). The most frequently involved muscles include the extra-

ocular and eyelid muscles. Except for the facial muscles (frontalis, orbicularis oculi, or platysma), cranial muscles cannot be tested by repetitive electrical stimulation of their respective motor nerves. Ischemia and regional curare tests are obviously not applicable to these or the proximal limb muscles.

Because the proximal limb and girdle muscles seem to be involved more often and more severely than are distal limb muscles, extension of the repetitive stimulation test to these muscles such as the deltoid and biceps has been advocated (Ozdemir and Young, 1971, 1976). Abnormal decrements have been seen in these muscles where none were seen in the distal muscles of the limbs in response to repetitive supramaximal stimulation alone or repetitive stimulation combined with exercise of the muscles (Ozdemir and Young, 1976; Desmedt and Borenstein, 1976a, 1977).

It is not clear whether the greater yield of repetitive stimulation tests as applied to proximal muscles reflects more severe involvement of the end-plates in these in relation to the distal muscles, or whether these differences simply reflect the higher safety factors for neuromuscular transmission in the normally cooler distal muscles. This is one reason why careful attention must be paid to the temperature of the muscles being tested, the diagnostic yield in warmed distal muscles being as a rule, much higher than when these same muscles are cool. The frequent involvement of the extraocular and levator palpebrae muscles relative to other muscles probably reflects their tonic activity in the awake state.

Relative Value of Repetitive Stimulation and Other Tests in Myasthenia Gravis

Repetitive Stimulation

In a critical survey of 80 patients with MG, Ozdemir and Young (1976) made several important observations. Among these were:

1. Whether or not an abnormal decrement was detected depends on which muscles were tested. Abnormal decrements were more common in the deltoid than in the oribicularis oculi or abductor digiti minimi muscles (Table 10.5).
2. Abnormal decrements were seen in at least one muscle in 95 percent of myasthenic patients, exceptions being those with pure ocular myasthenia or in whom the disease was mild and generalized.
3. There was poor correlation between the degree of muscle weakness and the presence or absence of a decrement. Thus clinically normal muscles commonly had a decrement and abnormal muscles, on clinical examination, might not have.

It is worth recalling that the decrements as measured with this test occur within the first few potentials in the train, and those occurring so early (within the first 2 seconds) would not be apparent in any clinical assessment of power where the firing frequencies are much higher and the discharges go on for much longer times (5 or more seconds usually). Clinical weakness probably corresponds better with the phenomenon of PTE, although this remains to be proved conclusively.

4. The pattern of decrement was important, certain ones being more characteristic of MG than others. The most common pattern was a progressive decline in the negative peak amplitude of the maximum M-potential, which was maximum by the fourth or fifth M-potential in the train. The decrement was followed by a progressive increment in the negative peak amplitude to levels that sometimes exceeded the initial M-response. This pattern was best seen at stimulus frequencies of 1 to 3 per second.

Less common patterns included the absence of any subsequent increment in the amplitude of the M-potential or a maximum decrement that was apparent by the second potential, not the fourth or fifth in the train. Sometimes actual incremental responses were seen, especially at the higher stimulus frequencies, and in clinically stronger muscles. This increment could be substantial and as much as 100 to 350 percent (Mayer and Williams, 1974).

In contradistinction to other disorders where decrements may also be seen, such as in the myotonias (Aminoff, Layzer, Satya-Murti, and Faden, 1977) or peripheral neuropathies, in MG the decrements, where present, were already apparent by the second potential in the train. Continuous and progressive decrements were rare in MG, unlike the situation in myotonia. Ozdemir and Young also stressed the value of exercise as a means of increasing the sensitivity of these tests. There were no comparable experiences with the regional curare test or SF-EMG to report at that time.

The value of the two-step and regional curare tests still has not been clearly shown to be better than repetitive stimulation alone or especially when the latter is combined with exercise and includes the testing of at least one proximal muscle. The most important requirement in all the repetitive stimulation tests and their modifications is careful attention to proper techniques to avoid artifacts and thereby misleading conclusions.

The pros and cons of repetitive stimulation test and its modifications include:

TABLE 10.5. Percentage of Muscles that Had an Abnormal Decrement in Response to Repetitive Stimulation

Muscle Tested	Percentage of Muscles with Abnormal Decrement
Orbicularis oculi	63
Deltoid	82
Abductor digiti minimi	59

From Ozdemir and Young (1976).

1. With respect to distal muscles: the main technical advantages here include better control of movement to avoid induced artifacts. Moreover, in such studies the stimulus can easily be confined to the desired motor nerve without extension to other nearby motor nerves. The prime disadvantage is that these muscles often showed less decrement than more proximal muscles, even though the chance of demonstrating a decrement in the distal muscles can be improved by warming, prior exercise, and possibly, ischemia.

2. With respect to proximal limb muscles: the most common method used in many laboratories is to stimulate the brachial plexus at Erb's point and record the maximum M-response of the deltoid muscle by surface electrodes. Such stimuli, however, in order to be supramaximal for the deltoid are also sufficiently intense to excite other parts of the brachial plexus. The latter may produce movements whose intensity varies with both minor changes in intensity of the stimulus and even slight shifts in the position of the stimulating electrodes. The motor responses in muscle may all contribute to some degree to the potential recorded over the deltoid through volume conduction.

    It is impossible to test strong proximal contractions with the same degree of control as in the hand muscles. Moreover, such coarse movements of the limb can displace the stimulating electrode sufficiently for the stimulus to become submaximal and evoke submaximal M-responses or increase the deltoid recorded potential if the stimulus spreads to excite more completely other nearby muscles. These problems, plus the fact that such stimulation is distressing even at lower stimulus frequencies of 1 and 3 per second, limit the value of this technique somewhat. Other possibilities include recording maximum M-potentials of the biceps brachialis muscles evoked by stimulation of the musculocutaneous nerve or the trapezius muscle in response to stimulation of the accessory nerve. These are clearly better ways of testing proximal muscles, because the stimulus can be confined to a single motor nerve and there is no stimulus spread to other motor axons, as when stimulating the brachial plexus at Erb's point.

3. With respect to cranial muscles: earlier, the possibility of testing various facial muscles was alluded to and indeed, repetitive stimulation techniques can be applied to the frontalis, orbicularis oculi, and platysma (Krarup, 1977a, 1977b). These tests, in our experience, produce moderate distress because supramaximal stimulation of the seventh cranial nerve is required, but they are said to be sensitive indicators of neuromuscular transmission abnormalities in MG (Ozdemir and Young, 1976; Krarup, 1977a, 1977b). We have found that application of repetitive stimulation to these muscles (orbicularis oculi or frontalis) has not been nearly so sensitive as SF-EMG applied to the same muscles.

4. With respect to combining repetitive stimulation with tetanic stimulation or ischemia: such protocols are more time consuming, and it is questionable whether these rather complicated protocols are any better indicators of neuromuscular disorders than the use of repetitive stimulation alone applied to more proximal muscles. The use of a brief period of voluntary contraction is, however, a very convenient way to enhance the value of repetitive stimulation applied not only to the intrinsic muscles of the hand, but to proximal muscles as well, where tetanic stimulation of motor nerves would be too distressing for many patients. Combining

exercise with repetitive stimulation also makes it possible to look for PTF and PTE.

5. With respect to combining repetitive stimulation with the regional curare test: regional curarization carries with it the risk of respiratory or bulbar muscle paralysis on release of the tourniquet, because the curare may reach the systemic circulation at this point (Hertel, Ricker, and Hirsch, 1977). Also, this test has not been shown to be any better than repetitive stimulation combined with exercise, especially when muscles are properly warmed and two or more muscle groups, including a proximal muscle, are tested.

Other Tests of Neuromuscular Transmission in Myasthenia Gravis

Repetitive Stimulation as Applied to Single Motor Axons

By carefully grading the intensity of an electrical stimulus delivered to a motor nerve, single motor axons can be excited without others being excited by the same stimulus (Bergmans, 1970; Desmedt and Borenstein, 1970; Kadrie and Brown, 1978a, 1978b). This makes it possible to test neuromuscular transmission in single thenar (T), hypothenar (HT), or extensor digitorum brevis (EDB) motor units. Changes in the p-p amplitude and duration of single MUPs as recorded by surface electrodes positioned over the respective muscles in response to stimulation at various frequencies in normal persons have shown:

1. An increment in the p-p voltage amplitude and reciprocal shortening in the p-p duration at frequencies between 1 and 10 stimuli per second, the largest changes being seen at 10 per second (Figure 10.12). These changes in the surface-recorded M-potential are paralleled by a progressive

reduction in the intervals between the discharge times of the component MF action potentials in the same MUP as seen when these were recorded by an SF-EMG electrode (Figure 10.13).

2. In the occasional MUP that exhibited a decrement at stimulus frequencies of 1, 3, or 10 per second, the decrement was usually maximum by the fifth potential in the train and never exceeded 10 percent.

One important advantage with single axon stimulation was the very much lower stimulus intensities required (one-half or less of supramaximal intensity); hence the stimuli were better tolerated by the subject. There was also no appreciable movement produced by the actions of single MUs.

When this technique was applied to MG, the more important observations included:

1. Not all MUs exhibited an abnormal decrement in the amplitude of their MUPs in response to repetitive stimulation. The proportion of affected MUs varied between 0 and 90 percent, and also, severity of the decrements varied considerably among different MUPs (Figures 10.14 and 10.15).

2. Decrements in individual MUPs were most pronounced in the fifth potential in the train, although less often the maximum decrements were seen in the fourth or sixth potential.

3. Decrements in single MUPs often exceeded the decrement in the maximum M-potential at the same stimulus frequency. This was not unexpected in view of the fact that the maximum M-potential represents the compound sum of the responses of all the component MUPs, some of which are normal in their response while others are variably abnormal.

4. MUPs with the lowest amplitudes recorded by surface electrodes over the

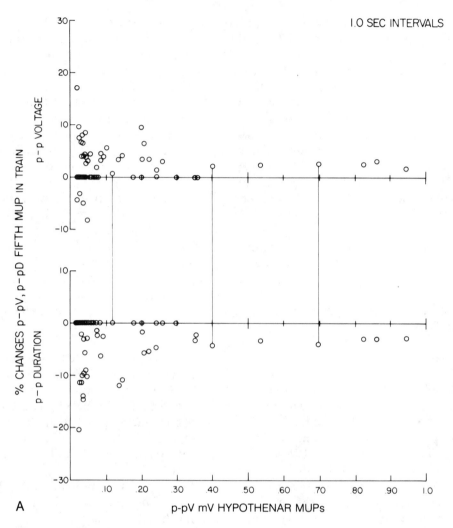

FIGURE 10.12.   Changes in peak-to-peak voltage (p-pV) and peak-to-peak duration (p-pD) of single hypothenar MUPs recorded with surface electrodes. Changes are expressed as a percentage in the fifth compared to the first MUP in a train at stimulus intervals of 1.0 (A), 0.3 (B), and 0.1 (C) second. Vertical bars connect changes in amplitude and duration in representative single MUPs. The sizes of the MUPs (p-p) in millivolts are indicated by the X axis. Note the reciprocal increases in p-p amplitude and reductions in p-pD, especially at the shorter-stimulus intervals. From Kadrie and Brown (1978a, figure 9).

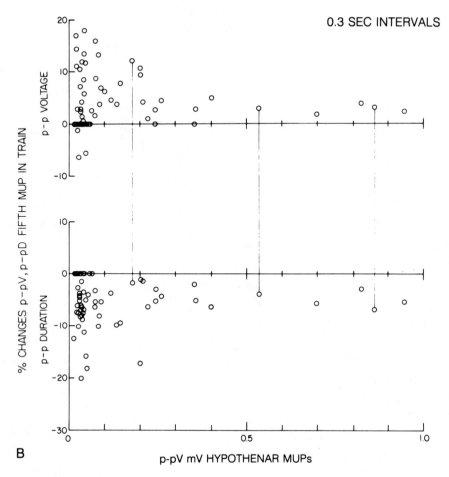

FIGURE 10.12.   *(continued)*

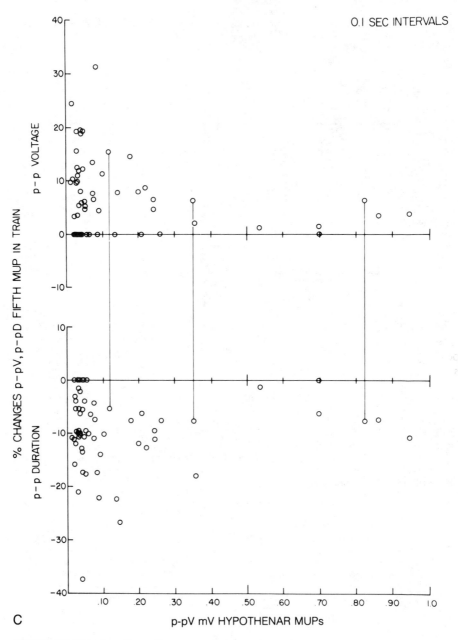

C

FIGURE 10.12.   (continued)

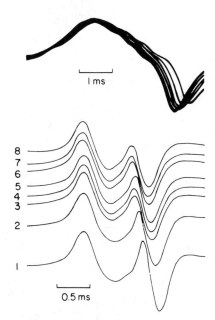

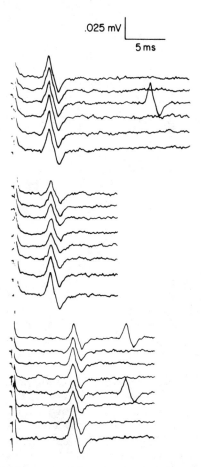

FIGURE 10.13.   (Top) Changes in the size and shape of the surface-recorded potential of a single motor unit in response to stimuli adjusted to exceed threshold for this one motor axon alone. Stimuli were delivered at a rate of 10 per second.

(Bottom) The corresponding changes in the interspike period between two muscle fiber potentials belonging to the same motor unit shown above; successive responses to the train of stimuli being numbered from below, upward. Note the progressive reduction in the interspike period.

From Kadrie and Brown (1978a, figure 10).

FIGURE 10.14.   Changes in the size of a single MUP (here thenar) as recorded with surface electrodes in response to stimulation at the level of the wrist (top and middle) and elbow (bottom) at frequencies of 1 per second (top) and 3 per second (middle and bottom). There was no decrement at 1 per second, but at 3 per second there was a 44 percent reduction in peak-to-peak amplitude maximum in the fourth potential in the train that was identical in magnitude, as it should be when elicited by stimulation at the elbow and wrist. Note the F-response in the same MUPs seen both with stimulation at the wrist (top) and elbow (bottom).

muscle most often displayed the greatest decrements (Figure 10.15). In view of the fact that the amplitude of the surface-recorded MUP is proportional to the force generated by the MU, it seems reasonable to conclude, based on the greater decrements seen in the lower-amplitude MUPs, that neuromuscular transmission is most abnormal in those MUs generating the least force. This hypothesis has yet to be proved directly.

Several explanations are possible for the above hypothesis. For example, there may be important differences in the safety factors for neuromuscular transmission among MUs even in the normal state.

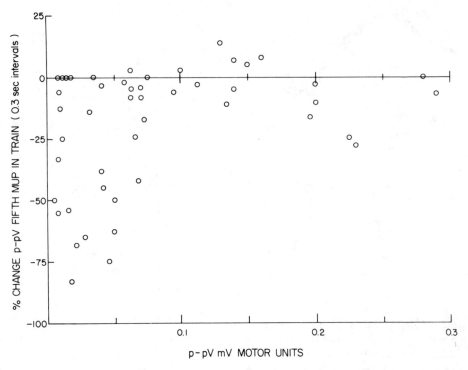

FIGURE 10.15.   Plot of the percentage changes in the peak-to-peak voltage (p-pV) of the fifth compared to the first MUP in the train elicited by stimulation at 0.3-second intervals (top) in myasthenia gravis and the p-pV in millivolts of the respective MUPs indicated by the scale on the X axis.

There were larger decrements in amplitude of the smaller- compared to the relatively higher-amplitude MUPs.

From Kadrie and Brown (1978a, figure 6).

Hence in the presence of a disease affecting neuromuscular transmission such as MG, those MUs with the lowest margin for safe transmission would be affected first and exhibit the most abnormal neuromuscular transmission. The circumstantial evidence suggests that these MUs would tend to be those generating the lowest force. This hypothesis receives some support from recent studies that have shown that the safety factor for neuromuscular transmission is lower in red than in white muscles (Gertler and Robbins, 1978).

Mayer (1982) used intramuscular microstimulation to isolate the contractile and electrical responses in single motor units in the first dorsal interosseus muscle of myasthenic subjects. He showed that while decrements are seen in both fast- (F) and slow- (S) twitch motor units, the potential decrements tended to be greater in the former.

5. The abnormal decrements did not all reverse with edrophonium chloride (Tensilon). The reason for this is unknown.

6. PTE could be shown in many MUPs by this technique (Figure 10.16).

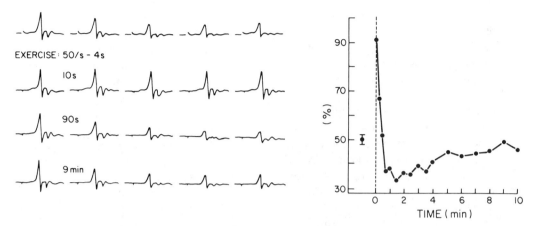

FIGURE 10.16.   Posttetanic exhaustion in a single myasthenic MUP (here in abductor pollicis brevis) as recorded by surface electrodes. Stimuli were delivered to the median nerve at 3 per second and were supramaximal for this motor axon alone. Note that after a period of exercise induced by repetitive stimulation at 50 per second for four seconds, the magnitude of the decrement in this MUP was initally reduced 10 seconds after the tetanus but by 90 seconds the size of the decrement was clearly increased (posttetanic exhaustion). The percentage decrements in the peak-to-peak amplitude of this MUP at various times following the tetanus are shown on the right. From Desmedt and Borenstein (1970).

Whatever the type of MU tested by this technique, the method clearly possesses advantages. Because of the lower stimulus intensities, it is better tolerated by patients, and clearly abnormal decrements are demonstrable in single MUPs where they can be shown in the maximum M-potentials in response to supramaximal stimulation. The technique is not, however, without its problems. For example, it takes experience to select single motor axons by incremental stimulation, and the technique is really only applicable in distal limb muscles such as the hypothenar, first dorsal interosseus, thenar, extensor digitorum brevis, and possibly, tibialis anterior muscles, but not in proximal limb muscles. Normal results have sometimes been seen in ocular myasthenics where clear abnormalities using the SF-EMG technique in the orbicularis oculi muscle were demonstrable. In the original reported studies there was no attempt to warm the muscles to be tested, and possibly prior warming would

have increased the proportion of abnormal MUPs and the severity of these abnormalities.

Single-Fiber EMG

The theoretical basis and basic techniques of SF-EMG have been described in Chapter 7. Unlike repetitive stimulation and other methods that depend on transmission block occurring at enough neuromuscular junctions for reductions in the M-potential to become apparent, SF-EMG can detect neuromuscular transmission abnormalities prior to the development of conduction block. The characteristics in MG (Stålberg and Ekstedt, 1973; Stålberg, Ekstedt, and Broman, 1974; Schwartz and Stålberg, 1975b; Sanders, Howard, and Johns, 1978; Stålberg, Trontelj, and Schwartz, 1976; Stålberg and Trontelj, 1979) include:

1. An increase in fiber density in some patients. This probably results from the collateral reinnervation of MFs functionally

denervated through destruction of their end-plates.

2. Increased jitter. This may vary widely between fiber pairs within the same muscle and even within the same MU (Figure 10.17).

3. Impulse block. This is most apparent at junctions exhibiting the most jitter, and both tend to be the most abnormal in MUPs with the highest innervation ratios. These abnormalities are most easily seen among the first few MUPs recruited at each recording site.

The abnormal jitter and sometimes block may be seen in clinically normal muscles where no abnormal decrement may have been demonstrable in response to repetitive stimulation of the motor nerve, or in the limb muscles of patients with ocular myasthenia.

4. Improvement in the degree of jitter and blocking may be seen following the administration of edrophonium chloride. This is not true at all end-plates, however, because at others the edrophonium chloride may actually increase both. It turns out that most of these patients were taking anticholinesterase drugs at the time of the test. The paradoxical effect of edrophonium chloride in these instances is probably explained by the production or aggravation of a cholinergic block at "overtreated" end-plates (Stålberg, Trontelj, and Schwartz, 1976; Stålberg, 1980).

5. SF-EMG was never normal in a muscle showing an abnormal decrement in response to repetitive stimulation.

In patients with various types of myasthenia, the relative percentage of positive test results using SF-EMG, repetitive stimulation, and measurement of ACh-R antibody titers are compared in Table 10.6.

In the above study it is clearly apparent that SF-EMG offered the best chance of detecting

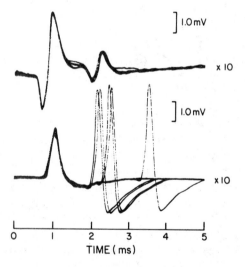

FIGURE 10.17. Representative single-fiber electrode recordings of pairs of fibers in normal (top) and myasthenic extensor digitorum communis muscles. The jitter values between the muscle fiber potentials in the normal pair did not exceed 50 ms, whereas in the myasthenic pair illustrated here, the jitter value exceeded 1,000 ms and impulse blocking was common.

TABLE 10.6.   Percentages of Positive Results Using Three Techniques

Subgroups of Myasthenia	SF EMG	RS ADM	RS Biceps Brachii/ Deltoid	ACh R- Ab
Restricted ocular	85	4	19	76
Generalized				
Mild	96	31	68	76
Moderate	100	68	89	88
Remission	69	0	0	

Based on Stålberg and Sanders (1981). See also Konishi, Hishitani, Matsubara, and Ohta (1981).

RS—repetitive stimulation.

ACh R-A.b—acetylcholine receptor–antibodies.

ADM—adductor digiti minimi.

an abnormality in the restricted ocular group, a group in which the responses to repetitive stimulation is more often normal, and about one-third had no detectable ACh-R antibody. The SF-EMG was sometimes negative in situations where ACh-R antibody was detectable. Thus it appears to be a very sensitive way of revealing abnormalities in neuromuscular transmission. These abnormalities are not specific for MG, however, and can also be seen in other neuromuscular disorders such as in the case of diseases of the lower motor neuron, peripheral neuropathies and even primary myopathies, especially polymyositis (Stålberg, 1980).

Muscle Twitches

The force of a muscle contraction may be measured by recording the isometric tensions generated by a maximum voluntary contraction, or in response to trains of stimuli or a single stimulus delivered to the motor nerve. In MG, the maximum twitch tension evoked by a single stimulus delivered to the motor nerve is usually in the normal range, although there may be some reduction in patients with moderate to severe disease (Lambert, Rooke, Eaton, and Hodgson, 1961; Slomić, Rosenfalck, and Buchthal, 1968). Even repeated short maximum voluntary contractions may be well maintained. When these are repeated after one or more minutes, however, a substantial reduction in force may occur that may last 5 to 15 minutes. This is probably the mechanical equivalent of post-tetanic exhaustion.

The positive staircase has been reported to be absent or reduced in many myasthenic patients, even those receiving anticholinesterase drugs (Slomić, Rosenfalck, and Buchthal, 1968; Desmedt and Borenstein, 1970). This was seen both in the distal muscles of the upper limb (Slomić, Rosenfalck, and Buchthal, 1968; Desmedt and Borenstein, 1970) and in the platysma (Krarup, 1977b).

The *staircase phenomenon* is characterized by a change in the force of twitches evoked by a series of stimuli delivered at a frequency low enough to allow complete relaxation between single twitches. It is best seen when stimuli are delivered at 0.1 to 3 per second, higher frequencies producing partial fusion of the twitches. The staircase may be positive (increase in force) or negative (decrease in force). In healthy subjects, positive staircase is the general rule. It is maximum at stimulus frequencies between 1 and 2 per second. The maximum increase at 2 per second (180 stimuli in the train) is of the order of 5 percent, but can exceed 100 percent in some subjects. A negative staircase that is less pronounced and precedes the positive staircase occurs in about half of healthy subjects (Slomić, Rosenfalck, and Buchthal, 1968; Desmedt and Borenstein, 1970).

The cause of the staircase phenomenon is not known for certain. The phenomenon is apparently not the result of any change in the numbers of active MFs and hence dependent on neuromuscular transmission; nor is it the result of repetitive discharges in the MFs, although this may occur in myasthenic patients taking anticholinesterase drugs. In the latter, the force and duration of the twitch evoked by single supramaximal nerve stimuli may be increased despite the absence of any evidence of an increase in peak-to-peak amplitude of the maximum M-potential (Desmedt, 1961).

The staircase phenomenon may be produced by a decay of the active state in muscle (Slomić, Rosenfalck, and Buchthal, 1968). There is also the special problem of identifying and quantifying the staircase potentiation in MG because the forces generated are also a function of the number of MFs generating the tension. This in turn depends on the state of neuromuscular transmission at all the endplates in the muscle. Post-tetanic exhaustion, for example, could substantially reduce the number of MFs contributing to the tension.

Even so, in some cases of myasthenia a positive staircase phenomenon may yet be clearly recognized (Desmedt and Borenstein, 1970).

Measurements of Ocular Movement

Techniques are available for measuring the velocity of ocular movement for certain angular displacements (Baloh and Keesey, 1976; Yee, Cogan, Zee, Baloh, and Honrubia 1976). In some myasthenics, these methods have been able to show reduced eye movement velocities, abnormal fatigability of these eye movements, and partial reversal of these abnormalities with edrophonium chloride (Baloh and Keesey, 1976). The methods are attractive because electrical stimulation is not necessary and the extraocular muscles are among the earliest and most common to be involved in MG; however, they do require a patient's attention. In our own limited experience with this test, abnormalities could be shown in all patients with MG, even those with mild disease, including those with ocular myasthenia only, although these may not reverse with edrophonium chloride.

Stapedius Test

The acoustic impedance of the tympanic membrane can be altered by changes in the activity of the stapedius muscle (Blom and Zakrisson, 1974; Morioka, Neff, Boisseranc, Hartman, and Cantrell, 1976; Warren, Gutmann, Cody, Flowers, and Segal, 1977; Kramer, Ruth, Johns, and Sanders, 1980; Stålberg and Sanders, 1981). The stapedius muscle in turn contracts in response to auditory stimuli through a polysynaptic brainstem reflex.

Pulsed auditory stimuli have been shown in MG to produce a characteristic decremental pattern in the impedance of the tympanic membrane that often improves in response to edrophonium chloride. The stapedius test offers a diagnostic yield that is very close to that of SF-EMG, but unlike the latter, it is much easier to carry out. Therefore it promises to be of considerable diagnostic value in MG, as well as in monitoring the response to treatment (Kramer, Ruth, Johns, and Sanders, 1980; Stålberg and Sanders, 1981).

Summary of Neuromuscular Tests in Myasthenia Gravis

There is now available a wide variety of techniques and test protocols for assessing neuromuscular transmission in MG. Unfortunately, there are only a few studies that directly compare the relative values of the techniques and test protocols for the detection of abnormalities in neuromuscular transmission (Desmedt, 1970; Desmedt and Borenstein, 1976a; Ozdemir and Young, 1976; Horowitz, Jenkins, Kornfeld, and Papatestas, 1976; Stålberg, 1980; Stålberg and Sanders, 1981; Oh, Eslami, Nishihira, Sarala, Kuba, Elmore, Sunwoo, and Ro, 1982; Kelly, Daube, Lennon, Howard, and Younge, 1982).

The major problems are presented by the distress that sometimes attends repetitive supramaximal stimulation, especially at frequencies much in excess of 10 per second and when this type of stimulation is delivered to the brachial plexus, and the relative insensitivity of repetitive stimulation alone when applied to the intrinsic hand muscles (Oh, Eslami, Nishihira, Sarala, Kuba, Elmore, Sunwoo, and Ro, 1982). Based on my view of others' and our own experience in MG, the protocol used in the laboratory is outlined in Table 10.7. Prior to any testing, when possible, the anticholinesterase medication is reduced or withdrawn altogether for a period of 4 to 6 hours before the test. Also, especially where the intrinsic hand muscles are tested, the muscle is warmed to at least 35°C before the test is begun. Our experience with the relative values of repetitive stimulation and SF-EMG closely parallels that of Stålberg, whose results are presented in Table 10.6.

Table 10.7 outlines the protocol currently followed in our laboratory for testing neuromuscular transmission in patients with myasthenia gravis.

Our laboratory has no appreciable experience with the stapedius test, which seems to be both sensitive and acceptable to patients because it does not involve electrical stimulation of peripheral nerves. The tests of ocular angular displacement and velocity of movement, although very sensitive, are technically more difficult to carry out than the stapedius test.

OTHER DISORDERS OF NEUROMUSCULAR TRANSMISSION

Other disorders of neuromuscular transmission are listed in Table 10.1 (see also the review by Swift, 1981). The most common are

TABLE 10.7. Suggested Protocol for Detecting Abnormalities in Neuromuscular Transmission in MG

Begin—Supramaximal motor nerve stimulation and measurement of changes in the amplitude of the maximum M-potential in the intrinsic hand muscles (hypothenar or thenar group)

Test trains at 1, 3, and 10 per second

If the maximum M-potential amplitude is normal and there is not abnormal decrement in the amplitude, proceed to exercise.

Exercise—Maximum contraction for 20–30 seconds

Following this, repeat test train (10 stimuli at 3/s) at 10 seconds and 2, 4, and 6 minutes to look for post-tetanic facilitation or post-tetanic exhaustion

If normal, repeat above sequence for a proximal muscle such as, biceps, brachialis—stimulate musculocutaneous nerve

Trapezius—accessory nerve

If normal, switch to SF-EMG examination of the extensor digitorum communis

If jitter values are in normal range, switch to the orbicularis oculi muscle

those that are seen in motoneuronal and axonal diseases, especially in the more rapidly advancing varieties. Aside from MG, the remaining disorders of neuromuscular transmission are for the most part, quite rare, although they may be seen at some time in an active neurological center.

Eaton-Lambert (Myasthenic) Syndrome

The Eaton-Lambert syndrome is often associated with a small cell carcinoma of the lung, especially in males. There is evidence now, however, that it too, like MG, may be an autoimmune disorder (Gwilt, Lang, Newsom-Davis, and Wray, 1981; Lang, Newsom-Davis, Wray, Vincent, and Murray, 1981). The Eaton-Lambert syndrome may also be seen in association with Sjögren's syndrome, pernicious anemia, and thyroid disease, and may even rarely be associated with MG in the same patient. The antibodies in this disorder are probably directed against components in the presynaptic terminal axon membrane, perhaps the intramembranous particles that may be the calcium channels in the membrane (Fukunaga, Engel, Osame, and Lambert, 1982). In keeping with such an autoimmune hypothesis at least for the non-neoplastic variety of myasthenic syndrome, is evidence that plasma exchange and corticosteroids improve the condition (Lang, Newsom-Davis, Wray, Vincent, and Murray, 1981; Streib and Rothner, 1981).

The most characteristic structural abnormalities in the Eaton-Lambert syndrome include degenerative changes and atrophy in some of the motor axon terminals, demyelination and remyelination in some of the intramuscular preterminals, but normal numbers of vesicles per unit area of motor terminal and axon terminal areas. The major postsynaptic abnormalities are characterized by striking increases in the numbers and complexities

of the postsynaptic folds and increased variability of the widths of the primary and secondary synaptic clefts (Engel and Santa, 1971;
Santa, Engel, and Lambert, 1972; Santa and
Engel, 1973) (Figure 10.18).

The above morphological studies point to
the presence of a presynaptic disorder in which
there is destruction and degeneration of some
motor terminals and reductions in the numbers of release sites of ACh in the presynaptic
axon terminal; possibly through antibodies directed against the intramembranous particles
in the active zones, although as yet there is
no direct evidence of this. The suggestion of
a presynaptic defect in ACh release is borne
out by the physiological characteristics of this
disease.

For example, in vitro biopsy studies
(Elmqvist and Lambert, 1968; Elmqvist, 1973)

clearly show that the EPP amplitudes and EPP
quantal contents are well below normal values in response to single presynaptic stimuli.
The failure of many of the EPPs to reach requisite threshold levels for generating action
potentials in their MFs explains the weakness
in this disease. The presynaptic defect is also
underlined by the failure of an increase in the
concentration of extracellular potassium ions
to increase the frequency of the MEPPs. The
transmembrane potentials of the MFs and amplitudes of the quantal components of the EPP
and MEPP are all normal. The MEPP frequency, however, is about double that seen
at normal end-plates, for unknown reasons.

Characteristically, repetitive stimulation increases the quantum content and amplitudes
of the EPPs and restores suprathreshold synaptic transmission at most end-plates (Figure

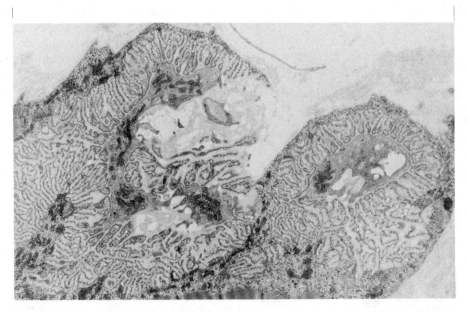

FIGURE 10.18.   Electronic micrograph of an end-plate in a patient with the myasthenic
syndrome. In this section of an end-plate the two adjacent axon terminals are surrounded by overly abundant junctional folds in the postsynaptic membrane, whose
total area may thereby be substantially increased. The vesicle content of the presynaptic
terminals is, however, normal. (Magnification × 9200)
From Engel and Santa (1971, figure 6).

10.19). Morphological and physiological studies therefore point clearly to a primary abnormality in the release of ACh, possibly through the destruction of release sites for the ACh in the presynaptic axonal membrane. In keeping with this hypothesis, studies have not shown any defect in ACh synthesis or storage in the Eaton-Lambert syndrome (Molenaar, Newsom-Davis, Rolak, and Vincent, 1982).

The explanation for hypertrophy of the postsynaptic membrane is not at all clear at this time. Increasing the number of ACh-R sites could help to overcome the reduced presynaptic release of ACh by providing many more potential sites for bonding for whatever ACh is released.

The basic biological mechanism behind the disease has not been established. Extracts of tissue taken from small cell carcinomas of the lung have been shown to reduce the quantum content of EPPs in frog muscle (Ishikawa, Engelhandt, Fujisawa, Okamoto, and Katsuki, 1977). Also, similar presynaptic defects in neuromuscular transmission can be shown in unselected intercostal biopsies from patients with lung carcinomas (Teräräinen and Larsen, 1977).

There is also the recent evidence that physiological abnormalities in neuromuscular transmission can be passively transferred to mice by IgG taken from affected patients (Gwilt, Lang, Newsom-Davis, and Wray, 1981). This observation suggests the possibility that autoantibodies may be present in the patients, directed, as pointed out earlier, against the presynaptic membrane.

Clinical tests of neuromuscular transmission in the myasthenic syndrome show equivalent though less direct abnormalities such as:

1. Very low amplitudes of the maximum M-potentials in response to single supramaximal nerve stimuli.

2. Dramatic increases in the amplitude of the maximum M-potentials to near normal or normal values in response to trains of stimuli delivered at 20 pulses per second. At stimulus frequencies of 3 per second, actual decrements can occur between the second and tenth M-potentials in the train. These decrements can mimic those seen in MG, although in the myasthenic syndrome the amplitudes of the M-responses are much lower than in MG.

3. The above two abnormalities are seen in 100 percent of distal limb muscles in the Eaton-Lambert syndrome.

4. Changes in the twitch tension parallel

FIGURE 10.19.   Recordings from a patient with the Eaton-Lambert syndrome. Effects of repetitive stimulation on the amplitude of the hypothenar maximum M-potential as recorded with surface electrodes in response to supramaximal stimulation of the ulnar nerve at frequencies of 1, 20, and 40 per second. Note the very substantial increase in amplitude of the maximum M-potential, especially at 40 per second.

An equivalent change in the intercostal muscles was seen as well.

From Elmqvist and Lambert (1968, figure 1).

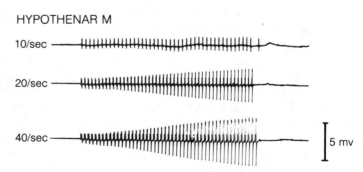

HYPOTHENAR M

10/sec

20/sec

40/sec

5 mv

those in the amplitude of the M-response except at frequencies of stimulation of 20 per second or more. Here a disproportionate increase in the tension develops that exceeds the amplitude increment in the maximum M-potential. This is because not only do more EPPs become suprathreshold and their MFs add their tension to the total generated, but individual twitches begin to fuse into a tetanus.

5. Exercise lasting as much as 10 to 30 seconds will increase the amplitude of the maximum M-potential when retested within 3 seconds of the end of the exercise period. By 1 minute, however, the amplitude has generally returned to preexercise values.

6. The maximum motor conduction velocities and residual latencies are well within the normal range. In addition, there is no evidence of abnormal spontaneous activity within the muscle to suggest the presence of denervation.

7. Like MG, intramuscularly recorded MUPs often show considerable fluctuation in their amplitudes because of variabilities in the safety factors for neuromuscular transmission at their various end-plates.

8. Anticholinesterase drugs are relatively ineffective in changing the amplitudes of the maximum M-potentials or in the tension development in the muscle. Improvements in these two values may, however, occur in vivo and in vitro with the use of quinidine hydrochloride.

The keys to electrophysiological diagnosis of this disease are the very low amplitudes of the initial M-potentials to single nerve stimuli and the subsequent dramatic increments in these amplitudes in response to trains of stimuli delivered at frequencies that exceed 15 pulses per second. It is well to remember here that occasionally, similar dramatic increases may be seen in the amplitudes of the maximum M-potential in MG at similar frequencies of stimulation (Ozdemir and Young, 1971).

Single-fiber EMG studies in the Eaton-Lambert syndrome may show increases in jitter and impulse block, but these, in contradistinction to MG, improve with repetitive activity and become more abnormal with rest (Schwartz and Stålberg, 1975a). Furthermore, no improvements develop in response to edrophonium chloride. In patients with Eaton-Lambert syndrome in whom quantitative oculography showed slowed ocular movement, improvements in ocular speed have recently been shown to follow administration of edrophonium chloride (Dell' Osso, Ayyar, Daroff, and Abel, 1983).

CONGENITAL MYASTHENIC SYNDROMES

In recent years several new though rare types of congenital myasthenia have become recognized. These characteristically appear in early life with fluctuating ptosis, sometimes ophthalmoparesis, and often feeding difficulties. They may present as excessive fatigability into adult life. At least four types have now been recognized.

Familial Congenital Myasthenic Syndrome Possibly due to Defective ACh Synthesis

In this disorder (Hart, Sahashi, Lambert, Engel, and Lindstrom, 1979; Engel, 1980; Lambert, 1982), which is most common in the newborn, but with which older patients have been seen, in vitro studies reveal:

1. Normal structure of the motor axon terminals, numbers of ACh-Rs, AChE content, and end-plates, although increases in densities of the vesicles in the terminals has been described

2. Normal EPP and MEPP amplitudes
3. Normal quantum content of the EPP
4. Marked decrement in the amplitudes of EPPs and MEPPs at 10-Hz stimulation
5. Normal stores of immediately releasable ACh in the motor nerve terminals

There is a striking decrement in the amplitudes of MEPPs as well as EPPs in response to repetitive stimulation. This points toward a possible disorder of ACh synthesis in a manner similar to that of hemicholinium-treated neuromuscular functions (Elmqvist and Quastel, 1965).

Clinical EMG studies reveal no decrement in the maximum M-potential to repetitive stimulation at 2 Hz when the muscle has been rested. Following exercise or a tetanic stimulus, however, obvious decrements become apparent.

Myasthenic Syndrome—Associated with a Deficiency of AChE, Reduced ACh Release, and Small Nerve Terminals (Engel, Lambert, and Gomez, 1977)

The one published case of this disorder appeared in infancy with fluctuating ptosis and has continued into adolescence with generalized fatigability not responding to anticholinesterase treatment. In vitro studies in this case have shown:

1. Normal MEPP amplitudes, although MEPP frequencies were reduced
2. A remarkable prolongation of the time courses of individual MEPPs
3. Reduced quantum contents of the EPP
4. Reduced immediately available stores of ACh
5. No increase in extrajunctional sensitivity to ACh
6. Total absence of AChE at the end-plates

7. Normal numbers of ACh-Rs
8. Small nerve terminals

There seems little doubt that the absence of AChE accounts for the prolonged durations of MEPPs and the repetitive firing of some MFs in response to a single presynaptic nerve stimulus. It is not known whether the small nerve terminals are related to the low quantum content of the EPP. Whatever the basic cause, it is probably fortunate, in view of the absence of AChE, that the amount of ACh released per synaptic impulse is less than normal.

Clinical electromyographic abnormalities include characteristic repetitive discharges seen in the M-potential following single motor nerve stimuli, and decrements in the M-potential at all frequencies of stimulation. No fibrillation potentials have been seen.

Vincent and others (Vincent, Cull-Candy, Newsom-Davis, Trautman, Molenaar, and Polak, 1981) have also described another probably presynaptic variety of congenital myasthenia in which marked reductions in MEPP amplitudes were accompanied by much higher quantum contents of the EPP (5 to 6 times) and decrements in response to 5-Hz stimulation.

Congenital Myasthenic Syndrome— Attributable to a Prolonged Open Time of the ACh-R-associated Ion Channels

This disorder may arise in infancy or adult life and characteristically involves the extraocular, cervical scapular, and forearm finger extensor muscles (Engel, Lambert, Mulder, Torres, Sahashi, Bertorini, and Whitaker, 1981; Engel, 1980). In vitro studies reveal:

1. Very prolonged EPPs and MEPPs
2. Very prolonged miniature end-plate currents

3. Normal quantum content of the EPP
4. Reduced amplitudes of MEPPs
5. Normal readily available stores of ACh
6. Decrease in nerve terminal size and increase in densities of vesicles in the terminals
7. Abundant AChE activity
8. Focal degeneration of the postjunctional folds
9. Reduction in the numbers of ACh-Rs
10. Small groups of atrophic MFs
11. Degenerative changes in the MFs

Clinical EMG studies in this disorder reveal repetitive discharges in response to single presynaptic stimuli. This is readily explained by the greatly prolonged EPP seen in this disease that could reexcite the MFs. Also, decrements in the amplitudes of the maximum M-potential may be seen in response to 2-Hz stimulation.

Here the prolonged EPPs and MEPPs are not a result of the absence of AChE, but possibly a prolonged opening time of the ACh-R-associated ion channels. This would explain the prolonged extracellularly recorded miniature end-plate currents, which are a function of the number of open channels and the times these channels are open.

Degenerative changes in the MFs in this syndrome have been attributed to the accumulation of calcium within the junctional folds of the MFs through the action of the end plate current. The prolonged channel openings would have the effect of greatly increasing the influx of calcium into the MFs. These local accumulations of calcium ions could in turn inhibit mitochondrial function, activate proteases, and produce breakdowns in intramuscular cytoskeletal elements. Calcium deposits in the postsynaptic regions have been shown in this disease (Engel, Lambert, Mulder, Torres, Sahashi, Bertorini, and Whitaker, 1981).

Familial Congenital Myasthenic Syndrome—with Possible Abnormalities in the Synthesis of ACh-R or Its Insertion into the Postsynaptic Membrane

This disorder has been recognized in two brothers (Lambert, 1982). The special features of in vitro studies include:

1. Normal MEPP durations and frequencies
2. Reduced MEPP amplitudes
3. Normal quantum content of the EPP
4. Normal readily available store of ACh
5. Reduced numbers of ACh-Rs with no evidence of ACh-R antibodies or immunoglobulin complexes at the end-plate

Clinical studies reveal electrophysiological abnormalities very similar to those in MG. The reduced numbers of ACh-R probably explain the physiological abnormalities, but the reasons for the loss of ACh-R are not known. Perhaps ACh-Rs are synthesized more slowly, their insertion in the membrane is faulty, or they break down more rapidly.

Cases 2, 4, and 5 reported by Vincent and associates (1981) may be similar in that the MEPP amplitudes were also reduced in company with clear reductions in the numbers of α-bungarotoxin binding sites. In these three cases SF-EMG was abnormal in all. Case 3 of the study may be unique in that severe reductions in MEPP amplitudes were not accompanied by much loss of α-bungarotoxin binding sites.

DRUG-INDUCED DISORDERS OF NEUROMUSCULAR TRANSMISSION

D-Penicillamine-induced Myasthenia

Penicillamine may induce a reversible myasthenic-like syndrome when used to treat rheumatoid arthritis, scleroderma, or Wilson's disease. The myasthenic disorder is indistinguishable clinically and electrophysiologically from autoimmune MG, and in the vast majority, ACh-R antibodies can be shown (Bucknall, Dixon, Glick, Woodland, and Ztschi, 1975; Masters, Dawkins, Zilko, Simpson, Leedman, and Lindstrom, 1977; Stålberg and Trontelj, 1979; Vincent, Newsom-Davis, and Martin, 1978; Fawcett, McLachlan, Nicholson, Argov, and Mastaglia, 1982).

Antibiotics

Some antibiotics may cause apnea and paralysis of extraocular, bulbar, and limb muscles, especially in patients who have a preexisting disorder of neuromuscular transmission (i.e., MG) or those with severe renal disease. Weakness may last several hours to several days and in some instances at least, may be improved by increasing the concentration of extracellular calcium ions and by the use of anticholinesterase drugs.

The nature of the neuromuscular transmission disorder depends on the antibiotic. Some, such as *tetracycline* and *oxytetracycline,* act like tubocurarine, as competitive blockers with ACh for the ACh-R. Others block ACh-Rs noncompetitively, such as the *polymyxin group. Neomycin,* one of the *aminoglycosides* (others include *streptomycin* and *kanamycin)* reduces both the amplitudes and the quantum contents of the EPPs with variable increases in both following stimulation at 40 per second (Daube and Lambert, 1973).

In vivo, low maximum M-potential amplitudes may be seen with increments in these amplitudes, as well as PTE in response to high-frequency stimulation (about 40 per second). At lower frequencies (0.1 per second) decrements in the amplitudes of the maximum M-potentials are seen. These studies and those of others (Elmqvist and Josefsson, 1962) show

that there is a presynaptic defect in the mobilization or release of ACh, defects that can be substantially reversed by tetanic stimulation and treated by increasing the calcium ion concentrations.

In humans, despite the documented instances of apnea and paralysis in patients receiving one or more of these "risk" antibiotics, there are few comprehensive studies of neuromuscular transmission. One exception is the case reported by McQuillen, Cantor, and O'Rourke (1968). Their patient was paraplegic with a history of repeated urinary tract infections. The patient was treated on the last admission with kanamycin and subsequently developed extraocular, bulbar, respiratory, and limb paralysis. Amplitudes of the maximum M-potentials were well below normal values in response to a single supramaximal stimulus delivered to the motor nerve. In addition, no increments in the M-potential occurred in response to trains of stimuli delivered at 0.1 to 50 pulses per second, and PTF and PTE were not seen. A dramatic (7 to 8 times) increment in the maximum M-potential did occur, however, following intravenous infusion of calcium, suggesting that the neuromuscular block was partially reversible by increasing the concentration of extracellular calcium ions. The patient unfortunately died, and no examination of the end-plates or peripheral nerves were available.

Another ten patients underwent transurethral prostatectomy under spinal anesthesia and were given kanamycin (Wright and McQuillen, 1971). No clinical weakness developed, nor were any abnormal responses to repetitive stimulation seen in these men.

Abnormalities produced by *colistin* are characterized by reduced MEPP amplitudes and, as in neomycin toxicity, reduced quantum contents of the EPP (McQuillen and Engbaek, 1975).

The *monobasic amino acid* antibiotics such

as lincomycin and clindamycin reduce spontaneous and stimulus-evoked ACh release, but in addition reduce the postjunctional sensitivity to ACh.

Anticholinesterase Toxicity

Anticholinesterase toxicity may be produced through the use of insecticides (organophosphates and carbamate), nerve gases, or simply overtreatment with anticholinesterase drugs. The results in all cases are greatly to prolong the actions of whatever ACh is released, producing repetitive discharges in MFs and decrements with repetitive stimulation because of the cholinergic block.

Anticonvulsants

Phenytoin and trimethadione may both produce myasthenia. Phenytoin is known to impair stimulus-evoked quantum release, although enhancing spontaneous ACh. There is some question as to whether desensitization at the end-plate accounts for some of the reductions in MEPP amplitude.

β-Adrenergic Blocking Agents

β-Adrenergic blocking agents such as propranolol may aggravate MG and in so doing exert presynaptic and postsynaptic actions at the neuromuscular junction.

Lithium

Lithium reduces both spontaneous and stimulus-evoked ACh release as well as the number of ACh-Rs.

Curare

In vitro, the primary action of curarine is postjunctional. Curare combines with ACh-Rs and prevents their interaction with ACh. Despite the controversy over a possible prejunctional effect of curarine (Galindo, 1970; Hubbard and Wilson, 1973), curare does not reduce the amount of ACh released (Fletcher and Forrester, 1975), the quantum content of the EPP, or MEPP frequency (Auerbach and Betz, 1971), or alter the binding time of ACh and ACh-Rs (Katz and Miledi, 1973). Curare does, however, reduce the number of possible interactions between ACh and ACh-Rs by reducing the number of available ACh-Rs. Amplitudes of EPP and MEPP are therefore reduced primarily through postjunctional blockade of ACh-Rs, evidence for a possible accompanying minor prejunctional effect of ACh and possible presynaptic ACh-Rs notwithstanding (Miyamoto, 1978).

In humans, curare in nonparalytic doses increases the amount of jitter present and may cause impulse block, especially when jitter values exceed 70 μsec, at which time diplopia and slight ptosis may be seen (Ekstedt and Stålberg, 1969). In these studies, there were no accompanying alterations in the conduction velocities of MFs. Fractionation of MUPs has been observed with curarization (Locke and Henneman, 1960). The explanation for this phenomenon is not known.

Procainamide and Quinidine

Procaine blocks neuromuscular transmission partly through a curare-like interaction with the ACh-Rs, the strength of this combination being a function of the transmembrane potential (Kordas, 1970). Both may also produce some block of presynaptic axons. Procainamide has been shown to exert a predominately postsynaptic inhibitory action on neuromuscular transmission, an effect which is reversible. As well, procainamide has been shown to reduce the quantal content of the EPP and the amplitude of MEPPs (Lee, Kim, Liu, and Johns, 1983).

CATION-INDUCED NEUROMUSCULAR DISORDERS

Magnesium

Increases in the extracellular concentration of magnesium ions produce a reduction in MEPP frequency, and neuromuscular transmission may be blocked through reductions in the amplitudes and quantum contents of the EPPs. Magnesium ions competitively interact with calcium ions. Hence increases in the extracellular concentration of calcium ions can partially reverse the effects of increasing the magnesium concentration (see Hubbard, 1961; Hubbard, Jones, and Landau, 1968; Hubbard, Llinás, and Quastel, 1969).

Calcium

Some spontaneous quantal release occurs even in the total absence of calcium; however, normal ACh release depends on normal calcium ion concentrations just outside the axon terminals. Calcium ions must be present just prior to depolarization of the nerve terminal by the presynaptic nerve impulse. Both the quantal content of the EPP and frequency of the MEPP are direct functions of the concentration of extracellular calcium ions (Hubbard, 1973; Llinás, 1982).

TOXIN-INDUCED NEUROMUSCULAR DISORDERS

Botulism

Botulism is a rare disorder caused by neurotoxins—types A and B and rarely type E—elaborated by the *Clostridium botulinum* bacterium. The clinical disorder is characterized by development of paralysis 10 to 36 hours after ingestion of the toxin (Cherington 1973, 1974; Pickett, 1982; Cornblath, Sladky, and Sumner, 1983). The paralysis primarily involves the extraocular, bulbar, respiratory, trunk, and limb muscles; in most patients the pupils are spared. It is a serious disorder carrying a fatality rate of about 25 percent.

The basic mechanisms in botulinum poisoning have been the subject of several in vitro experiments (Lambert, Engel, and Cherington, 1974; Cull-Candy, Lundh, and Thesleff, 1976; Kao, Drachman, and Price, 1976; Lundh, Leander, and Thesleff, 1977). Morphological changes at the end-plate have been described by Duchen (1971a, 1971b).

In vitro studies of botulinum toxin-poisoned end-plates clearly show reductions in the quantum content of the EPPs, sometimes to such a severe extent that the EPP consists of only a few quanta or fails to occur at all in response to a single stimulus. The quantal contents of such EPPs may be increased by repetitive stimulation of the presynaptic nerve, increasing the extracellular calcium ion concentration, or exposure of the affected end-plates to tetraethylammonium (TEA). The last, by blocking potassium conductance in the nerve terminal and prolonging the duration of the action potential, increases the entry of calcium into the axon terminal (Katz and Miledi, 1967), thereby increasing the release of acetylcholine from the nerve terminal and possibly restoring conduction at the neuromuscular junction. The improvement in acetylcholine release by measures increasing Ca^{++} ion influx into the nerve terminal strongly suggests that the botulinum toxin produces its defect at least partially through blocking Ca^{++} ion channels in the axon terminals.

Strategies designed to increase the influx of Ca^{++} ions into the presynaptic terminal, for example, increasing the concentrations of extracellular K^+ and Ca^{++} ions, do not, however, restore the very reduced frequencies of MEPPs at poisoned end-plates. Moreover, amplitudes of MEPPs are often higher and their time courses significantly slower compared to the EPPs at affected neuromuscular junctions (Thesleff, 1982). Thesleff suggests that the latter may represent ACh release possibly in nonquantal form, or exocytosis of giant vesicles or clusters of vesicles outside the active zone.

Despite the fact that increases in concentrations of extracellular K^+ or Ca^{++} ions do not increase MEPP frequencies, repetitive presynaptic stimulation (at 20 to 100 Hz) when accompanied by the addition of black widow spider venom does dramatically increase both the amplitude and frequencies of the MEPPs (Harris and Miledi, 1971; Cull-Candy, Lundh, and Thesleff, 1976). This venom is known to facilitate acetylcholine release through mechanisms apparently independent of Ca^{++} ion entry into the axon terminal.

In this respect it is of interest that calcium ionophores (carboxylic antibiotics), which are known to increase the permeability of the membrane to calcium and increase quantum release at normal neuromuscular junctions, fail to do the same to botulinum toxin-treated neuromuscular junctions unless the extracellular calcium ion concentration is increased at the same time (Cull-Candy, Lundh, and Thesleff, 1976).

The above collective evidence suggests that calcium channels in botulinum toxin-poisoned axon terminals may indeed be blocked or destroyed in some way, thus preventing entry of calcium ions into the nerve terminals. The de-

fect can be overcome somewhat by increasing the concentration of extracellular calcium ions, using calcium ionophores to increase the terminal membrane permeability to calcium, repetitive nerve stimulation, or by TEA. All these strategies increase intracellular concentration of calcium ions. These measures all increase the amplitude of MEPPs, although they do not alter MEPP frequencies.

Quinidine, TEA, and 4-aminopyridine (4-AP) will each restore neuromuscular transmission to botulinum toxin-poisoned end-plates (Lundh, Leander, and Thesleff, 1977). Quinidine and TEA both require concomitant increases in the extracellular calcium ion concentrations to 4 mmole or more, whereas 4-AP, the most potent agent, is able sometimes to restore in vivo neuromuscular transmission to normal at extracellular concentrations of calcium ions as low as 2 mmole.

In addition to prolonging the duration of the presynaptic action potential and increasing thereby Ca^{++} ion influx into the axon terminal, 4-AP may alter intracellular calcium ion binding to organelles. Despite the theoretical attractiveness of 4-AP as a potentially helpful drug for the treatment of botulism and the Eaton-Lambert syndrome, it has turned out to be associated with adverse side effects that prohibit its use (Murray and Newsom-Davis, 1981).

Clinical Electromyographic Abnormalities in Botulism

The most characteristic physiological abnormalities in clinical botulinum toxin poisoning (Cherington, 1974, 1982; Gutmann and Pratt, 1976; Oh, 1977) include:

1. Reduced amplitudes of the maximum M-potentials, especially in severe cases.
2. Decrements in amplitude of maximum M-potentials at low frequencies of stimulation (1 to 5 stimuli per second) (such decrements may be absent in mild cases).

3. Increments (over 50 percent) in the maximum M-potential in response to higher-frequency stimulation (10 to 50 stimuli per second) in over 90 percent of mild cases. Such increments are much less common in severe cases. Reductions in the amplitudes of maximum M-potentials are neither as marked nor as uniformly present in all muscles in botulinum poisoning as they are in the Eaton-Lambert syndrome. Similarly, the incremental responses are not as dramatic or as common as in Eaton-Lambert, and PTE has been seen in botulism.

4. Fibrillation potentials may be seen after the initial two-week period.

5. Fasciculations have occasionally been seen.

6. Motor nerve conduction velocities are usually normal, although mild reductions in conduction velocity may be seen in some patients.

7. Increased jitter and impulse blocking improve as the firing frequency of the MUs increase (Schiller and Stålberg, 1976).

8. Abnormalities in sensory conduction have been documented in at least one case report.

In summary, botulinum toxin binds to nerve membranes and must, in some way, block calcium ion influx or interfere with the intracellular binding of calcium ions and in motor axon terminals. In this way they block ACh release (Simpson, 1973; Oh, 1977). The explanation for the abnormalities in peripheral sensory nerve fibers is not, however, known. Structural abnormalities at end-plates exposed to botulinum toxin have been described by Duchen (1971b, 1971c).

Tetanus

Tetanus is caused by *Clostridium tetani*. In man, the disorder is characterized by intense tonic contraction of skeletal muscle, the result of abnormal spontaneous firing of motoneurons. Such firing may be caused by impaired inhibitory mechanisms in the spinal cord (Brooks, Curtis, and Eccles, 1957). In addition, however, tetanus toxin impairs cholinergic transmission in both skeletal muscle and in the autonomic nervous system. In vitro, the neuromuscular block in tetanus (Duchen and Tonge, 1973) is characterized by:

1. Blocking of neuromuscular transmission; EPPs are either absent or their amplitudes very reduced.

2. Reduced MEPP frequencies and disproportionate increases in the number of low-amplitude MEPPs.

3. No increases in MEPP frequency in the presence of increases in the extracellular calcium ion concentration, and only minimally accelerated MEPP frequency with exposure to increases in potassium ion concentrations. Repetitive nerve stimulation does, however, increase MEPP frequency, especially that of the larger-amplitude MEPPs.

4. Fibrillation potentials develop in the soleus (a slow muscle) but not in the extensor digitorum longus (a fast muscle). Within days, sprouting develops with the subsequent formation of new end-plates in the soleus muscle.

These abnormalities point to presynaptic defects in neuromuscular transmission and degeneration of axons, although the cause of these changes is not known.

Tick Paralysis

Tick bites can cause an areflexic paralysis in association with normal cerebrospinal fluid. The paralysis may not resolve unless the engorging tick is found and removed. Characteristic electrophysiological abnormalities in these patients (Cherington and Snyder, 1968; Swift and Ignacio, 1975) include:

1. Reduced amplitudes of maximum M-potentials that subsequently increase as recovery proceeds.
2. No dramatic decrements or increments in response to stimulation or exercise and no PTF or PTE.
3. Reduced maximum motor conduction velocities, at least in the beginning, which may reflect the loss of the faster-conducting motor axons or motor units.
5. Normal latencies and amplitudes of peripheral sensory nerve action potentials, although slight reductions in maximum sensory conduction velocities have been observed.

The evidence to date has not established whether or not there is a true disorder of neuromuscular transmission in tick paralysis. It seems more likely on the evidence, that conduction block, perhaps at the level of the motor nerve terminals or preterminals, in motor axons is responsible for the weakness.

In vitro studies (Cooper and Spence, 1976) have shown that the quantal content of the EPP may be reduced and that it was very dependent on environmental temperature. Thus dramatic falls in the amplitudes and quantal contents of the EPPs may develop as the temperature increases. This demonstration of neuromuscular transmission abnormalities was based on the toxin produced by the *Ixodes holocyclus* type of tick; whereas the quantal content of the EPP is said to be normal in the presence of the toxin produced by *Dermacentor variabilis* tick, the cause of tick paralysis in North America. The basic defect and cause of the paralysis may therefore critically depend on the species of tick causing the paralysis.

Black Widow Poisoning

Black widow spiders *(Latrodectus mactans)* elaborate a toxin (α-latrotoxin) that affects both the central and peripheral nervous systems. It causes cramp in the trunk and limb muscles. The toxin has been shown greatly to increase ACh release to the point of depletion at the end-plate, and can act in the absence of calcium ions. It may possibly insert itself into the presynaptic membrane, forming its own ion channels. The brown widow *(Latrodectus geometricus)* has a similar action.

Scorpion Poisoning

The toxin(s) elaborated by the scorpion produce repetitive firing in motor axon terminals, increasing the release of ACh. This action is produced through delays in the inactivation of sodium channels. Effects are seen in MF as well as axonal membranes in which the resulting prolonged action potentials cause repetitive discharges.

DISORDERS OF NEUROMUSCULAR TRANSMISSION IN ASSOCIATION WITH MOTONEURON DISEASES, MULTIPLE SCLEROSIS, PERIPHERAL NEUROPATHIES, AND MUSCLE DISEASES

Amyotrophic Lateral Sclerosis

Abnormalities of neuromuscular transmission in amyotrophic lateral sclerosis (ALS) have been recorded by many investigators (Lambert and Mulder, 1957; Mulder, Lambert, and Eaton, 1959; Simpson, 1966; Lambert, 1969; Miglietta, 1971; Brown and Jaatoul, 1974; Norris, 1975; Carleton and Brown, 1979). The most characteristic of these consist of abnor-

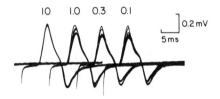

FIGURE 10.20.   Decrement in a single thenar MUP from a patient with amyotrophic lateral sclerosis. Stimulus intervals were 10, 1.0, 0.3, and 0.1 ms from left to right. A 22 percent decrement in peak-to-peak amplitude was already apparent at 1.0 ms, and there was not much increase at interstimulus periods of 0.3 or 0.1 ms.

mal decrements in amplitudes of the maximum M-potential, even at low frequencies of stimulation (less then 1 Hz) and only partial reversal of these decrements by anticholinesterase medication. Decrements in single ALS motor unit potentials are greatest in those with the lowest amplitudes as recorded with surface electrodes (Carleton and Brown, 1979) (Figures 10.20 and 10.21).

Structural abnormalities at ALS end-plates are many, although in the most recent investigation, there was no correlation between the degree of these and motor disability or rate of clinical progression of the disease (Bjornskov, Dekker, Norris, and Stuart, 1975). In two recent electrophysiological studies, however, decrements in the maximum M-potentials were more common in more rapidly progressive cases of ALS (Bernstein and Antel, 1981) and in studies of single MUPs, the later stages of involvement of particular muscles (Carleton and Brown, 1979). Factors that may contribute to the magnitude of the decrement in ALS include:

1. Neuromuscular transmission abnormalities at end-plates that are undergoing degeneration. Probably not all end-plates in an MU fail at the same time, or have equivalent safety factors for neuromuscular transmission.

2. There may be intermittent axonal conduction block, particularly at higher frequencies of stimulation (i.e., over 10 Hz).

3. Immature end-plates may be present where the safety factors for neuromuscular transmission are probably below normal. These end-plates are a product of the collateral sprouting and reinnervation of denervated muscle fibers. Structural abnormalities at ALS end-plates have been the subject of a number of investigations (Wohlfart, 1957; Coërs and Woolf, 1959; Zacks, 1964; Woolf, Alberca-Serrano, and Johnson, 1969; Bjornskov, Dekker, Norris, and Stuart, 1975) and the reader is encouraged to look at these sources.

All of these factors may contribute to the observed decrements in ALS, especially at stimulus frequencies that exceed 10 Hz. Axonal block is an unlikely source of decrements at stimulus frequencies of 3 Hz or less. At the level of single fibers, abnormal increases in the jitter and impulse blocking are particularly common in the complex MU potentials; these abnormalities being more common in the more rapidly advancing cases (Stålberg, Schwartz, and Trontelj, 1975). Evidence of neurogenic blocking was seen in 5 to 10 percent of potentials in ALS (Stålberg and Thiele, 1972).

Following experimental section of the motor nerve (Miledi and Slater, 1970), the end-plate continues to transmit normally for a period whose duration is a function of the length of the nerve stump distal to the section. Neuromuscular transmission then fails abruptly, usually accompanied by termination of the MEPP at about the same time. In most clinical disorders of the motoneurons or axons, however, the progression to failure at end-plates is probably much more gradual, perhaps extending from normal presynaptic func-

FIGURE 10.21.   Changes in motor unit (MU) potential peak-to-peak voltage (p-pV) in millivolts in response to repetitive stimulation at 0.3-second intervals in control hypothenar MUPs (top) and MUPs of subjects with amyotrophic lateral sclerosis (bottom) in whom the amplitude of the maximum M-potential was less than the 2-SD lower limit of control subjects. All changes in MUP amplitude are shown with respect to the p-pV amplitude of the first MUP in the train as recorded with surface electrodes, as well as with respect to the adjusted latency of the MU (see Chapter 3).

Note the absence of any decrement in the fifth compared to the first MUP in any of the control MUPs, and the wide range in the amplitudes of these MUPs (see Chapter 6). (Bottom) In contrast, many of the MUPs here exhibited decrements in their amplitude, such decrements on the whole being more common and more pronounced in those MUPs whose amplitudes were at the lower end of the amplitude range. Notice also the relatively greater proportion of larger amplitude (surface-recorded) MUPs relative to the lower amplitude MUPs in this disease.

From Carleton and Brown (1979, figure 3).

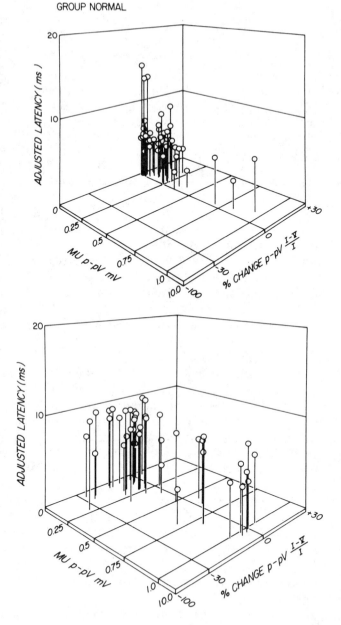

tion to failed neuromuscular transmission (subthreshold EPP) over several weeks or even several months, although there is no direct evidence for this hypothesis. It is worthwhile remembering, too, that even in otherwise healthy muscle, degeneration and regeneration of motor nerve terminals continually takes place (Barker, 1966). Hence there are probably a few immature end-plates present, even in healthy muscle, their numbers being too few to be revealed as an abnormal decrement with repetitive stimulation. In the first few weeks of life, decrements in excess of those seen in adults may be present in response to repetitive stimulation, especially at the higher stimulus frequencies as well as PTE (Churchill-Davidson and Wyse, 1963). In this context it is worth pointing out that in experimental disuse of muscle, even though MEPP frequencies and amplitudes remain unchanged, minor changes in the quantal contents of EPPs may be seen.

Reinnervation

Following crush or section of a peripheral nerve where all the motor axons to a muscle are interrupted, motor axons may regenerate and contact the denervated muscle fibers. Unlike the innervation of developing muscle, where only one synapse per MF survives despite multiple reinnervations in earlier periods (Bennett and Pettigrew, 1974a, 1974b), in older animals multiple or dual reinnervation may persist (Guth, 1962; Bennett, McLaughlin, and Taylor, 1973; Bennett, Florin and Woog, 1974). The MEPPs appear before the EPPs and the amplitudes of the earliest EPPs are subthreshold. Unlike the more mature pattern, the amplitudes of EPPs at immature neuromuscular junctions tend to increase in response to short trains of presynaptic stimuli. The more usual pattern, a depression of EPP amplitudes by trains of stimuli, begins only once the amplitudes of EPPs reach suprathreshold levels for the generation of action potentials in MFs (Bennett, Florin, and Woog, 1974). There is some evidence even prior to the establishment of synaptic connections that regenerating axon tips can release ACh (Decino, 1981).

In the human, in the early period following reinnervation, abnormal decrements in the amplitudes of MUPs in response to repetitive

stimulation are common. Also common are abnormal increases in jitter and the incidence of impulse blocking, especially in the longer-latency spike components of the MUP. These abnormalities no doubt reflect the immature state of the newly formed neuromuscular junctions where the safety factor for neuromuscular transmission would be reduced compared to normal. The lower quantum contents and amplitudes of the EPPs that are characteristic of newly formed end-plates could be explained by:

1. Smaller stores of ACh being available for release.
2. Impaired ACh release mechanisms.
3. Conduction block in presynaptic axon terminals or preterminal branches. If the block occurs close enough to the terminal to allow for some albeit reduced depolarization of the terminal through electronic conduction, a reduced amount of ACh may be released. This is because the amount of ACh is a function of the magnitude of the shift of the transmembrane potential of the motor axon terminals.

Whatever mechanisms operate at newly formed end-plates, these may be expected to contribute to the overall muscular transmission defects seen in any disorder of neuromuscular transmission, the motoneuron, or axon where axonal regeneration and reinnervation of MFs takes place.

Peripheral Neuropathies

Abnormal decrements in the maximum M-potentials of various muscles in response to repetitive stimulation have been reported in diabetic, Guillain-Barré, and post-herpes zoster motor neuropathy, and in chronic polyneuritis (Simpson and Lenman, 1959; Simpson, 1966). Thiel and Stålberg (1975), however, in a more recent study, were not able to show abnormalities in neuromuscular transmission in uremic or diabetic neuropathies. The same authors were able to show abnormal increases in jitter values and impulse blocking as well as an increase in fiber density in alcoholic neuropathy.

How much these decrements in response to repetitive stimulation are a result of abnormal neuromuscular transmission and how much the result of neurogenic blocking is not known. A variety of structural abnormalities at the end-plates and presynaptic neural apparatus has been described in many of the motoneuronal and axonal neuropathies (Coërs and Woolf, 1959).

Multiple Sclerosis

In multiple sclerosis (MS), abnormal decrements in the maximum M-response to repetitive stimulation has been reported, together with partial improvement in these decrements and clinical fatigue with the use of anticholinesterase drugs (Patten, Hert, and Lovelace, 1972). This earlier evidence has received support from others (Eisen, Yufe, Trop, and Campbell, 1978). Jitter is increased at some end-plates at MS muscle, and abnormalities in single MU potentials may be present that suggest the presence of patchy denervation and reinnervation (Weir, Hansen, and Ballantyne, 1979, 1980). These electrophysiological abnormalities find some support in histological evidence of abnormalities in myelination seen in teased myelinated nerve fibers on biopsy in MS (Pollock, Calder, and Allpress, 1977).

In short, there is evidence of abnormal neuromuscular transmission in MS. This should not be too surprising in view of the fact that sometimes the plaques involve the ventral horn regions, and although not common, muscle atrophy not accounted for by the cachexia, malnutrition, or mechanical injuries to the peripheral nerve, is well recognized.

NEUROMUSCULAR TRANSMISSION IN PRIMARY DISORDERS OF MUSCLE

Single-fiber EMG has shown increased fiber densities, abnormal increases in jitter and impulse blocking in a variety of dystrophic disorders. These abnormalities probably reflect the formation of new and immature neuromuscular junctions with relatively low safety factors for neuromuscular transmission. This proposal is supported by the high incidence of late linked potentials in these disorders (Stålberg, 1977; Buchthal, 1977; Borenstein and Desmedt, 1973; Desmedt and Borenstein, 1976b) at which time the jitter was usually most pronounced.

In the myotonic disorder, abnormal decrements in amplitudes of the maximum M-potentials in response to repetitive stimulation have been described by several observers (Ozdemir and Young, 1976; Aminoff, Layzer, Satya-Murti, and Faden, 1977). Decrements were seen in all varieties of myotonia including myotonia congenita, myotonic dystrophy, and paramyotonia with hyperkalemic periodic paralysis. They were not seen in all such patients, nor were they related to the presence or absence of weakness or the degree of myotonia. The decrements could be distinguished from those in MG because in the myotonias, they developed later in the stimulus train, not as early as the second or third potential in the train as is characteristic of MG. Moreover, the decrements in myotonia characteristically increase as the stimulus frequency increases, may occur with direct muscle stimulation, and are absent at 3 per second when the muscle is warm (Desmedt, 1977). The fact that they are present in response to direct as well as indirect stimulation is important in that it establishes their origin as not at the neuromuscular junction, but in progressive reductions in amplitudes of the extracellularly recorded action potentials of MFs. Such amplitude reductions are no doubt explained by the progressively increasing interspike depolarization produced by repetitive stimulation.

Except for those abnormalities in neuromuscular transmission secondary to the formation of new end-plates, there is no evidence for primary abnormalities of neuromuscular transmission in the experimental muscular dystrophies, where the quantal sizes and contents of the EPPS are normal and the incidence of such failures is very low.

References

Aminoff MJ, Layzer RB, Satya-Murti S, Faden AI. The declining electrical response of muscle to repetitive nerve stimulation in myotonia. Neurology 1977;27:812–16.

Auerbach A, Betz W. Does curare affect transmitter release? J Physiol 1971;213:691–705.

Baloh RW, Keesey JC. Saccade fatigue and response to edrophonium for the diagnosis of myasthenia gravis. Ann NY Acad Sci 1976; 274:631–41.

Barker D. Sprouting and degeneration of mammalian motor axons in normal and de-afferented skeletal muscle. Proc R Soc Biol (Lond) 1966;163:538–54.

Bennett MR, Florin T, Woog R. The formation of synapses in regenerating mammalian striated muscle. J Physiol 1974;238:79–92.

Bennett MR, McLaughlin EM, Taylor R. The formation of synapses in reinnervated and cross-reinnervated adult avian muscle. J Physiol 1973;230:331–57.

Bennett MR, Pettigrew AG. The formation of synapses in striated muscle during development. J Physiol 1974a;241:515–45.

Bennett MR, Pettigrew AG. The formation of synapses in reinnervated and cross-reinnervated striated muscle during development. J Physiol 1974b;241:547–73.

Bergmans J. The physiology of single human nerve fibers. Louvain, Belgium: Vander, 1970.

Bernstein LP, Antel JP. Motor neuron disease: decremental responses to repetitive nerve stimulation. Neurology 1981;31:202–4.

Bjornskov EK, Dekker NP, Norris FH, Stuart ME.

End-plate morphology in amyotrophic lateral sclerosis. Arch Neurol 1975;32:711–12.

Blom S, Zakrisson JE. The stapedius reflex in the diagnosis of myasthenia gravis. J Neurol Sci 1974;21:71–76.

Borenstein S, Desmedt JE. Electromyographical signs of collateral reinnervation. In: Desmedt JE, ed. New developments in electromyography and clinical neurophysiology. Basel: Karger, 1973:130–40.

Borenstein S, Desmedt JE. Temperature and weather correlates of myasthenic fatigue. Lancet 1974;2:63–66.

Borenstein S, Desmedt JE. Local cooling in myasthenia. Arch Neurol 1975;32:152–57.

Brooks VB, Curtis DR, Eccles JC. The action of tetanus toxin on the inhibition of motoneurones. J Physiol 1957;135:655–72.

Brown JC, Charlton JE, White DJK. A regional technique for the study of sensitivity to curare in human muscle. J Neurol Neurosurg Psychiatry 1975;38:18–26.

Brown WF, Jaatoul N. Amyotrophic lateral sclerosis electrophysiological study (number of motor units and rate of decay of motor units). Arch Neurol 1974;30:242–48.

Bucknall RC, Dixon AStJ, Glick EN, Woodland J, Ztschi DW. Myasthenia gravis asssociated with penicillamine treatment for rheumatoid arthritis. Br Med J 1975;1:600–2.

Buchthal F. Diagnostic significance of the myopathic EMG. In: Rowland LP, ed. Pathogenesis of human muscular dystrophies. Proceedings of the Fifth International Scientific Conference of the Muscular Dystrophy Association, Durango, Colorado. Amsterdam, Oxford: Excerpta Medica, 1977:205–18.

Campbell WW Jr, Leshner RT, Swift TR. Plasma exchange in myasthenia gravis: electrophysiological studies. Ann Neurol 1980;8:584–89.

Carleton SA, Brown WF. Changes in motor unit populations in motor neurone disease. J Neurol Neurosurg Psychiatry 1979;42:42–51.

Ceccarelli B, Hurlbut WP. Vesicle hypothesis of the release of quanta of acetylcholine. Physiol Rev 1980;60:396–441.

Cherington M. Botulism: electrophysiological and therapeutic observations. In: Desmedt JE, ed. New developments in electromyography and clinical neurophysiology. Basel: Karger, 1973:375–79.

Cherington M. Botulism. Ten-year experience. Arch Neurol 1974;30:432–37.

Cherington M. Electrophysiological methods as an aid in diagnosis of botulism: a review. Muscle Nerve 1982;5:S28–S29.

Cherington M, Snyder RD. Tick paralysis: neurophysiologic studies. N Engl J Med 1968; 278:95–97.

Churchill-Davidson HC, Wyse RP. Neuromuscular transmission in the newborn infant. Anaesthesiology 1963;24:271–78.

Coërs C, Woolf AL. The innervation of muscle: a biopsy study. Oxford: Blackwell, 1959.

Cooper BJ, Spence I. Temperature-dependent inhibition of evoked acetylcholine release in tick paralysis. Nature 1976;263:693–95.

Cornblath DR, Sladky JT, Sumner AJ. Clinical electromyography of infantile botulism. Muscle Nerve 1983;6:448–52.

Cull-Candy SG, Lundh H, Thesleff S. Effects of botulinum toxin on neuromuscular transmission in the rat. J Physiol 1976;260:177–203.

Dahlbäck O, Elmqvist D, Johns TR, Radner S, Thesleff S. An electrophysiological study of the neuromuscular junction in myasthenia gravis. J Physiol 1961;156:336–43.

Daube JR, Lambert EH. Post activation exhaustion in rat muscle. In: Desmedt JE, ed. New developments in electromyography and clinical neurophysiology. Basel: Karger, 1973:343–49.

Decino P. Transmitter release properties along regenerated nerve processes at the frog neuromuscular junction. J Neurosci 1981;1:308–17.

Dell' Osso LF, Ayyar DR, Daroff RB, Abel LA. Edrophonium test in Eaton-Lambert syndrome: quantitative oculography. Neurology 1983; 33:1157–63.

Desmedt JE. Neuromuscular defect in myasthenia gravis. Electrophysiological and histological evidence. In: Viets H, ed. Myasthenia gravis. Springfield, Ill.: Charles C Thomas, 1961:150–76.

Desmedt JE, Borenstein S. The testing of neuromuscular transmission. In: Vinken PJ, Bruyn GW, eds. Handbook of clinical neurology. Amsterdam: Elsevier North-Holland, 1970:104–15.

Desmedt JE, Borenstein S. Diagnosis of myasthenia gravis by nerve stimulation. Ann NY Acad Sci 1976a;274:174–88.

Desmedt JE, Borenstein S. Regeneration in Duchenne muscular dystrophy. Arch Neurol 1976b;33:642–50.

Desmedt JE, Borenstein S. Double-step nerve stimulation test for myasthenic block: sensitization of post-activation exhaustion by ischemia. Ann Neurol 1977;1:55–64.

Duchen LW. An electron microscopic comparison of motor end-plates of slow and fast skeletal muscle fibers of the mouse. J Neurol Sci 1971a;14:37–45.

Duchen LW. An electron microscopic study of the changes induced by botulinum toxin in the motor end-plates of slow and fast skeletal muscle fibers of the mouse. J Neurol Sci 1971b;14:47–60.

Duchen LW. Changes in the electron microscopic structures of slow and fast skeletal muscle fibers of the mouse after the local injection of botulinum toxin. J Neurol Sci 1971c;14:61–74.

Duchen LW, Tonge DA. The effects of tetanus toxin on neuromuscular transmission and on the morphology of motor end-plates in slow and fast skeletal muscle of the mouse. J Physiol 1973; 228:157–72.

Eisen A, Yufe R, Trop D, Campbell I. Reduced neuromuscular transmission safety factor in multiple sclerosis. Neurology 1978;28:598–602.

Ekstedt J, Stålberg E. The effect of non-paralytic doses of D-tubocurarine on individual motor end-plates in man, studied with a new electrophysiological method. Electroencephalogr Clin Neurophysiol 1969;27:557–62.

Ellisman MH, Rash JE, Staehelin LA, Porter KR. Studies of excitable membranes. II. A comparison of specialization of neuromuscular junctions and non-junctional sarcolemmas of mammalian fast- and slow-twitch muscle fibers. J Cell Biol 1976;68:752–74.

Elmqvist D. Neuromuscular transmission defects. In: Desmedt JE, ed. New developments in electromyography and clinical neurophysiology. Basel: Karger, 1973:229–40.

Elmqvist D, Hofmann WW, Kugelberg J, Quastel DMJ. An electrophysiological investigation of neuromuscular transmission in myasthenia gravis. J Physiol 1964;174:417–34.

Elmqvist D, Josefsson JO. The nature of the neuromuscular block produced by neomycine. Acta Physiol Scand 1962;54:105–10.

Elmqvist D, Lambert EH. Detailed analysis of neuromuscular transmission in a patient with the myasthenic syndrome sometimes associated with bronchogenic carcinoma. Mayo Clin Proc 1968;43:689–713.

Elmqvist D, Quastel DMJ. Presynaptic action of hemicholinium at the neuromuscular junction. J Physiol 1965;177:463–82.

Engel AG. Morphologic and immunopathologic findings in myasthenia gravis and in congenital myasthenic syndromes. J Neurol Neurosurg Psychiatry 1980;43:577–89.

Engel AG, Lambert EH, Gomez MR. A new myasthenic syndrome with end-plate acetylcholinesterase deficiency, small nerve terminals and reduced acetylcholine release. Ann Neurol 1977;1:315–30.

Engel AG, Lambert EH, Howard FM. Localization of acetylcholine receptors, antibodies and complement at end-plates of patients with myasthenia gravis. Mayo Clin Proc 1977;52:267–80.

Engel AG, Lambert EH, Mulder DM, Torres CF, Sahashi K, Bertorini TE, Whitaker JN. A newly recognized congenital myasthenic syndrome attributed to a prolonged open time of the acetylcholine-induced ion channel. Ann Neurol 1981;11:553–69.

Engel AG, Lindstrom JM, Lambert EH, Lennon VA. Ultrastructural localization of the acetylcholine receptor in myasthenia gravis and in its experimental autoimmune model. Neurology 1977;27:307–15.

Engel AG, Santa T. Histometric analysis of the ultrastructure of the neuromuscular junction in myasthenic gravis and in the myasthenic syndrome. Ann NY Acad Sci 1971;183:46–63.

Engel AG, Tsujihater M, Lambert EH, Lindstrom EH, Lennon VA. Experimental autoimmune myasthenia gravis: a sequential and quantitative study of the neuromuscular junction ultrastructure and electrophysiological correlations. J Neuropathol Exp Neurol 1976;35:569–87.

Eusebi F, Miledi R. Divalent cations and temperature-dependent block of impulse propagation at the frog neuromuscular junction. Muscle Nerve 1983;6:602–5.

Fambrough DM. Control of acetylcholine receptors in skeletal muscle. Physiol Rev 1979;59:165–227.

Fambrough DM, Drachman DC, Satyamurti S. Neuromuscular junction in myasthenia gravis: decreased acetylcholine receptors. Science 1973; 182:293–95.

Fardeau M. Normal ultrastructural aspect of human motor end-plate and its pathologic modifications. In: Pearson CM, Mostof FK, eds. The striated muscle. International Academy of Pathology Monograph. Baltimore: Williams & Williams, 1973.

Fatt P, Katz B. An analysis of the end-plate potential recorded with an intracellular electrode. J Physiol 1951;115:320–70.

Fawcett PRW, McLachlan SM, Nicholson LVB, Argov Z, Mastaglia FL. D-Penicillamine-associated myasthenia gravis: immunological and electrophysiological studies. Muscle Nerve 1982;5:328–34.

Fletcher P, Forrester T. The effect of curare on the release of acetylcholine from mammalian motor nerve terminals and an estimate of quantum content. J Physiol 1975;251:131–44.

Fukunaga H, Engel AG, Osame M, Lambert EH. Paucity and disorganization of presynaptic membrane active zones in the Lambert-Eaton myasthenic syndrome. Muscle Nerve 1982;5:686–97.

Gage PW. Generation of end-plate potentials. Physiol Rev 1976;56:177–247.

Galindo A. Prejunctional effect of curare: its relative importance. J Neurophysiol 1970;34:289–301.

Gauthier GF. The motor end-plate: structure. In: Landon DN, ed. The peripheral nerve. London: Chapman & Hall, 1976:464–94.

Gertler R, Robbins N. Differences in neuromuscular transmission in red and white muscles. Brain Res 1978;142:160.

Guth L. Neuromuscular function after regeneration of interrupted nerve fiber into partially denervated muscle. Exp Neurol 1962;10:236–50.

Gutmann L, Pratt L. Pathophysiological aspects of human botulism. Arch Neurol 1976;33:175–79.

Gwilt M. Lang B, Newsom-Davis J, Wray D. Electrophysiological studies on the myasthenic (Eaton-Lambert) syndrome passively transferred from man to mouse. J Physiol 1981;324:29P.

Harris AJ , Miledi R. The effect of type D botulinum toxin on frog neuromuscular junctions. J Physiol 1971;217:497–515.

Hart ZH, Sahashi K, Lambert EH, Engel AG, Lindstrom JM. A congenital, familial myasthenic syndrome caused by a presynaptic defect of transmitter resynthesis or mobilization. Neurology 1979;29:556–57.

Harvey AM, Masland RL. A method for the study of neuromuscular transmission in human subjects. Bull Johns Hopkins Hosp 1941a;68:81–93.

Harvey AM, Masland RL. The electromyogram in myasthenia gravis. Bull Johns Hopkins Hosp 1941b;69:1–13.

Hatt H, Smith DO. Synaptic depression related to presynaptic axon conduction block. J Physiol 1976;259:367–93.

Hertel G, Ricker K, Hirsch A. The regional curare test in myasthenia gravis. J Neurol 1977;24:257–65.

Heuser JE, Reese TS. Structure of the synapse. In: Kandel ER, ed. Handbook of physiology. The nervous system. Vol. 1. Cellular biology of neurons. Bethesda, Md.: American Physiological Society, 1977:261–94.

Heuser JE, Reese TS. Structural changes from transmitter release at the frog neuromuscular junction. J Cell Biol 1981;88:564–80.

Heuser JE, Reese TS, Dennis MJ, Jan Y, Jan L, Evans L. Synaptic vesicle exocytosis captured by quick freezing and correlated with quantal transmitter release. J Cell Biol 1979;81:275–300.

Horowitz SH, Jenkins G, Kornfeld P, Papatestas AE. Regional curare test in evaluation of ocular myasthenia. Arch Neurol 1975;32:83–88.

Horowitz SH, Jenkins G, Kornfeld P, Papatestas AE. Electrophysiologic diagnosis of myasthenia gravis and the regional curare test. Neurology 1976;26:410–17.

Hubbard JI. The effect of calcium and magnesium on the spontaneous release of transmitter from mammalian motor nerve endings. J Physiol 1961;159:507–17.

Hubbard JI. Repetitive stimulation at the mammalian neuromuscular junction, and the mobilization of transmitter. J Physiol 1963;169:641–62.

Hubbard JI. Microphysiology of vertebrate neuromuscular transmission. Physiol Rev 1973;53:674–725.

Hubbard JI, Jones SF, Landau EM. On the mechanism by which calcium and magnesium effect the spontaneous release of transmitter from mammalian motor nerve terminals. J Physiol 1968;194:355–80.

Hubbard JI, Llinás R, Quastel DMJ. Electrophysiological analysis of synaptic transmission. London: Edward Arnold, 1969.

Hubbard JI, Schmidt RF. An electrophysiological investigation of mammalian motor nerve terminals. J Physiol 1963;166:145–67.

Hubbard JI, Willis WD. The effects of depolarization of motor nerve terminals upon the release of transmitter by nerve impulses. J Physiol 1968;194:381–405.

Hubbard JI, Wilson DF. Neuromuscular transmission in a mammalian preparation in the absence of blocking drugs and the effect of d-tubocurarine. J Physiol 1973;228:307–25.

Ishikawa K, Engelhardt J, Fujisawa T, Okamoto T, Katsuki H. A neuromuscular transmission block provided by a cancer tissue extract derived from a patient with the myasthenic syndrome. Neurology 1977;27:140–43.

Ito Y, Miledi R, Vincent A, Newsom-Davis J. Acetylcholine receptors and end-plate electrophysiology in myasthenia gravis. Brain 1978; 101:345–68.

Kadrie HA, Brown WF. Neuromuscular transmission in human single motor units. J Neurol Neurosurg Psychiatry 1978a;41:193–204.

Kadrie HA, Brown WF. Neuromuscular transmission in myasthenic single motor units. J Neurol Neurosurg Psychiatry 1978b;41:205–14.

Kao I, Drachman DB. Myasthenic immunoglobulin accelerates acetylcholine receptor degradation. Science 1977;29:527–29.

Kao I, Drachman DB, Price DL. Botulinum toxin: mechanism of presynaptic blockade. Science 1976;193:1256–58.

Katz B. Nerve, muscle and synapse. New York: McGraw-Hill, 1966.

Katz B. The release of neural transmitter substances. Liverpool: Liverpool University Press, 1969.

Katz B, Miledi R. Propagation of electrical activity in motor nerve terminals. Proc R Soc Lond Biol 1965;161:453–82.

Katz B, Miledi R. A study of synaptic transmission in the absence of nerve impulses. J Physiol 1967;192:407–36.

Katz B, Miledi R. The role of calcium in neuromuscular facilitation. J Physiol 1968;195:481–92.

Katz B, Miledi R. The statistical nature of the acetylcholine potential and its molecular components. J Physiol 1972;224:665–99.

Katz B, Miledi R. The binding of acetycholine to receptors and its removal from the synaptic cleft. J Physiol 1973;231:549–74.

Katz B, Miledi R. Transmitter leakage from motor nerve endings. Proc R Soc Lond Biol 1977;196:59–72.

Kelly JJ, Daube JR, Lennon VA, Howard FM Jr, Younge BR. The laboratory diagnosis of mild myasthenia gravis. Ann Neurol 1982;12:238–42.

Kelly JJ Jr, Lambert EH, Lennon VA. Acetylcholine release in diaphragm of rats with chronic experimental autoimmune myasthenia gravis. Ann Neurol 1978;4:67–72.

Konishi T, Hishitani H, Matsubara MS, Ohta M. Myasthenia gravis: relation between jitter in single fiber EMG and antibody to acetylcholine receptor. Neurology 1981;31:386–92.

Kordas M. The effect of procaine on neuromuscular transmission. J Physiol 1970;209:689–99.

Kramer LD, Ruth RA, Johns ME, Sanders DB. A comparison of stapedial reflex fatigue with repetitive stimulation and single-fiber EMG in myasthenia gravis. Ann Neurol 1980;9:531–36.

Krarup C. Electrical and mechanical responses in the platysma and in the adductor pollicis muscle: in normal subjects. J Neurol Neurosurg Psychiatry 1977a;40:234–40.

Krarup C. Electrical and mechanical responses in the platysma and in the adductor pollicis muscle: in patients with myasthenia gravis. J Neurol Neurosurg Psychiatry 1977b;40:241–49.

Kuffler SW, Nicholls JG. From neuron to brain. Sunderland, Mass.: Sinauer Associates, 1976.

Kuffler SW, Yoshikami D. The number of transmitter molecules in a quantum: an estimate from iontophoretic application of acetylcholine at the neuromuscular synapse. J Physiol 1975;251:465–82.

Kuno M, Turkanis SA, Weakly JN. Correlation between nerve terminal size and transmitter release at the neuromuscular junction of the frog. J Physiol 1971;213:545–56.

Lambert EH. Defects of neuromuscular transmission in syndromes other than myasthenia gravis. Ann NY Acad Sci 1966;135:367–84.

Lambert EH. Electrography in amyotrophic lateral sclerosis. In: Norris FH Jr, Kurland LT, eds. Motor neuron diseases. New York: Grune & Stratton, 1969:135–53.

Lambert EH. Electrophysiological studies of the myasthenic syndrome and congenital neuromuscular syndromes. In: Didactic Programme, Twenty-ninth Annual Meeting American Association of Electromyography and Electrodiagnosis, Minneapolis, October 1982.

Lambert EH, Engel AG, Cherington M. End-plate potentials in botulism. Third International Congress on Muscle Diseases, Newcastle-on-Tyne. Amsterdam: International Congress Series no. 334. Excerpta Medica, 1974:65.

Lambert EH, Mulder DW. Electrographic studies in amytrophic lateral sclerosis. Mayo Clin Proc 1957;32:441–46.

Lambert EH, Okihiro M, Rooke ED. Clinical physiology of the neuromuscular transmission. In: Paul WM, Daniel EE, Kay CM, Monckton G, eds. Muscle. New York: Pergamon Press, 1965:487–99.

Lambert EH, Rooke ED, Eaton LM, Hodgson CH. Myasthenic syndrome occasionally with bronchial neoplasm. Neurophysiological studies. In: Viets HR, ed. Myasthenia gravis. Springfield, Ill.: Charles C Thomas, 1961:362–410.

Lang B, Newsom-Davis J, Wray D, Vincent A, Murray N. Autoimmune aetiology for myasthenia (Eaton-Lambert) syndrome. Lancet 1981;2:224–26.

Lee DC, Kim YI, Liu HH, Johns TR. Presynaptic and postsynaptic actions of procainamide on neuromuscular transmission. Muscle Nerve 1983;6:442–47.

Lester HA. The response to acetylcholine. Sci Am 1977;236:107–17.

Liley AW. An investigation of spontaneous activity at the neuromuscular junction of the rat. J Physiol 1956a;132:650–66.

Liley AW. The effects of presynaptic polarization in the spontaneous activity at the mammalian neuromuscular junction. J Physiol 1956b; 134:427–43.

Lindstrom J, Dau P. Biology of myasthenia gravis. Ann Rev Pharmacol Toxicol 1980;20:337–62.

Lindstrom J, Lambert EH. Content of acetylcholine receptor and antibodies bound to receptor in myasthenia gravis, experimental autoimmune myasthenia gravis and Eaton-Lambert syndrome. Neurology 1978;28:130–38.

Llinás RR. Calcium in synaptic transmission. Sci Am 1982;247:56–65.

Locke S, Henneman E. Fractionation of motor units by curare. Exp Neurol 1960;2:638–51.

Lundh H, Leander S, Thesleff S. Antagonism of the paralysis produced by botulinum toxin in the rat. J Neurol Sci 1977;32:29–43.

Martin ARA. A further study of the statistical composition of the end-plate potential. J Physiol 1955;130:114–22.

Martin ARA. Quantal nature of synaptic transmission. Physiol Rev 1966;46:51–66.

Martin ARA. Junctional transmission. II. Presynaptic mechanisms. In: Kandel ER, ed. Handbook of physiology. The nervous system. Vol. 1. Cellular biology of neurones. Bethesda, Md.: American Physiological Society, 1977:329–55.

Masters CL, Dawkins RL, Zilko PJ, Simpson JA, Leedman RJ, Lindstrom J. Penicillamine-associated myasthenia gravis, anti-acetylcholine receptor and antistriational antibodies. Am J Med 1977;63:689–94.

Mayer RF. Neuromuscular transmission in single motor units in myasthenia gravis. Muscle Nerve 1982;5:S46–S49.

Mayer RF, Williams IR. Incrementing responses in myasthenia gravis. Arch Neurol 1974;31:24–26.

McComas AJ, Sica REP, Brown JC. "Myasthenia gravis": evidence for a "central" defect. J Neurol Sci 1971;13:107–13.

McQuillen MP, Cantor HE, O'Rourke JR. Myasthenic syndrome associated with antibiotics. Arch Neurol 1968;18:402–14.

McQuillen MP, Engbaek L. Mechanism of colistin-induced neuromuscular depression. Arch Neurol 1975;32:235–38.

Miglietta OE. Myasthenic-like response in patients with neuropathy. Am J Phys Med 1971;50:1–16.

Miledi R. Transmitter release induced by injection of calcium ions into nerve terminals. Proc R Soc Lond Biol 1973;183:421–25.

Miledi R, Slater CR. On the degeneration of rat neuromuscular junctions after nerve section. J Physiol 1970;207:507–28.

Morioka WT, Neff PA, Boisseranc TE, Hartman PW, Cantrell RW. Audiotympanometric findings in myasthenia gravis. Arch Otolaryngol 1976;102:211–13.

Miyamoto MD. The actions of cholinergic drugs on motor nerve terminals. Pharmacol Rev 1978;29:221–47.

Molenaar PC, Newsom-Davis J, Rolak RL, Vincent A. Eaton-Lambert syndrome: acetylcholine and choline acetyltransferase in skeletal muscle. Neurology 1982:32:1062–65.

Mulder DW, Lambert EH, Eaton LM. Myasthenic syndrome in patients with amyotrophic lateral sclerosis. Neurology 1959;9:627–31.

Murali K, Pagala D, Tada S, Namba T, Grob D. Neuromuscular transmission in neonatal mice injected with serum globulin of myasthenia gravis patients. Neurology 1982;32:12–17.

Murray NMF, Newsom-Davis J. Treatment with oral 4-aminopyridine in disorders of neuromuscular transmission. Neurology 1981;31:265–71.

Norris FH. Adult spinal motor neuron disease. Progressive muscular atrophy (Aran's disease) in relation to amyotrophic lateral sclerosis. In: Vinken PJ, Bruyn GW, eds. Handbook of clinical neurology. Amsterdam: Elsevier North-Holland, 1975:1–56.

Oda K, Korenaga S, Ito Y. Myasthenia gravis: passive transfer to mice of antibody to human and mouse acetylcholine receptor. Neurology 1980; 31:282–87.

Oh SJ. Botulism: electrophysiological studies. Ann Neurol 1977;1:481–85.

Oh SJ, Eslami N, Nishihira T, Sarala PK, Kuba T, Elmore RS, Sunwoo IN, Ro YI. Electrophysiological and clinical correlation in myasthenia gravis. Ann Neurol 1982;12:348–54.

Ozdemir C, Young RR. Electrical testing in myasthenia gravis. Ann NY Acad Sci 1971;183:287–302.

Ozdemir C, Young RR. The results to be expected from electrical testing in the diagnosis of myasthenia gravis. Ann NY Acad Sci 1976;274:203–22.

Padykula HA, Gauthier GF. The ultrastructure of the neuromuscular junctions of mammalian red, white and intermediate skeletal muscle fibers. J Cell Biol 1970;46:27–41.

Pagala MKD, Tada S, Namba T, Grob D. Neuromuscular transmission in neonatal mice injected with serum globulin of myasthenia gravis patients. Neurology 1982;32:12–17.

Patten BM, Hert A, Lovelace R. Multiple sclerosis associated with defects in neuromuscular transmission. J Neurol Neurosurg Psychiatry 1972;35:385–94.

Peter K, Bradley RJ, Dreyer F. The acetylcholine receptor at the neuromuscular junction. Physiol Rev 1982;62:1271–1340.

Pickett JB. Infant botulism — the first five years. Muscle Nerve 1982;5:S26–S27.

Pollock M, Calder C, Allpress S. Peripheral nerve abnormality in multiple sclerosis. Ann Neurol 1977;2:41–48.

Pumplin DW, Reese TS, Llinás R. Are the presynaptic membrane particles calcium channels? Proc Natl Acad Sci USA 1981;78:7210–13.

Ricker K, Hertel G, Stodieck S. Influence of temperature on neuromuscular transmission in myasthenia gravis. J Neurol 1977;216:273–82.

Roses AD, Olanow CW, McAdams MW, Lane RJM. No direct correlation between serum antiacetylcholine receptor antibody levels and clinical state of individual patients with myasthenia gravis. Neurology 1981;3:220–24.

Rowland LP, Aranow H, Hoefer PFA. Observations on the curare test in the differential diagnosis of myasthenia gravis. In: Viets HR, ed. Myasthenia gravis. Springfield, Ill.: Charles C Thomas, 1961:411–34.

Sahashi K, Engel AG, Lindstrom JM, Lambert EH, Lennon VA. Ultrastructural localization of immune complexes (IgG and C3) at the end-plate in experimental autoimmune myasthenia gravis. J Neuropathol Exp Neurol 1978;37:212–23.

Sanders DB, Howard JF, Johns TR. Single-fiber electromyography in myasthenia gravis. Neurology (Minneap) 1978;29:68–76.

Santa T, Engel AG. Histometric analysis of neuromuscular junction ultrastructure in rat red, white and intermediate muscle fibers. In: Desmedt JE, ed. New developments in electromyography and clinical neurophysiology. Basel: Karger, 1973:41–54.

Santa T, Engel AG, Lambert EH. Histometric study of neuromuscular junction ultrastructure. II. Myasthenic syndrome. Neurology 1972;22:370–76.

Satyamurti S, Drachman DB, Slone F. Blockade of acetylcholine receptors: a model of myasthenia gravis. Science 1975;187:955–57.

Schiller HH, Stålberg E. Human botulism studied with single-fiber electromyography. Arch Neurol 1976;35:346–49.

Schwartz MS, Stålberg E. Myasthenic syndrome studied with single-fiber electromyography. Arch Neurol 1975a;32:815–17.

Schwartz MS, Stålberg E. Single-fiber electromyographic studies in myasthenia gravis with repetitive nerve stimulation. J Neurol Neurosurg Psychiatry 1975b;38:678–82.

Simpson JA. Disorders of neuromuscular transmission. Proc R Soc Med 1966;59:993–98.

Simpson JA. Myasthenia gravis and myasthenic syndromes. In: Walton J, ed. Disorders of voluntary muscle. Edinburgh: Churchill Livingstone, 1981:585–624.

Simpson JA, Lenman JAR. The effect of frequency of stimulation in neuromuscular disease. Electroencephalogr Clin Neurophysiol 1959;11:604–5.

Simpson LL. The neuroparalytic and hemagglutinating activities of botulinum toxin. In: Simpson LL, ed. Neuropoisons. New York: Plenum Press, 1973:303–23.

Slomić A, Rosenfalck A, Buchthal F. Electrical and mechanical responses of normal and myasthenic muscle. Brain Res 1968;10:1–74.

Stålberg E. Electrogenesis in human dystrophic

muscle. In: Rowland LP, ed. Pathogenesis of human muscular dystrophies. Proceedings of the Fifth International Scientific Conference of the Muscular Dystrophy Association, Durango, Colorado. Amsterdam, Oxford: Excerpta Medica, 1977:570–89.

Stålberg E. Clinical electrophysiology in myasthenia gravis. J Neurol Neurosurg Psychiatry 1980;43:622–33.

Stålberg E, Ekstedt J. Single-fiber EMG and microphysiology of the motor unit in normal and diseased human muscle. In: Desmedt JE, ed. New developments in electromyography and clinical neurophysiology. Basel: Karger, 1973:113–29.

Stålberg E, Ekstedt J, Broman A. Neuromuscular transmission in myasthenia gravis studied with single-fiber electromyography. J Neurol Neurosurg Psychiatry 1974;37:540–47.

Stålberg E, Sanders DB. Electrophysiological tests of neuromuscular transmission. In: Stålberg E, Young RR, eds. Clinical neurophysiology. Woburn, Mass.: Butterworth's, 1981:88–116.

Stålberg E, Schwartz MS, Trontelj JV. Single-fibre electromyography in various processes affecting the anterior horn cell. J Neurol Sci 1975;24:403–15.

Stålberg E, Thiele B. Transmission block in terminal nerve twigs: a single-fiber electromyographic finding in man. J Neurol Neurosurg Psychiatry 1972;35:52–59.

Stålberg E, Trontelj JV. Single-fiber electromyography. Surrey, England: Mirvalle Press, 1979.

Stålberg E, Trontelj JV, Schwartz MS. Single-muscle-fiber recording of the jitter phenomenon in patients with myasthenia gravis and in members of their families. Ann NY Acad Sci 1976; 274:189–202.

Streib EW, Rothner AD. Eaton-Lambert myasthenic syndrome: long-term treatment of three patients with prednisone. Ann Neurol 1981;10:448–53.

Swift TR. Disorders of neuromuscular transmission other than myasthenia gravis. Muscle Nerve 1981;4:334–53.

Swift TR, Ignacio OJ. Tick paralysis: electrophysiologic studies. Neurology 1975;25:1130–33.

Takeuchi A. Junctional transmission. I. Postsynaptic mechanisms In: Kandel ER, ed. Handbook of physiology. The nervous system. Vol. 1. Cellular Biology of Neurones. I. Bethesda, Md.: American Physiological Society, 1977:295–327.

Tauc L. Nonvesicular release of neurotransmitter. Physiol Rev 1982;62:857–93.

Teräräinen H, Larsen A. Some features of the neuromuscular complications of pulmonary carcinoma. Ann Neurol 1977;2:495–502.

Thesleff SW. Spontaneous transmitter release in experimental neuromuscular disorders of the rat. Muscle Nerve 1982;5:S12–S16.

Thiele B, Stålberg E. Single-fiber electromyography findings in polyneuropathies of different etiology. J Neurol Neurosurg Psychiatry 1975;38:881–89.

Tindall RS. Humoral immunity in myasthenia gravis: biochemical characterization of acquired antireceptor antibodies and clinical correlations. Ann Neurol 1981;10:437–47.

Vincent A, Cull-Candy SG, Newsom-Davis J, Trautman A, Molenaar PC, Polak RL. Congenital myasthenia: end-plate acetylcholine receptors and electrophysiology in five cases. Muscle Nerve 1981;4:306–18.

Vincent A, Newsom-Davis J. Anti-acetylcholine receptor antibodies. J Neurol Neurosurg Psychiatry 1980;43:590–600.

Vincent A, Newsom-Davis J, Martin V. Anti-acetylcholine receptor antibodies in D-penicillamine-associated myasthenia gravis. Lancet 1978;1:1254.

Warren WR, Gutmann L, Cody RC, Flowers P, Segal AT. Stapedius reflex decay in myasthenia gravis. Arch Neurol 1977;34:496–97.

Weir A, Hansen S, Ballantyne JP. Single-fiber electromyographic jitter in multiple sclerosis. J Neurol Neurosurg Psychiatry 1979;42:1146–50.

Weir A, Hansen S, Ballantyne JP. Motor unit potential abnormalities in multiple sclerosis: further evidence for a peripheral nervous system defect. J Neurol Neurosurg Psychiatry 1980;43:999–1004.

Wohlfart G. Collateral regeneration from residual motor nerve fibers in amyotrophic lateral sclerosis. Neurology 1957;7:124–34.

Woolf AL, Alberca-Serrano R, Johnson AG. The intramuscular nerve endings and muscle fibers in amyotrophic lateral sclerosis—a biopsy study.

In: Norris FH, Kurland LT, eds. Motor neuron diseases. New York: Grune & Stratton, 1969: 166–77.

Wright EA, McQuillen MP. Antibiotic-induced neuromuscular blockade. Ann NY Acad Sci 1971;183:358–68.

Yee RD, Cogan DG, Zee DS, Baloh RW, Honrubia V. Rapid eye movements in myasthenia gravis. Arch Ophthalmol 1976;94:1465–72.

Zacks SI. The motor end-plate. Philadelphia: WB Saunders, 1964.

11 ELECTROMYOGRAPHY AND THE CRANIAL NERVES

The most important cranial nerves for electromyographers to be familiar with are the fifth, seventh, accessory (eleventh), and hypoglossal (twelfth) nerves. These may be involved at their origin, in their courses through the brainstem, outside the brainstem but within the intracranial cavity, at the base of the skull, or in their peripheral courses. Electromyographers with a working knowledge of the anatomy and physiology of these nerves may, in some instances, be able to provide important aid in detecting and localizing lesions within and outside the central nervous system (CNS) that involve these nerves or their synaptic connections. This chapter reviews some of the more important aspects of the anatomy and physiology of these nerves, and the electrophysiological methods now available for testing them. The discussion begins with the fifth cranial nerve.

TRIGEMINAL (FIFTH) NERVE

The Jaw Jerk

The fifth nerve is of interest to electromyographers primarily because of the localizing value of its reflex connections within the brainstem. Recording and measuring the latencies of the jaw jerk (JJ) is one way of testing the integrity of the latter connections and disclosing lesions in the brainstem, especially when these are not apparent through computed tomography or clinical examination. Important anatomical points to remember about the underlying reflex pathway include:

1. The primary sensory neurons for spindle stretch receptors in the masseter and temporalis muscles are not located in the gasserian ganglion along with other trigeminal primary sensory neurons, but in the mesencephalic nucleus of the midbrain tegmentum (Figure 11.1). Collaterals of these primary stretch afferents connect to motoneurons in the trigeminal pontine motor nucleus to complete the stretch reflex arc. Not all neurons in the mesencephalic nucleus are the cell bodies of muscle stretch receptors; others mediate pressure sense from the teeth and peridontium and thus may play a role in adjusting the force of a bite (Johansson and Olsson, 1976; Brodal, 1981). Cell bodies of Golgi tendon organs for jaw closure muscles are located in the gasserian ganglion.

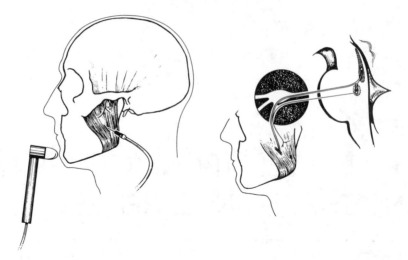

FIGURE 11.1.   One method of recording the jaw jerk. (Left) The reflexly elicited EMG potentials in the masseter muscle are recorded by an intramuscular electrode because frequently, the resultant EMG discharge is so small as to be barely detectable by surface electrodes over the masseter muscle. On the right is shown the reflex pathway. The cell bodies of primary afferents of spindle receptors in the masseter are located in the mesencephalic nucleus of the midbrain and these neurons are monosynaptically connected to trigeminal motoneurons in the pons.

This anatomical arrangement is based on studies in the cat. See Szentágothai (1948).

2. There is some uncertainty about the route taken by muscle stretch afferent originating in the jaw closure muscles to reach the brainstem. In the cat, evidence suggests that unlike the Golgi tendon organ afferents, primary spindle afferents from these muscles reach the brainstem by way of the motor root of the trigeminal nerve (Szentágothai, 1948). McIntyre and Robinson (1959) claimed this was true in man as well, but more recently Ferguson (1978) and Ongerboer de Visser (1982a, 1982b) have pointed to ipsilateral absence of the JJ in patients where the sensory root was sectioned or the prolonged latencies of the JJ were prolonged ipsilateral to where thermocoagulation of the gasserian ganglion has been carried out. Whether these two procedures also produced partial conduction block in the motor root sufficient to abolish the JJ without producing detectable denervation in the motor root is an open question. The weight of the evidence at this time, however, favors the recent claims of Ferguson and Ongerboer de Visser.

3. Unlike the spindle afferents in the limbs, Godaux and Desmedt (1975a) have suggested that primary spindle afferents from the masseter muscle exert no direct inhibitory influence on the antagonistic muscles (jaw opening).

The above points suggest some anomalous features of the trigeminal complex; namely, the location of some of the primary sensory neurons within the CNS, the possible separation of peripheral afferent pathways for the spindle and Golgi tendon organ afferents, and perhaps some difference in the central connectivities of these afferents in relation to agonist and antagonist muscles. The latter two points are of more physiological than clinical interest, but the mesencephalic location of the spindle afferent neurons is of clear parctical importance.

For example, Ongerboer de Visser (1982a, 1982b) and others (McIntyre and Robinson, 1959; McIntyre, 1951; Goodwill, 1968; Hufschmidt and Spuler, 1962) have clearly shown that the JJ may be absent ipsilateral to lesions restricted to the midbrain tegmentum, lesions that could be expected to interrupt the central afferent connection and perhaps destroy the afferent neurons themselves.

The JJ EMG responses may be recorded by surface electrodes by placing the stigmatic electrode over the motor point of the masseter muscle and the reference electrode on the neck (Godaux and Desmedt, 1975a), or by using intramuscular electrodes (Yates and Brown, 1981a) (Figures 11.1 and 11.2). The latter provide better-defined latencies, especially when they are inserted near the innervation zone. Taps delivered to the chin tangentially to the radius of action of the jaw evoke a brisk stretch of the masseter muscles, and they provide a contact trigger pulse to the recording equipment to signal onset of the stimulus and a zero point from which to measure the latencies to the EMG discharges (Yates and Brown, 1981a) (Figure 11.3).

By means of this method, absent or delayed JJs have been documented in multiple sclerosis (Goodwill and O'Tuama, 1969; Kimura, Rodnitzky, and Van Allen, 1970; Yates and Brown, 1981a) and in a variety of other lesions involving the peripheral and central connections related to JJ (Kimura, Rodnitzky, and Van Allen, 1970; Ongerboer de Visser and Goor, 1974, 1976; Goor and On-gerboer de Visser, 1976; Ongerboer de Visser, 1982a, 1982b).

The H-reflex equivalent of the JJ can be elicited by graded stimulation of the mandibular nerve (Godaux and Desmedt, 1975a) (Figure 11.4). Unlike the soleus H-reflex or the Achilles tendon reflex, where vibration of the muscle reduces the reflex EMG discharge, vibration of the jaw muscles facilitates the masseter reflex. This result suggests the absence of any reciprocal inhibitory connections to the jaw-closing muscles. This contrasts with the situation in the limbs where the vibratory stimulus spreads to antagonistic muscles and possibly even more distant muscles that have reciprocal inhibitory (presynaptic) influences on the excitatory afferent inputs to the agonist muscles. Such presynaptic inhibition could reduce the size of the EMG response in the agonist muscles (Godaux and Desmedt, 1975a).

SEVENTH CRANIAL NERVE

Anatomy

The cell bodies of the seventh motoneurons are located in the tegmentum of the pons just medial to the spinal tract of the fifth cranial nerve. Their motor axons loop around the nucleus of the sixth cranial nerve to exit through the ventrolateral aspect of the brainstem. From here the seventh cranial nerve crosses the angle between the pons and cerebellum and in company with the eighth cranial nerve enters the internal auditory meatus and thence the facial canal. Within the facial canal, the nerve occupies about 20 to 50 percent of the lumen.

The nerve innervates all the facial muscles as well as the platysma, posterior digastric, stapedius, and stylohyoid muscles. There are about 7,000 motor axons in the seventh nerve and those comprise about 60 percent of the total nerve fiber population in that nerve (VanBuskirk, 1945; Kullman, Dijck, and Cody, 1971).

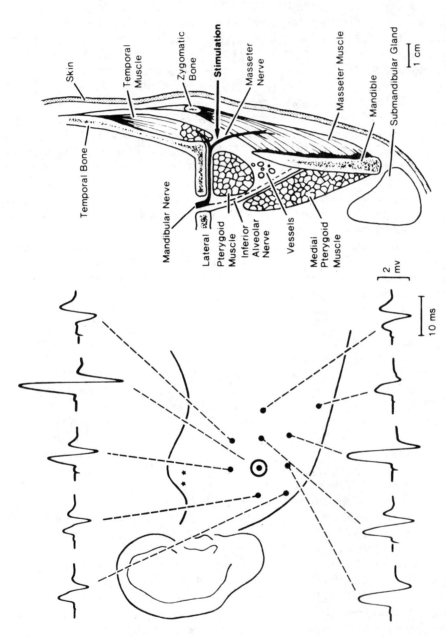

FIGURE 11.2.   (Left) Various shapes and sizes of surface-recorded potentials over the masseter muscle (reference electrode, the neck) elicited in response to single supramaximal shocks delivered to the masseter nerve. The motor point of the masseter is indicated by the circled dot.

Frontal section shows the anatomical relationship of the mandibular nerve in relation to the zygomatic bone. Electrical stimulation of ths nerve may be used to study the H-reflex in the masseter muscle.

From Godaux and Desmedt: Human masseter muscle: H and tendon reflexes. Arch Neurol 1975;32:229–234. Figure 1. Copyright 1962–75–75, American Medical Association.

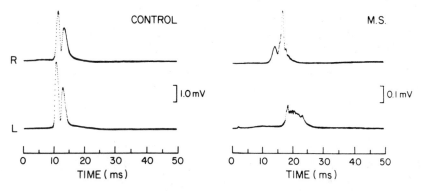

FIGURE 11.3. EMG discharges as recorded in both the right (R) and (L) masseter muscles by standard concentric needle electrodes. The potentials were full-wave rectified and averaged. Recordings from a healthy subject are shown on the left and from a patient with multiple sclerosis on the right. Note the obviously prolonged latency (normal 8.7 + 1.0 ms; 1 SD) in the subject with MS.
From Yates and Brown (1981a, figure 3).

Facial Muscles

There are in the human, about 7,000 to 10,500 motoneurons in the seventh nerve nucleus. Facial motor units on the average have very small innervation ratios (about 25 muscle fibers, or MFs, per motoneuron in the platysma) (Feinstein, Lindegård, Nyman, and Wohlfart, 1954). Whether the innervation ratios in other facial muscles are similar is unknown. The durations of motor unit potentials (MUPs) in the facial muscles are short in comparison to those in limb muscles (Jasper and Ballem, 1949; Petersen and Kugelberg, 1949; Buchthal and Rosenfalck, 1955; Buchthal, 1965). The shorter durations and to some extent lower amplitudes are probably explicable by the low innervation ratios of facial muscles. In addition, however, facial muscles are so thin that the concentric needle electrode may act more as a bipolar electrode because the area of the cannula contacting the muscle would be much less than in thicker muscles elsewhere. The effect would be to reduce the durations of MUPs as well as their amplitudes.

The contraction times of facial muscles are short. Type II (fast) motor units (MUs) predominate, at least in the cat (Lindquist and Mårtennson, 1970; Edström and Lindquist, 1973; Lindquist, 1973a, 1973b) (Table 11.1).

Facial motoneurons differ from spinal motoneurons in that there is no recurrent inhibition because Renshaw cells do not exist. Little is known presently about the nature of peripheral feedback and the importance of muscle and cutaneous afferents in adjusting the activities of facial motoneurons.

In some facial muscles there are clear func-

TABLE 11.1. Contraction Times and Percentages of Type II (Myofibrillar ATPase) Muscle Fibers in Cat Facial Muscles

Muscle	Contraction Time (ms)	Percentage of Type II Muscle Fibers
Orbicularis oculi	8.5	90
Orbicularis oris	33.0	85
Depressor conchae	25.0	70

From Lindquist (1973a, 1973b).

FIGURE 11.4. (Top) Normal H-reflex in the masseter muscle of a 22-year-old man. Shown are belly tendon recordings of the electrical potentials from the masseter muscle in response to increasingly intense stimulation of the masseter nerve beginning at the lowest intensity in (A) and increasing to supramaximal levels by (F). Note the typical H-reflex characteristics in both the direct recordings and the plotted sizes of the direct and late (H-reflex) potentials. Amplitude is shown in millivolts.

(Bottom) Size in mV of the H (*dots*) and M (*circles*) potentials as a function of the relative intensity of the stimulus delivered to the masseter nerve. The value 1.0 represents the stimulus intensity eliciting a maximum M-potential one-half of its maximum value. The symbols represent mean values of 10 successively recorded responses.

From Godaux and Desmedt. Human masseter muscle: H and tendon reflexes. Arch Neurol 1975; 32:229–234. Copyright 1962–75–75, American Medical Association.

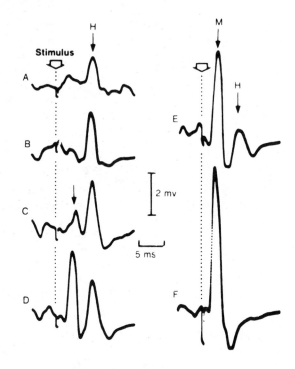

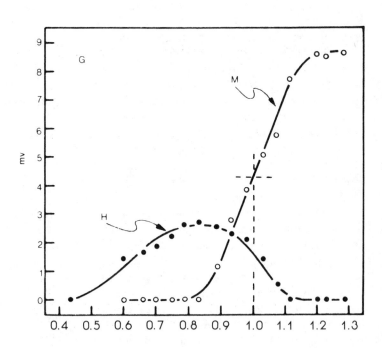

tional subdivisions. For example, in the orbicularis oculi, three main subdivisions exist; there being orbital, pretarsal, and preseptal subdivisions of the palpebral division of this muscle (Gordon, 1951; Hoyt and Loeffler, 1965). The orbicularis oculi MUs participating in the spontaneous and stimulus-evoked blinks are primarily pretarsal and epitarsal. These MUs fire at high frequencies (over 40 Hz). Motor units participating in voluntary eye closure (sustained closure) are primarily orbital and do not, as a rule, participate in spontaneous blinks. A third group of MUs is more intermediate in their physiological characteristics between the previous two groups. They are recruited with more difficulty than the orbital MU voluntary eye closures, but are activated in spontaneous blinks (Gordon, 1951).

The maximum conduction velocities of facial motor axons in the cat range between 25 and 75 m/s (Kitai, Tanaka, Tsukahara, and Yu, 1972). In man, the maximum velocity is reported to be 46 ± 3 m/s (Willer and Lamore, 1977), but the lower limit of motor conduction velocities in the seventh nerve in man is not known.

Stretch Receptors in Facial Muscles

The nature of the stretch receptors and of proprioceptive feedback from the facial muscles is an area of controversy at the present time. In other muscles there are spindle receptors to signal changes in the length and the rate of change of length in muscles. Their afferent inputs serve to adjust the output of their respective motoneurons in response to anticipated and unanticipated changes in length.

Facial muscles are unique, however, in that there are no unexpected changes in the loads imposed on them or their lengths, unlike most other muscles in the body. Because of this there may be no real need for sensory feedback from the facial muscles. Facial movements may be entirely preprogrammed in the central nervous system. Alternatively, some type of peripheral feedback may be necessary, but perhaps other peripheral receptors, for example cutaneous mechanoreceptors, are able to serve the equivalent proprioceptive role of muscle stretch receptors for these muscles.

Although muscle spindles have been seen in the platysma, stylohyoid, and stapedius muscles and at least in some of the mimetic muscles (Kadanoff, 1956; Cooper, 1960; Matthews, 1972), no definite spindles or Golgi tendon organs have been seen in the orbicularis oculi. This muscle is thin and large, however, and possibly spindles and spindlelike structures may have been missed in the search.

Available physiological evidence provides no direct support for the presence of muscle spindles in the orbicularis oculi muscle. For example:

1. Stretching or tapping the orbicularis oculi when this muscle has been freed of its overlying skin evokes no reflex contraction, as it should if there were stretch receptors in the muscle. Such experiments presuppose careful preservation of the nerve supply of the muscle including the motor innervation from the seventh cranial nerve and possible afferents originating in the orbicularis oculi muscle but traveling in various branches of the trigeminal nerve. In the same experiments, stimulation of the skin regularly elicited contractions in the orbicularis oculi (see Lindquist and Mårtennson, 1970; Shahani and Young, 1973).

2. Nerve fiber discharges could not be detected in filaments of either the fifth or seventh nerves when the orbicularis oculi muscle was stretched or after intravenous succinylcholine was administered (a drug known to excite spindle receptors; Granit, Skoglund, and Thesleff, 1953). On the

other hand, tapping the overlying skin evoked large discharges in the fifth nerve afferents (Lindquist and Mårtennson, 1970).

3. In the human at least, no true silent period exists in the blink reflex. The thresholds for the early (R1) and late (R2) reflexes are similar (Figure 11.5) and the conduction velocities of fifth nerve afferents mediating the R1 and R2 are in the range of the cutaneous afferents (Shahani and Young, 1973).

4. Fluctuations in the latencies of some individual MUPs in the R1 exceed the value of MUPs in known H-reflexes elsewhere (Trontelj, 1968). In some cases, however, the latency fluctuations in R1 MUPs are much lower (0.4 to 2.5 ms) and of an order that suggests a possible monosynaptic reflex for some of the MUP components in the R1 (Brown and Rushworth, 1973).

Minimal fluctuations in the latencies of reflex discharges of single MUPs do not by themselves establish the central connections as monosynaptic, and even less that the afferents involved are necessarily spindle afferents. Such minimal latency fluctuations do, however, suggest that the central synaptic connections involve no more than, at the most, two synapses.

5. In the cat, the central delay for the R1 is too long for a single synapse only. The same central delay in man is only 1.5 ms (Bynke, 1971), and therefore must in-

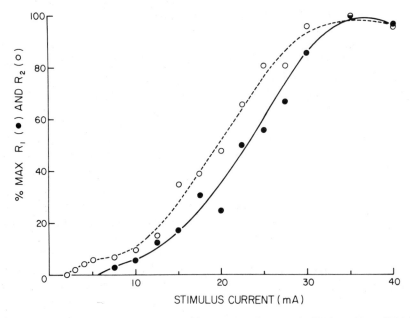

FIGURE 11.5.   Comparative growth in the size of the early (R1) and late (R2) blink reflexes in the orbicularis oculi muscle in response to percutaneous stimulation of the supraorbital nerve in a healthy subject. Note that in this subject it was the R2 response that had the lowest threshold (about one-half that of the R1). The growth of the two responses, however, was basically similar. The R1 and R2 reached their maximum values at stimulus intensities 15 to 5 times their respective threshold intensities.

volve only one or at the most two synapses. Such short central delays do not themselves establish the R1 as monosynaptic and therefore equivalent to the H-reflex in the lower limb, but suggest only that the synaptic linkages for whatever afferents are involved are tight.

The above evidence bearing on the question of spindles in the orbicularis oculi muscle is all indirect. It suggests that if there are muscle spindles, these are few in number and possibly their functions are met by other afferents, such as cutaneous mechanoreceptors, that could transmit their proprioceptive messages to the CNS by the fifth cranial nerve.

Other Afferents to the Seventh Motor Nucleus

In addition to skeletomotor efferents, the seventh nerve contains visceral efferents and afferents, most of the latter of which are gustatory in origin. There are also some somatic afferents originating in the external ear canal or behind the ear (Foley and DuBois, 1943; Brodal, 1981). Because of the importance of the blink reflexes (BR) to EMG, it is important to examine the nature of the afferents mediating the blink responses in the orbicularis oculi muscle.

There are high-threshold afferents, possibly equivalent to the small-diameter (1 to 6 μ) nerve fibers reported by Bruesch (1944) in the seventh nerve that when excited, evoke a late response in the orbicularis oculi muscle. The latency of the response exceeds by 5 ms or more the late blink response (R2) to stimulation of the supraorbital nerve (Lindquist and Mårtennson, 1970).

Lower-threshold and faster-conducting afferents are also present in the seventh nerve that are disynaptically or multisynaptically linked to seventh motoneurons. These, while present in the peripheral portions of the sev-

enth nerve, are transmitted to the brainstem by way of the fifth cranial nerve through peripheral interconnections between seventh and fifth nerves. Stimulation of the central cut ends of such transected peripheral branches of the seventh nerve has been shown monosynaptically to excite trigeminal spinal sensory neurons. These same afferents originating from the seventh nerve have rapid conduction velocities and are connected through one or more interneurons to seventh motoneurons in the brainstem (Kitai, Tanaka, Tsukahara, and Yu, 1972; Iwata, Kitai, and Olson, 1972). Van-Hasselt (1976) has shown in the cat that stimulation of peripheral branches of the seventh nerve elicited reflex discharges in the orbicularis oculi whose latencies were much shorter than the R2 response (10 to 13 ms vs 25 ms for the R2). These earlier-occurring reflex discharges had some H-reflex characteristics and were abolished by section of the third division of the trigeminal nerve. The last suggested that the transfer of the afferents in the seventh nerve was to the third division of the trigeminal nerve.

In man, Willer and Lamore (1977) have shown that there are afferents in the seventh nerve whose conduction velocities (51 ± 2 m/s) exceed the maximum conduction velocities of motor fibers in the same nerve (46 ± 3 m/s). Both these compare with the slightly slower conducting afferents in the supraorbital nerve (33 to 34 m/s) mediating the R1 (Shahani, 1970). In Willer and Lamore's study (1977), stimulation of the seventh nerve in the periphery elicited reflex discharges in the orbicularis oculi whose latencies (25 to 38 ms) just exceeded the R2 response to stimulation of the supraorbital nerve (20 to 33 ms), both being enhanced by attention.

It is not known whether reflex discharges in the orbicularis oculi evoked by stimuli delivered to the peripheral branches of the seventh nerve in man are mediated by afferents that cross to the trigeminal nerve prior to entering the base of the skull in a manner similar to that seen in the cat (Iwata, Kitai, and Olson, 1972).

In summary, there are small-diameter somatic afferents in the seventh nerve, some of which apparently end on blood vessels (Bruesch, 1944). The electrical thresholds of these fibers are high and they could possibly mediate some of the long-latency reflexes seen in the cat and man. Also, there is support for the presence of other larger-diameter and faster-conducting afferents in the seventh nerve whose peripheral sites of origin (skin or muscle) and the locations of whose cell bodies are unknown. Some or all of these afferents may pass by way of connecting branches to the fifth nerve prior to reaching the brainstem and their synaptic connection to trigeminal neruons. Such afferents could mediate reflex discharges in the facial muscles in response to electrical stimulation of peripheral branches of the seventh nerve, and they deserve to be investigated further.

Presynaptic Input to Seventh Motoneurons

There are direct cortico-motoneuronal projections from the motor cortex to seventh nerve motoneurons on the opposite side (Kuypers, 1958). There are also bilateral cortico-motoneuronal projections to facial motoneurons supplying the muscles about and above the eye. Other projections to the seventh nerve nucleus originate in the red nucleus, mesencephalic reticular formation, superior colliculus, superior olive, the trigeminal sensory nuclei, both the main and spinal divisions, the nucleus of the solitary tract, and even the spinal cord.

Blink Reflex

The orbicularis oculi muscle contracts and the subject blinks in response to a variety of stimuli, including touching the cornea, electrically stimulating the supraorbital nerve (or other trigeminal sensory branches), light and sound (Figure 11.6). This is not unexpected in view of the known input connections to the facial motor nucleus and the probable protective nature of this reflex. The latencies of these reflex blink responses vary depending on the type and site of the stimulus, and all except the earliest (R1) blink response to electrical stimulation of the supraorbital nerve (SO-BR) demonstrate so-called habituation (Rimpel, Geyer, and Hopf, 1982). This is a progressive reduction in the size of the reflex response to repeated stimulation, which is again not unexpected in view of the multisynaptic connections mediating these reflexes (except for the R1 a bisynaptic or possibly monosynaptic reflex) (Figure 11.7). Reductions in habituation in patients with Huntington's chorea have been reported (Ferguson, Lenman, and Johnston, 1978), but this probably has little clinical diagnostic value.

The central connections mediating the BR are not all known at this time. In the case of the various trigeminal BRs, much more is known because of the development of extensive correlative electrophysiological and neuropathological evidence.

The *trigeminal stimulus-evoked blink reflex* (T-BR) and *light stimulus-evoked blink reflexes* (L-BR) are valuable tools for the localization of lesions in the related peripheral and central connections. The *auditory stimulus-evoked blink reflex* (A-BR) is much less valuable because it often requires click stimuli that exceed 100 db; even so, it is often absent in healthy subjects. The latency of the S-BR is between 23 and 30 ms (Rushworth, 1962, 1966; Yates and Brown, 1981b; Säring and VonCramon, 1981).

Trigeminal Facial Reflex

Blink reflexes may be evoked by mechanical stimuli such as tapping the skin lightly about the eyes or touching the cornea, or by electrical stimulation of trigeminal cutaneous nerves such as the supraorbital nerve (Figure

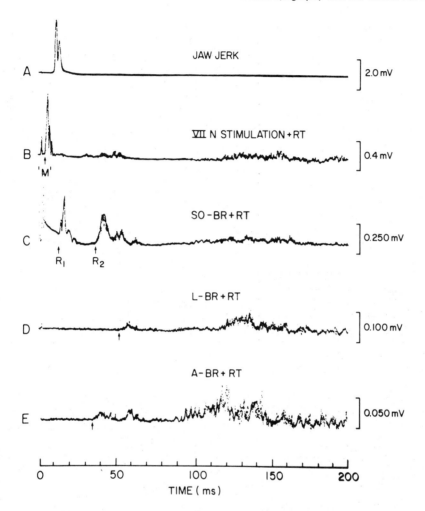

FIGURE 11.6.   Illustration in a healthy subject of the comparative latencies of:

(A) The jaw jerk as recorded in the masseter muscle.

(B) The direct M-response and late responses in the orbicularis oculi (O. Ocu) evoked in response to percutaneous stimulation of the seventh cranial nerve just below the ear. As in (C), (D), and (E), the subject was instructed to close the eye as soon as possible following the stimulus (reaction time = RT).

(C) The supraorbital nerve stimulus-evoked blink reflex (SO-BR) in the O. Ocu showing the early (R1) and late (R2) blink reflexes.

(D) The light stimulus-evoked blink reflex (L-BR) in the O. Ocu.

(E) The auditory click-elicited blink reflex (A-BR) response in the O. Ocu muscle.

All EMG recordings were full-wave rectified and electronically averaged.

Note the shorter latency of the A-BR (just over 30 ms) compared to the L-BR (just over 50 ms) and the correspondingly longer RT for the L-BR.

FIGURE 11.7. Presumed central connections sub-
serving the trigeminal stimulus (corneal touch or supraorbital nerve stimulus) evoked blink reflexes in
the orbicularis oculi. In the case of the corneal blink
reflex (C-BR), there is no early blink reflex equivalent to the early (R1) blink reflex response to supraorbital nerve stimulation. Hence the corneal reflex does not apparently utilize the more direct
central pathway from trigeminal main sensory nucleus to facial nucleus (at least one interposed interneuron) and blocking of impulses in the spinal
trigeminal tract or complex could delay the blink
reflexes on both sides (afferent delay). Blocking
crossing impulses near the midline would likely
abolish blink responses contralateral to the side of
stimulation, but would not alter the ipsilateral blink
responses.
Abbreviations: V N. = trigeminal nerve; Vm =
trigeminal motor nucleus; Vp = trigeminal principle
sensory nucleus; sp V tr = spinal trigeminal tract; sp
V co = spinal trigeminal complex; VI = abducens
nucleus; VII = facial nucleus; VII N. = facial nerve;

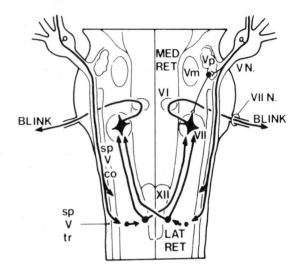

XII = hypoglossal nucleus; MED RET = medial reticular formation; and LAT RET = lateral reticular
formation.
From Ongerboer de Visser (1981a, figure 7).

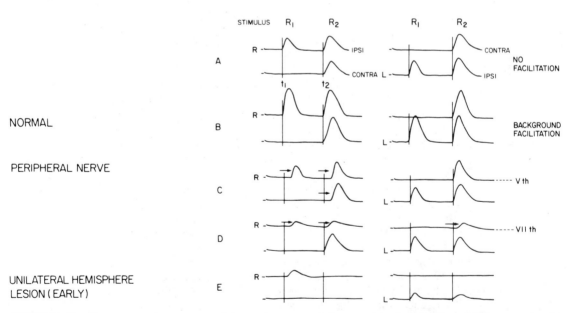

FIGURE 11.8. Diagrammatic summary of the major types of abnormalities in the supraorbital nerve stimulus
evoked blink reflexes (SO-BR) produced through lesions in the central and peripheral nervous systems. The
early (R1) and late (R2) blink reflexes in the orbicularis oculi muscles ipsilateral and contralateral to the side
of stimulation (indicated by the R or L) are shown. The t1 and t2 denote upper limits of normal for latencies
of R1 and R2 respectively.

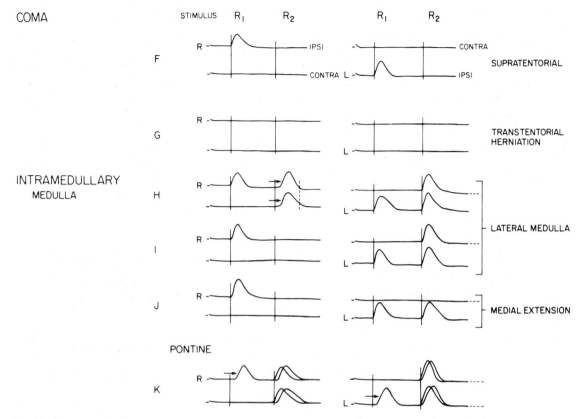

FIGURE 11.8. *(continued)*

(A) and (B) SO-BR in a normal subject. (A) An early (R1) and late (R2) blink response is present in the orbicularis oculi ipsilateral to the stimulus, and a late (R2) response is seen contralateral to the side of the supraorbital nerve stimulated. The latter stimulus is shown delivered on the right (left column) and left (right column) sides. (B) An enhancing effect on the size of the EMG discharge occurs upon instructing the subject to make a weak steady contraction of the orbicularis oculi muscles.

(C) and (D) Delays *(arrows)* in the SO-BR as caused by R fifth nerve (afferent) lesion in (C) and a right seventh (efferent) lesion (see text).

(E) Here is demonstrated the effect sometimes seen on the SO-BR of a lesion in the unilateral hemisphere, here considered to be on the left side. Note preservation of R1 but abolition of the contralateral R2 on both sides and ipsilateral R2 on the side contralateral to the lesion.

(F) and (G) The effects sometimes seen of supratentorial lesions (F) and transtentorial herniation (G) on the SO-BR. Note abolition of both R1 and R2 reflexes in the case of transtentorial herniation and the absence (common) of all R2 reflexes, both ipsilateral and contralateral to the stimulus and to the lesion in some supratentorial lesions.

(H), (I), (J) The variety of alterations in R1 and R2 with respect to lesions of the medulla affecting the lateral medulla—(H) and (I). The R2 reflexes ipsilateral and contralateral, in this case, to a right lateral medullary lesion were delayed or abolished when the attempt was made to elicit them by a stimulus on the affected side, both R1 and R2 reflexes being normal when stimulation was carried out on the normal (left) side.

(J) The lesion extended medially in the medulla and in so doing abolished the R2 both ipsilateral and contralateral to the lesion as well as the R2 contralateral to stimulation on the unaffected side.

(K) In pontine lesions the R1 may be abolished or delayed. The R2 reflex both ipsilateral and contralateral to the lesion may also be delayed or in other cases remain unaffected.

11.8 A, B). These stimuli, except for the corneal stimulus, evoke two EMG discharges; early (R1) and late (R2) responses. The R2 is seen on both sides but the R1 only on the side ipsilateral to the stimulus. Although evoked with the lowest threshold by taps about the eye and in particular over the orbicularis oculi muscle, stronger taps delivered to widely separate facial regions will also evoke BRs (Kugelberg, 1952).

The latencies of R1 and R2 produced by electrical stimulation of the supraorbital nerve are listed in Table 11.2. They are about 1 to 3 ms shorter than the corresponding responses evoked by tapping the skin because the latter must be mediated through direct excitation of the receptors and the more asynchronous nature of the afferent volley.

The two main BR components, early R1 and later R2, have distinctive physiological characteristics (Table 11.3). The R2 usually lasts longer and has a higher amplitude than the R1 because larger numbers of MUPs contribute to the R2. Frequently, individual MUPs discharge two or three times in the course of the R2. Cutaneous afferents are probably the dominant afferents mediating the R1 and R2 responses, although—at least in the cat—deep, possibly muscle afferents may contribute to the afferent volley (Lindquist and Mårtennson, 1970).

Figure 11.7 illustrates that for the R1, there is one interneuron interposed between the primary trigeminal sensory inputs and the seventh nerve motoneurons on the same side only. In the case of the R2, there are two and possibly more interneurons interposed between the sensory inputs and the seventh motoneurons, here on both sides. For the R2, collaterals of *primary trigeminal afferents* to the main sensory nucleus descend in the *descending tract of the trigeminal nerve* in the medulla and make connections to the *descending nucleus of the trigeminal nerve,* and these neurons in turn connect to neurons in the *lateral reticular formation* of the brainstem. The latter, through ascending projections, connect to seventh motoneurons on the same side or cross at the lower medulla before ascending to project to the opposite seventh motor nucleus (Ongerboer de Visser and Kuypers, 1978).

The SO-BRs are especially valuable because they are relatively easy to elicit and thus provide a ready means of assessing the integrity of the pons and medulla. Their latencies are also affected by rostral lesions, disorders affecting consciousness, and the presence of certain drugs. Figure 11.8 illustrates patterns of abnormalities in the SO-BRs seen with lesions at various levels of the neuraxis as well as in the presence of peripheral lesions affecting the trigeminal and facial nerves.

Unilateral Trigeminal Nerve

In unilateral lesions affecting the trigeminal nerve (Figure 11.8C), latencies of the ipsilateral R1 and R2 as well as the contralateral R2 BR are increased because these share the same afferents. Conduction through these afferents may be slowed or blocked by the lesions. The BRs all have normal latencies when the stimulus is applied to the opposite side because afferent conduction on this side is normal and efferent conduction is normal on both sides.

TABLE 11.2. Latencies of the Early (R1) and Late (R2) Blink Reflex Responses to Supraorbital Nerve Stimulation ($\pm$ 1 SD)

Side of Stimulation		R1 (ms)	R2 (ms)
R	Ipsilateral	9.8 ± 0.7	30.1 ± 3.6
	Contralateral	—	31.0 ± 3.9
L	Ipsilateral	9.8 ± 0.7	30.2 ± 3.3
	Contralateral	—	31.6 ± 4.4

TABLE 11.3.   Characteristics of the Early (R1) and Late (R2) Blink Reflex Responses to Electrical Stimulation of the Supraorbital Nerve

	R1	R2
Peripheral receptors and afferents	Probably cutaneous mechanoreceptors belonging to fifth cranial nerve, CVs 30–40 m/s ± muscle receptors of facial muscles	Same
	Present ipsilaterally only	Present both sides
Latency variations, single MUPs	Some 0.4–2.5 ms, others >2.5 ms	Characteristically >2.5 ms
Repetitive MUP discharges	Not common	Common
Least central delay	1.5 ms	
Central connections	Probably at least one interneuron (pontine); possibly some monosynpatic connections	2 or more interneurons in the medulla
Threshold	Similar to R2; lowest for mechanical stimulation over O. oculi and electrical stimulation of supraorbital nerve	Same; characteristically diminished by stress, calculation, random stimuli
Habituation	Less than R2	
Effect of background contraction of O. oculi	Enhances	Enhances

Unilateral Seventh Cranial Nerve

The R1 and R2 latencies are increased or the responses absent ipsilateral to the lesion because conduction is blocked, slowed, or absent in the involved seventh nerve (Figure 11.8D). The opposite R2 response would be normal, however, because both the ipsilateral afferent input and contralateral efferent pathways are intact (Boongird and Vejjajiva, 1978).

Stimulation of the supraorbital nerve on the normal side would evoke normal R1 and R2 responses on that side, but the R2 response on the opposite side, which is mediated through the abnormal seventh nerve, could be expected to be delayed or absent. Needle electrode recordings from the affected facial muscles may also reveal evidence of denervation and reduced recruitment, depending on the nature of the lesion.

The above pattern is seen in the acute traumatic and nontraumatic facial palsies. In the case of the latter, Schenck and Manz (1973) have claimed that the clinical outcome is better where the R1 persists or returns early, or when its latency on the affected side does not exceed the latency on the nonaffected side by more than 6 ms.

Combined Trigeminal and Seventh Nerve Lesions

Commonly, tumors in the cerebellopontine angle involve both the fifth and seventh cranial nerves (Eisen and Danon, 1974; Rossi, Buonaguidi, Muratorio, and Tusini, 1979). This is true also in the peripheral neuropathies such as Charcot-Marie-Tooth and Guillain-Barré neuropathies, where the involvement is also bilateral and all the latencies of the SO-BRs may be prolonged.

LESIONS IN THE BRAINSTEM

Mesencephalic Lesions

There are no changes in the R1 or R2 with mesencephalic lesions (Tokunaga, Oka, Murao, Yokoi, Okumura, Hirata, Miyashita, and Yoshitatsu, 1958); however, the JJ on the ipsilateral side may be lost (see earlier section).

Pons

Unilateral lesions involving the mid to lower pons (Figure 11.8K) may abolish or increase the latency of the R1 on the same side, the latency of the R2 on the same side, and the R2 on the opposite side. The SO-BRs evoked by stimulation on the normal side should be normal, including the R2 on the involved side, unless the lesion extends to involve seventh motoneurons or their axons in the lower pons (Kimura, 1970).

Medulla

In the medulla (Figure 11.8H, I, J), the patterns of the abnormalities depend on whether the lesion involves the lateral or medial medulla (Kimura and Lyon, 1972; Ongerboer de Visser and Kuypers, 1978; Ongerboer de Visser and Moffie, 1979).

When the lesion involves the lateral medulla, the ipsilateral and contralateral R2 responses may be absent or their latencies prolonged because the descending connections (descending tract of the trigeminal nerve) of the fifth nerve are involved. The SO-BRs in response to stimulation on the normal side would be normal, however, including the R2 ipsilateral and contralateral to the stimulus, because the para-midline ascending crossed connections to the seventh nucleus are intact. Where the lesion involves the medial medulla and hence the crossed ascending connections to the seventh nuclei (Figure 11.11), not only are the ipsilateral and contralateral R2 responses elicited on the side of the lesion absent or their latencies prolonged, but the R2 on the affected side evoked by stimulation on the normal side may be absent or its latency prolonged.

Cerebral Hemisphere: Unilateral Lesions

There are very important supranuclear projections to the fifth and seventh neurons, some originating in the cerebral cortex and other suprabrainstem structures (Figure 11.8E). These can alter the excitabilities of fifth and seventh neurons as well as their related interneurons within the brainstem. In acute hemispheric lesions, the R1 latencies elicited contralateral to the lesion may be increased only to return to normal with time. The R2 responses also may be lost in the unilateral hemispheric lesions. These observations emphasize both the importance of these hemispheric projections of the brainstem neurons mediating the BR, and the point that the SO-BRs may be abolished or their latencies increased in the absence of intrinsic brainstem lesions (Oliver, 1952; Ross, 1972; Fisher, Shahani, and Young, 1979; Ongerboer de Visser and Moffie, 1979). Lesions involving the lower postcentral region (Ongerboer de Visser, 1981a) are also associated with abnormalities in the *corneal blink reflex* (C-BR).

Disorders of Consciousness

The R1 and R2, especially R1, may be lost or hard to obtain in stages III and IV of normal sleep (Ferrari and Messina, 1972). In coma secondary to supratentorial structural diseases, the R2 responses are commonly absent (Figure 11.8F, G) (Lyon, Kimura, and McCormick, 1972; Serrats, Parker, and Merino-Cañas, 1976; Buonaguidi, Rossi, Sartucci, and Ravelli, 1979). The R1 is usually lost only with transtentorial progression and subsequent direct involvement of the brainstem.

Both the R1 and R2 may also be lost in metabolic encephalopathies and in barbiturate and glutethimide intoxications. Thus the SO-BRs cannot be used to distinguish between structural and metabolic causes of coma. Both the R1 and R2 may also be absent in awake subjects who are taking diazepam.

The preceding examples demonstrate the value and some of the limitations of the trigeminal-facial reflex in clinical neurology. Both the SO-BR and L-BR are valuable ways of testing the integrity of their related peripheral and central connections, and possibly localizing lesions within this system. These tests are not, however, very valuable for recognizing or localizing tumors or vascular lesions within the brainstem. For the latter, computed tomography, nuclear magnetic resonance, or posterior fossa myelography is a better procedure. The main value of SO-BRs at the present includes:

1. Detecting lesions not evident in clinical or computed tomographic studies of patients with multiple sclerosis. With the advent of nuclear magnetic scanning techniques, these and other electrophysiological procedures may turn out to be less valuable.

2. Localizing lesions of the fifth and seventh peripheral nerves.

CORNEAL BLINK REFLEX

Testing the reflex blink response to touch stimulation of the cornea is part of the general neurological examination. Its electrophysiology is therefore of special interest to clinical neurologists (Ongerboer de Visser, 1980, 1981a, 1981b, 1982b).

The receptors in the cornea are free nerve endings and their afferents in the long ciliary nerve are all small myelinated and unmyelinated nerve fibers (Lele and Weddell, 1959). In other sensory branches of the trigeminal nerve, however, such as the supraorbital nerve, contain larger myelinated nerve fibers and these, no doubt, mediate both the R1 and R2 responses to electrical stimulation of the respective nerves or mechanical taps delivered to the skin in the trigeminal territory. Whatever the differences between the afferents responsible for the SO-BR late response (R2) and the C-BR, the medullary brainstem pathways mediating the two are probably very similar. Hence lesions within the medulla and pons affecting, for example, the R2 responses to electrical stimulation of the supraorbital nerve are likely to affect the C-BR responses in a similar way (Ongerboer de Visser and Moffie, 1979; Ongerboer de Visser, 1980). Whether this conclusion is justified all the time remains to be tested.

The C-BR may be impaired in lesions affecting the cerebral hemisphere, particularly those lesions involving the lower postcentral region (Figure 11.9). Abnormalities include

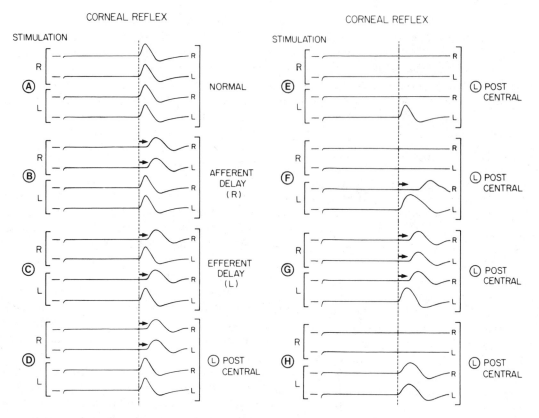

FIGURE 11.9.   Diagrammatic representation of the types of abnormalities in the corneal stimulus-evoked blink reflexes (C-BR) to be seen in various peripheral and central lesions.

(A) Normal blink EMG responses in both the ipsilateral and contralateral orbicularis oculi muscles in response to touching the cornea. The side of corneal stimulation and sides of recording are indicated on the left and right respectively.

(B) In lesions affecting the trigeminal nerve, both ipsilateral and contralateral C-BRs are delayed when the cornea is stimulated on the affected side, but are normal when the normal side is stimulated.

(C) In the case of lesions affecting the seventh nerve, the C-BR responses mediated through the abnormal efferent path are delayed irrespective of the side of stimulus, whereas those mediated by the normal seventh nerve are normal.

In (D), (E), (F), (G), and (H) are shown the various types of abnormalities in the C-BR in lesions of the postcentral region. Commonly, the C-BRs as elicited on the side opposite the lesion are delayed or absent contralateral to the lesion, whereas those elicited by corneal stimulation on the same side of the lesion may be normal, delayed, or absent contralateral to the lesion and normal on the same side.

Summary based on studies of Ongerboer de Visser (1981a, 1981b).

absent or delayed C-BRs evoked by corneal stimulation on the side opposite to the cerebral lesion, as well as absence or delay of the consensual C-BR to corneal stimulation on the side of the lesion. In every case, the direct C-BR to ipsilateral corneal stimulation is normal (Ongerboer de Visser, 1981a, 1981b, 1982b).

Because the latencies of the C-BR may vary

widely among individuals (35 to 65 ms), little importance can be attached to differences in them from one person to another. There should, however, be no more than a 10-ms difference between the direct and consensual C-BRs evoked by stimulation on the two sides.

Light Stimulus-evoked Blink Reflex

Brief intense light stimuli delivered to both eyes together or one eye alone evokes EMG discharges in the orbicularis oculi muscles on both sides (Figures 11.7, 11.10, and 11.11). The latencies depend somewhat on the intensity of the light stimulus at the source and, related to this, the distance between the light source and the eye. We have used a stroboscopic light source (Grass P.S. 22 photostimulator) with which the least latencies of the L-BR were 51 ± 4.0 ms (1 SD) (Figure 11.14). The L-BR habituates, and to reduce the effect of this as much as possible, the stimuli must be delivered randomly and at inter-

stimulus periods of at least 5 seconds. The subjects should be dark-adapted as well.

When tested for in the above manner, the L-BR is present in almost all control subjects under 60 years of age but may more often be absent occasionally in apparently healthy older persons. When absent or hard to obtain at rest, it can sometimes be brought out by weak background contraction of the orbicularis oculi muscle. Prior instruction to subjects to blink briskly as soon as they see the flash will also bring out a *reaction time* response whose latency (84.0 ± 6.5 ms) is invariably prolonged, where the L-BR latency is prolonged or the L-BR is absent in lesions involving the brainstem or optic nerves.

That the L-BR does not depend on the integrity of the occipital regions is suggested by its persistance in one case examined here, where both occipital lobes were infarcted and the patient was cortically blind. The pathways mediating the L-BR within the brainstem unfortunately, however, remain unknown at the present time.

FIGURE 11.10. Method for eliciting the light stimulus-evoked blink reflex. The EMG response in the orbicularis oculi muscle may be recorded by surface or intramuscular electrodes (the latter here). The light stimulus is delivered by a stroboscopic light source positioned about 200 mm in front of the subject. Stimuli are delivered randomly (least interval 2 seconds) to avoid habituation as much as possible. Monocular stimulation is obtained through covering one eye. The pathway (interrupted line in brainstem) central to the lateral geniculate body is not known, but probably does not involve the occipital cortex, since the reflex is preserved in occipital lesions.

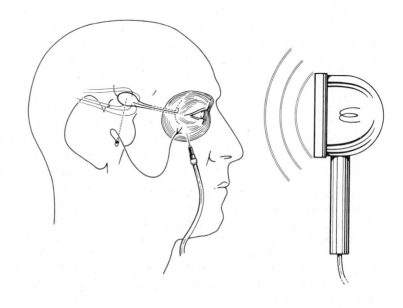

In multiple sclerosis, the L-BR and corresponding reaction times are often prolonged (Lowitzsch, Kuhnt, Sakmann, Maurer, Hopf, Schott, and Thater, 1976) and the L-BR itself may be absent (Yates and Brown, 1981b). Prolonged latencies or absence of the L-BR in response to monocular stimulation provides a good indication of the presence of a unilateral optic nerve lesion in MS (Figure 11.11). Both correlate nicely with other indications of monocular optic nerve involvement such as the presence of a central scotoma and monocular abnormalities of the pattern visual evoked response. Sometimes the occurrence and latency of the L-BR are dependent on the temperature of the subject in multiple sclerosis (Figure 11.12).

FUNCTIONAL ABNORMALITIES OF SEVENTH MOTONEURONS AND AXONS

Functional abnormalities of seventh motoneurons may occur in disorders of the upper mo-

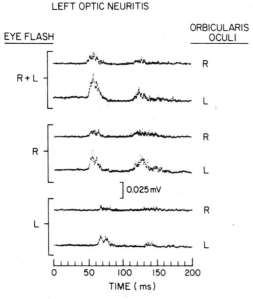

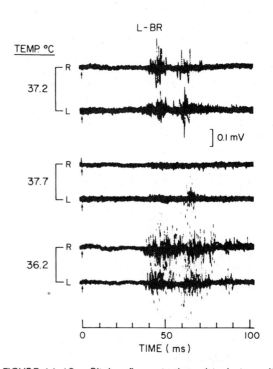

FIGURE 11.11.   Patient with recent left optic neuritis. Light stimulus-evoked blink reflex as recorded in the right (R) and left (L) orbicularis oculi muscles in response to stimulation of both eyes together (R + L) or either eye independently. The EMG recordings have been full-wave rectified and averaged. Note the delay in the early and late EMG discharges in response to light flashes delivered to the L eye alone compared to the normal latencies as elicited by R eye or R and L eye stimulation (top). The basis of the second discharge at about 100 to 110 ms is not known, but occurs even in the absence of any instruction to blink on receipt of the stimulus.

FIGURE 11.12.   Blink reflexes in the orbicularis oculi muscles elicited by light flashes (L-BR) delivered to both eyes. The recordings from the right and left orbicularis oculi muscles are shown in the top and bottom traces respectively of each pair of recordings at various temperatures. Note the almost complete absence of L-BR at 37.7°C, its return at 37.2°C, and the even larger response at 36.2°C. The absolute latencies of the L-BR in all recordings were in the normal range. This patient has multiple sclerosis and had noted reduction in his vision when in hot baths or in the course of exercise. The temperatures were oral recordings.

toneuron or basal ganglia. Also, lesions in the lower pons or upper medulla can directly destroy the nuclear and infranuclear structures of the seventh nerve and cause denervation and paralysis in the facial muscles, something that is common in tumors and vascular and other lesions in this region. Sometimes such involvement of the seventh nerve is not apparent clinically, but demonstrated only by needle electromyographic demonstration of fibrillation potentials and positive sharp waves in the facial muscles, such as may be seen sometimes in multiple sclerosis.

Acute Idiopathic Facial Nerve Palsy (Bell's Palsy)

Lesions such as idiopathic acute facial palsy (Bell's palsy) are common and produce a characteristic pattern of electrophysiological abnormalities. Because these have been studied in detail serially throughout the clinical course of the neuropathy, they are of special importance for the electromyographer (Olson, 1975; Esslen, 1977), not only for their own sake but because they serve as models for other acute focal nerve injuries in man.

Bell's palsy is an acute facial palsy the exact cause of which has not been established. Only in a minority is there a concomitant proved viral infection such as herpes zoster. In the remainder, direct evidence of a viral neuritis is usually never established, although there is some experimental support for a viral hypothesis in idiopathic acute facial palsy (Davis, 1981).

Surgical exposure of affected seventh nerve proximal to the facial canal in the acute phase of Bell's palsy usually reveals a swollen nerve in which the intraneural vessels are engorged and intraneural hemorrhages may be present. The nerve becomes constricted at the entrance to the facial canal. Beyond the canal entrance the nerve may abruptly fill and bulge out of the canal when an opening is made in

the bony roof over the canal (Figure 11.13). Compression of the swollen nerve within the facial canal and possibly ischemia are probably the most important causes of the functional and structural abnormalities in the nerve, although experimental evidence bearing on the relative importance of these two mechanisms is inconclusive (Devriese, 1974). The site at which the nerve enters the facial canal is the most constant site for conduction block (Esslen, 1977).

Early and later sequelae of this seventh nerve lesion are determined by:

1. The proportion of seventh nerve fibers that undergo degeneration distal to the site of compressive or ischemic injury
2. The extent to which the connective tissue framework of the nerve, especially the Schwann cell basement membranes, is destroyed
3. The proportion of nerve fibers whose impulses are blocked although their axons remain intact
4. The extent to which sites of ectopic impulse generation, ephaptic transmission, or abnormal regeneration patterns develop in the nerve

As with proximally situated lesions in the peripheral nervous system where the affected regions are, generally speaking, inaccessible to direct studies of conduction, so also here, conduction in the seventh nerve cannot be assessed directly within its intratemporal course. The level of the injury to the nerve can only be assessed indirectly by testing, for example, the functions of the various component branches such as lacrimation for the greater superficial petrosal nerve, the stapedius reflex for the motor nerve to stapedius, and taste for the chorda tympani branch provide this information (see Olson, 1975 for review).

To estimate the relative numbers of degenerated or blocked nerve fibers in the facial nerve, the maximum M-potentials of the fron-

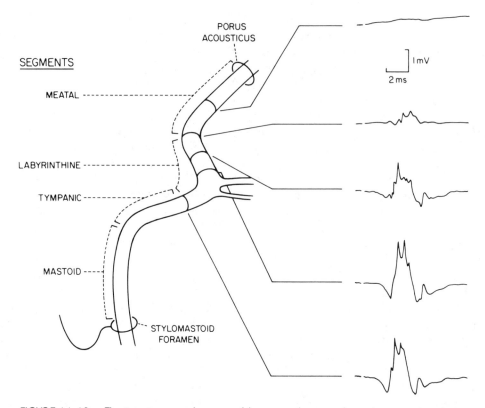

FIGURE 11.13.   The intratemporal course of the seventh nerve shows its successive major divisions—meatal segment, labyrinthine segment, horizontal (or tympanic) segment, and vertical (mastoid) segment—as well as the sites of stimulation of the nerve exposed operatively in the acute phase. Concentric needle electrodes were used to record the resultant maximum M-potentials in the perioral muscles. Representative recordings are shown on the right. In this case the major change in amplitude occurred between the midpoint of meatal segment (S1) and just proximal to the geniculate ganglion (S3). Overall, the most consistent localization of the conduction block was just distal to the entrance to the eustachian tube.
From Esslen (1977, figure 4) and reprinted with the permission of the publisher, Springer-Verlag.

talis, orbicularis oris, or triangularis muscles as recorded by surface electrodes in response to supramaximal stimulation of the seventh nerve distal to the stlomastoid foramen may be measured and compared to their respective values on the uninvolved side and known control values (Figure 11.14). The catch here is that it may take about three to five days for

facial nerve fibers distal to a transection to become inexcitable, as these fibers undergo degeneration (Gilliatt and Taylor, 1959; Gilliatt, Fowler, and Rudge, 1975). Following this period (allowing up to ten days for any continuing injury to the nerve to take place) the amplitude of the maximum M-potential on the abnormal side comes more truly to reflect the

FIGURE 11.14.   M-potentials as recorded with surface electrodes from the frontalis muscle and elicited by stimulation of the facial nerve. The contralateral midfrontalis electrode serves here as the reference electrode.

Note on day 1 of an acute idiopathic facial palsy, the similar amplitudes of the frontalis M-potentials on the two sides. At 10 days the amplitude on the affected side was relatively much reduced (all recordings shown at the same gain). Fibrillation potentials and positive sharp waves began to appear at this time and subsequently became much more common in all facial muscles on the affected side.

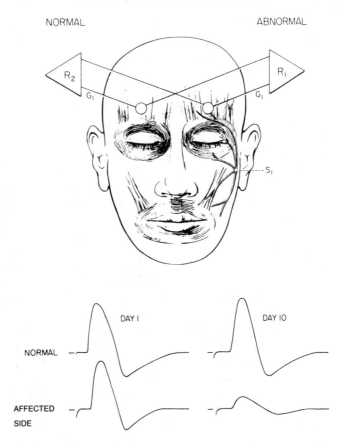

proportion of facial motor axon population that has not undergone degeneration. This provides no clue, however, to that proportion of motor fiber population in which transmission is blocked somewhere proximal to the site of stimulation (the stylomastoid foramen). This can be roughly estimated by comparing the numbers of facial MUPs that can be recruited by a maximum voluntary contraction to the amplitude of the maximum M-potential. The maximum conduction velocity in the seventh nerve remains normal up to the time nerve fibers become inexcitable (Gilliatt and Taylor, 1959).

In the acute idiopathic facial palsies where the primary lesions are proximal to the stylomastoid foramen, there may be no apparent change in the excitability or the terminal latencies to the facial muscles unless the lowest-threshold and shortest-latency facial motor axons undergo degeneration. The latter fibers may, however, be preferentially damaged by compression of the nerve (Leksell, 1945; Gelfan and Tarlov, 1956; Sunderland, 1978) within the facial canal, and their loss may account for the apparent increases in threshold (diminished excitability) and prolonged motor terminal latencies on the involved side seen in some patients. In such cases, these changes reflect only the normal excitabilities and conduction times of the remaining higher-threshold and slower-conducting fibers, once the lower-threshold and faster-conducting fibers have undergone degeneration. In this respect it is well to recall that there is a threefold range in the conduction velocities of seventh motor axons in the cat and probably about a twofold range in the human.

Evidence of denervation in facial muscles in the form of fibrillation potentials and positive sharp waves develops by about ten days, but the occurrence and numbers of fibrillating MFs have no apparent predictive value as far as the prognosis for recovery is concerned. End-plate degeneration may not become apparent until about 5 to 10 days after a nerve is transected (Adams, Denny-Brown, and Pearson, 1962), and although fibrillation potentials may be seen as early as 4 days after onset of a facial palsy, they are not usually seen until 7 to 21 days (Tavener, 1955).

Reinnervation of the facial muscles may develop in two ways. First, sprouts of intact motor axons may reinnervate nearby denervated MFs and second, with resolution of the acute destructive lesions in the nerve the motor axons may regenerate and reaching the muscles, proceed to establish new end-plates. Collateral sprouting and reinnervation begin early following denervation (Wohlfart, 1960; Coërs and Woolf, 1959). Collateral reinnervation is probably, however, able to reinnervate only those MFs in the immediate vicinity of intact motor axon terminals and preterminal branches. Early collateral reinnervation probably explains the slight increase in the duration and amplitude of facial MUPs seen early following the onset of the palsy, as well as proportion of abnormally complex MUPs seen within one to three weeks after onset of the palsy (Olson, 1975).

Where damage to the seventh nerve has been more severe, and especially where large numbers of nerve fibers have undergone degeneration, there may be too few surviving motor axons available to reinnervate all the denervated MFs. Further recovery probably depends on whether and in what numbers the facial motor axons are able to regenerate and

subsequently reach the facial muscles. To reach the facial muscles takes at least three months based on the most favorable estimated rates of regeneration of about 1 to 3 mm per day. The regenerative process may be complicated by:

1. The failures of many motor axons to regenerate
2. The development of faulty reinnervation patterns, such that the same motor axons come to supply MFs in two or more facial muscles not normally functionally related, for example, the platysma and perioral or orbicularis oculi muscles and possibly the lacrimal gland

Destruction of the basement membranes of the Schwann cells or growth of regenerating nerve fibers down incorrect basement membrane tubes probably accounts for many of the failures of nerve fibers to regenerate properly and reach their correct destinations in the periphery. The development of faulty reinnervation patterns, however, is not a reliable indication of the severity of the original nerve injury, because some evidence of faulty reinnervation is common even in facial palsies with otherwise excellent functional recovery (Olson, 1975).

Largely based on serial measurements of the amplitudes of the surface-recorded maximum M-potentials in the facial muscles, the prognosis of an acute facial palsy has been predicted (Olson, 1975; Esslen, 1977) (Table 11.4). In Esslen's (1977) study, the presence or absence of fibrillation potentials or positive sharp waves had no predictive value, although prolonged motor terminal latencies in the seventh nerve, higher apparent thresholds in the nerve, and the absence of voluntarily recruited MUs on the abnormal side all tended to suggest that recovery would be delayed and incomplete. The most reliable predictor of time and completeness of eventual recovery

TABLE 11.4.   The Prognosis of Acute Facial Palsy Based on the Amplitude of the Maximum M-Potential on the Abnormal Side

$\dfrac{\text{Max M-amplitude} - \text{abnormal side}}{\text{Max M-amplitude} - \text{normal side}} \times 100$	Prognosis
>50%	Very good; time required for recovery 6–7 weeks.
10–50%	Some had some residual paralysis; recovery time was 3 times longer than above.
2–10%	Time required 6 mo–1 yr; despite prolonged recovery time, few showed ultimately poor recovery and in some the recovery was excellent.
<2%	In most the recovery was poor, but in some the eventual recovery was surprisingly good.

From Esslen (1977).

was the amplitude of the maximum M-potential in the facial muscles.

In the above studies, some evidence of wallerian degeneration in the form of fibrillation potentials or positive sharp waves occurred in all patients, even in those who later experienced excellent and early recovery. In Chapter 2, it was pointed out that it was hard to compress a nerve sufficiently hard to produce severe conduction block without at the same time causing some wallerian degeneration in the compressed nerve (Rudge, Ochoa, and Gilliatt, 1974).

Needle electromyographic changes in acute facial palsy reflect the early degenerative and later recovery processes. For example, early reductions in the number of recruitable MUs in maximum voluntary contractions reflect the numbers of motor axons still able to conduct impulses through the site of the injury. Denervation of MFs is indicated by the development of fibrillation potentials and positive sharp waves in the facial muscles. Even in patients with a residual severe facial palsy, abnormal spontaneous activity in muscle fibers

is uncommon six months after onset of the palsy.

Early increases in the durations and amplitudes of facial MUPs as well as in the proportions of abnormally complex motor unit potentials reflect the processes of collateral sprouting and reinnervation. Beyond six months, the mean MUP durations, numbers of abnormally complex MUPs, and the degree of temporal dispersion in the maximum M-response may all actually decrease because of the continuing maturation of the new sprouts and better synchronization in the sum of the component MF action potentials in the MUP (Olson, 1975).

Less than complete recruitment patterns may indicate losses of axons even in patients with apparently satisfactory clinical recovery. In addition, sometimes MUPs can be recruited voluntarily, even though the related motor axons are not apparently excitable by direct seventh nerve stimulation. This is probably because their thresholds are so high that the patient cannot tolerate the stimulus intensities necessary to excite them.

Ectopic generation of impulses and ephaptic transmission (see Chapter 9) probably develop in the seventh nerves of patients with Bell's palsy. Evidence of such abnormal impulse generation is based on clinical observation of active tonic contractions of the facial muscles and the abnormal associated movements sometimes seen. Tonic contraction of the facial muscles is indicated by narrowing of the palpebral fissure, retraction of the mouth, and deepening of the nasolabial fold. The EMG reveals steady discharges in a few MUs in the related facial muscles in these cases. Both the discharges and tonic contractions may be abolished by local anesthetic block of the seventh nerve (Tavener, 1955).

Associated movements (synkinesis) are characterized by coactivation of facial muscles that normally do not act in concert. Possible explanations include abnormal nerve fiber regeneration whereby fibers branch to innervate widely separate muscles or ephaptic transmission between motor axons at or near the original level of the nerve injury. The latter is probably very common in Bell's palsy, even in some patients who otherwise appear to have recovered completely (Olson, 1975).

Bell's palsy was chosen to illustrate the sequence of changes in nerves and muscle resulting from a localized injury to the nerve. In review, the most important of these points are:

1. Nerve fibers undergoing degeneration lose their conductivity over a period of two to ten days following the injury.

2. Some estimate of the proportion of motor axons that did not undergo degeneration may be made by comparing the amplitudes of surface-recorded maximum M-potentials on the affected and unaffected sides. The inability voluntarily to recruit many of the MUPs, which together sum to account for the residual maximum M-potential on the affected side, provides an indication of the proportion of these remaining motor axons in which conduction is blocked proximally to the site of stimulation of the seventh nerve just distal to the stylomastoid foramen.

3. The recovery process is reflected in the changes in amplitude of the maximum M-potential and in the durations and amplitudes of the MUPs as well as the proportion of complex MUPs. These considerations regarding MUPs are important reflections both of early processes of collateral sprouting and reinnervation, and the later regeneration of motor axons and still later maturational changes in MUPs.

4. Abnormal spontaneous and synkinetic activities are probably caused by the ectopic spontaneous generation of impulses, ephaptic transmission, and possibly, faulty regeneration patterns in the nerve fibers.

ACCESSORY (ELEVENTH) CRANIAL NERVE

The accessory nerve is rarely involved by itself, but is important because through its cranial (nucleus ambiguus) and spinal (C2–6) origins, it innervates the trapezius and sternocleidomastoid muscles. Sometimes the accessory nerve is directly injured just proximal or distal to the innervation to the sternocleidomastoid muscle, and the electromyographer can help by looking for evidence of denervation and reinnervation in one or both of these muscles.

THE TWELFTH CRANIAL NERVE

The twelfth cranial nerve is included in this discussion for two reasons. First, needle electromyographic demonstration of denervation in the tongue provides evidence of degeneration of twelfth montoneurons or their motor axons as may happen in Werdnig-Hoffmann disease, amyotrophic lateral sclerosis, or syringomyelia, where such denervation may only be suspected on clinical examination alone.

Second, the tongue muscles and their nervous innervation are another example of the sometimes peculiar nature of the cranial nerves. For example, only a few typical spindles have been seen in the tongue (Cooper, 1960). The nature of the proprioceptive feedback from the tongue has not been determined either in terms of types and numbers of peripheral receptors or the peripheral route(s) by which afferents reach the brainstem. Local anesthetic block of the lingual nerve is said to block proprioception originating in the anterior two-thirds of the tongue (Weddell, Lambley, and Young, 1940; Brodal, 1981). Alternatively, these and other afferents may travel within the hypoglossal nerve itself.

Hypoglossal motoneurons probably have direct cortico-motoneuronal connections from the opposite precentral cortex as well as other inputs from the trigeminal system, the reticular formation, and the nucleus of the tractus solitarius. No true H-reflex in the tongue, however, can be elicited by stimulation of the twelfth nerve.

References

Adams RD, Denny-Brown D, Pearson CM. Diseases of muscle. London: Kimpton, 1962.

Boongird P, Vejjajiva A. Electrophysiologic findings and prognosis in Bell's palsy. Muscle Nerve 1978;1:461–66.

Brodal A. Neurological anatomy. Oxford: Oxford University Press, 1981.

Brown WF, Rushworth G. Reflex latency fluctuations in human single motor units. In: Desmedt JE, ed. New developments in electromyography and clinical neurophysiology. Basel: Karger, 1973:660–65.

Bruesh SR. The distribution of myelinated afferent

fibers in the branches of the cat's facial nerve. J Comp Neurol 1944;81:169–91.

Buchthal F. Electromyography in paralysis of the facial nerve. Arch Otolaryngol 1965;81:463–69.

Buchthal F, Rosenfalck P. Action potential parameters in different human muscles. Acta Psychiatr Neurol Scand 1955;30:125–31.

Buonaguidi R, Rossi B, Sartucci F, Ravelli V. Blink reflex in severe traumatic coma. J Neurol Neurosurg Psychiatry 1979;42:470–74.

Bynke O. Facial reflexes and their clinical uses. Lancet 1971;1:137–38.

Coërs C, Woolf AL. The innervation of muscle. Oxford: Blackwell, 1959.

Cooper S. Muscle spindles and other receptors. In: Bourne, GH, ed. Structure and function of muscle. New York: Academic Press, 1960:381–420.

Davis LE. Experimental viral infections of the facial nerve and geniculate ganglion. Ann Neurol 1981;9:120–25.

Devriese PP. Compression and ischemia of the facial nerve. Acta Otolaryngol 1974;77:108–18.

Edström L, Lindquist C. Histochemical fiber composition of some facial muscles in the cat in relation to their contraction properties. Acta Physiol Scand 1973;89:491–503.

Eisen A, Danon J. The orbicularis oculi reflex in acoustic neuromas: a clinical and electrodiagnostic evaluation. Neurology 1974;24:306–11.

Esslen E. The acute facial palsies. New York: Springer-Verlag, 1977.

Feinstein B, Lindegård B, Nyman E, Wohlfart G. Morphologic studies of motor units in normal human muscles. Acta Anat (Basel) 1954;23:127–42.

Ferguson IT. Electrical study of jaw and orbicularis oculi reflexes after trigeminal nerve surgery. J Neurol Neurosurg Psychiatry 1978;41:819–23.

Ferguson IT, Lenman JAR, Johnston BB. Habituation of the orbicularis oculi reflex in dementia and dyskinetic states. J Neurol Neurosurg Psychiatry 1978;41:824–28.

Ferrari E, Messina C. Blink reflexes during sleep and wakefulness in man. Electroencephalogr Clin Neurophysiol 1972;32:55–62.

Fisher MS, Shahani BT, Young RR. Assessing

segmental excitability after acute rostral lesions. Neurology 1979;29:45–50.

Foley JO, DuBois F. An experimental study of the facial nerve. J Comp Neurol 1943;79:79–105.

Gelfan S, Tarlov IM. Physiology of spinal cord, nerve root and peripheral nerve compression. J Neurophysiol 1956;18:217–29.

Gilliatt RW, Fowler TJ, Rudge P. Peripheral neuropathy in baboons. In: Meldrum BS, Marsden CD, eds. Advances in neurology. New York: Raven Press, 1975:253–72.

Gilliatt RW, Taylor JC. Electrical changes following section of the facial nerve. Proc R Soc Med 1959;52:1080–83.

Godaux E, Desmedt JE. Exteroceptive suppression and motor control of the masseter and temporalis muscles in normal man. Brain Res 1975a;85:447–58.

Godaux E, Desmedt JE. Human masseter muscle: H and tendon reflexes. Arch Neurol 1975b; 32:229–34.

Goodwill CJ. The normal jaw reflex: Measurement of the action potential in the masseter muscles. Ann Phys Med 1968;9:183–88.

Goodwill CJ, O'Tuama L. Electromyographic recording of the jaw reflex in multiple sclerosis. J Neurol Neurosurg Psychiatry 1969;32:6–10.

Goor C, Ongerboer de Visser BW. Jaw and blink reflexes in trigeminal nerve lesions. Neurology 1976;26:95–97.

Gordon G. Observations upon the movements of the eyelids. Br J Ophthalmol 1951;35:339–51.

Granit R, Skoglund S, Thesleff S. Activation of muscle spindles by succinylcholine and decamethonium. The effects of curare. Acta Physiol Scand 1953;28:134–51.

Hiraoka M, Shimamura M. Neural mechanisms of the corneal blinking reflex in cat. Brain Res 1977;125:265–75.

Hoyt WF, Loeffler JD. Neurology of the orbicularis oculi. Anatomic, physiologic and clinical aspects of lid closure. In: Smith JL, ed. Neuro-ophthalmology. St. Louis: CV Mosby, 1965:167–205.

Hufschmidt HJ, Spuler H. Mono- and polysynaptic reflexes of the trigeminal muscles in human sclerosis. J Neurol Neurosurg Psychiatry 1962; 25:332–35.

Iwata N, Kitai ST, Olson S. Afferent component of the facial nerve: its relation to the spinal trigeminal and facial nucleus. Brain Res 1972; 43:662–67.

Jasper HH, Ballem G. Unipolar electromyograms of normal and denervated human muscle. J Neurophysiol 1949;12:231–44.

Johansson RS, Olsson KA. Microelectrode recordings from human oral mechanoreceptors. Brain Res 1976;118:307–11.

Kadanoff D Von. Die sensibelen nervenendigungen in der minischen muskulatur des menschen. Z Mikrosk Anat Forsch 1956;62:1–15.

Kimura J. Alteration of the orbicularis oculi reflex by pontine lesions. Arch Neurol 1970;22:156–61.

Kimura J. The blink reflex as a test for brainstem and higher central nervous function. In: Desmedt JE, ed. New developments in electromyography and clinical neurophysiology. Basel: Karger, 1973:682–91.

Kimura J. Effect of hemisphere lesions on the contralateral blink reflex. Neurology 1974;24:168–74.

Kimura J. Electrically elicited blink reflex in diagnosis of multiple sclerosis. Review of 260 patients over a seven-year period. Brain 1975; 98:413–26.

Kimura J, Lyon LW. Orbicularis oculi reflex in the Wallenberg syndrome: alteration of the late reflex by lesions of the spinal tract and nucleus of the trigeminal nerve. J Neurol Neurosurg Psychiatry 1972;35:228–33.

Kimura J, Powers M, Van Allen MW. Reflex responses of orbicularis oculi muscle to supraorbital nerve stimulation. Arch Neurol 1969; 21:193–99.

Kimura J, Rodnitzky RL, Van Allen MW. Electrodiagnostic study of trigeminal nerve. Neurology 1970;20:574–83.

Kitai ST, Tanaka T, Tsukahara N, Yu H. The facial nucleus of cat: antidromic and synaptic activation and peripheral nerve representation. Exp Brain Res 1972;16:161–83.

Kugelberg E. Facial reflexes. Brain 1952;75:385–96.

Kullman GL, Dijck PJ, Cody DTR. Anatomy of the mastoid portion of the facial nerve. Arch Otolaryngol 1971;93:29–33.

Kuypers HGJM. Cortico-bulbar connections to the

pons and lower brainstem in man. An anatomical study. Brain 1958;81:364–88.

Leksell L. The action potential and excitatory effects of the small ventral root fibers to skeletal muscle. Acta Physiol Scand 1945;10(suppl 131):37.

Lele PP, Weddell G. Sensory nerves of the cornea and cutaneous sensibility. Exp Neurol 1959; 1:334–59.

Lindquist C. Contraction properties of cat facial muscles. Acta Physiol Scand 1973a;89:482–90.

Lindquist C. Reflex organization and contraction properties of facial muscles. Acta Physiol Scand 1973b;suppl 393:3–15.

Lindquist C, Mårtennson A. Mechanisms involved in the cats' blink reflex. Acta Physiol Scand 1970;80:149–59.

Lowitzsch K, Kuhnt U, Sakmann C, Maurer K, Hopf HC, Schott D, Thater K. Visual pattern evoked responses and blink reflexes in assessment of MS diagnosis. J Neurol 1976;213:17–32.

Lyon LW, Kimura J, McCormick WT. Orbicularis oculi reflex in coma: clinical electrophysiological and pathological correlations. J Neurol Neurosurg Psychiatry 1972;35:582–88.

Matthews PBC. Muscle receptors. London: Edward Arnold, 1972.

McIntyre AK. Afferent limb of the myotactic reflex arc. Nature 1951;168:168–69.

McIntyre AK, Robinson RG. Pathway for the jaw-jerk in man. Brain 1959;82;468–74.

Mehta AJ, Seshia SS. Orbicularis oculi reflex in brain death. J Neurol Neurosurg Psychiatry 1976;39:784–87.

Oliver LC. The supranuclear arc of the corneal reflex. Acta Physiol Scand 1952;27:329–33.

Olson PZ. Prediction of recovery in Bell's palsy. Acta Neurol Scand 1975;suppl 61:52.

Ongerboer de Visser BW. The corneal reflex: electrophysiological and anatomical data in man. In: Kerkut GA, Phillis JW, eds. Progress in neurobiology. Oxford: Pergamon Press, 1980:71–83.

Ongerboer de Visser BW. Corneal reflex latency in lesions of the lower post central region. Neurology 1981a;31:701–7.

Ongerboer de Visser BW. Recorded reflexes passing through the trigeminal system: a review of the anatomical data in man. In: Desmedt JE, ed. Motor control mechanisms in man. New York: Raven Press, 1981b.

Ongerboer de Visser BW. Afferent limb of the human jaw reflex: electrophysiologic and anatomic study. Neurology 1982a;32:563–66.

Ongerboer de Visser BW. Anatomical and functional organization of reflexes involving the trigeminal system in man: jaw reflex, blink reflex, corneal reflex, and exteroceptive suppression. In: Desmedt JE, ed. Brain and spinal mechanisms of movement control in man: new developments and clinical applications. New York: Raven Press, 1982b.

Ongerboer de Visser BW, Goor C. Electromyographic and reflex study in ideopathic and symptomatic trigeminal neuralgias: latency of the jaw and blink reflexes. J Neurol Neurosurg Psychiatry 1974;37:1225–30.

Ongerboer de Visser BW, Goor C. Jaw reflexes and masseter electromyograms in mesencephalic and pontine lesions: an electrodiagnostic study of Wallenberg's syndrome. Brain 1978; 101:285–94.

Ongerboer de Visser BE, Kuypers HGJM. Late blink reflex changes in lateral medullary lesions. An electrophysiological and neuroanatomical study of Wallenberg's syndrome. Brain 1978;101:285–94.

Ongerboer de Visser BW, Melchelse K, Megens PHA. Corneal reflex latency in trigeminal nerve lesions. Neurology 1977;27:1164–67.

Ongerboer de Visser BW, Moffie D. Effects of brainstem and thalamic lesions on the corneal reflex: an electrophysiological and anatomical study. Brain 1979;102:595–608.

Petersen J, Kugelberg E. Duration and form of action potential in normal human muscle. J Neurol Neurosurg Psychiatry 1949;47:65–71.

Rimpel J, Geyer D, Hopf HC. Changes in the blink responses to combined trigeminal, acoustic and visual repetitive stimulation, studied in the human subject. Electroencephalogr Clin Neurophysiol 1982;54:552–60.

Ross RT. Corneal reflex in hemisphere disease. J Neurol Neurosurg Psychiatry 1972;35:877–80.

Rossi, B, Buonaguidi R, Muratorio A, Tusini G. Blink reflexes in posterior fossa lesions. J Neurol Neurosurg Psychiatry 1979;42:465–69.

Rudge P, Ochoa J, Gilliatt RW. Acute peripheral nerve compression in the baboon. J Neurol Sci 1974;23:403–20.

Rushworth G. Observations on blink reflexes. J Neurol Neurosurg Psychiatry 1962;25:93–108.

Rushworth G. Some functional properties of deep facial afferents. In: Andrew BL, ed. Control and innervation of muscle. Edinburgh: Livingstone, 1966:125–33.

Saring W, VonCramon D. The acoustic blink reflex: stimulus dependence, excitability and localizing value. J Neurol 1981;224:243–52.

Schenck E, Manz F. The blink reflex in Bell's palsy. In: Desmedt JE, ed. New developments in electromyography and clinical neurophysiology. Basel: Karger, 1973:678–81.

Serrats AF, Parker SA, Merino-Cañas AV. The blink reflex in coma and recovery from coma. Acta Neurochirurg 1976;34:79–97.

Shahani BT. The human blink reflex. J Neurol Neurosurg Psychiatry 1970;33:792–800.

Shahani BT, Young RR. Blink reflexes in orbicularis oculi. In: Desmedt JE, ed. New developments in electromyography and clinical neurophysiology Basel: Karger, 1973:641–48.

Sunderland S. Nerves and nerve injuries. Edinburgh: Churchill Livingstone, 1978.

Szentágothai J. Anatomical considerations of monosynaptic reflex arcs. J Neurophysiol 1948;11:445–54.

Tavener D. Bell's palsy. A clinical and electromyographic study. Brain 1955;78:209–27.

Tokunaga A, Oka M, Murao T, Yokoi H, Okumura T, Hirata T, Miyashita Y, Yoshitatsu S. An experimental study on facial reflex by evoked electromyography. Med J Osaka Univ 1958;9:397–411.

Trontelj JV. H-reflex of single motoneurones in man. Nature 1968;220:1043–44.

VanBuskirk C. The seventh nerve complex. J Comp Neurol 1945;82:303–33.

Van Hasselt P. Facial reflexes evoked by electrical stimulation of peripheral-facial nerve branches in the cat: experiments of the auriculotemporal-facial nerve anastomoses. Exp Neurol 1976;51:407–13.

Weddell G, Harpman JA, Lambley DG, Young L. The innervation of the musculature of the tongue. J Anat (Lond) 1940;74:255–67.

Willer JC, Lamore Y. Electrophysiological evidence for a facio-facial reflex in facial muscles in man. Brain Res 1977;119:459–64.

Wohlfart G. Clinical significance of collateral sprouting of remaining motor nerve fibers in partially denervated muscles. J Exp Med Sci 1960;3:128–33.

Yates SK, Brown WF. The human jaw jerk: electrophysiological methods to measure the latency, normal values and changes in multiple sclerosis. Neurology 1981a;31:632–34.

Yates SK, Brown WF. Light-stimulus-evoked blink reflex: methods, normal values, relation to other blink reflexes and observations in multiple sclerosis. Neurology 1981b;31:272–81.

12 ELECTROMYOGRAPHY AND DISORDERS OF THE CENTRAL NERVOUS SYSTEM

In previous chapters, most of the attention has been directed toward diseases of the peripheral nervous system, neuromuscular junction, and muscle, and the characteristic types of abnormalities seen in the EMG in these disorders. Electromyography, however, also has a place in the physiological analysis of central nervous system (CNS) disorders. For example, lesions in the CNS can alter the recruitment patterns of motor units (MUs), the central excitabilities of motoneurons, electrical and mechanical properties of MUs and muscles, and of course, central conduction in the somatosensory pathways.

In the last two to three decades, the central and peripheral basis of motor control has been the subject of several excellent reviews (Granit, 1970; Brooks and Stoney, 1971; Matthews, 1972; Desmedt, 1973; Porter, 1973; Shahani, 1976; Wiesendanger, 1972, 1981; Phillips and Porter, 1977; as well as volumes 4, 5, 8, and 9 of the *Progress in Clinical Neurophysiology* series, edited by Desmedt, 1978a, 1978b, 1978c, 1978d; and the *Handbook of Physiology* series, parts 1 and 2 on motor control, edited by Brooks, 1981 and Freund, 1983)

and need not be repeated here. The main objective of this chapter is to cover areas of special interest to electromyographers that have not been dealt with in the preceding reviews. In this category are the physiological and morphological changes in hemiplegia and paraplegia and the Babinski response.

Other subjects such as transcortical reflexes have been included because of the enormous interest in this area over the last ten years and the need to make available to electromyographers a summary of the basic concepts involved and the evidence to date. Tremor has also been included because the electromyographer may occasionally be able to aid clinicians in the recognition and correct labeling of some tremors, and because tremors and other central motor disturbances that are sometimes associated with them may alter MU recruitment patterns. The H-reflex, introduced in Chapter 3, is covered here again; this time in combination with the tendon reflex (TR) and tonic vibration reflex (TVR), in order to discuss briefly the alterations in motoneuron excitability and connectivity and their asessment following spinal transection.

PYRAMIDAL SYNDROME

One of the most common and important sequelae of central lesions interrupting descending projections to motoneurons is the so-called *pyramidal syndrome*. This syndrome, as it is so conveniently but incorrectly labeled, is characterized by weakness in a particular distribution, certain postural changes, increased tendon reflexes, spasticity, Babinski responses (extensor plantar responses), and abnormalities in some cutaneous reflexes.

The weakness in the arms is most apparent in shoulder abduction and external rotation, elbow extension, forearm supination, wrist and digit extension, and in the actions of the intrinsic hand muscles. In the lower limbs, weakness is generally most pronounced in hip flexion and abduction, knee flexion, and foot dorsiflexion and eversion, rather than in the corresponding hip extensors, knee flexors, or ankle and toe plantar flexors. The affected limbs often assume a posture in which the arm is internally rotated and adducted at the shoulder, the elbow flexed, the forearm pronated, and the fingers and wrist flexed; while in the lower limb the hip is adducted and extended, the knee extended, and the foot plantar flexed and inverted. The spasticity, which usually accompanies the above but which is often quite variable in degree, does not always match the distribution of the weakness.

The pyramidal syndrome may be confined to one region such as facial or bulbar area, upper or lower limbs, or in its even most limited expression, to particular groups of muscles such as the forearm, finger, and thumb extensor and intrinsic hand muscles in the upper limb, or the dorsiflexor and everter muscles of the foot in the leg. Meticulous examination in such cases often reveals a more widespread distribution of the motor abnormalities. Sometimes the weakness, postural changes, and alterations in tendon reflexes or tone are not all apparent to the same degree.

Indeed, there may be important dissociations among the features. For example, extensor plantar responses may be present even though the tendon reflexes and tone are normal or reduced. Conversely, increased tone and increased tendon reflexes may be associated with flexor plantar responses.

Even though entrenched in the clinical neurological literature, the term pyramidal syndrome is strictly speaking incorrect as applied to humans, because naturally occurring lesions affecting pyramidal fiber systems are almost never restricted to the pyramid alone; other cortical and subcortical descending projections almost invariably being involved as well (Brodal, 1981). Use of the covering term pyramidal is therefore misleading because it implies that the motor disturbances are solely attributable to the interruption of fiber systems passing through the pyramid.

Lesions restricted to the pyramid in subhuman primates do not lead to spasticity or increases in tendon reflexes in the affected limbs (Patton and Amassian, 1960; Wiesendanger, 1969, 1981; Phillips, 1973; Lawerance and Hopkins, 1976; Brodal, 1981; Asanuma, 1981), but do produce several distinct changes in motor performance (Patton and Amassian, 1960; Wiesendanger, 1969; Wiesendanger, 1973; Brodal, 1981; Asanuma, 1981) (Table 12.1). Loss of the ability to make discrete movements is not confined to the distal muscles in the limb, but extends to involve proximal muscles as well (Kuypers, 1981). It probably reflects the loss of cortico-motoneuronal pathways that allow for more direct selection of motoneurons in motor tasks. For example, in monkeys whose pyramids are intact, single-pulse cortical stimuli are able to evoke well-synchronized and short-latency EMG responses in contralateral distal muscles of the limbs. Such stimuli fail to evoke any response in the presence of partial pyramid sections, although more intense trains of stimuli will evoke longer-latency and more asynchronous

TABLE 12.1.   Consequences of Pyramid Section

Permanent loss of independent digit movements[1,2,3]
Slowness in the initiation of movements[4,5,6]
Hypotonia and reduced tendon reflexes[7,8]
Loss of superficial reflexes, i.e., abdominal and cremasteric[7,8]
Appearance of a Babinski response (extensor plantar reflex)[7,8]
Atrophy in the affected limbs[7,8]

---

[1]Lawerance and Hopkins (1976).
[2]Asanuma (1981).
[3]Kuypers (1981).
[4]Hepp-Reymond and Wiesendanger (1972).
[5]Hepp-Reymond, Trouche, and Wiesendanger (1974).
[6]Wisendanger (1973).
[7]Tower (1940).
[8]Tower (1949).

EMG responses in the same muscles (Felix and Wiesendanger, 1971).

Loss of the *direct cortico-motoneuronal* (DCM) projections that are transmitted through the pyramid probably accounts for the above loss of the lowest-threshold EMG responses in contralateral limb muscles to direct cortical stimulation (Felix and Wiesendanger, 1971). Such DCM projections are more dense in the chimpanzee than in the monkey and are especially abundant in man (Kuypers, 1981). Thus in the absence of these DCM projections to motoneurons, longer temporal summation times are required to recruit motoneurons. The slower initiation of movements probably also reflects not only reductions in the numbers of MUs that can be recruited, but in the ability of subjects to maintain the discharges of these MUs in motor tasks (Wiesendanger, 1973b).

Unfortunately for electromyographers, these early physiological and anatomical studies in lower primates of the effects of pyramid section (see reviews by Patton and Amassian, 1960; Wiesendanger, 1969, 1981; Asanuma, 1981) included no electromyographic (EMG) studies to look for denervation in the affected muscles nor did they study possible changes

in the physiological properties and numbers of MUs within the affected muscles. Indeed, only the studies of Tower (1940) and Travis (1955), the latter made following precentral ablations, commented on changes in muscle bulk in the affected limbs following the central lesions.

The Babinski response and the loss of independent digit movements (Lawerance and Hopkins, 1976) and other discrete motor actions in the absence of paralysis of these muscles are probably consequences of interruption of fiber systems passing through the pyramid.

The spasticity, hyperreflexia, and to an unknown extent, weakness, probably depend more on the interruption of other descending cortically or subcortically originating fiber systems that do not pass through the pyramid. Extrapolations based on studies of even higher primates may be somewhat misleading, however, because of the enormous increase in the quantitative importance of the DCM projections in man (Kuypers, 1981).

MU RECRUITMENT IN HEMIPARETIC HUMANS

Recruitment of MUs is changed in hemiparetic subjects (Freund, Dietz, Wita, and Kapp, 1973). For example, in affected muscles, subjects often experience difficulties recruiting even those MUs normally recruited with the least effort. Difficulties may also be experienced maintaining steady discharges in these same MUs. Sometimes there may even be apparent reversals of the normal order of recruitment (Grimby, Hannerz, and Ranlund, 1972; Grimby and Hannerz, 1973; Freund, Dietz, Wita, and Kapp, 1973). In such instances, proprioceptive and other inputs may help to restore the normal recruitment order. Whether there is any true alteration in the absolute thresholds at which MUs are recruited or just increases in the subject's sense of effort in recruiting these MUs is unknown. Nor is it known whether the difficulties experienced recruiting MUs preferentially involve certain MUs or extend equally to all types.

In controls, double discharges in MUs are especially common when subjects try to maintain steady and constant contractions (Andreassen and Rosenfalck, 1979). The intervals between such double discharges are generally less than one-half the mean interval between the discharges in a steady contraction and may be as short as 5 ms. Such double discharges can produce "catchlike" increases in tension (Burke, Rodomin, and Zajac, 1976) and are characteristically absent in upper motoneuron lesions.

PATHOGENESIS OF ATROPHY AND THE QUESTION OF DENERVATION IN HEMIPLEGIA AND PARAPLEGIA

Atrophy in limb muscles on the side opposite cerebral lesions has been well documented in subhuman primates (Winkelman and Silverstein, 1932, 1935; Fulton, 1936; Tower, 1940, 1949; Travis, 1955; Patton and Amassian, 1960) and hemiplegic atrophy in man is a long-established observation (see reviews of Critchley, 1953; Silverstein, 1955). Indeed, as early as 1879 Charcot described degenerative changes in motoneurons following contralateral intracerebral hemorrhage.

In humans, lesions in the cerebral hemisphere interrupting descending projections to brainstem and spinal motoneurons may be associated with a variety of structural and physiological changes within the spinal cord and muscles (Table 12.2).

Charcot's (1879) and others' (Brissaud, 1879; Schaffer, 1897; Kiss, 1929) early observations of so-called degenerative changes in spinal motoneurons contralateral to lesions in the cerebral hemisphere need to be reexamined. Such examinations would require quan-

TABLE 12.2.   Changes in the Spinal Cord, Peripheral Nerves, and Muscle Contralateral to Lesions in the Cerebral Hemisphere

Possible degenerative changes in motoneurons[1]
Possible losses of MUs[2]
Appearance of denervation potentials in the affected muscles[3,4]
Physiological changes in MUs[5]
    Increases in twitch contraction times of fast MUs
    Increases in mean tensions of slow-twitch MUs
    Increases in the proportion of fatigable MUs
Morphological changes in muscle[6-9]
    Type I fiber hypertrophy
    Type II fiber atrophy
    Fiber type grouping
    Grouped fiber atrophy
    Angular fibers
Reductions in amplitudes of maximum M-potential[2]
Increases in mean MU potential amplitudes[2]
Maintenance of near normal maximum twitch tensions[2]
Possible abnormalities in neuromuscular transmission[2]
Possible changes in peripheral nerve conduction
    Slowing of motor conduction[10,11]
    No change in motor conduction[3,7,9,12]
    Prolongation of motor terminal latencies[2]
    Slowing of sensory conduction[12]

[1]Charcot (1879).
[2]McComas, Sica, Upton, and Aguilera (1973).
[3]Goldkamp (1967).
[4]Bhala (1969).
[5]Young and Mayer (1982).
[6]Brook and Engel (1969).
[7]Edstrom (1970).
[8]Chokroverty, Reyes, Rubino, and Barron (1976).
[9]Segura and Sahgal (1981).
[10]Panin, Paul, Policoff, and Eson (1967).
[11]Shigeno (1972b).
[12]Namba, Schuman, and Grob (1971).

titative assessments of the numbers of ventral horn cells as well as whatever reactive changes may be present in those same neurons, especially in the spinal segments and regions of the ventral horn most likely to show the changes; for example, in the case of the arm in the C7-T1 cervical segments and the lateral regions of the ventral horn where the forearm and hand motoneurons are located (see Chapter 5). Based on the timing of the appearance and disappearance of denervation activity (Goldkamp, 1967) in hemiparetic muscles, reactive changes in motoneurons should be most pronounced in the early weeks following the cerebral event. The extent to which descending pathways to the spinal cord have been interrupted should also be an important factor. If transsynaptic degeneration were an important pathogenetic mechanism producing dysfunctional changes in the motoneurons, this might be expected to be linked quantitatively to the extent and abruptness of the central denervation. By analogy with the peripheral nervous system, such interruptions should be most effective in denervating the motoneurons where the descending axons underwent actual degeneration rather than functional interruption through conduction block alone.

The appearance of denervation activity, namely, fibrillation activity and positive sharp waves in upper motoneuron lesions, is another area of sharp controversy. Not all investigators agree as to the frequency of this activity in hemiplegic or paraplegic (spinal cord origin) muscles. In an electromyographic study of 116 hemiplegic patients, Goldkamp observed fibrillation potentials and sometimes positive sharp waves in about two-thirds of the patients in the hemiplegic muscles. The denervation was most common in more distal muscles (Table 12.3).

In Goldkamp's investigation, fibrillation potentials were most common in the forearm and intrinsic hand muscles. Studies in the lower limb were too limited in scope to make useful comment about the distribution of the denervation. Fibrillation potentials and positive sharp waves were not seen in the first week, but were most common between four and five weeks. Unfortunately, the precise locations or sizes of the central lesions causing the hemiplegia were not included in the report in the series of hemiplegics studied by Bhala (1969)

TABLE 12.3. Distribution of Fibrillation Potentials in Hemiplegic Muscles

Muscle(s)	Percentage of Patients with Fibrillation Potentials
Deltoid	36
Biceps	20
Triceps	27
Forearm extensor	47
Forearm flexor	38
Opponens pollicis	50
Hypothenar	39
First dorsal interosseus	45
Quadriceps	22
Tibialis anterior	16
Peroneus longus	15
Gastrocnemius	21

From Goldkamp (1967).

who, like Goldkamp, also reported a similar distribution and frequency of denervation in hemiplegic limbs (Table 12.4).

TABLE 12.4. Distribution of Denervation in Hemiplegic Muscle

Muscle(s)	Percentage of Patient Population with Fibrillation Potentials or Positive Sharp Waves in Muscles
Deltoid	27
Biceps	27
Triceps	8
Brachioradialis	4
Forearm extensor (EDC)	46
Forearm flexor (FCR)	39
Abductor pollicus brevis	19
Quadriceps	15
Tibialis anterior	23
Peroneus longus	4
Gastrocnemius	23

From Bhala (1969).

These two investigations and other evidence (Krueger and Waylonis, 1973; Johnson, Denny, and Kelley, 1975; Petty and Johnson, 1980; Segura and Sahgal, 1981; Spaars and Wilts, 1982) suggests that denervation is indeed common in hemiplegic muscles.

Abnormal spontaneous activity is not, however, seen in all hemiplegic subjects. It has been alternatively suggested that pressure on peripheral nerves and perhaps traction injuries to the brachial or lumbosacral plexuses may explain some or all of the denervation (Chokroverty and Medina, 1978), although Segura and Sahgal (1981) were unable to confirm such a possibility in their well-studied case.

Alterations in the physiological properties of single MUs in hemiparetic muscles have only recently been studied (Young and Mayer, 1982). The authors described early, slight increases in the mean contraction times of fast MUs. In hemiparesis of longer duration there were increases in the mean tension of slow MUs and in the proportion of fatigable MUs. At all stages, the three main types (FF, FR, and S) (see Chapter 5) of MUs could still be recognized by their fatigue and characteristics of twitch contractions. Some of the apparent increases in the mean tension of S-MUs may have represented changes of some fast-twitch MUs into slow-twitch units, a possibility supported by the finding that some S fatigable MUs also demonstrated the "sag" property (see Chapter 5), a property normally of fast- but not slow-twitch MUs. The increased twitch tensions of S-MUs could also be explained by the type I MF hypertrophy known to occur in spastic hemiplegia (Edstrom, 1970). In addition, Young and Mayer claimed that the mean twitch tension of fast MUs was increased also in well-established hemiplegia. This may have reflected sampling errors in these MUs, because type II fibers are said to atrophy, not hypertrophy, in hemiplegic muscles (Brooke and Engel, 1969; Edstrom, Grimby, and Han-

nerz, 1972). These increases in tensions of both fast- and slow-twitch MUs, if they are a product of an increase in the innervation ratio of these MUs or hypertrophy of the muscle fibers (MFs) or both, could well be the mechanical equivalent of the higher mean amplitudes of motor unit potentials (MUPs) in hemiplegic muscles reported by McComas, Sica, Upton, and Aguilera (1973). Unfortunately, Young and Mayer failed to record the surface amplitudes of these MUs in hemiplegia and their study provided no indication of the numbers of MUs in the hemiplegic muscles.

Losses of about one-half the normal number of MUs and increases in the mean MUP amplitudes in hemiplegic muscles have been reported by McComas, Sica, Upton, and Aguilera (1973), although frank morphological evidence of denervation and reinnervation in hemiplegic muscles has been seen only in the study of Segura and Sahgal (1981). These losses of MUs in McComas's study were curiously not apparent for the first eight weeks following the appearance of hemiplegia; curious because fibrillation in the affected muscles usually appears much earlier (three to five weeks), based on Goldkamp's study (1967). These apparent MU losses in hemiplegic muscles need to be confirmed by other techniques because of the fundamental importance of the claim that they occur presumably through transsynaptic degeneration, as originally announced (McComas, Sica, Upton, and Aguilera, 1973).

One stumbling block to such studies, however, may well be the selection of muscles for biopsy because tissues from the distal limb muscles are not readily taken for this purpose. This is especially true in the upper limbs, which show the most denervation and are among those most likely to suffer presumably from the loss of their dense DCM connections (see review by Kuypers, 1981). More detailed electrophysiological studies of the latter muscles are needed, though it should not be assumed that the more usual patterns of collateralization, reinnervation, and indication of fiber grouping will be seen as in peripheral neurogenic disorders (Chapter 8).

The reductions in the maximum M-potentials could be produced by any factors that reduce the total membrane currents generated in the muscles. This could happen through disuse atrophy, the loss of MFs through denervation, or alterations in membrane conductances through changes in the densities and properties of ion channels in the sarcolemmal membranes. Atrophy of subcutaneous tissues would also bring the active membranes nearer to the recording surface electrodes and would tend to increase the amplitude of the potentials recorded.

The maximum twitch tensions in McComas's study (1973) were said to be near normal or normal; however, too few subjects were studied to make any comment about the changes, especially in the early period when denervation activity is most frequent. In keeping with other studies of single MUs in hemiplegia (Young and Mayer, 1982) where the twitch contraction times of MUs were increased, the contraction time of the maximum twitch is prolonged in hemiplegia (McComas, Sica, Upton, and Aguilera, 1973).

The questions of changes in motor and sensory conduction are just as controversial in hemiplegia (Table 12.2). Reductions in the maximum motor conduction velocities in hemiplegic limbs have been reported (Panin, Paul, Policoff, and Eson, 1967; Shigeno, 1972b), but others have not been able to substantiate this claim (Goldkamp, 1967; Namba, Schuman and Grob, 1971; McComas, Sica, Upton, and Aguilera, 1973; Segura and Sahgal, 1981; Young and Mayer, 1982). Prolonged motor terminal latencies were noted by McComas and co-workers (1973) and preferential slowing in the slower-conducting motor nerve fibers was reported by Namba,

Schuman, and Grob (1971). The latter also concluded there were reductions in maximum sensory conduction velocities as well on the hemiplegic side, although why these should be slowed and not the faster-conducting motor fibers was not clear.

It can, of course, be argued that the slower velocities seen in hemiplegic limbs were accounted for by the slightly lower temperatures in the hemiplegic limbs or possibly inadvertent trauma to various peripheral nerves on the hemiplegic side (Chokroverty and Medina, 1978).

Abnormal decrements in the maximum M-potential seen at stimulus frequencies of 30 Hz by McComas, Sica, Upton, and Aguilera (1973) possibly correlate with the sometimes abnormally complex and enlarged subneural apparatuses reportedly present in hemiplegic muscles (Chokroverty, Reyes, Rubino, and Barron, 1976). Abnormalities in neuromuscular transmission would be expected to be most prominent in the early weeks when denervation activity is said to be most active.

It was pointed out earlier that atrophy contralateral to experimental pyramid section and ablation of areas 4 and 6 (Fulton, 1936; Tower, 1940, 1949; Patton and Amassian, 1960; Travis, 1955) has been well documented. Whether such changes are products of disuse atrophy, compressive or traction injuries to the peripheral nerves, or transsynaptic degeneration of motoneurons is unknown. That transsynaptic degeneration does occur in the CNS has long been appreciated, examples being the medial geniculate body following enucleation of the eye (Cook, Walker, and Barr, 1951; Goldby, 1957), the inferior olive after section of the central tegmental tract (Torvik, 1956), and Clarke column cells and even motoneurons following section of the dorsal roots (Warrington, 1898, 1899; Young, 1966; Young and Rowley, 1970; Goldberger, 1974, 1980).

Moreover, we were recently able to show

that hemisection of the macaque spinal cord in the thoracic region resulted in the loss of about 20 percent of the ventral horn cells at the level of the lumbosacral cord (Brown, Milner-Brown, Ball, and Girvin, 1978). Such hemisections could be expected to interrupt all the descending projections, direct and indirect, to the motoneurons. It must therefore be accepted, at least in circumstances where a major part of the input to motoneurons has been interrupted (Young and Rowley, 1970; Brown, Milner-Brown, Ball, and Girvin, 1978), that degeneration of motoneurons may take place. It is not known at this time whether this is simply a product of the quantitative extent of the loss of inputs or is in some way related to the specific sources of those inputs, some of which exert hypothetically unique trophic influence over the motoneurons, a form of "central disuse" in which the motoneurons atrophy or become dysfunctional for lack of synaptic drive, or other reasons. Nor is it known whether the MUs (FF, FR, and S) are all equally vulnerable. In the author's opinion, in view of the impressive quantitative increase in DCM projections with ascent through the evolutionary scale to man (Kuypers, 1981), it is not unreasonable to suggest that loss of these quantitatively important direct inputs may be especially significant in the genesis of the dysfunctional and degenerative changes in motoneurons for which there now seems to be some experimental and clinical evidence.

Transsynaptic degeneration of motoneurons could clearly explain the losses of MUs and appearance of denervation in hemiplegia, changes that disuse alone would not be expected to produce. Disuse can produce muscle atrophy and changes in the contractile properties of MUs, although not in the histochemical mosaic patterns in muscles that are experimentally immobilized (Mayer, Burke, Toop, Hodgson, Kanda, and Wolmsley, 1981). In man, disuse atrophy may produce marked type I MF atrophy (Edstrom, 1970; Sargeant, Davies, Edwards, Maunder, and Young, 1977).

The presence of denervation in hemiplegic muscles has alternatively been explained, as alluded to earlier, as a product of injuries to various peripheral nerves and possible plexuses because of the imposed immobility and greater liability to compressions of nerves at vulnerable sites such as the elbow for the ulnar nerve, common peroneal nerve at the fibular head, or possibly radial nerve in its retrohumeral course. Concomitant sensory loss, inattention, or disordered consciousness could compound the problem. Traction injuries of the brachial plexus could well add to the extent of the trauma to the peripheral nerves. No doubt all the above, at one time or another, may contribute to the motor abnormalities and denervation, and there has been no concerted effort in any of the studies to date to exclude them by systematic clinical or electrophysiological studies designed to recognize such factors except the report of Segura and Sahgal (1981). Nonetheless, peripheral injuries cannot account for the widespread denervation noted by Goldkamp (1967) and Bhala (1969).

Equivalent electrophysiological abnormalities in hemiplegic limbs have been reported in lower limb muscles well below the level of spinal cord injuries. For example, fibrillation potentials and sometimes positive sharp waves have been seen in muscles in the lower limb after spinal cord injuries as high as the cervical region (VanAlphen, Lammers, and Walder, 1962; O'Hare and Abbot, 1967; Rosen, Lerner, and Rosenthal, 1969; Nyboer and Johnson, 1971; Spielholz, Sell, Gold, Rusk, and Greens, 1972; Taylar, Kewalramani, and Fowler, 1974; Onkelinx and Chantraine, 1975; Brandstater and Dinsdale, 1976). We too have seen frequent fibrillation potentials and positive sharp waves in the trunk and lower limb muscles beginning as early as three weeks following an acute complete cervical cord transection. In general, the denervation in lower limb muscles is said to be more severe following lesions of the thoracic or high lumbosacral cord than after those of the cervical cord.

Of course, in the absence of direct pathological examination of the spinal cords in such cases, it is impossible to exclude the possibility that the lesions may extend many segments below the upper clinical level and thus directly isolate or damage anterior horn cells many segments below. It is not well appreciated, for example, that posttraumatic cavities in the syringomyelus can extend many segments below the clinical level.

Whatever the pathogenesis of denervation turns out to be in hemiplegia and paraplegia, it is important for electromyographers to be aware of its possible occurrence, the controversies involved, and the functional changes in MUs and MU recruitment patterns in the resultant upper motoneuron (pyramidal) syndrome.

TRANSCORTICAL REFLEXES

Based on evidence that motor cortical neurons can exert powerful excitatory effects on cervical motoneurons (see review by Phillips and Porter, 1977) and the demonstration that activity in pyramidal tract neurons increases with increasing resistance to movements (Evarts, 1968), Phillips (1969) postulated the existence of a transcortical stretch reflex that would serve to adjust the output of motor cortical neurons in response to changes in load imposed on movements. This hypothesis generated a wealth of studies designed to establish whether or not the necessary anatomical substrate existed to support such a reflex, and to investigate the possible physiological roles for such a presumed reflex.

One important avenue by which such presumed transcortical stretch reflexes have been

investigated has been through analysis of the successive bursts of EMG activity that occur at various early, intermediate, and later latencies (by convention labeled M1, M2 and M3 by Tatton, Bawa, Bruce, and Lee, 1978), in response to the abrupt imposition of an increase in load (resistance) or stretch in the course of a steady muscle contraction.

For example, in 1956 Hammond, Merton, and Sutton noted that when healthy subjects were instructed to flex the elbow and maintain a steady force contraction, two EMG bursts were seen in the biceps when the muscle was abruptly stretched (elbow extended). The earliest (M1) burst of EMG activity began at about 15 to 20 ms, a latency quite appropriate for the segmental stretch reflex. This was followed by a second burst (M2), whose latency was almost double that of the earlier discharge. They reasoned that the second burst (the M2 now, by convention) was too short to be voluntary because prior instruction to flex the elbow the instant the perturbation (here a stretch) was applied evoked an EMG discharge whose earliest components were much later (90 ms or more). This last voluntary component (or M3) is as might be expected, very dependent on the intent of the subject. The latencies of M1 and M2 in various muscles are shown in Table 12.5.

The identity of this intermediate burst (M2) and its subcomponents in some studies (Marsden, Merton, Morton, and Adam, 1978; Marsden, Merton, Morton, Adam, and Hallett, 1978) has been the source of enormous physiological interest and debate over the last decade (Desmedt, 1978c; Wiesendanger, 1978; Wiesendanger and Rüegg, 1978; Conrad and Meyer-Lohmann, 1980; Evarts and Fromm, 1981; Wiesendanger and Miles, 1982). Because of the possible utility of this late response in the EMG analysis of central motor disorders (see reviews by Wiesendanger and Rüegg, 1978; Desmedt, 1978; Wiesendanger and Miles, 1982), the current controversies

TABLE 12.5. Comparative Latencies of Segmental and Intermediate and Late EMG Responses to Stretch (in ms)

Muscle	M1 Spinal Response	M2 Intermediate Response	Latency Difference M2–M1	M3 Late Response
Jaw muscles				
(masseter and temporalis)	7,8	12,14	4,7	
Infraspinatus	13–15	40	25	
Pectoralis major	12	40	25	
Biceps	15	50 ±	35	90
Flexor pollicis longus	20–25	40–50	15–20	
Quadriceps	21	68	47	117
Gastrocnemius	37	108	73	157

Based on Marsden, Merton, and Morton (1976) and Chan, Melvill-Jones, Kearney, and Watt (1979).

over the identities of these responses are reviewed here.

Possible causes for the intermediate (M2) EMG responses to muscle stretch are seen in Table 12.6.

The evidence in support of a transcortical basis for the M2 is impressive. First, there is now clear evidence that both spindle primaries and secondaries project to other sensorimotor cortex (Phillips, Powell, and Wiesendanger, 1971; Wiesendanger, 1973a and 1973b). Second, the timing of the M2 response is quite appropriate for the known latencies from the periphery to the cortex and

TABLE 12.6. Basis for the Intermediate (M2) Response to Muscle Stretch

Central origin
  Transcortical reflex
  Subcortical—spino-bulbo-spinal reflex
  Spinal reflex
Peripheral origin
  Reflex response to more slowly conducting afferents
  Stretch-induced mechanical oscillations in the muscle
  Double segmental reflex loop

again from the cortex to the respective muscles (Table 12.7). Based on studies in which percutaneous stimulation of the cerebral cortex and spinal cord were done in awake volunteers, Marsden, Merton, and Morton (1982) have estimated the conduction velocities in the pyramidal pathway to cervical and lumbosacral (tibialis anterior) motoneurons to be 48 and 47 m/s respectively.

Moreover, as might be expected in such a hypothetical transcortical stretch reflex, lesions at various stations along the path including the dorsal columns, precentral and postcentral cortex, as well as the internal capsule have been shown to abolish or reduce the M2 response (Tatton, Forner, Gerstein, Chambers, and Lin, 1975; Lee and Tatton, 1975; Marsden, Merton, Morton, and Adam, 1977a, 1977b). Cooling of the precentral cortex has also been shown reversibly to block the M2 response (Wiesendanger, Rüegg, and Lachat, 1978; Chofflon, Lachat, and Rüegg, 1982) (Figure 12.1). Third, there are striking correlations between the timing and appropriateness of cortical neuron discharges and the M2 (Conrad, Meyer-Lohmann, Matsunami, and Brooks, 1975; Evarts and Fromm, 1981; Cheney and Fetz, 1978).

Also in keeping with the proposed stretch

TABLE 12.7.   Recorded or Estimated Latencies in Man:
Periphery to Cerebral Cortex and Cerebral Cortex to Periphery

	Periphery to Cortex (in ms)	Cortex to Periphery (in ms)	
Upper limb			
Median nerve stimulation (wrist)	19–20[1]	Direct cortical stimulation to	
		Facial muscles	10
		Biceps muscles	10
		Thenar muscles	17–20[2]
		Adductor pollicis muscle	23[5]
FPL to cortex	19[3]	Hand muscles	22.5[6]
Lower limb			
FHL to cortex (estimate)	41–47[3]	Tibialis anterior	34[5]
Cortical potential evoked by foot flexion	37[4]		35[6]

[1]See Chapter 5.
[2]Milner-Brown, Girvin, and Brown (1975); Brown, Milner-Brown, Ball and Girvin (1978).
[3]Marsden, Merton, and Morton (1976a).
[4]Starr, McKeon, Skuse, and Burke (1981).
[5]Merton, Morton, Hill, and Marsden (1982).
[6]Marsden, Merton, and Morton (1982).
FPL = flexor pollicis longus.
FHL = flexor hallucis longus.

reflex value of the M2, both its amplitude and the amplitude of known segmental stretch reflex, the M1, have been shown to be dependent on the amplitude and velocity of the imposed stretch. Prior instruction to the subject to resist or let go the moment the perturbation is imposed will, however, somewhat alter the amplitude of the M2 but not of the M1.

The possibility that the sensorimotor cortex could act as servo loop superimposed on the segmental stretch reflex is a very attractive hypothesis that was originally proposed by Phillips (1969). This concept has received much experimental support in the studies of the input-output relationships in the sensorimotor cortex and the firing patterns of corticospinal neurons in relation to movements, especially in response to imposed loads (see review of Wiesendanger and Miles, 1982). That the late M2 component or the EMG response to stretch is solely explicable on the basis of the proposed train cortical reflex is now, however, in growing doubt.

For example, in the cat, torque motor stretch of the triceps evokes three distinct EMG bursts. Both the M1 and M2 presumed equivalents in this animal have been shown to persist despite spinal transsection at C2–3 or decerebration (Ghez and Shinoda, 1978). It was also shown even earlier that stimulation of motor or, for that matter, cutaneous nerves in the cat evoked not only segmental reflex EMG responses but later EMG discharges, some of which were of spino-bulbo-spinal reflex origin and persisted in the decerebrate preparations (Shimamura and Akert, 1965; Shimamura, Mori, and Yamauchi, 1967). Hence it is obvious that even allowing for spe-

FIGURE 12.1. Effect of cooling the motor cortex on the H-reflex (M1) and probable equivalent of the M2 response in the monkey. In these studies the monkey was trained to maintain a steady, weak contraction of the soleus muscle. The H-reflexes were then elicited in the soleus muscle by stimuli delivered to the posterior tibial nerve (three pulses at 300-ms intervals), which intensities were submaximal for any direct M-potential. Such stimuli probably stimulated group Ia afferents more or less selectively.

At intervals following the conditioning H-reflex stimulus a second (test) stimulus was delivered. Its timing was altered in respect to the conditioning stimulus so as to assess the early and later excitability changes induced in the motoneurons at various times following the preceding conditioning afferent volleys.

Under these conditions, two periods of enhanced excitability of the motoneuron were seen, one, M1, occurring at H-latency and the second, M2, beginning at 45 ms and peaking by about 75 ms, a period of reduced excitability separating these two facilitory periods.

Following cooling of the precentral hind-limb cortical cortex, however, the late M2 response was abolished without apparently altering the earlier facilitation.

Each set of three traces represents the mean + SE obtained from three monkeys in 10 sessions each.

From Chofflon, Lachat, and Rüegg (1982, figure 3).

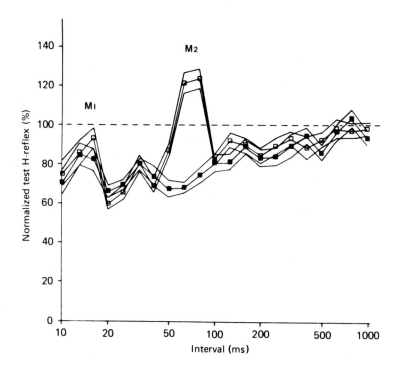

cies differences, impulses originating in muscle stretch afferents can evoke dramatic and long-lasting changes in motoneuron excitability, especially when these motoneurons operate unchecked by supraspinal control (Wiesendanger, 1978). These changes in excitabilities of motoneurons in response to cutaneous and motor afferent peripheral sensory inputs are a product of the convergence of influences originating at segmental and intersegmental spinal levels as well as possibly at the sensorimotor and cerebellar cortical levels.

More recently, in the monkey it has been shown that intermediate-latency responses persist in the presence of a variety of lesions or cold blocks in structures on the presumed transcortical pathway (Miller and Brooks, 1981) as well as in the spinal preparation (Tracey, Walmsley, and Brinkman, 1980). Whether or not these persisting intermediate responses are truly equivalent to the intermediate responses in the intact cervical spine remains in question because there may be subcortical changes in the "gating" of various reflex pathways in the presence of central lesions.

In man, the M2 response in the lower limb is lost following spinal transections between T2 and T12, although it is preserved in the upper limb above the section (Chan, Melvill-Jones, Kearney, and Watt, 1979). Further in contradistinction to experimental studies in cats and lower animals, lesions on the probable transcortical loop path in man do abolish the M2 as noted earlier (see Marsden, Merton, Morton, and Adam, 1977a, 1977b; Lee and Tatton, 1978; Chan, Melvill-Jones, Kearney, and Watt, 1979).

There is now, however, compelling evidence that the peripheral afferent volley may have much to do with generation of the intermediate response. For example, grouped spindle afferent discharges with a timing quite appropriate for generating the various grouped EMG responses to abrupt imposed stretches have been clearly shown to be present in man (Hagbarth, Hägglund, Wallin, and Young, 1981). These may be caused simply by mechanical oscillations in the limb imposed by the sudden impact imparted to the limb by the perturbing stimulus (Eklund, Hagbarth, Hägglund, and Wallin, 1982a, 1982b).

The peripheral afferents involved in the production of the intermediate EMG response may involve not only spindles but cutaneous and joint receptor afferents as well, with respect to the flexor pollicis longus muscle at least, based on the clear reduction in M2 in this muscle produced by local anesthesia or ischemia-induced block of thumb afferents. These procedures leave the flexor pollicis longus afferents in the forearm intact (Marsden, Merton, and Morton, 1977).

The possibility that more slowly conducting afferents account for the intermediate responses seems unlikely in view of the fact that the differences between the M1 and M2 latencies for proximal muscles are not less, but more than those for the distal limb muscles where the latency differences imposed by differently conducting afferents would be expected to be greater (Table 12.7).

Another possibility is that the stretch, by activating spindle secondaries, would activate the homonymous gamma motoneurons, thereby driving the spindle primaries, which in turn would activate the motoneurons through a sort of double segmental loop as suggested recently (Appleberg, Johannsson, and Kalistratov, 1977; Noth and Thilmann, 1980). Other peripheral mechanisms have also been suggested (see Wiesendanger and Miles, 1982) but their importance, like that of the above, is not established.

In summary, there is good physiological and anatomical evidence to support a transcortical reflex, but whether the gain through this loop is sufficient to account for the M2 in man is not known at this time. The fact that lesions in man along the appropriate pathway abolish the M2 does not itself establish the presence of a transcortical loop. The reported results could equally be explained by removal of a cortical or subcortical facilitation of a lower-level pathway within the spinal cord or through the brainstem. More troublesome for the transcortical hypothesis is the clear demonstration that mechanical vibration of the limb by the perturbing device itself may account for periodic motoneuron activity through repetitive activation of the spindle or possibly other receptors. Relevant experiments will have to be repeated in conditions where such mechanically evoked oscillations are substantially reduced.

At present, it must be said that until the preceding controversies are cleared up, the late EMG responses to muscle stretch are unlikely to have much clinical value in the investigation of central motor disorders.

TREMOR

Tremor is an important subject in clinical EMG because the electromyographer may be able to help distinguish among varieties of tremor by recording and quantifying the frequency and amplitude of the mechanical oscillations themselves, the accompanying MU discharges, and the effects of strategies designed to alter the tremors (see reviews by Marsden, 1978; Shahani and Young, 1978; Stein and Lee, 1981). In this chapter emphasis is placed on physiological, essential, neurogenic, and parkinsonian tremors because these are the most commonly encountered in the majority of EMG laboratories.

Tremors are involuntary rhythmic oscillations. Because the body has the twin physical properties of a spring and mass, external energy inputs to this mechanical system can induce regular oscillations. The resonant frequencies of such a mechanical system depend on the stiffness of the spring and the mass of its parts. Hence the resonant frequency (see Stiles and Randall, 1967; Joyce and Rack, 1974) of the finger is higher than that of the wrist (9 Hz) or elbow (2 Hz).

Physiological tremor (Marsden, 1978; Stein and Lee, 1981) is present in most healthy subjects. It is absent at rest, and is most easily seen in the outstretched fingers where its frequency is between 8 and 12 Hz. It is seen in other muscle groups and body parts as well, such as the tongue, or lower limbs, the frequency tending to be somewhat lower in more proximal massive components of the limbs than in distal parts. The amplitude of the tremor is increased by fatigue, anxiety, the parenteral injection of β-adrenergic agonists, diseases or conditions where there is increased endogenous catecholamine production, as well as by increases in the force of muscle contraction (Sutton and Sykes, 1967a, 1967b; Joyce and Rack, 1974).

The cause of physiological tremor is not known. Marsden (1978) has estimated, however, that the heartbeat contributes less than 10 percent to the tremor in the outstretched fingers, although the role of the heartbeat and its harmonics is suggested by the persistence of some tremor in paralyzed limbs (Marsden, 1978).

Clearly, any tendency toward grouping together of the discharges of motoneurons could impose an oscillation in muscles. Except in conditions of fatigue and isometric training (Milner-Brown, Stein, and Lee, 1975), however, MUs normally discharge asynchronously. It has been suggested, that the unfused twitches of the larger-tension MUs normally recruited only by moderate or stronger contractions could evoke noticeable mechanical oscillations in a muscle (Dietz and

Allum, 1975). This seems an unlikely mechanism in the majority of contractions where several muscles are coactivated. Contracting muscles because of the prolonged duration of individual twitches, do act as low-pass filters, tending to filter out the higher-frequency components of tremors.

The role of the stretch reflex in physiological tremor is uncertain. Lippold (1970) showed that perturbations applied to the outstretched fingers produce oscillations at about 10 Hz associated with grouped MU potential discharges in phase with the oscillation. This suggested that the stretch reflex here behaved as an undamped servosystem. Such tremor, however, may persist when the limb has been deafferented (Marsden, Meadows, Lange, and Watson, 1967; Marsden, 1978). Moreover, the tremor frequency is apparently not altered when the conduction velocities are slowed in peripheral neuropathies or by differences in the reflex loop time, which would be significantly shorter for proximal muscles and would be expected to support faster frequencies for these as compared to distal muscles in the limbs. The converse turns out to be the case, the frequency of tremor in the proximal muscles being less, not higher than for distal muscles. The higher frequencies possible for proximal muscles through the shorter loop times may be more than compensated for by the damping effect of the much greater mass of the proximal limb.

Marsden has drawn attention to the possible importance of intramuscular β-adrenergic receptors in the genesis of physiological tremor. The intraarterial injection of isoproterenol into a limb increases the tremor in that limb and this effect is abolished by intraarterial injection of β-adrenergic blocking agents such as propranolol into the same limb. β-Adrenergic agonists may act directly on muscle spindle sensitivity (Hodgson, Marsden, and Meadows, 1969).

Thus, although the precise cause of physiological tremor is unknown, the firing patterns of MUs, stretch reflex, peripheral β-adrenergic receptors within the muscle, and the mechanical properties all seem to play a role.

Benign Essential Tremor

This tremor, about 4 to 8 Hz in older persons and higher (8 to 10 Hz) in younger adults in the outstretched fingers, is like physiological tremor: absent at rest and brought out when muscles are posturally active, such as when the arms and hands are outstretched, or when the head is erect in subjects with a prominent head tremor. It may also be accentuated in point-to-point movements such as finger-nose testing, this often being described as an intention component to the tremor.

There is often a strong family history of this tremor, which, although it may begin in early life, frequently becomes more apparent (larger amplitude) in the later decades. In some older subjects, the head, speech, or limb components of tremor may become very coarse and troublesome.

The tremor is improved by alcohol and, like physiological tremor, is aggravated by β-adrenergic agonists and improved by propranolol. Unlike physiological tremor, intraarterial propranolol apparently does not suppress tremor in the limb in which the injection is made (Young, Growdon, and Shahani, 1975).

The EMG recordings show that MUPs tend to discharge in bursts sometimes, although not always synchronously in agonists and antagonists, and demonstrate instantaneous firing frequencies of 20 to 50 Hz, very comparable with those seen in ballistic contractions.

A role for the peripheral reflex in essential tremor is suggested by the observation that as in physiological tremor, peripheral perturbations can alter the phase of the tremor (Stein, Lee, and Nichols, 1978; Lee and Stein, 1981).

Parkinsonian Tremor

Classically, parkinsonian tremor occurs at 4 to 7 Hz and is present at rest, but not in action. Not uncommonly, however, it may persist and even increase in amplitude in the course of movements.

A broader frequency range (4 to 9 Hz) in parkinsonian tremor has been described by Stiles and Pozos (1976), the frequency varying inversely with amplitude. Muscle contraction generally increases the apparent frequency of the tremor (Rondot and Bathien, 1978). The EMG records high instantaneous discharge frequencies lasting two to three impulses in the bursts that accompany the tremor (Shahani and Young, 1978). These EMG bursts tend to alternate in agonist and antagonist muscles, although this is not invariably the case (Stein and Lee, 1981). The rank order of recruitment of MUs in Parkinson's disease is not altered, but the onset frequencies of the MUs are usually lower (4 to 6 Hz) than normal (Milner-Brown, Fisher, and Weiner, 1979).

Incidentally, these three authors also showed that in Parkinson's disease, MU recruitment is altered in other ways, namely, there are long delays sometimes between the beginning of the effort and recruitment of the first MUs (20 to 180 ms). Patients may experience great difficulties maintaining steady discharges even among the lower-threshold MUs, some discharges ceasing despite the patient's persistent efforts for up to 3 minutes.

THE H-REFLEX

The general characteristics of the H-reflex and one method of eliciting it were outlined in Chapter 3 (see Figure 3.30). In this chapter our primary concern is with the recovery cycle of the H-reflex and its subsequent use to evaluate changes in the excitability of motoneurons in central motor disorders.

Recovery Cycle of the H-reflex

Following the discharges of motoneurons in the H-reflex, the excitabilities of the motoneurons are altered for up to 5 seconds. The degree of such facilitation or depression of motoneuron excitability may be assessed by measuring the changes in the amplitude of an H-reflex induced by a *test stimulus* delivered at various times following a preceding *conditioning H stimulus* to the motor nerve. The recovery cycle so studied passes through several phases (see review by Wiesendanger, 1972).

First, there is early facilitation that reaches its peak by about 10 ms. This is followed by a depression (early depression), lasting about 10 ms, followed in turn by an interval of partial but incomplete recovery of motoneuron excitability. This reaches its maximum at about 200 ms and is followed by still a later depression. The whole cycle may not be complete for as long as 5 seconds.

Explanations for these phases are all speculative at this time. Such changes in the excitabilities of motoneurons in the wake of motoneuron discharges induced by H-reflexes could, however, be produced as follows:

Early events:

1. Early monosynaptic excitatory postsynaptic potentials, in some cases terminated and followed by disynaptically induced inhibitory postsynaptic potentials.
2. Afterpotentials as a direct consequence of the spikes in the motoneurons
3. Possible recurrent inhibition of the Renshaw cells of the motoneurons
4. Central effects of other more slowly conducting cutaneous and deeper afferents that may also have been excited by the stimulus

Later events:

1. Late excitability changes produced by intersegmental spinal and spino-bulbo-spinal reflexes
2. Peripheral muscle contraction-induced afferent volleys in various muscle and tendon receptors

Once above motor threshold, antidromic impulses in motor axons may directly invade the soma of the motoneurons producing long-lasting afterpotentials, regenerative spikes, and possibly, recurrent inhibition and direct and indirect excitation of neighboring motoneurons (see Chapter 3).

Whatever the explanation, the important point is that for practical use, the H-reflex should not be elicited at intervals of much less than 2 seconds to avoid depression of the response.

At stimulus intensities exceeding motor threshold, the late response is a combination of H- and F-responses. The only certain way to separate the two is by section of the dorsal roots to interrupt the reflex arc on which the H-response depends, leaving the F-response intact (Gassel and Wiesendanger, 1965).

Synaptic Basis of the H-reflex

In the cat, impulses in single Ia afferents produce unitary excitatory postsynaptic potentials (EPSPs) in motoneurons, whose amplitudes are of an order of about 0.1 mV. To exceed threshold for spike generation in motoneurons the compound EPSP must exceed 5 to 10 mV. Hence, to generate postsynaptic spikes in motoneurons, impulses in close to 50 to 100 Ia afferents must reach the motoneuron membrane at more or less the same time (Henneman and Mendell, 1971; Henneman and Mendell, 1981). In man, by indirect

methods, it has been learned that about 60 unitary (single) Ia EPSPs are necessary to depolarize the motoneuronal membrane beyond threshold and generate impulses in soleus motoneurons (McComas, Mirsky, Velho, and Struppler, 1979). In this muscle, the number of spindles has been estimated to be about 300 (McComas, 1977). Thus in the human, orthodromic impulses in at least 20 percent or more of the population of soleus Ia afferents would be needed to generate postsynaptic spikes in soleus motoneurons.

The amplitudes of the compound EPSPs in single motoneurons produced by the afferent inputs in the H-reflex are probably close to and often just barely exceed the thresholds for spike generation on the respective motoneurons. This, and slight fluctuations in the times to peak of the compound EPSPs, is probably responsible for variations in latencies of motoneuron spikes and MUPs from impulse to impulse. These fluctuations in latency exceed by two to three times the variability in latency of single MUs in the F- and direct M-response (Trontelj, 1973; also see Chapter 3). Buchthal and Schmalbruch (1970) have suggested that it is the slower-twitch MUs that preferentially participate in the human soleus H-reflex.

Whether or not the H-reflex is obtainable and the amplitude of the H-reflex may depend not only on the strength of the afferent volley in the spindle afferents, but possibly in some cases on the central effects of other afferents excited by the peripheral electrical stimulus. Electrical stimuli even near threshold for the H-reflex may excite Golgi tendon organs as well, and more intense stimuli could also excite group II muscle and cutaneous mechanoreceptor nerve fibers within the nerve trunk. Percutaneous stimuli may also excite cutaneous and subcutaneous nerve fibers deep and just within the skin as well as in the underlying nerve trunk itself. Theoretically, however, central events of these other afferents should follow, not precede, the actions of the primary spindle afferents because of the latter's faster conduction velocities (Diamantopoulos and Gassel, 1965; Gassel and Diamantopoulos, 1965, 1966). Whether conduction velocities of spindle afferents are in all instances faster than those of other afferents in man remains to be established. Until this is known it is not safe to assume that other afferents play no part in the central excitation or depression of motoneurons in the H-reflex.

The excitability of motoneurons and thus the amplitude of the H-reflex could also be expected to be altered by changes in some other segmental, intersegmental, and suprasegmental influences on motoneurons (see discussion to follow on the tendon reflex). Other factors influencing the H-reflex are shown in Table 12.8.

Use of the H-reflex to Assess Central Excitability of Motoneurons

The H-reflex may be altered by lesions of the cerebral hemisphere. Such alterations include:

1. The H-reflex may be elicited in muscles where normally it is seldom seen, such as in the biceps intrinsic muscles of the hand, tibialis anterior, extensor digitorum longus, or peroneal or foot muscles.
2. There may be an increase in the ratio of the amplitude of the H- to the M-potentials indicating a larger proportion of MUs participating in the H-reflex.

These changes probably are indications of increased central excitabilities of the motoneurons.

3. The late period of facilitation may begin earlier and be enhanced.

TABLE 12.8.   Factors Altering the H-Reflex

Sleep	Sleep reduces the amplitude of the H-reflex.
Vibration	Vibration, through occlusion or presynaptic inhibition reduces the amplitude of the H-reflex (Hagbarth and Eklund, 1966a, 1966b; Lance, Gail, and Nielson, 1966).
Contraction of muscles	Agonist contractions facilitate H-reflexes when the contractions are moderate; as the contractions become stronger, the amplitude of the H-reflex may be reduced. The latter also may be produced through contraction of antagonist muscles (Wiesendanger, 1972). Moderate contraction of the agonist muscle may facilitate the H-reflex, whereas stronger contractions may actually reduce the H-reflex amplitude, an effect also produced by contraction of antagonist muscles (Wiesendanger, 1972).
Drugs	For discussion of the effects of various drugs on the H-reflex, see Gassel (1973) and Brunia (1973).
Jendrassik maneuver	This may facilitate the H-reflex somewhat, but not as much as the corresponding facilitation of the tendon reflex. Sometimes the Jendrassik maneuver may even reduce the H-reflex (see Wiesendanger, 1972).

4. Subjects may experience difficulty potentiating the H-reflex on the affected side.

In healthy subjects, voluntary contractions of muscles superimposed on supramaximal electrical stimuli delivered to the motor nerve enhances the late EMG potential seen at H and F latencies. Such facilitation is seen in both the upper limb (thenar and hypothenar) muscles and in the lower limb (tibialis anterior) muscle (Upton, McComas, and Sica, 1971; Sica, McComas, and Upton, 1971). These authors reported that 16 of 17 patients who had mild upper motoneuron deficits were only partially able or sometimes completely unable to potentiate the late response (Figure 12.2).

These changes are complex because such late EMG discharges are probably primarily made up of recurrent F-responses and not H-reflex potentials. Such supramaximal stimuli could be expected to all but abolish the H-reflex volley through collision of the reflex volley with the antidromic volley.

As a final point, in normal muscles, vibration reduces the amplitude of the H-reflex possibly through a combination of occlusion and presynaptic inhibition. In the presence of hemisphere lesions, the degree of such suppression of the H-reflex by vibration is apparently reciprocally related to the degree of spasticity in the muscles. This may be related somehow to impairment of the supraspinal regulation of presynaptic inhibition of group Ia afferents as has been suggested by Delwaide (1970).

Relationship Between the H-reflex and Tendon Reflex

The tendon jerk (TJ) is the clinical equivalent of the H-reflex, both being mediated by activation of motoneurons by the primary spindle afferents. Beyond this, however, there are important distinctions between the TJ and H-reflex (see Table 3.12; also see Gassel and Diamantopoulos, 1966). For example, the TJ depends on a tendon tap to stretch abruptly the intramuscular spindle receptors. Stretching the spindles evokes a burst of impulses in the spindle primary and secondary afferents, the primaries producing monosynaptically induced discharges in the related motoneurons.

The sensitivity of the spindle to stretch may be altered by changing the level of fusimotor activity. Enhanced fusimotor activity lowers the threshold of the spindle organ to imposed stretches and increases the size of resultant discharges in the spindle afferents, especially those exhibiting the greatest dynamic sensitivity, namely, the spindle primaries (see Matthews, 1972, 1981). Recent studies suggest that when muscles are relaxed, gamma motor activity is absent (Burke, McKeon, and Skuse, 1981a). Indeed, there is some indication that the Jendrassik maneuver used by clinicians to facilitate TRs exerts its facilitory effects not through enhanced fusimotor drive to the spin-

FIGURE 12.2. (Top) Early direct and late M-responses recorded from the thenar muscles in response to supramaximal median nerve stimulation at the wrist when the patient was relaxed. Shown are responses on both the normal (left) and hemiparetic sides (right).
(Bottom) Maximal voluntary contraction. Note failure to potentiate the late EMG response on the hemiparetic side.
From Sica, McComas, and Upton (1971, figure 1).

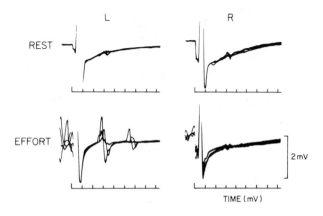

dles, thus increasing the dynamic sensitivity of the spindles to imposed stretch, but rather through more direct central increases in the excitabilities of the motoneurons (Burke, McKeon, and Skuse, 1981b). Alterations in the amplitude of TJ produced through pain, changes in attention, or the Jendrassik maneuver are not apparently accompanied by any change in the activities of spindle afferents. Such central facilitation of the TJ does not explain the lack of equivalent facilitation of the H-reflex by the same maneuver (Wiesendanger, 1972).

The temporally dispersed nature of the afferent volley evoked by tendon taps in comparison to the much more synchronous volley in the H-reflex is explained by the activation of the afferents through their receptor endorgans in the former and the bypassing of these receptors through activation of the afferents at one site in the latter. For example, the spindle receptors in the quadriceps muscles are widely dispersed throughout these expansive muscles. Because of this there are appreciable differences in conduction distances among various receptors and the related spinal cord segments. Also, these spatially dispersed receptors are not all activated at the same time because it requires a finite time for the tendon tap-induced traveling stretch wave to reach the receptors because of the viscoelastic properties of the tendons and muscles. These two factors account for the temporally dispersed nature of the afferent volley (Delwaide, 1970). Also, many afferents repetitively fire in response to such a stimulus. Even in smaller muscles, where differences in activation times of the stretch receptors should be less and their conduction distances to the spinal cord more uniform, the centripetal volley may be appreciably temporally dispersed.

The rise times of the compound EPSPs in soleus motoneurons evoked in response to Achilles tendon taps are long—8.3 ms ± 2.5 ms (1 SD)—when compared to those of the much less temporally dispersed group Ia compound EPSPs (3.5 to 5.5 ms) temporally evoked by electrical stimulation of the posterior tibial nerve in the popliteal fossa (Homma and Nakajima, 1979). The longer durations and slower rise times characteristic of the EPSPs evoked by tendon tap help to explain their longer latencies and the greater variabilities in the latencies of single MUPs in the tendon jerk versus the H-reflex-induced EMG discharges. Indeed, the compound EPSPs evoked by tendon taps are sufficiently dispersed in time to suggest that disynaptic and trisynaptic connections to the motoneurons may contribute to the EMG discharges evoked by the tendon taps. Both disynaptic and trisynaptic group Ia connections to homonymous motoneurons have been described in the cat (Watt, Stauffer, Taylor, Reinking, and Stuart, 1976) and may also exist in man. Single taps may, as well, trigger repetitive discharges in the spindle afferents.

The longer latency of the TJ in relation to the H-reflex is probably explained by the longer afferent paths (receptors to spinal cord), the necessary prior activation of the receptors, and the extra times required because of the temporally dispersed nature of the afferent volley to generate a large enough compound EPSP amplitude to generate spikes in the motoneurons. For example, the latency of the knee jerk (18 ms) is about 4 ms longer than the comparable H-reflex latency in the rectus femoris muscle.

The amplitude of EMG discharges produced by the H-reflex usually exceeds those in the TJ, possibly because tendon taps may also activate Golgi tendon organs with a consequent disynaptic inhibition of homonymous motoneurons.

Both the H-reflex and tendon reflexes have a place in EMG. The TJ is the easiest way to assess central conduction times in certain muscle groups such as the biceps or triceps, or other muscles where the motor nerves are less conveniently stimulated or H-reflexes are normally hard to obtain (Diamantopoulos and Gassel, 1965). The H-reflexes, however, have the advantage that their latencies are more constant and reproducible and the fusimotor and receptor mechanisms are bypassed.

TONIC VIBRATION REFLEX

One interesting development in clinical neurophysiology has been the introduction of vibration to the investigation of muscle tone. In the human, vibration of a muscle or tendon through the skin at amplitudes exceeding 1 mm (about 100 times that required by vibratory stimuli applied directly to the muscle or tendon in experimental preparations) at a frequency of about 100 Hz evokes an initial phasic EMG burst. This burst is followed by a silent period lasting about 100 ms that is in turn followed by a slowly increasing EMG discharge and mounting tension in the muscle, reaching a maximum in about 1/2 to 1 minute. This last tonic vibration response is enhanced by voluntary contraction, the Jendrassik maneuver, and passive lengthening of the muscle. The tonic vibration reflex (TVR) response may be reduced by cerebral lesions, and in patients with cord transections no TVR may be observed (Lance, Burke, and Andrews, 1973).

The TVR response is probably mediated through selective excitation of muscle stretch receptors and the subsequent activation of motoneurons by direct and multisynaptic (Ia) connections (Hagbarth and Eklund, 1968; Marsden, Meadows, and Hodgson, 1969; Delwaide, 1973). The absence of the TVR response seen shortly after supraspinal lesions is perhaps explained by hyperpolarization of the motoneurons (Barnes and Pompeiano, 1970a, 1970b), and possible increases in the thresholds to monosynaptic EPSPs seen at this time (McCouch, Liu, and Chambers, 1966).

The tendon and H-reflexes and the TVRs have all been used to investigate the various functional abnormalities that occur following spinal cord lesions (see review by Ashby and Verrier, 1975). These may be divided according to time following the functional transections of the spinal cord. For example, in the immediate period following spinal transection, the H-reflexes may be normal but the tendon reflexes hard to evoke, perhaps because of transient reductions in the amount of fusimotor drive. Within days, however, the tendon reflexes may recover and even become enhanced, whereas the TVR is reduced or absent and continues to remain so. The reason for the latter is not at all clear but may result from reduced multisynaptic Ia drives to the motoneurons. The fact that vibration may reduce the H-reflex even more following spinal cord transections compared to normal suggests that presynaptic inhibition may somehow be enhanced following cord transection. The latter effect can last several months.

Recently, Nelson and colleagues have demonstrated increases in the amplitudes of Ia monosynaptic EPSPs on spinal motoneurons below a cord transection that appeared within hours following the transection (Nelson, Collatos, Niechaj, and Mendell, 1979; Nelson and Mendell, 1979). Such changes occur too early for a mechanism such as collateral sprouting to account for the enhancement of EPSP amplitude. They could indicate immediate changes in the postsynaptic membrane response to the presynaptic inputs or, more likely, enhancement of the presynaptic release at individual boutons or perhaps the recruitment into action of boutons of Ia afferents previously silent. Longer-term increases in EPSP amplitude may, of course, also reflect expanded innervation by Ia afferents of the motoneurons through collateral sprouting to occupy regions of the motoneurons vacated because of the loss of central projections to the motoneuron severed by the original lesion. There is also some indication that repetitive stimulation of dorsal root afferents may produce enlargement of spinal cord synapses (Illis, 1969).

After a variable period the tendon reflexes may become enhanced even though muscle tone may continue to be reduced. There may also be reduction in the degree of apparent presynaptic inhibition thought to be present at this stage.

These physiological changes that follow spinal cord transections or lesions in the cerebral hemisphere cannot be interpreted solely on the basis of the known normal central connections and functional relations. There may be important remodeling of the central reflex pathways and input connections to motoneurons (McCouch, Austin, Liu, and Liu, 1958; Goldberger and Murray, 1978; Bernstein, Wells, and Bernstein, 1978; Goldberger, 1980; Liu and Chambers, 1980; Bernstein and Bernstein, 1980; Veraa and Grafstein, 1981). Such changes include:

1. The degeneration of presynaptic connections to motoneurons. Fiber system projecting to motoneurons may be interrupted by rostral lesions. Their terminals may subsequently degenerate with consequent loss of their contributions to the excitability of the motoneuron.
2. The development of denervation hypersensitivity in motoneurons.
3. Central reinnervation by collateral sprouting. There is now considerable evidence that terminal and preterminal sprouts originating in other preserved presynaptic connections to neurons may occupy regions of the neuronal membrane vacated by degenerated terminals of other input connections to the neuron interrupted by various lesions (Goldberger, 1974).

   The enhancement of the stretch reflex often seen following transection of the spinal cord may be partially explained by

denervation hypersensitivity. Motoneurons and their related interneurons, deprived of their connections to more rostral neurons may become abnormally sensitive to the normal segmental inputs of muscle stretch receptors. As collateral sprouts of dorsal root afferents come to occupy regions of the motoneuronal membrane vacated by the degenerated terminals of the supraspinal connections, the reflex response to these segmental inputs may become enhanced, thereby altering the pattern of reflex activity through establishment of these new synaptic connections.

4. Activation of other, previously marginal inputs. Possibly through collateral sprouting as well as direct alterations in the excitabilities of the motoneuronal membrane, previously marginal inputs may become quantitively more important and more powerful synaptic drives to the motoneurons.

The above mechanisms together with other possible changes in central connections produced through training and conditioning may well explain many of the functional changes that follow supraspinal or spinal lesions.

THE BABINSKI REFLEX

The subject of spasticity (see Bishop, 1977; Clemente, 1978; Lance and McLeod, 1981) is excluded from this review of the central motor disorders in EMG. The Babinski reflex, however, is included because it is one of the most important signs in neurology, and EMG may be of value in its detection and confirmation.

The Babinski response (see review by Brodal, 1981) is elicited by stroking the ball and hollow of the sole of the foot with a key, pin, or other noxious mechanical stimulus. This stimulus provokes flexion of the first toe and

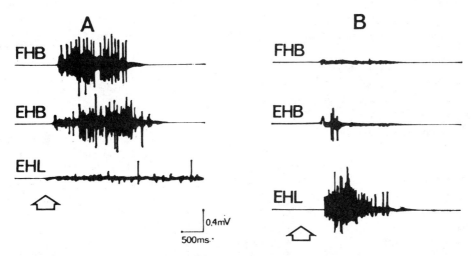

FIGURE 12.3.   Reflex activity in the flexor hallucis brevis (FHB), extensor hallucis brevis (EHB), and extensor hallucis longus (EHL) as elicited by mechanical stimulation at the times indicated by arrows in a normal subject (A) and patient with a Babinski sign (B). Note the enhanced activity in EHL and accompanied by diminished activity in the FHB and EHB muscles.
From VanGijn (1975, figure 1).

possible flexion of the other toes in the healthy subject. The reflex varies and is critically dependent on the regions stimulated. Thus noxious stimulation of the pads of the toes evokes dorsiflexion of the first toe as part of a normal general flexion reflex response, which includes plantar flexion of the toes and flexion at the ankle, knee, and hip. In the abnormal situation, the same noxious stimulus delivered to the ball or hollow of the foot evokes dorsiflexion of the first toe and possible abduction or fanning of the other toes.

Electrophysiological studies reveal several points:

1.   In normal subjects, stroking the skin along the plantar arch and border of the foot evokes EMG activity in the extensor hallucis brevis (EHB) and flexor hallucis brevis (FHB) but not the extensor hallucis longus (EHL).
2.   In those patients with the Babinski sign

EMG activity in EHL exceeds that in EHB and is synchronous with EMG activity in other flexor muscles, including the tensor fasciae latae and hamstring muscles (Figure 12.3).
3.   Mechanical stimulation is a more reliable way of eliciting normal and abnormal plantar responses than electrical stimuli delivered to the skin.
4.   EMG, by recording from active muscles, can improve the clinical interpretation of equivocal plantar responses (VanGijn, 1975, 1976).

From his clinical and EMG experience, VanGijn suggests certain criteria for a pathological plantar response. These include:

1.   Dorsiflexion of the first toe is abnormal only when it is the result of activity in EHL.
2.   EHL contraction is abnormal only when

synchronous EMG activity is seen in other flexor muscles, such as the hamstrings and tensor fasciae latae.

3. Voluntary withdrawal lasts longer than the pathological extensor plantar response, but voluntary retraction is diminished, lost, or inconstant with repeated stimulation, whereas the flexion reflex remains constant.

Transection of the pyramidal tract in the higher primates does produce an extensor plantar response (Wiesendanger, 1969); similarly, lesions in area 4 in the high primates produce extensor plantar responses (Fulton, 1936). In man, however, there is no instance of a confirmed lesion restricted to the pyramidal tract with which to compare the observations in the lower primates (Wiesendanger, 1973; Brodal, 1981). Moreover, there is evidence that the Babinski sign may be present with sparing of the cortical spinal tract (lateral) in the spinal cord and conversely, absent with lesions in the latter (Nathan and Smith, 1955), disagreements notwithstanding (Walsch, 1956). The question then remains whether interruption of the pyramidal tract or fiber projections exclusive to it at other levels of the neuraxis for the Babinski response to occur.

The Babinski sign occupies a special place in clinical neurology. If its importance as a sign can be equated with the time spent debating its presence or absence in particular patients, it assumes an extraordinary importance indeed. It may be absent, however, in cases where the descending motor tracts are clearly affected as evidenced by spasticity, hyperreflexion, and even weakness (see earlier discussion in this chapter).

The role of the electromyographer in the resolving debates as to whether a true Babinski sign is present is limited. The studies of VanGijn help in that they suggest that the true Babinski as opposed to a withdrawal response is signaled by activity in EHL when accompanied by activity in other flexor muscles as well.

References

Andreassen, S, Rosenfalck A. Recording from a single motor unit during strong effort. IEEE Trans Biomed Eng 1979;6:501–08.

Appleberg B, Johannsson H, Kalistratov G. The influence of group II muscle afferents and low threshold skin afferents on dynamic fusimotor neurons to the triceps of the cat. Brain Res 1977;132:153–58.

Asanuma H. The pyramidal tract. In: Brooks VB, ed. Handbook of physiology. The nervous system, Vol. 2. Motor control. Bethesda, Md.: American Physiological Society, 1981:203–33.

Ashby P, Verrier M. Neurophysiological changes following spinal cord lesions in man. Can J Neurol Sci 1975;2:91–100.

Barnes CD, Powpeiano O. Inhibition of monosynaptic extensor reflex attributable to presynaptic depolarization of group Ia afferent fibers produced by vibration of flexor muscle. Arch Ital Biol 1970a;108:233–58.

Barnes CD, Powpeiano O. Presynaptic and postsynaptic effects in the monosynaptic pathway to extensor motoneurons following vibration of synergic muscles. Arch Ital Biol 1970b;108:259–94.

Bernstein JJ, Bernstein ME. Plasticity in the damaged spinal cord. In: Windle WF, ed. The spinal cord and its reaction to traumatic injury. New York: Marcel Dekker, 1980:237–47.

Bernstein JJ, Wells MR, Bernstein ME. Spinal cord regeneration synaptic renewal and neurochemistry. In: Cotman CW, ed. Neuronal plasticity. New York: Raven Press, 1978:49–72.

Bhala RP. Electromyographic evidence of lower motor neuron involvement in hemiplegia. Arch Phys Med Rehabil 1969;50:632–38.

Bishop B. Spasticity: its physiology and management. Phys Ther 1977;57:371–401.

Brandstater ME, Dinsdale SM. Electromyographic studies in the assessment of spinal cord lesions. Arch Phys Med Rehabil 1976;57:70–74.

Brissaud E. De' l'atrophie musculaire dans l'hemi-plegie. Rev Mensalle Med Chir 1879;616–25.

Brodal A. Neurological anatomy in relation to clinical medicine. 3rd ed. Oxford: Oxford University Press, 1981.

Brooke MH, Engel WK. The histographic analysis of human muscle biopsies with regard to fiber types. II. Diseases of the upper and lower motor neurons. Neurology 1969;19:378–93.

Brooks VB. The nervous system. In: Brooks VB, ed. Handbook of physiology. The nervous system. Vol. 2. Motor control. Bethesda, Md.: American Physiological Society, 1981.

Brooks VB, Stoney SD. Motor mechanisms: the role of the pyramidal system in motor control. Ann Rev Physiol 1971;33:337–92.

Brown WF, Milner-Brown HS, Ball M, Girvin JP. Control of the motor cortex on spinal motoneu-rones in man. In: Desmedt JE, ed. Cerebral motor control in man: long loop mechanisms. Progress in Clinical Neurophysiology. Vol. 4. Basel: Karger, 1978:246–62.

Brunia AHM. The influence of diazepam and chlorpromazine on the Achilles tendon and H reflexes. In: Desmedt JE, ed. New developments in electromyography and clinical neurophysiology. Vol. 3. Basel: Karger, 1973:367–70.

Buchthal F, Schmalbruch H. Contraction times of twitches evoked by H reflexes. Acta Physiol Scand 1970;80:378–82.

Burke D, McKeon B, Skuse NF. The irrelevance of fusimotor activity to the Achilles tendon jerk of relaxed humans. Ann Neurol 1981a;10:547–50.

Burke D, McKeon B, Skuse NF. Dependence of the Achilles tendon reflex on the excitability of spinal reflex pathways. Ann Neurol 1981b;10:551–56.

Burke RE, Rodomin P, Zajac FE. The effect of activation history on tension production by in-dividual muscle units. Brain Res 1976;109:515–29.

Chan CWY, Melvill-Jones G, Kearney RE, Watt DGD. The "late" electromyographic response to limb displacement in man. I. Evidence for supraspinal contribution. Electroencephalogr Clin Neurophysiol 1979;46:173–81.

Charcot JM. Lectures on disease of the nervous system. Translated and edited by G Sigerson. Philadelphia: Lea & Febiger, 1879.

Cheney PD, Fetz EE. Functional properties of primate corticomotoneuronal cells. Soc Neurol Sci Abst 1978;4:393.

Chofflon M, Lachat JM, Rüegg DG. A transcortical loop demonstrated by stimulation of low-threshold muscle afferents in the awake monkey. J Physiol 1982;323:393–402.

Chokroverty S, Medina J. Electrophysiological study of hemiplegia. Arch Neurol 1978;35:360–63.

Chokroverty S, Reyes MG, Rubino FA, Barron KD. Hemiplegic amyotrophy muscle and motor point biopsy study. Arch Neurol 1976;33:104–10.

Clemente C. Neurophysiologic mechanisms and neuroanatomic substrates related to spasticity. Neurology 1978;28:40–45.

Conrad B, Meyer-Lohmann J. The long loop transcortical load compensating reflex. Trends Neurosci 1980;1:269–72.

Conrad B, Meyer-Lohmann J, Matsunami K, Brooks VB. Precentral unit activity following torque pulse injection into elbow movements. Brain Res 1975;94:219–36.

Cook WH, Walker JH, Barr ML. A cytological study of transneuronal atrophy in the cat and rabbit. J Comp Neurol 1951;94:267–91.

Critchley M. The parietal lobes. London: Edward Arnold, 1953.

Delwaide PJ. Etude expérimentale de l'hyper ré-flexie tendineuse en clinique neurologique. Brussels: Thèse Arsia, 1970.

Delwaide PJ. Human monosynaptic reflexes and presynaptic inhibition. An interpretation of spastic hyper reflexia. In: Desmedt JE, ed. New developments in electromyography and clinical neurophysiology. Vol. 3. Basel: Karger, 1973:508–22.

Desmedt, JE. Human reflexes, pathophysiology of motor systems, methodology of human reflexes. In: Desmedt JE, ed. New developments in electromyography and clinical neurophysiology. Vol. 3. Basel: Karger, 1973.

Desmedt JE, ed. Cerebral motor control in man: long loop mechanisms. Progress in clinical neurophysiology. Vol. 4. Basel: Karger, 1978a;

Desmedt JE. Physiological tremor, pathological

tremors and clonus. In: Desmedt JE, ed. Progress in clinical neurophysiology. Basel: Karger, 1978b.

Desmedt JE. Motor control in man: suprasegmental and segmental mechanisms. In: Desmedt, JE, ed. Progress in clinical neurophysiology. Vol. 8. Basel: Karger, 1978c.

Desmedt JE. Recruitment patterns of motor units and the gradation of muscle force. In: Desmedt JE, ed. Progress in clinical neurophysiology. Vol. 9. Basel: Karger, 1978d.

Diamantopoulos E, Gassel MM. Electrically induced monosynaptic reflexes in man. J Neurol Neurosurg Psychiatry 1965;28:496–502.

Dietz V, Allum JHJ. Physiological tremor and its relationship to single motor unit discharges. Pflugers Arch 1975;355(suppl R84).

Edstrom L. Selective changes in the sizes of red and white muscles fibers in upper motor lesions and Parkinsonism. J Neurol Sci 1970;11:537–50.

Edstrom L, Grimby L, Hannerz J. Correlation between recruitment order of motor units and muscle atrophy pattern in upper motoneurone lesion—significance of spasticity. Experientia (Basel) 1972;29:560–61.

Eklund G, Hagbarth KE, Hägglund JV, Wallin EU. Mechanical oscillations contributing to the segmentation of the reflex electromyogram responses to muscle stretch. J Physiol 1982a; 326:65–77.

Eklund G, Hagbarth KE, Hägglund JV, Wallin EU. The "late" reflex responses to muscle stretch: the "resonance hypothesis" versus the "long-loop hypothesis." J Physiol 1982b;326:79–90.

Evarts EV. Relation of pyramidal tract activity to force exerted during voluntary movement. J Neurophysiol 1968;31:14–27.

Evarts EV, Fromm C. Transcortical reflexes and servo control of movements. Can J Physiol Pharmacol 1981;59:757–75.

Felix D, Wiesendanger M. Pyramidal and non-pyramidal motor cortical effects on distal fore-limb muscles of monkeys. Exp Brain Res 1971;12:81–91.

Freund H. Motor unit and muscle activity in voluntary motor control. Physiol Rev 1983;63:387–436.

Freund HJ, Dietz V, Wita CW, Kapp H. Discharge characteristics of single motor units in normal subjects and patients with supraspinal motor disturbances. In: Desmedt JE, ed. New developments in electromyography and clinical neurophysiology. Vol. 3. Basel: Karger, 1973:242–50.

Fulton JF. The interrelation of cerebrum and cerebellum in the regulation of somatic and autonomic functions. Medicine 1936;15:247–306.

Gassel MM. An objective technique for the analysis of the clinical effectiveness and physiology of action of drugs in man. In: Desmedt JE, ed. New developments in electromyography and clinical neurophysiology. Vol. 3. Basel: Karger, 1973:349–59.

Gassell MM, Diamantopoulos E. Nerve potential recording during electrically and mechanically evoked monosynaptic reflexes in man. Nature (London) 1965;208:1004–05.

Gassel MM, Diamantopoulos E. Mechanically and electrically elicited monosynaptic reflexes in man. J Appl Physiol 1966;21:1053–58.

Gassel MM, Wiesendanger M. Recurrent and reflex discharges in plantar muscles of the cat. Acta Physiol Scand 1965;65:138–42.

Ghez C, Shinoda Y. Spinal mechanisms of the functional stretch reflex. Exp Brain Res 1978; 32:55–68.

Goldberger ME. Recovery of movement after CNS lesions in monkeys. In: Stein DG, Rosen JJ, Butters N, eds. Plasticity and recovery of function in the central nervous system. New York: Academic Press, 1974:265–337.

Goldberger ME. Motor recovery after lesions. Trends Neurosci 1980;3:288–91.

Goldberger ME, Murray M. Recovery of movement and axonal sprouting may obey some of the same laws. In: Cotman CW, ed. Neuronal plasticity. New York: Raven Press, 1978:73–96.

Goldby F. A note on transneuronal atrophy in the human lateral geniculate body. J Neurol Neurosurg Psychiatry 1957;20:202–7.

Goldkamp O. Electromyography and nerve conduction studies in 116 patients with hemiplegia. Arch Phys Med 1967;48:59–63.

Granit R. The basis of motor control. London: Academic Press, 1970.

Grimby L, Hannerz J. Tonic and phasic recruitment order of motor units in man under normal and pathological conditions. In: Desmedt JE, ed. New developments in electromyography and clinical neurophysiology. Vol. 3. Basel: Karger, 1973:225–33.

Grimby L, Hannerz J, Ranlund T. Disturbances in the voluntary recruitment order of anterior tibial motor units in spastic paraparesis upon fatigue. J Neurol Neurosurg Psychiatry 1972; 37:40–46.

Hagbarth KE, Eklund G. Motor effects of vibratory stimuli in man. In: Granit Nobel symposium I. Muscle afferents and motor control. Stockholm: Almqvist and Wiksell, 1966a:177–86.

Hagbarth KE, Eklund G. Tonic vibration reflexes (TVR) in spasticity. Brain Res 1966b;2:201–3.

Hagbarth KE, Eklund G. The effects of muscle vibration in spasticity, rigidity and cerebellar disorders. J Neurol Neurosurg Psychiatry 1968; 31:207–13.

Hagbarth KE, Hägglund JV, Wallin EU, Young RR. Grouped spindle and electromyographic responses to abrupt wrist extension movements in man. J Physiol 1981;312:81–96.

Hammond PH, Merton PA, Sutton GG. Nervous gradation of muscular contraction. Br Med Bull 1956;12:214–18.

Henneman E, Mendell LM. Functional organization of motor neuron pool and its inputs. In Brooks VB, ed. Handbook of physiology. The nervous system. Vol. 2. Motor control. Bethesda, Md.: American Physiological Society, 1981:423–507.

Hepp-Reymond MC, Trouche E, Wiesendanger M. Effects of unilateral and bilateral pyramidotomy on a conditioned rapid precision grip in monkeys (Macaca fascicularis). Exp Brain Res 1974;21:519–27.

Hepp-Reymond MC, Wiesendanger M. Unilateral pyramidotomy in monkeys: effect on force and speed of conditioned precision grip. Brain Res 1972;36:117–31.

Hodgson HJF, Marsden CD, Meadows JC. The effect of adrenaline on the response to muscle vibration in man. J Physiol 1969;202:98–99.

Homma S, Nakajima Y. Coding in human stretch reflex analyzed by phase-locked spikes. Neurol Sci Lett 1979;11:19–22.

Illis LS. Enlargement of spinal cord synapses after repetitive stimulation of a single posterior root. Nature 1969;233:76–77.

Johnson EW, Denny ST, Kelley JP. Sequence of electromyographic abnormalities in stroke syndrome. Arch Phys Med Rehabil 1975;56:468–73.

Joyce GC, Rack PMH. The effects of load and force on tremor at the normal human elbow joint. J Physiol 1974;240:375–96.

Kiss J. Uber die cerebrale muskelatrophie des nervensystems. Berl Klin Wochenschr 1929;31:421–35.

Krueger KC, Waylonis GW. Hemiplegia: lower motor neuron electromyographic findings. Arch Phys Med Rehabil 1973;54:360–64.

Kuypers HGJM. Anatomy of the descending pathways. In: Brooks VB, ed. Handbook of physiology. The nervous system. Vol. 2. Motor control. Bethesda, Md.: American Physiological Society, 1981:597–666.

Lance JW, Burke D, Andrews CJ. The reflex effects of muscle vibration. In: Desmedt JE. ed. New developments in electromyography and clinical neurophysiology. Vol. 3. Basel: Karger, 1973:444–62.

Lance, JW, Gail P, Nielson PD. Tonic and phasic spinal cord mechanisms in man. J Neurol Neurosurg Psychiatry 1966;29:535–44.

Lance JW, McLeod JG. A physiological approach to clinical neurology. 3rd ed. London: Butterworth's, 1981.

Lawerance DG, Hopkins DA. The development of motor control in the rhesus monkey: evidence concerning the role of corticomotoneuronal connections. Brain 1976;99:235–54.

Lee RG, Stein RB. Resetting of tremor by mechanical perturbations: a comparison of essential tremor and Parkinsonian tremor. Ann Neurol 1981;10:523–31.

Lee RG, Tatton WG. Motor responses to sudden limb displacements in primates with specific CNS lesions and in human patients with motor system disorders. Can J Neurol Sci 1975;2:285–93.

Lee RG, Tatton WG. Long loop reflexes in man: clinical applications. In: Desmedt JE, ed. Cerebral motor control in man: long loop mechanisms. Progress in Clinical Neurophysiology. Vol. 4. Basel: Karger, 1978:320–33.

Lippold OCJ. Oscillation in the stretch reflex arc

and the origin of the rhythmical 8-12 c/s component of physiological tremor. J Physiol 1970;206:359–82.

Liu CN, Chambers WW. Intraspinal sprouting of dorsal root axons. Arch Neurol Psychia 1958;79:46–61.

Marsden CD. The mechanisms of physiological tremor and their significance for pathological tremors. In: Desmedt JE, ed. Physiological tremor, pathological tremors and clonus. Progress in Clinical Neurophysiology. Vol. 5. Basel: Karger, 1978:1–16.

Marsden CD, Meadows JC, Hodgson HJ. Observation of the reflex response to muscle vibration and its voluntary control. Brain 1969;92:829–46.

Marsden CD, Meadows JC, Lange GW, Watson RS. Effect of deafferentation on human physiological tremor. Lancet 1967;2:700–2.

Marsden CD, Merton PA, Morton HB. Servoaction and stretch reflex in human muscle and its apparent dependence in peripheral sensation. J Physiol 1971;21P–22P.

Marsden CD, Merton PA, Morton HB. Servoaction in the human thumb. J Physiol 1976a;257:1–44.

Marsden CD, Merton PA, Morton HB. Stretch reflex and servoaction in a variety of human muscles. J Physiol 1976b;259:531–60.

Marsden CD, Merton PA, Morton HB. The sensory mechanism of servoaction in human muscle. J Physiol 1977;265:521–35.

Marsden CD, Merton PA, Morton HB. Percutaneous stimulation of spinal cord and brain: pyramidal tract conduction velocities in man. J Physiol 1982;328:6.

Marsden CD, Merton PA, Morton HB, Adam JE. The effect of posterior column lesions on servoresponses from the human long thumb flexor. Brain 1977a;100:185–200.

Marsden CD, Merton PA, Morton HB, Adam JE. The effect of lesions of the sensorimotor cortex and the capsular pathways on servoresponses from the human long thumb flexor. Brain 1977b;100:503–26.

Marsden CD, Merton PA, Morton HB, Adam JE. The effect of lesions of the central nervous system on long-latency stretch reflexes in the human thumb. In: Desmedt JE, ed. Cerebral motor control in man: long loop mechanisms.

Progress in Clinical Neurophysiology. Vol. 4. Basel: Karger, 1978:334–41.

Marsden CD, Merton PA, Morton HB, Adam JE, Hallett M. Automatic and voluntary responses to muscle stretch in man. In: Desmedt JE, ed. Cerebral motor control in man: long loop mechanisms. Progress in Clinical Neurophysiology. Vol. 4. Basel: Karger, 1978:167–77.

Matthews PBC. Mammalian muscle receptors and their central actions. London: Edward Arnold, 1972.

Matthews PBC. Muscle spindles: their messages and their fusimotor supply. In: Brooks VB, ed. Handbook of physiology. The nervous system. Vol. 2. Motor control. Bethesda, Md.: American Physiological Society, 1981;189–228.

Mayer RF, Burke RE, Toop J, Hodgson JA, Kanda K, Wolmsley B. The effect of long-term immobilization on the motor unit population of the cat medial gastrocnemius muscle. Neuroscience 1981;6:725–39.

McComas AJ. Neuromuscular function and disorders. Woburn, Mass.: Butterworth's, 1977.

McComas AJ, Mirskey M, Velho F, Struppler A. Soleus motoneurone excitability in man: an indirect approach for obtaining quantitative data. J Neurol Neurosurg Psychiatry 1979;42:1091–99.

McComas AJ, Sica REP, Upton ARM, Aquilera N. Functional changes in motoneurones of hemiparetic patients. J Neurol Neurosurg Psychiatry 1973;36:183–93.

McCouch GP, Austin GM, Liu CN, Lin CY. Sprouting as a cause of spasticity. J Neurophysiol 1958;21:205–16.

McCouch GP, Liu CN, Chambers WW. Descending tracts and spinal shock in the monkey (Macaca mulatta). Brain 1966;89:359–76.

Mendell LM, Henneman E. Terminals of single Ia fibers: location, density and distribution within a pool of 300 homonymous motoneurons. J Neurophysiol 1971;34:171–87.

Merton PA, Hill DK, Morton HB, Marsden CD. Scope of a technique for electrical stimulation of human brain, spinal cord and muscle. Lancet 1982;2:597–600.

Miller AD, Brooks VB. Late muscular responses to arm perturbations persist during supraspinal dysfunctions in monkeys. Exp Brain Res 1981;41:146–58.

Milner-Brown HS, Fisher MA, Weiner WJ. Electrical properties of motor units in Parkinsonism and a possible relationship with bradykinesia. J Neurol Neurosurg Psychiatry 1979;42:35–41.

Milner-Brown HS, Girvin JP, Brown WF. The effects of motor cortical stimulation on the excitability of spinal motoneurones in man. Can J Neurol Sci 1975;2:245–53.

Milner-Brown HS, Stein RB, Lee RG. Synchronization of human motor units: possible roles of exercise and supraspinal reflexes. Electroencephalogr Clin Neurophysiol 1975;38:245–54.

Namba T, Schuman MH, Grob D. Conduction velocity in the ulnar nerve in hemiplegic patients. J Neurol Sci 1971;12:177–86.

Nathan PW, Smith MC. The Babinski response: a review and new observations. J Neurol Neurosurg Psychiatry 1955;18:250–59.

Nelson SG, Collatos TC, Niechaj A, Mendell LM. Immediate increase in Ia-motoneuron synaptic transmission caudal to chronic spinal cord transection. J Neurophysiol 1979;21:655–64.

Nelson SG, Mendell LM. Enhancement in Ia-motoneuron synaptic transmission caudal to chronic spinal cord transection. J Neurophysiol 1979; 42:642–54.

Noth J, Thilmann A. Autogenic excitation of extensor motoneurones by group II muscle afferents in the cat. Neurol Sci 1980;17:23–26.

Nyboer VJ, Johnson HE. Electromyographic findings in lower extremities of patients with traumatic quadriplegia. Arch Phys Med Rehabil 1971;52:256–59.

O'Hare VM, Abbot GH. Electromyographic evidence of lower motor neuron injury in cervical spinal cord injury. Proc Ann Clin Spinal Cord Inj Cent 1967;17:25–35.

Onkelinx A, Chantraine A. Electromyographic study of paraplegic patients. Electromyogr Clin Neurophysiol 1975;15:71–81.

Panin N, Paul BJ, Policoff LD, Eson ME. Nerve conduction velocities in hemiplegia. Arch Phys Med Rehabil 1967;48:606–10.

Patton HD, Amassian VE. The pyramidal tract: its excitation and functions. In: Field J, ed. Handbook of physiology and neurophysiology. Washington, D.C.: American Physiological Society, 1960:837–61.

Petty J, Jr, Johnson EW. In: Johnson EW, ed. Practical electromyography. Baltimore: Williams & Wilkins, 1980:276–89.

Phillips CG. Motor apparatus of the baboon's hand. Proc R Soc Lond Biol 1969;173:141–74.

Phillips CG. Pyramidal apparatus for control of the baboon hand. In: Desmedt, JE, ed. New developments in electromyography and clinical neurophysiology. Vol. 3. Basel: Karger, 1973: 136–44.

Phillips CG, Porter R. Corticospinal neurons: their role in movement. London: Academic Press, 1977.

Phillips CG, Powell TPS, Wiesendanger M. Projection from low-threshold muscle afferents of hand and forearm to area 3a of baboon's cortex. J Physiol 1971;217:419–46.

Porter R. Functions of the mammalian cerebral cortex in movement. In: Kerkut GA, Phillis JW, eds. Progress in neurobiology. Oxford: Pergamon Press 1973;1–51.

Rondot P, Bathien N. Pathophysiology of Parkinsonian tremor. A study of the patterns of motor unit discharges. In: Desmedt JE, ed. Physiological tremor, pathological tremors and clonus. Progress in Clinical Neurophysiology. Vol. 5. Basel: Karger, 1978;5:138–49.

Rosen JS, Lerner IM, Rosenthal AM. Electromyography in spinal cord injury. Arch Phys Med Rehabil 1969;50:271–73.

Sargeant AJ, Davies CTM, Edwards RHT, Maunder CA, Young A. Functional and structural changes after disease of human muscle. Clin Sci Molec Med 1977;52:337–42.

Schaffer K. Zur lehre der cerebralen muskel atrophie nebst beitrag zur trophie der neuroven. Monatsschr Psychiatr Neurol 1897;2:30.

Segura RP, Sahgal V. Hemiplegic atrophy: electrophysiological and morphological studies. Muscle Nerve 1981;4:246–48.

Shahani M. The motor system: Neurophysiology and muscle mechanisms. Amsterdam: Elsevier North-Holland, 1976.

Shahani BT, Young RR. Action tremors: a clinical neurophysiological review. In: Desmedt JE, ed. Physiological tremor, pathological tremors and clonus. Progress in Clinical Neurophysiology. Vol. 5. Basel: Karger, 1978:129–37.

Shigeno K. Hemiplegic amyotrophy and motor nerve conduction velocity in hemiplegic patients. I. Hemiplegic amyotrophy: its clinical and etiological considerations. Keio J Med 1972a; 21:73–88.

Shigeno K. Hemiplegic amyotrophy and motor nerve conduction velocity in hemiplegic patients. II. Motor nerve conduction velocity of the ulnar nerves in hemiplegic patients. Keio J Med 1972b;21:89–104.

Shimamura M, Akert K. Peripheral nervous relations of propriospinal and spino-bulbo-spinal reflex systems. Jpn J Physiol 1965;15:638–47.

Shimamura M, Mori S, Yamauchi T. Effects of spino-bulbo-spinal reflex volleys on extensor motoneurons of hind limbs in cats. J Neurol Physiol 1967;30:319–32.

Sica REP, McComas AJ, Upton ARM. Impaired potentiation of H-reflexes in patients with upper motoneurone lesions. J Neurol Neurosurg Psychiatry 1971;34:712–17.

Silverstein A. Diagnostic localizing value of muscle atrophy in parietal lobe lesions. Neurology 1955;5:30–55.

Spaans F, Wilts G. Denervation due to lesions of the central nervous system. J Neurol Sci 1982;57:291–305.

Spielholz NI, Sell GH, Gold J, Rusk HA, Greens SK. Electrophysiological studies in patients with spinal cord lesions. Arch Phys Med Rehabil 1972;53:558–62.

Starr A, McKeon B, Skuse N, Burke D. Cerebral potentials evoked by muscle stretch in man. Brain 1981;104:149–66.

Stein RB, Lee RG. Tremor and clonus. In: Brooks VB, ed. Handbook of physiology. The nervous system. Vol. 2. Motor control. Bethesda, Md.: American Physiological Society, 1981:325–43.

Stein RB, Lee RG, Nichols TR. Modification of ongoing tremor and locomotion by sensory feedback. Electroencephalogr Clin Neurophysiol 1978;34:511–19.

Stiles RN, Pozos RS. A mechanical reflex oscillator hypothesis for parkinsonian hand tremor. J Appl Physiol 1976;40:990–98.

Stiles RN, Randall JE. Mechanical factors in human tremor frequency. J Appl Physiol 1967;23:324–30.

Sutton GG, Sykes K. The effect of withdrawal of visual presentation of errors upon the frequency spectrum of tremor in a manual task. J Physiol 1967a;190:281–93.

Sutton GG, Sykes K. The variation in hand tremor with force in healthy subjects. J Physiol 1967b;191:699–711.

Tatton WG, Bawa P, Bruce IC, Lee RG. In: Desmedt JE, ed. Cerebral motor control in man: long loop mechanisms. Progress in Clinical Neurophysiology. Vol. 4. Basel: Karger, 1978.

Tatton WG, Forner SD, Gerstein GL, Chambers WW, Lin CN. The effect of post central lesions on motor responses to sudden upper limb displacement in monkeys. Brain Res 1975;96:108–13.

Taylar RG, Kewalramani LS, Fowler WM. Electromyographic findings in lower extremities of patients with high spinal cord injury. Arch Phys Med Rehabil 1974;55:16–23.

Torvik A. Transneuronal changes in the inferior olive and pontine nuclei in kittens. J Neuropathol Exp Neurol 1956;15:119–45.

Tower SS. Pyramidal lesion in the monkey. Brain 1940;63:36–90.

Tower SS. The pyramidal tract. In: Bucy P, ed. The precentral motor cortex. Urbana: University of Illinois Press, 1949:149–72.

Tracey DJ, Walmsley B, Brinkman J. "Long-loop" reflexes can be obtained in spinal monkeys. Neuroscience 1980;18:59–65.

Travis AM. Neurological deficiencies after ablation of the precentral motor area in *Macaca mulatta*. 1955;78:155–73.

Trontelj JV. A study of the F-response by single-fiber electromyography. In: Desmedt JE, ed. New developments in electromyography and clinical neurophysiology. Vol. 3. Basel: Karger, 1973:318–22.

Upton ARM, McComas AJ, Sica REP. Potentiation of "late" responses evoked in muscles during effort. J Neurol Neurosurg Psychiatry 1971;34:699–711.

VanAlphen HA, Lammers HJ, Walder HAD. On remarkable reaction of motor neurons of lumbosacral region after traumatic cervical transection in man. Neurochirurgie 1962;8:328.

VanGijn J. Babinski response: stimulus and effector. J Neurol Neurosurg Psychiatry 1975;38:180–86.

VanGijn J. Equivocal plantar responses: a clinical and electromyographic study. J Neurol Neurosurg Psychiatry 1976;39:275–82.

Veraa RP, Grafstein B. Cellular mechanisms for recovery from nervous system injury; a conference report. Expt Neurol 1981;71:6–75.

Walsh FMR. The Babinski plantar response, its

forms and its physiological and pathological significance. Brain 1956;79:529–56.

Warrington WB. On the structural alterations observed in nerve cells. J Physiol 1898;23:112–29.

Warrington WB. Further observations on the structural alterations in nerve cells. J Physiol 1899; 24:464–78.

Watt DG, Stauffer EK, Taylor A, Reinking RM, Stuart DG. Analysis of muscle receptor connections by spike-triggered averaging. I. Spindle primary and tendon organ afferents. J Neurophysiol 1976;39:1375–92.

Wiesendanger M. The pyramidal tract: recent investigations on its morphology and function. Ergeb Physiol 1969;61:73–135.

Wiesendanger M. Pathophysiology of tone. Berlin: Springer-Verlag, 1972.

Wiesendanger M. Input from muscle and cutaneous nerves of the hand and forearm to neurons of the precentral gyrus of baboons and monkeys. J Physiol 1973a;2281:203–19.

Wiesendanger M. Some aspects of pyramidal tract functions in primates. In: Desmedt JE, ed. New developments in electromyography and clinical neurophysiology. Vol. 3. Basel: Karger, 1973b; 159–74.

Wiesendanger M. Comments on the problem of transcortical reflexes. J Physiol (Paris) 1978;74:325–30.

Wiesendanger M. The pyramidal tract, its structure and function. In: Towe AL, Luschei ES, eds. Handbook of behavioral neurobiology. New York: Plenum Press, 1981:401–91.

Wiesendanger M, Miles TS. Ascending pathway of low-threshold muscle afferents to the cerebral cortex and its possible role in motor control. Physiol Rev 1982;62:1234–70.

Wiesendanger M, Rüegg DG. Electromyographic assessment of central motor disorders. Muscle Nerve 1978;1:407–12.

Wiesendanger M, Rüegg DG, Lachat JM. The role of proprioceptive afferents in motor cortical output in contemporary clinical neurophysiology. In: Cobb WA, Van Duijn H, eds. EEG supplement no. 34. Amsterdam: Elsevier North-Holland, 1978.

Winkelman NW, Silverstein A. Localization of function in the cerebral cortex. Res Nerv Ment Dis Proc 1932;13:485–528.

Winkelman NW, Silverstein A. Am J Syphilis Neurol 1935;19:58–76.

Young J. Morphological and histochemical studies of partially and totally deafferented spinal cord segments. Exp Neurol 1966;14:238–48.

Young JI. Rowley WF. Histochemical alterations of ventral horn cells resulting from chronic hemispherectomy or chronic dorsal root section. Exp Neurol 1970;26:460–81.

Young JI, Rowley WF. Physiological alterations of motor units in hemiplegia. J Neurol Sci 1982; 54:401–12.

Young RR, Growdon JG, Shahani BT. Beta-adrenergic mechanisms in action tremor. N Engl J Med 1975;293:950–53.

INDEX